V. Schulz · R. Hänsel · M. Blumenthal · V.E. Tyler

Rational Phytotherapy

A Reference Guide for Physicians and Pharmacists

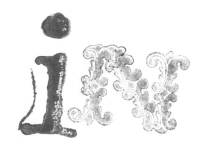

VOLKER SCHULZ · RUDOLF HÄNSEL

MARK BLUMENTHAL · VARRO E. TYLER[†]

Rational Phytotherapy

A Reference Guide for Physicians and Pharmacists

Fifth edition, fully revised and expanded

With 97 figures and 53 tables

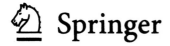 Springer

Prof. Dr. med. Volker Schulz
Oranienburger Chaussee 25
13465 Berlin, Germany

Prof. Dr. rer. nat. Rudolf Hänsel
formerly Institut für Pharmakognosie und
Phytochemie der Freien Universität Berlin
Private address:
Westpreußenstraße 71
81927 München, Germany

Mark Blumenthal
Founder & Executive Director
American Botanical Council
P.O. Box 144345
Austin, TX 78714-4345, USA

Prof. em. Varro E. Tyler, Ph. D., Sc. D. †

Translator: Terry C. Telger, 6112 Waco Way, Fort Worth, TX 76133, USA

ISBN 3-540-40832-0 Springer Berlin Heidelberg New York

Library of Congress Control Number: 2003070714

Springer is a part of Springer Science+Business Media

springeronline.com

© Springer-Verlag Berlin Heidelberg 2004

Printed in Germany

Editor: Dr. Thomas Mager, Heidelberg
Developing Editor: Susanne Friedrichsen, Heidelberg
Production Editor: Frank Krabbes, Heidelberg
Typesetting: wiskom e.K., Friedrichshafen
Cover design: design & production GmbH, Heidelberg
Printed on adic-free paper   SPIN 10869228   14/3109 - 5 4 3 2 1 0

The demand for accurate, reliable information on the various benefits and potential risks of herbs and phytomedicinal products has never been greater. In the past few years, health professionals throughout the world – in both developing and developed countries – have been exposed to a virtual avalanche of research papers on various toxicological, pharmacological, and clinical properties of numerous botanical preparations. These herbal preparations are usually termed phytomedicines in Europe, "dietary supplements" in the United States, or "natural health products" in Canada under a new regulatory system currently being implemented. Articles have appeared in numerous peer-reviewed journals, many that support the clinical efficacy of a particular phytomedicinal preparation, and some that find little or no efficacy, at least under the parameters of the particular studies.

Various articles and editorials in English-language medical journals have questioned the appropriateness of herbal preparations for quality, safety, and/or efficacy, often calling for more strict regulation of these products – particularly in the United States, where their regulation as dietary supplements has been a matter of considerable confusion among health professionals and members of the media. The result has been the dissemination of the myth that herbs are "unregulated" – a message that has a profoundly negative impact on the perception of their potential beneficial roles in clinical medicine by health professionals and their potential benefits for self-care among consumers. This has resulted in a general trend to reduce the standing of herbs and phytomedicines among many professionals and consumers, and the market has responded with lower sales for herbal products in the past few years, at least in the mainstream retail channels of trade. As is so often the case in these matters, the truth is elusive.

The regulatory and media morass regarding herbs and phytomedicines in North America contrasts sharply with the situation in Western Europe, particularly Germany, where herbs and phytomedicines are afforded a greater degree of respect and legitimacy by the regulatory system, in medical education and clinical practice, and among consumers. Germany has traditionally led the way in the development of high quality herbal medicinal products, manufactured according to a high level of quality control in accordance with good manufacturing practices (GMPs) by phytomedicine companies who view their business as the natural medicine component of a larger medical culture. It should be of no surprise then that at least until very recently, when the U.S. government began to fund clinical trials on herbal products through the National Center for Complementary and Alternative Medicine at the National Institutes of Health, Germany has been the world leader in the publication of controlled clinical trials to document the safety and efficacy of a variety of phytomedicines.

What's more, unlike the majority of clinical trials in the U.S. which are public funded, most of the German trials have been sponsored by particular phytomedicine manufacturers and the trials have been conducted on specific proprietary phytomedicinal preparations, many of which are chemically-defined extracts. This raises the question of phytoequivalence, i.e., whether the research conducted on such preparations can be extrapolated to other, more generic, herbal products that probably have a significantly or even slightly different chemical profile, and hence, potentially different pharmacological effects.

It is therefore a welcome development that this book is now available in English. The first four editions of this publication (only the last two being translated from the German into English) presented some of the most lucid discussions of the clinical trials published at the time on the leading herbs and phytomedicinal products in Germany. This edition continues in that tradition, providing insightful comments on clinical trials on the majority of the most widely used botanical preparations employed in German clinical practice. In addition, it contains discussions of botanicals that have yet to become popular or widely adapted in the U.S. However, in light of some of the compelling data from published trials discussed in this volume on some of these relatively more obscure botanicals, it is highly likely that their acceptance and popularity will increase both in the general marketplace where self-medication products are sold, as well as in modern clinical practice. The ultimate beneficiary of such information is, of course, the consumer or patient, many of whom continue to express their desire for safe, natural, low-cost, effective medicines.

As explained more eloquently in the following pages, the concept of "rational phytotherapy" presupposes the use of reason and thus the evaluation of all forms of evidence to support the safety and efficacy of herbs and phytomedicinal preparations. Recent events in the international herbal arena have raised questions about how "rational"some regulatory actions might be. For example, the banning of the sale of kava in more than eight nations based on reports of adverse hepatic reactions have been viewed by numerous herbal experts as premature, precipitous and irrational, particularly since several detailed toxicological evaluations of the adverse event reports in which kava has been implicated do not support the conclusion that kava is inherently hepatotoxic.

On another subject, the banning of dietary supplements containing the controversial herb ephedra and/or any ephedrine alkaloids by the U.S. Food and Drug Administration in February 2004 followed a long process of evaluation of the safety of ephedra and an independent safety analysis of all the clinical, pharmacological, and toxicological literature on ephedra, as well as the adverse event reports associated with the herb. While not concluding that ephedra was definitely causally related to serious adverse events (heart attack, stroke, death), the report concluded that these serious events were "sentinel events" – a conclusion that is viewed by many as almost an indictment of causality, but not stepping over the line. Nevertheless, in rational phytotherapy, ephedra is still seen as a safe and effective remedy for short-term treatment of respiratory disorders, just as it has been used in traditional Chinese medicine for several thousand years, and as the ephedrine alkaloids are still employed in conventional medicine.

Rational phytotherapy employs various levels of empirical and scientific evidence with sound reasoning to determine the most appropriate ways to apply the benefits of herbs and phytomedicinal products to human health. As our esteemed colleague, the late Professor Varro E. Tyler, the American editor of the two previous editions of this book, stated repeatedly, the official German Commission E's process of evaluation of the benefits and indications for herbs and phytomedicines was conducted using a "doctrine of reasonable certainty." Accordingly, the herbal preparations discussed in this book will provide a "reasonably certain" benefit to the health of those patients whose physicians chose to employ these safe, relatively low-cost, natural therapeutic agents.

Austin, Texas, April 2004
MARK BLUMENTHAL

Herbal medicines have a special tradition in Germany. Since the fourth edition of this book was published, however, physicians have been prescribing more synthetic drugs in place of phytomedicines. One result of this has been a sharp rise in overall drug costs. At the same time, this substitution has had more negative than positive effects from a public health standpoint. One explanation for this trend is that for the typical applications of herbal medicines, it is common to overestimate the importance of pharmacology alone in determining the therapeutic response. This belief, which is also applied to other traditional remedies and is very widespread, is the subject of detailed discussions that appear mainly in the revised and expanded portions of this edition: Sections 1.5, 2.1.8, 2.2.7, 4.1, and 6.3.

Approximately two-thirds of phytomedicine prescriptions written by German doctors are for single-herb products, i.e., products that contain only one medicinal herb. But ten herbs accounted for approximately 80 % of these prescriptions, and 20 herbs accounted for more than 90 %. This is surprising when we consider that Commission E of the former German Health Agency evaluated the therapeutic use of some 400 medicinal herbs from 1982 to 1994 and recommended approximately 250 of them. Clearly, the prescriptions written by physicians today no longer reflect the rich historical diversity of herbal remedies. Of course, family doctors also counsel their patients in self-medication, and this more than doubles the yearly consumption of the leading phytomedicines. Nevertheless, the total number of medicinal herbs that are still used to a significant degree in modern medicine are but a fraction of the traditional botanicals that have been described in classic textbooks of herbal medicine.

Despite being called an "alternative therapy" in a 1976 German drug law, phytotherapy is actually a scientifically tested and proven treatment modality to which modern pharmacotherapy can trace its roots. As with any medication, our knowledge on the safety and efficacy of a phytomedicine improves as the medicine is used more frequently. For this reason, one of our main concerns in all editions of this book has been to focus attention on the plant constituents and products whose safety and efficacy have been tested by modern scientific methods. We have added considerable material since the fourth edition in 1999, including new results on clinical aspects, pharmacology, and toxicology, especially for extracts of ginkgo leaves, St. John's wort, kava rhizome, hawthorn, myrtol, pelargonium root, butterbar, peppermint and caraway oil, saw palmetto berries, agnus castus, and rhodiola. Chapter 4 (Respiratory System) and Chapter 5 (Digestive System) have been trimmed and updated to reflect modern diagnostic and therapeutic advances.

Combination products consisting of several medicinal herbs are more difficult to test and evaluate. Many of these products are derived from traditional herbal medicine.

With few exceptions, we cannot draw conclusions on the additive or potentiating effects of their individual constituents based on comparative clinical studies. But theoretical considerations aside, we gave due regard to practical physician experience with these multi-herb products and, as in previous editions, included products that are among the 100 most commonly prescribed herbal medications listed in Table A3 of the Appendix.

We express special thanks to Dr. Wiltrud Juretzek of Karlsruhe for her helpful corrections and additions. We also thank our wives, who served as patient "copyreaders" during the course of our work.

Berlin and Munich, July 2003
V. Schulz   R. Hänsel

Table of Contents

1 Medicinal Plants, Phytomedicines, and Phytotherapy

1.1 Common Roots of Pharmacotherapy

From a historical perspective, the production of medicines and the pharmacologic treatment of diseases began with the use of herbs. In fact, the very word *drug* used to denote a medicinal preparation is derived from the old Dutch word *droog* meaning" to dry", as plants were dried to be used as medicines. Methods of folk healing practiced by the peoples of the Mediterranean region and Asia found expression in the first European herbal, *De Materia Medica*, written by the Greek physician Pedanios Dioscorides in the first century C.E. During the Renaissance, this classical text was revised to bring it more in line with humanistic doctrines. The plants named by Dioscorides were identified and illustrated with woodcuts, and some locally grown medicinal herbs were added. Herbals were still based on classical humoral pathology, which taught that health and disease were determined by the four bodily humors – blood, phlegm, black bile, and yellow bile. The humors, in turn, were associated with the elemental principles of antiquity: air, water, earth, and fire. The elements could be mixed in varying ratios and proportions to produce the qualities of cold, moist, dry, or warm – properties that also were associated with various proportions of the four bodily humors. Thus, if a particular disease was classified as moist, warm, or dry, it was treated by administering an herb having the opposite property (Jüttner, 1983). Plant medicines were categorized by stating their property and grading their potency on a four-point scale as "imperceptible," "perceptible," "powerful," of "very powerful." For example, opium, the classic drug derived from the opium poppy (*Papaver somniferum*), was classified as grade 4/cold. A line of association that linked sedation with "cooling" allowed the empirically known sedative and narcotic actions of opium to be fitted into the humoral system. Pepper (the black pepper of the historical spice trade, i.e., *Piper nigrum*, not to be confused with the red pepper of the genus *Capsicum*, which as introduced to medicine after the discovery of the New World, was classified as grade 4/dry and warming. The goal of all treatment, according to Hippocrates, was to balance the humors by removing that which is excessive and augmenting that which is deficient" (Haas, 1956). Humoral pathology obviously developed into one of the basic principles of conventional medicine.

The monographs that appeared in medieval and renaissance herbals typically consisted of an illustration of the healing plant, the name of the plant and its synonyms, its action (potency grade and property), and the indications for its use. Indications were not stated in the modern sense of disease entities but as symptoms. For example, cough, catarrh, and hoarseness were each considered separate illnesses. The monograph concluded with a detailed account of the various preparations that could be made from the herb. By and large, the authors of herbals were not laypersons but medical doctors trained in conventional medical schools. The herbals were written not just for doctors but also for the "common man," in some cases for the express purpose of serving as a guide "when the doctor is too expensive or too far away" (quoted in Jüttner, 1983).

Prior to 1800, when medicine entered the scientific age, traditional herbal medicine was the unquestioned foundation for all standard textbooks on pharmacology. It was not until the advent of modern chemistry and the development of modern pharmacotherapy and "medical science" that phytotherapy was relegated to the status of an alternative modality. From the historical perspective, however, it is incorrect to classify phytotherapy as a special or alternative branch of medicine. When we consider that the history of classical herbal medicine spans more than 2500 years from antiquity to modern times, it is reasonable to assume that many of the medicinal herbs used during that period not only have specific actions but are also free of hazardous side effects. Otherwise they would not have been passed down so faithfully through so many epochs and cultures. It would be frivolous and unscientific to dismiss the collective empirical experience of more than 50 generations of patients and physicians as simply a "placebo effect" (Benedum, 1998).

1.2 Making Medicines Safer by Isolating and Modifying Plant Constituents

In his famous *Account of the Foxglove* [published in 1785, William Withering described how he was called to the home of an itinerant salesman in Yorkshire. "I found him vomiting incessantly, his vision was blurred, and his pulse rate was about 40 beats per minute. On questioning, I learned that his wife had boiled a handful of foxglove leaves in a half pint of water and had given him the brew, which he swallowed in one draught to seek relief from asthmatic complaints. This good woman was well acquainted with the medicine of her region but not with the dose, for her husband barely escaped with his life."

Cardiac glycosides of the digitalis type (from foxglove leaf, *Digitalis purpurea* and *D. lanata*) have a very narrow range of therapeutic dosages. Exceeding the full medicinal dose by just about 50 % can produce toxic effects. The dosage problem is compounded by the large qualitative and quantitative variations that occur in the crude plant material. Depending on its origin, the crude drug may contain a predominance of gitoxin, which is not very active when taken orally, or it may carry a high concentration of the very [orally?] active compound digitoxin.

Thus, isolating the active constituents from herbs with a narrow therapeutic range (Fig. 1.1) and administering the pure compounds is not simply an end in itself. This scientific method of medicinal plant research is, rather, the means by which very potent constituents can be processed into safe medicinal products. The goal is not to concentrate the key active component but to obtain a pharmaceutical product that has a consistent, uniform composition. Processing the isolated constituent into pills, tablets, or

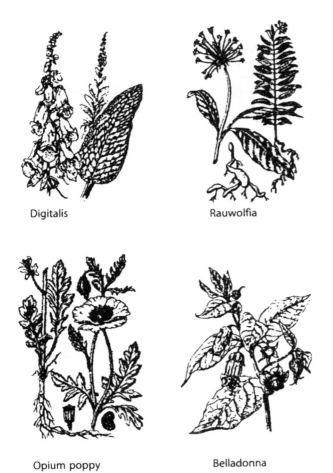

Figure 1.1. ◄ Potent medicinal plants whose active constituents are isolated for therapeutic use as conventional drugs.

Digitalis

Rauwolfia

Opium poppy

Belladonna

capsules results in a product that isdiluted by pharmaceutical excipients. For example, the concentration of digitoxin in a digitoxin tablet is approximately 10 times lower than in the original digitalis leaf.

With the development of the natural sciences and the scientific method in medicine beginning in the early 19th century, herbal remedies became an object of scientific analysis. The isolation of morphine from opium (1803–1806) marked the first time that relatively modern chemical and analytic methods were used to extract the active principle from a herb. It then became possible to perform pharmacologic and toxicologic studies on the effects of morphine in animals and humans. Various substances isolated from opium, including morphine, codeine, and papaverine, are still in therapeutic use today. In other cases efforts have been made to improve on the natural substance by enhancing its desired properties and minimizing its adverse side effects. One of the first examples of this approach was the development of acetylsalicylic acid from the salicin in willow bark (*Salix* spp.). In an effort to surpass the natural precursors, scientists would sometimes produce medicines with unexpected effects. Modifying the reserpine

Table 1.1.
Examples of plant constituents that are isolated for medicinal use. Naturally, these constituents do not occur alone in plants but as fractions accompanied by related chemical compounds. The isolated substances, which generally have strong, immediate actions, are not considered phytomedicines in the strict sense.

Constiuent/Drug	Plant	Action
Atropine	Belladonna leaves.& roots	Parasympatholytic
Caffeine	Coffee shrub	Analeptic, CNS stimulant
Cocaine	Coca leaves	Local anesthetic
Colchicine	Autumn crocus bulb	Gout remedy, antiinflammatory
Digoxin	Digitalis/Foxglove leaves	Cardiac remedy (positive inotropic)
Emetine	Ipecac root	Emetic
Ephedrine	Ephedra herb	Antihypotensive
Kawain	Kava root/.rhizome	Anxiolytic
Morphine	Opium poppy exudate	Analgesic
Physostigmine	Calabar bean	Cholinesterase inhibitor
Pilocarpine	Jaborandi leaves	Glaucoma remedy
Quinidine	Cinchona bark	Antiarrhythmic
Quinine	Cinchona bark	Antimalarial
Reserpine	Rauwolfia/Indian snakeroot	Antihypertensive
Salicin	Willow bark	Anti-inflammatory
Scopolamine	Datura spp./Jimson weed	Antispasmodic
Taxol®	Pacific yew bark	Cytostatic
Theophylline	Tea leaves	Bronchodilator

molecule (from the traditional Ayurvedic sedative plant Indian snakeroot, *Rauvolfia serpentina*) led to mebeverine, while modifying the atropine molecule (from belladonna, *Atropa belladonna* and related tropane alkaloid-containing plants in the nightshade family, Solanaceae) led to ipratropium bromide and the powerful meperidine group of analgesics. The development of cromolyn from khellin (from *Ammi visnaga*) is another instance where a plant constituent was modified to obtain a more useful medicine. Medicinal herbs from the New World were another source of important drug substances. The leaves of the coca shrub (*Erythoxylum coca*) yielded cocaine, the prototype for modern local anesthetics, while the bark of *Cinchona* species yielded quinine, a drug still important in the treatment of malaria. A recent example of an active compound successfully isolated from plants is artemisinin, an antimalarial agent derived from a species of Chinese wormwood (*Artemisia annua*). Resistance to this compound develops much more slowly than to synthetic antimalarial drugs. Taxol, and its analogs, which were initially derived from the bark of the Pacific yew tree (*Taxus brevifolia*), have demonstrated cytostatic properties in the treatment of malignant tumors.

A significant portion of all currently used medications are derived, either directly or indirectly, from active principles that have been isolated from plants. Some well-known examples are listed in Table 1.1. Most of these substances do not occur in plants individually but in groups of compounds, such as caffeine in the group of methylxanthines, digoxin in the group of cardiac glycosides, and morphine in the group of opium alkaloids. These isolated compounds and groups of compounds generally produce strong, immediate effects and are in the strict sense not classified as phytomedicines (phytomedicinals) but more appropriately as plant-derived drugs. Researchers have by no means exhausted the potential of these secondary plant constituents. The sheer number of plant alkaloids that could provide the basis for the development of future remedies is estimated at more than 20,000 (Cordell et al., 2002).

1.3   Medicinal Herbs, Preparations, and Extracts

Phytomedicines are medicinal products whose pharmacologically active components contain only preparations that are made from medicinal herbs (Keller, 1996). The term "medicinal herbs" or "plant drugs" generally refers to plants or plant parts that have been dried to yield a storable product. A medicinal herb or a preparation made from it is generally considered to be *one* active constituent, regardless of whether or not specific "main active constituents" are known (Note for Guidance, 1998). In Germany, the quality features of medicinal herbs, including the testing procedures that are used to monitor the pharmaceutical quality of the herbs and the medicinal products made from them, are defined in the German version of the *European Pharmacopeia* (*European Pharmacopeia*, 1997) and in the *German Pharmacopeia*. The European Pharmacopeia Commission based in Strasbourg and the German Pharmacopeia Commission based in Bonn review these volumes periodically to ensure that they are revised and current .

Thus, the efficacy and safety of phytomedicines are ensured mainly by quality specifications in the *Pharmacopeias*. The herbs form the basis of the preparations made from them, generally extracts, which are the active constituents of most phytomedicines. These preparations are multicomponent mixtures whose chemical compositions are usually known only to a very limited degree and are also subject to a certain range of biological variation. Besides the main active ingredients, which determine the type of effect that is produced, the preparations contain secondary constituents that can modify the effect of the main ingredients, e.g., by influencing their stability or bioavailability. Plant preparations also contain impurities that are pharmacologically inactive or that may even cause unwanted effects.

Another special feature of phytomedicines is the fact that preparations with different therapeutic properties can be made from the same herbal material, depending on the manufacturing process employed. Once a medicinal product has been officially approved (i.e., recognized as an official medicine by an appropriate governmental agency, as is the case, for example, in Germany and other Western European nations), then, neither the herbal preparation nor the manufacturing process should be varied or altered beyond strictly defined limits. In the U.S., there is little official recognition of benefit or efficacy of phytomedicinal preparations; nevertheless, the United States Pharmacopeia has developed standards monographs for the identity and purity of numerous botanical preparations, even though such standards do not constitute official approval for drug use. Since more than three-fourths of the dry weight of the initial herbal material usually consists of inert plant constituents such as cellulose, and starches that form the structural framework of the plant with no pharmacologic effects of their own, the majority of all phytomedicines today are produced from extracts. The therapeutic dosage of such products is often calculated based on the amount of the extract necessary to produce the desired biological effect; i.e., the entire extract serve as the active ingredient. Given the central importance of the active ingredients of herbal drug products, plant extracts will be described below in some detail.

The plant extracts that are marketed as approved medications in Germany have reached a relatively high level of pharmaceutical quality. For economic reasons further phytochemical characterization of the quality of extracts by defining additional herb-specific test parameters would be feasible only in cases where it could be definitely shown that the expanded control measures would yield a corresponding gain in efficacy and therapeutic safety (Gaedcke and Steinhoff, 2000).

Besides pharmaceutical quality, dosage is a critical concern in the prescription of herbal products. In most cases, it is reasonable to estimate that approximately 200–500 mg of extract (depending on the strength of the extract) is equivalent to the traditional single dose that is delivered in one cup of medicinal tea. Relatively large capsules, pills, tablets, etc. are often the only dosage forms that can accommodate these amounts of extract. This inevitably places limitations on combination products made from several medicinal herbs, and therefore these products must be viewed critically in terms of supplying an adequate dosage.

1.3.1 What are Extracts?

Extracts are concentrated preparations of a liquid, powdered, or viscous consistency that are ordinarily made from dried plant parts (the crude drug) by maceration or percolation. Most crude drugs have about a 20 % content of extractable substances, corresponding to a herb-to-extract ratio of 5:1. Fluidextracts are liquid preparations that usually contain a 1:1 ratio of fluidextract to dried herb (i.e., on a weight-to-weight [w/w] or volume-to-weight [v/w] basis). Ethanol, water, or mixtures of ethanol and water are used exclusively in the production of fluidextracts. Solid or powdered extracts are preparations made by evaporation of the solvent used in the production process (raw extract). Further details on pharmaceutical preparation and extraction techniques for herbal medications are shown in Fig. 1.2. The reader is also referred to the current (2002) edition of the *European Pharmacopeia*.

In some cases it is necessary to remove unwanted components from the raw extract and increase the concentration of the therapeutically active ingredients. Standardized ginkgo (*Ginkgo biloba*) powdered extract (50:1) is an example of this process. The 50:1 ratio means that, on average, 50 parts of crude drug (i.e., dried leaves) must be processed to yield 1 part extract. Potentially allergenic ginkgolic acids are also reduced from the extract along with pharmacologically inert substances.

Volatile oils are also concentrates of active plant constituents. They are generally obtained by direct distillation from the crude drug material or, less commonly, by

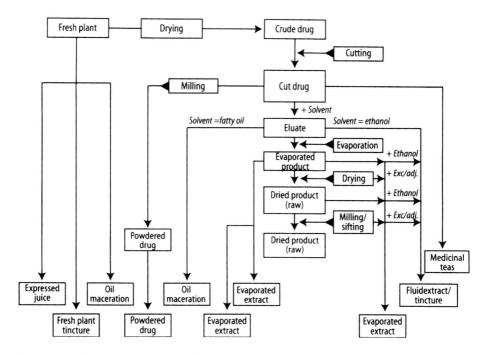

Figure 1.2. ▲ Technical processes involved in the production of phytomedicines (after Gaedcke and Steinhoff, 2000)

lipophilic (i.e., fat or oil soluble) extraction. The ration of herb to concentrate (known technically as the HER, or herb-to-extract ratio) for volatile oils is usually in the range of 50:1 to 100:1 (w/w), corresponding to a volatile oil content of 1–2 % in typical herbs that contain such oils.

1.3.2 Standardization of Extracts

Two key factors determine the internal composition of an extract: the quality of the herbal raw material and the production process (Fig. 1.2).

1.3.2.1 Quality of the Herbal Material

Herbs and botanical materials are natural products. Nature does not supply its products with a consistent, standardized composition. For example, we know from daily experience that there are different vintages of wines and different qualities of black teas, there are high-acid and low-acid coffees, and there are sweet and bitter types of fennel. Similarly, the constituents of medicinal herbs can vary greatly as a result of genetic factors, climate, soil quality, and other external factors. In general, the material derived from cultivated medicinal plants shows smaller variations in chemical constituents than material gathered from the wild. Another advantage of cultivation is that the increase in relevant constituents can be monitored during plant growth, making it possible to determine the optimum time for harvesting. Quality irregularities caused by variable growth conditions can be controlled in part by culling out materials that do not meet strict quality standards. This ensures that further processing is limited to plant materials that are sufficiently standardized in their relevant constituents. Thus, contrary to many popularly held misconceptions, standardization of the herbal extract is much more than simply a process of adjusting chemistry and begins with the cultivation, selection and mixing of the herbal raw materials. In fact, the standardization of herbs and herbal preparations actually begins with the current movement toward the development of Good Agricultural Practices (GAPs) wherein agronomic and horticultural parameters and practices for the commercial cultivation of medicinal plants is determined by national and international convention.

1.3.2.2 Production Methods

The nature of the solvent and of the extraction and drying processes critically affects the internal composition of the finished product. Polar compounds are soluble in water, while lipophilic constituents are soluble in alcohol. For example, an aqueous extract of valerian has a fundamentally different spectrum of constituents than a solid extract that has been processed with ethanol. Even when identical solvents are used, the extraction technique itself can yield extracts that have different chemical and pharmacologic actions. This principle can be further illustrated by a simple example:

A total of 107 volunteers were randomly assigned to 3 groups after a 3-week "run-in" phase. Group A drank 4–6 cups of coffee daily that had been brewed by boiling the coffee grounds (pharmaceutically, a decoction, filtered or decanted). Group B drank the same amount of coffee that had been brewed by filtering (pharmaceutically, a percolate), and Group C drank no coffee. The test period lasted a total of 9 weeks. The subjects in Group A showed a significant rise in serum cholesterol averaging 0.48 nmol/L. Their low-density lipoprotein (LDL) level also rose by 0.39 nmol/L. There was no significant difference between Groups B and C, and there were no significant changes in high-density lipoprotein (HDL)or apolipoprotein levels in any of the groups. Thus, adverse effects were associated with the consumption of coffee brewed by boiling but not with coffee brewed by filtering (Bak et al.; 1989).

This study illustrates that differences in the preparation process – in this case decoction versus percolation – can significantly alter the chemistry and therefore the action of the preparation in the human body. This particularly applies to commercially produced extracts, which are manufactured by a variety of processes using various solvents. All extracts are not the same!

Commercially available extracts vary greatly in their quality. Like many other products, plant extracts are sold in free markets and "spot markets" that offer surplus goods at a premium price. Strict standards usually are not applied to the phytochemical ingredients of these extracts, so there is no guarantee that processing of the extracts will yield an herbal medicine of consistent and acceptable quality (Hänsel and Trunzler, 1989; Gaedke and Steinhoff, 2000).

1.3.2.3 Adjustment of Quality

Another approach to achieving consistent pharmaceutical quality is to blend selected batches of the primary extracts together in a way that ensures a most consistent concentration of specific ingredients or groups of compounds. The ingredients selected for this "quality adjustment" process should be those that are important for the actions and efficacy of the product, to the extent that such constituents are known. If therapeutic efficacy is critically influenced by a single group of compounds (e.g., anthranoids in anthranoid-based stimulant laxatives, see Sect. 5.6.4), the quality adjustment can be accomplished with therapeutically inert excipients. With most phytomedicines, however, the contribution of specific components to therapeutic efficacy is either speculative or unknown. In these cases the extracts are adjusted to certain "marker compounds" to ensure pharmaceutical quality. Often these marker compounds are chemicals that are merely characteristic components of the herb in question, i.e., they can help ensure the identity or some other quality parameter of the botanical material. In many cases these substances have not been tested for their actions or therapeutic efficacy in pharmacologic test models or in clinical studies.

Since individual plant species are genetically determined, their chemical composition is also determined to some degree. It is reasonable to assume, then, that correlations exist between the marker compounds of plants and other therapeutically relevant ingredients that occur in whole extracts. The strength of these correlations is unknown for most phytomedicines, however, so the adjustment of whole plant extracts to improve their quality based solely on selected marker constituents remains questionable from a therapeutic standpoint. Technological means are needed to compensate for the biologic variability of herbal medicines.

1.3.2.4 Analytical Quality Control

Besides the controlled cultivation of herbs and the use of standardized production methods, chemical analysis is necessary to ensure the optimum homogeneity of plant extracts. This applies to the raw materials themselves (dried herbs and extracts) as well as the finished products. In contrast to the chemically defined constituents of synthetic drugs, which can be quantitatively measured, a lack of knowledge about the specific chemical constituents of phytomedicines requires the reliance on qualitative and semi-quantitative chromatographic methods of separation and analysis.

Figure 1.3 shows a typical profile of the ingredients in a St. John's wort (*Hypericum perforatum*) extract that was fractionated by high-performance liquid chromatography (HPLC). Depending on the technology and solvent used, this technique can generate

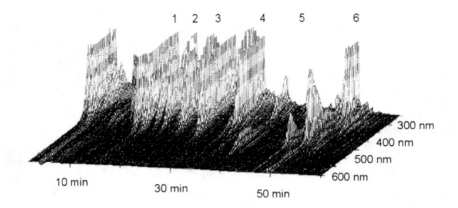

Figure 1.3. ▲ Segment of an HPLC fingerprint chromatogram of a commercially available St. John's wort extract. The constituents identified (here: 1 = hyperoside, 2 = quercitrin, 3 = quercetin, 4 = biapigenin, 5 = hypericin, 6 = hyperforin) must display the correct position and amplitude in tests for quality control.

chemical spectra that characterize the multicomponent active principle as uniquely as a fingerprint.

Covering a broad range of constituents, this "fingerprint chromatogram" can not only establish the identity of active plant constituents but can also test their constant internal composition by checking the "fingerprint" of a test batch against the electronically stored chromatogram of a standard reference sample.

1.4 Phytomedicines

1.4.1 Liquid Dosage Forms

Phytomedicines are drug products made from botanicals (herbs), whole extracts, or concentrates of active plant constituents. They are available in solid and liquid form. The liquid dosage forms include:

▶ Tinctures, glycerites, and related products
▶ Syrups
▶ Medicinal oils
▶ Medicinal spirits
▶ Plant juices.

1.4.1.1 Tinctures, Glycerites, and Related Products

Tinctures are alcoholic or hydroalcoholic solutions prepared from botanicals. If glycerol is used as a solvent, the preparation is known as a glycerite. Increasingly, extractions are performed with a mixture of glycerol, propylene glycol, and water instead of ethanol and water. Polyethylene glycol 400 has recently been used as a solvent. Glycerol is a biological substance, occurring as a component of natural glycerides. Propylene glycol is a form of glycerol in which one of the two terminal hydroxyl groups is absent. Polyethyleneglycol is a synthetic product, the number 400 indicating its average molecular weight. It is a clear, colorless liquid that preferentially extracts lipophilic compounds from the crude drug (usually, dried plant material).

The type of solvent used is indicated by the manufacturer; for example, it may appear on the package insert under the heading "Other Ingredients" or "Excipients." There are two methods of producing fixed combinations in tincture form: by mixing individual tinctures or by mixing the crude plant material and then performing the extraction. The difference is illustrated by two similar prescription formulas that are used in the treatment of indigestion:

Prescription 1:
Rx   Comp. cinchona tincture   100 mL
Directions: Take 30 drops, diluted with water,
             three times daily shortly before meals.

The preparation is made by extracting an herbal mixture composed of cinchona bark (12 parts), bitter orange peel (4 parts), gentian root (4 parts), and cinnamon bark(2 parts) with 70 % ethanol (v/v) (100 parts).

Prescription 2:
Rx   Cinchona tincture   60.0
            Bitter orange peel tincture   20.0
            Gentian tincture   20.0
            Cinnamon tincture   10.0
Directions: Take 30 drops, diluted with water,
             three times daily shortly before meals.

The compounding pharmacist makes up this preparation by mixing the ready-made tinctures. The preparation may become cloudy or form precipitates, but generally this will not alter its efficacy. One advantage of liquid dosage forms in general is that they provide an alternative for patients who have difficulty swallowing pills and capsules. One disadvantage is their shorter shelf life, which may be further reduced due to improper storage by the patient (open container, too much heat or moisture).

1.4.1.2 Syrups

Already known to ancient Arabic healers, medicinal syrups entered European medicine during the early Middle Ages. The word *syrup* is derived from the Arabic *sirab, scharab* or *scherbet*, meaning a sugary juice beverage. Syrups are viscous preparations for internal use containing at least 50 % sucrose and usually 60–65 %. The sugar content of syrups (about 66 %) is essential for extending their shelf life. Microorganisms cannot proliferate in saturated sugar solutions because highly concentrated solutions deprive the microbes of the water necessary for their development. Preservatives must be added to syrups with a lower sugar content to protect them from bacterial growth.

Syrups are used as flavoring agents, especially in pediatric medicine. Syrups made from marshmallow root, fennel seed), English plantain herb , and thyme herb are all commonly prescribed in German pediatrics.

1.4.1.3 Medicinal Oils

Medicinal oils are mostly fatty oils or liquid waxes containing solutions or extracts of drug substances. Medicinal oils are used both internally and externally. Examples of medicinal oils prepared by extraction of plant material are St. John's wort oil and garlic oil maceration. Oils containing dissolved drugs are exemplified by solutions of volatile oils in liquid jojoba (*Simmondsia chinensis*) wax, which are commonly used as massage oils, especially in aromatherapy.

1.4.1.4 Medicinal Spirits

A spirit or essence is al solution of a volatile substance in alcohol or in water and alcohol. Medicinal spirits are made either by dissolving the volatile oil in alcohol, as in the case of Peppermint Spirit BPC made with peppermint oil, or by distillation.

To produce a medicinal spirit by distillation, the crude drug is pulverized, mixed with alcohol, and allowed to stand until the volatile components have dissolved out of the herbal tissue (oil cells, oil glands, oil reservoirs). Finally these components are recovered by distillation.

There is an potential risk associated with the use of medicinal spirits as they may reactivate an old alcohol-related dependency or exacerbate an existing one.

1.4.1.5 Plant Juices

Freshly harvested plant parts are macerated in water and pressed. The shelf life of the expressed juice can be extended by conventional pasteurization or by rapid, ultra-high-temperature treatment (flash method). Plant juices are produced only from medicinal plants that do not contain highly potent chemicals. While expressed juices do contain the water-soluble components of the processed plant, they are free of lipophilic constituents. Little is known about the chemical composition of plant juices or their possible reactions in aqueous media. In Germany, plant juices are nonprespcription remedies that are used chiefly for self-medication.

Some common sources of plant juices are birch leaves, nettle, watercress, St. John's wort, garlic, dandelion, lemon balm, European mistletoe, radish, English plantain, and horsetail.

1.4.2 Solid Dosage Forms

Powdered extracts and concentrates must be protected from light, oxygen, and moisture. This is best accomplished by processing them into solid dosage forms such as granules, tablets, coated tablets, and capsules. Preparing medications in a form appropriate for their intended use also permits more accurate dosing. In addition to solid dosage forms, there are other forms such as tinctures of fluidextracts, ampoules, and semisolid preparations. This section deals exclusively with solid dosage forms. An herbal drug substance becomes a medication through the process of pharmaceutical formulation, in which excipients are added to the drug substance. In Europe, healthcare professionals can access product information to learn about the excipients that have been used in any given productSolid dosage forms must be taken with an adequate amount of liquid (100–200 mL) to avoid leaving drug residues that may harm the esophagus. This is a particular concern in the elderly and in patients with pre-existing damage to the esophageal mucosa (as in the case of excessive alcohol consumption).

1.4.2.1 Granules

Granules are aggregates of powdered material held together with binders. Their production involves the use of various excipients such as gelatin solution, methyl cellulose, simple syrup, lactose, and sucrose. Granules are usually processed into tablets but also may be used as a separate dosage form. Drug substances used in the treatment of gastrointestinal complaints are often produced in granulated form.

1.4.2.2 Uncoated Tablets

Tablets are made by the compression of powdered or granulated material (compressed tablets). Besides the active ingredients, which may amount o only a few milligrams, tablets may contain diluents, binders, lubricants, coloring and flavoring agents, and disintegrators to help the compressed tablet dissolve in an aqueous medium.

1.4.2.3 Coated Tablets

Coated tablets are compressed tablets covered with a coating of sugar, dyes, fat, wax, and/or protein. The function of the coating is to protect the medicinal core. Tablets can also be coated with film-forming agents, usually polymers (e. g., cellulose acetate phthalate), to produce a film-coated tablet (FCT). Several advantages of coated tablets are explained below:

▶ Release of the medication can be controlled or delayed (enteric-coated tablets, controlled-release tablets).
▶ Shelf life is extended, as the coating protects against external influences such as light, moisture, and mechanical stresses.
▶ They are easier to swallow than uncoated tablets; less chance they might adhere to oral or esophageal mucosa.
▶ The coating masks any unpleasant taste from the medicinal core.

1.4.2.4 Capsules

Hard gelatin capsules consist of a two-part cylindrical shell whose halves are fitted together after the medication – a powdered or granulated drug substance – has been placed inside. Besides gelatin, the capsule shell may contain either glycerin or sorbitol as a softening agent, water, aromatics, dyes, and antimicrobial additives. Volatile oils may be encapsulated by adding them first to a powdered excipient; the oils will subsequently be released in the gastrointestinal tract.

Soft gelatin capsules are spherical, oval, oblong, or teardrop-shaped capsules with a gelatin shell enclosing semisolid or liquid contents that must be free of water (e. g., oily garlic extracts or peppermint oil).

The material of the capsule shell can be designed to delay the release of the medicinal substance until the capsule has entered the stomach or intestine. A chemically modified cellulose, hydroxypropylene methylcellulose phthalate (HPMCP), makes an effective enteric (gastric-acid-resistant) coating. Insoluble while in the acidic milieu of the stomach, this compound dissociates when the pH rises above 7 and becomes soluble under physiologic conditions in the bowel.

Enteric coatings on capsules and tablets offer several advantages:

▶ They protect the drug substance from deactivation or decomposition by gastric juices.
▶ They shield the stomach lining from drug substances that could cause irritation or nausea (salicylates, emetine).
▶ They prevent dilution of the drug substance before it reaches the bowel (intestinal antispasmodics or antiseptics).

Enteric-coated capsules or tablets that release the drug substance after entering the bowel should never be taken during or after meals, but approximately 1 hour before meals.

Particles larger than 3 mm in diameter do not leave the stomach with the chyme; they are retained in the stomach until the subsequent interdigestive phase. One danger of enteric-coated capsules is that they may remain in the stomach for some time while the pH of the gastric juice rises, leading to premature release of the drug inside the stomach.

1.4.2.5 Lozenges

Lozenges (troches, pastilles) have a tablet-like appearance (round, oblong, etc.) but differ from tablets in that they are not made by compression but are molded or cut from pliable masses of varying composition. Lozenges are designed to release the active ingredient slowly into the oral cavity while sucked or chewed. The base is composed of sucrose (usually more than 90 %), acacia (about 7 %), gelatin, tragacanth, and water (e. g., Echinacea Capsettes).

1.4.3 Packaging

The package is an essential part of any medication. Packaging turns a pharmaceutical preparation into a product ready for consumer use. It encloses and protects the contents from the environment. The package is labeled to designate its contents and convey other information such as the expiration date and the batch number in case the product must be recovered or recalled. Package inserts provide detailed information on contents, actions, usage, indications, contraindications, and side effects. (Fig. 1.4).

In the United States where most botanical products are sold as dietary supplements, not as approved drugs, therapeutic claims cannot be made on the label or in the package insert (technically part of the labelling). A statement or claim can be made regarding the effect of the product on the structure or function of the body so long as the statement is truthful and not misleading, is supported by a reasonable amount of sci-

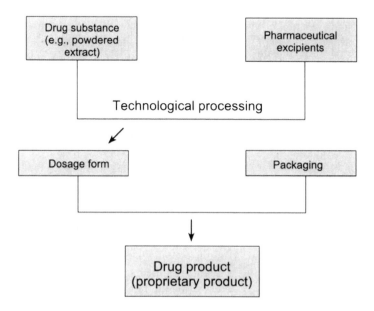

Figure 1.4. ▲ Relationship between drug substance, dosage form, and finished drug product.

entific evidence, and the manufacturer notifies the Food and Drug Administration (FDA) within 30 days that it has introduced the product with the stated claim. If such a claim is made, it must be followed by a disclaimer stating that the claim has not been approved by the FDA and that the product is not intended to diagnose, treat, cure, of prevent any disease.

1.4.4 Drug Approval

In Germany as elsewhere, drugs cannot be marketed until they have been approved by a competent federal agency. This applies to chemically-defined synthetic conventional drugs as well as to phytomedicines. Before a product is granted approval, it must be demonstrated that the product meets legally prescribed standards with regard to pharmaceutical quality, efficacy, and safety. The best way to do this is by conducting original pharmacologic, toxicologic, and clinical tests.

In some European countries data that have been published in the literature, including reports on clinical experience, can also be used for this purpose. This rule has been in force in Germany since 1978, when the German Drug Law of 1976 went into effect. One of its goals was to bring German drug laws into conformance with European laws. The German approval agency was unable to meet the 12-year transition deadline established by whom, the European Commission, with the result that traditional remedies having de facto approval" are currently on the market along with officially tested products. Pursuant to an intervention by the European Commission, it appears that the older products will either receive new approval or be pulled from the market in the near future.

In the original version of the 1976 German Drug Law, the manufacturers of known drug substances (including practically all phytomedicines) were required to document only the pharmaceutical quality of their products. They could demonstrate safety and efficacy by referral to published monographs. To make these monographs available, the German Health Agency (now called the Federal Institute for Drugs and Medical Devices) appointed expert commissions whose primary task was to review the pertinent literature. Commission E was appointed for phytotherapeutic agents. From 1983 to 1994, this commission reviewed a total of 380 monographs, 254 of which gave a positive therapeutic recommendation and 126 a negative recommendation (Gaedcke and Steinhoff, 2000). The negative recommendations were based on the evaluation that the particular herb was either too toxic to be sold as a non-prescription drug and/or that there was insufficient data to support a positive recommendation (Blumenthal et al., 1998).

The Commission E monographs mainly described single herbs and preparations made from them. The active ingredient of an herbal medication as defined by the German Drug Law is a preparation (e.g., a whole extract) that is made from one herb. If the product contains no additional plant ingredients, it is classified as a single-herb product. This type of product is preferred in the practice of rational phytotherapy. Nevertheless, a number of fixed combinations containing several active herbal ingredients are still being marketed in Germany1. The German Drug Law requires proof that each of these pharmacologically active ingredients makes its own contribution to the efficacy of the product. As a result, one of the tasks of Commission E was to identify effective combination patterns for this category of herbal products[1].

Commission E stopped gathering and reviewing monographs in 1994. A collected volume of the monographs that had appeared in the *Bundesanzeiger* up to that time was later published in English (Blumenthal et al., 1998). Commission E no longer updated these monographs after 1994, but they can still be used as corroborating data in German and European approval programs, in which applicants are obliged to document the current status of their products with original research, new contributions from the literature, and their evaluation by experts.

In Germany, which leads the phytomedicine market in Europe with about a 45 % share, an important change was made in the approval process in 1994. Since the change was enacted, proprietary herbal products can be approved either by citing original studies on efficacy and safety ("rational phytomedicines," see examples in Table 1.2) or by citing long-term experience with their therapeutic use ("traditional phytomedicines"). In the latter case, manufacturers are exempt from having to furnish their own proof of efficacy and safety for a list of designated herbal preparations. This exemption does not affect the manufacturers' obligation to guarantee the pharmaceutical quality of their products. The "traditionally" approved products must be specifically identified as such (e.g., with wording such as "mild acting," "for better health," "for more vigor," "for better organ function," etc.). Most of these products are used for minor health problems, and many are self-selected by patients. Generally, their costs are not covered by health insurance plans. Beyond general issues of patient counselling, the traditional phytomedicines are less important to prescribing physicians and therefore will be covered less fully in the chapters that follow.

The common Drug Law that has existed within the European Union (EU) since 1998 provides not only that phytomedicines shall retain their drug status in Germany but also that they shall be given that status in the other countries of the EU. The law further provides that the distinction between "rational" and "traditional" products that exists in Germany will be adopted in the other EU member nations as well (Keller, 1996; Gaedcke and Steinhoff, 2000; EU Commission, 2002). An essential prerequisite for establishing a European standard was the continuation and updating of monographs dealing with phytomedicines. This has been done chiefly by the European Scientific Cooperative on Phytotherapy (ESCOP), a coalition of all national phytotherapy soci-

---

[1] From an historical perspective, the penchant for multi-herb formulations in phytomedicine has different roots. One factor dating from antiquity is the "magic of numbers" principle. Galen (131–201 AD) taught that, while the nature and dosage of a remedy were important, it was also important to prescribe the correct number of medicines to achieve the desired curative effect (Haas, 1956). A later historical idea was the "theriaca" principle, which states that since we do not know what ingredient will work in any given case, we should pack as many drugs into a prescription as possible so that a potentially effective ingredient will not be missed. A theriaca was a mixture of 50–100 different substances; the theriaca dispensed by Valerius Cordus contained 65 ingredients (1511–1544). A theriaca with 12 ingredients was still listed in the *German Pharmacopeias* of 1882 and 1926 (including 1% opium). Theriaca-like mixtures are still being marketed today under various brand names ("Swedish Herbs").

Table 1.2.
Examples of phytomedicines that have undergone pharmacologic testing and whose efficacy has been further established by controlled studies and well-documented reports of physician experience.

Herb	Presumed-Active Compound(s)	Action	Indication
Ginkgo leaf extract (50:1)	Bilobalide, ginkgolides, flavonoids	anti-ischemic, antioxidative, PAF-antagonistic, hemorrhagic	Symptomatic treatment of cognitive deficiencies due to organic brain disease and peripheral arterial occlusive diseases
St. John's wort	Presumably hypericins and hyperforin and flavonoids	antidepressant	Mild to moderate depressive episodes (ICD-10: F32.0 and F 32.1)
Chamomile flowers	Presumably chamazulene, bisabolol, lipophilic flavonoids	anti-inflammatory, antispasmodic, carminative	Inflammatory disorders of the skin, airways, and gastrointestinal tract (see p. 251)
Kava rhizome	Methysticin and chemically related pyrones	local anesthetic, anticonvulsant, central muscle relaxant	States of nervous anxiety, tension, and restlessness
Garlic cloves	Presumably alliin, allicin, S-acetylcysteine	lowers lipid levels, inhibits platelet aggregation, fibrinolytic, antibacterial, antihypertensive	Prevention of general atherosclerosis
Milk thistle fruits (extract concentrated at 70–80% silymarin)	Silymarin, especially silybinin	antihepatotoxic; at the cellular level, promotes ribosome formation and protein synthesis	Dyspeptic complaints, toxic liver diseases
Horse chestnut extract	Aescin (triterpenoid saponins)	antiexudative, antiedemic	Complaints due to chronic venous insufficiency
Saw palmetto berries	Phytosterols	5α-Reductase inhibition, anti-inflammatory	Benign prostatic hyperplasia
Senna leaves	Sennosides, especially sennoside B	stimulates bowel motility, antiabsorptive, stimulates secretions	Constipation, or to cleanse the bowel before diagnostic procedures
Hawthorn leaf and flower extract	Presumably glycosyl flavonoids and proanthocyanidins	positive inotropic, positive chronotropic, improves hypoxic tolerance, reduces afterload	Mild heart failure (NYHA stage II)

eties in Europe (ESCOP, 2003). Another key function of these professional societies is to ensure that legal copyright protection is secured for significant scientific studies dealing with phytomedicines.

1.5 Phytotherapy

1.5.1 Applications of Phytomedicines

Phytomedicines are, with few exceptions (e.g., see Sect. 5.7.1.6), not appropriate for use in emergency or acute-care situations. They have only a minor role in the hospital setting. Phytomedicines are mainly prescribed by family doctors in office settings and certain specialists (e.g., Urologists who prescribe Serenoa etc., or OB-GYN's who prescribe Cimicifuga, or Psychiatrists who prescribe Hypericum) or are self-selected by patients according to their own regimens. A large percentage of patients treated with herbal medicines have relatively mild or ambiguous conditions that often defy a clear-cut diagnosis or can be diagnosed only by exclusion. These conditions include somatoform disorders, often associated with pain, as well as nervousness, sleep disorders, mild or moderate depressive episodes, and a number of chronic ailments and complaints.

The arrangement of the chapters in this book by organ systems reflects the most frequent applications of herbal medicines. This hierarchical arrangement by indications corresponds roughly to prescribing practice. The 100 most widely prescribed herbal medications in Germany in 2002 (see Appendix) can be broken down as follows according to their frequency of use for specific groups of indications:

- Diseases of the respiratory tract (25 products)
- Central nervous system disorders (25 products)
- Diseases of the stomach, bowel, liver, and bile (11 products)
- Urnary tract (11 products)
- Cardiovascular system (8 products)
- Dermatologic remedies and external anti-inflammatory agents (7 products)
- Nonspecific immune enhancers (4 products)
- Gynecologic remedies (4 products)
- Remedies for internal use in the treatment of rheumatic disorders and inflammatory conditions (5 products)

1.5.2 Patient Expectations

A well-known German institute of demographic research conducts regular opinion surveys to explore the attitudes of the German public toward natural remedies (IFD Survey 7016, 2002). In 2002 the institute surveyed a representative cross section of 2172 people ranging from 16 to 90 years of age. Thirty-five percent of the responders considered the prescription of natural remedies to be "very important," 41 % rated it as "important," and 13 % rated it as "not very important." This survey demonstrates the generally high regard in which phytomedicines are held by the German public. When asked whether these products were effective, 4 % said no, 38 % had no opinion, and 54 % were convinced that herbal remedies are effective. Most of the responders believed, however, that natural remedies worked differently from synthetic drugs.

Opinions on product safety were even more revealing: 82 % of those surveyed rated the risk of treatment with natural remedies as "low," while 84 % rated the risks of synthetic drugs as "moderate to high" (Fig. 1.5). This opinion was held about equally by devotees and opponents of natural remedies.

Thus, the demand of many patients, especially the elderly, for herbal remedies is rooted partly in the emotional perception that natural products are gentler and safer than chemical products. Beyond some very concrete evidence for certain active plant constituents, even a consultation with their doctor would be unlikely to shake patients from this preconceived notion. A more reasonable approach is to base the prescription and recommendation of herbal remedies on the way in which patients actually use these products, which presupposes that the products generally have a broad, safe therapeutic range. Potent plant-based medicines, such as preparations made from cardiac glycoside-containing plant parts like the foxglove (*Digitalis* spp.), tropane alkaloids from belladonna (*Atropa belladonna*), or colchicine from the autumn crocus (*Colchicum autumnale*) do not meet these safety criteria, and so it is best not to use the term "herbal" or "botanical" when referring to these products. For these indications it is better to prescribe pure "chemical" compounds such as digitalis glycoside, atropine, colchicine, etc. (see Table 1.1).

At the same time, confidence in a remedy is the best foundation for its successful use in selected therapeutic applications (see Sect. 1.5.3). Consequently, it would not be good medical practice to give such patients an academic lecture on pros and cons. Once the treatment decision has been made, it is better to bolster patients' confidence and their self-healing powers by educating them about the selected medication (and any associated risks!) in positive terms. The basic background information about a synthetic drug mainly involves its chemical structure, which is of little interest to most patients. But with an herbal medication, the patient can be shown a picture of the medicinal plant

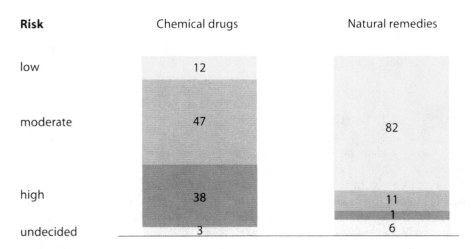

Figure 1.5. ▲ Results of a representative survey of 2172 German citizens on the risks of synthetic drugs versus natural remedies. The latter are believed to have a very large therapeutic range and a high safety margin (IFD Survey 7016, 2002).

and told its history, providing an excellent context for the treatment interview. Doctors who recommend plant-derived medicines, therefore, should become familiar with the plants from which they are derived. They should know about their botanical characteristics, the plant parts that are used medicinally, and their traditional therapeutic uses.

1.5.3 Drug Therapy and the "Doctor's Word"

The tools available to physicians in dealing with the sick are their senses, speech, hands, instruments, medications, and other aids. The emphasis in the choice of the various therapeutic modalities has changed many times during the past century. The initial decades were marked by epochal advances in medicine and especially in the use of drugs. This progress sparked a fondness for medical intervention, with a declining emphasis on the "doctor's word." The risks of drug treatment were also growing, and many patients had to learn about these risks by reading the package insert or experiencing them first-hand. This emphasis on chemistry and technology in physician services has become unacceptable to many patients. It has sparked a countermovement in which patients have strayed from orthodox medicine by the millions and turned to alternative fields of medicine. Doctors who offer natural healing services in their practices have bowed to this migration and are also helping in an important way to maintain the pre-eminence of orthodox medicine.

In almost half of the patients who see a general practitioner, a definitive diagnosis cannot be established in the doctor's office. The primary goal in these cases after the initial interview is to provide treatment that will allay the patient's discomfort, physical complaints, or specific symptoms (Mader and Weissgerber, 2003). To be successful despite an uncertain diagnosis, the treatment must take into account the basic attitudes of the patient, such as an aversion to synthetic drugs (see Sect. 1.5.2), as well as the risks and potential benefits of all available therapeutic modalities. The remedies prescribed by family doctors continue to rank highly in this regard. In Germany, general practitioners and internists in private practice write approximately two-thirds of all prescriptions, issuing most of them to patients over 60 years of age. But medical therapies in most older patients do not require the use of drugs that produce strong, acute effects with a rapid onset.

Today the therapeutic benefit of drugs is assessed mainly by outcome measures that were established in the artificial realm of clinical double-blind studies. In the official drug-approval process and in most evaluations for setting therapeutic guidelines, the efficacy of a pharmacologic treatment is considered equal to the difference between the true drug and the placebo. But comparisons of the actual and apparent pharmacodynamic effects of synthetic antidepressants in the wake of therapeutic studies with St. John's wort (Schulz, 2000, 2002 a, 2003 a; HDT Study Group, 2002; Timothy et al., 2002) show how misleading this standard can be when it is applied to whole classes of medications. A differentiated analysis of representative numbers from placebo-controlled studies has shown that the psychodynamic component of antidepressant therapy (the "herb doctor," measurable as the "placebo effect") accounts for between two-thirds and one-third of the overall effect relative to the pharmacodynamic component. This ratio holds equally true for synthetic and herbal antidepressants (Mulrow et al., 1999; Schulz, 2002a; Timothy et al., 2002). This means, however, that besides issues of drug tolerance and acceptance, the services rendered by the physician can have a greater impact on the patient's condition than the pharmacodynamic actions of the therapeutic agent itself.

This discovery is by no means limited to the treatment of depression. It is equally valid for a great many important indications in general medicine. This is proven by quantitative analyses of the placebo contribution to the overall efficacy of pharmacologic therapies in controlled clinical studies. As Fig. 1.6 shows, the pharmacodynamic properties of the active ingredients generally account for only about 20–40 % of the overall therapeutic effect for the indications shown (Kirsch and Sapirstein, 1998; Montgomery, 1999a,b; Nickel, 1998; Schulz, 2000; Weihrauch and Gauler, 1999). It is also noteworthy that the indications listed in Fig. 1.6 largely match the most common indications for the prescription of phytomedicines in Germany. This is consistent with the therapeutic impression of many physicians in private practice. Phytomedicines have properties that are particularly advantageous for these indications, such as good tolerance and a high degree of patient acceptance.

This also raises questions as to the clinical relevance and economy (see Sect. 1.5.4) of therapeutic studies in which the response component that is mediated by the sensitive guidance and conviction of the physician, which can stimulate the patient's self-healing powers, is either ignored altogether or dismissed as a placebo effect. This type of approach creates theoretical standards that are remote from the practical management of psychologically-related conditions such as depression, sleep disorders, and dementia (Schulz, 2002 b).

The opinion, especially prevalent in theoretical medicine, that only pharmacodynamically proven effects have a valid place in evidence-based medicine (EBM) should be modified for certain applications. This can even help to promote a broader acceptance of orthodox medicine. Placing greater emphasis on the interactive role of the physician in pharmacotherapeutic settings does not contradict the philosophy of EBM. The idea, rather, is to supplement the results of studies with experience gained from medical practice. The value of a therapy should be judged by its benefit for the patient, not by how the response is mediated solely according to statistical parameters. The patients themselves can best answer the question of whether diseases like those listed in Fig. 1.6 can be treated pharmacologically. The use of "folk medicines" for such indications cannot be prevented by administrative actions. Instead, we know from experience that these therapies are becoming increasingly widespread and, unfortunately, are occurring in areas from which orthodox medicine has partially excluded itself (Eisenberg et al., 1998; Ernst et al., 2001; Rees, 2001). It should also be noted that almost all "confirmed" efficacy findings for these indications come from controlled drug studies. (Controlled studies of nonpharmacologic treatment methods – e.g., massage therapy and other related modalities – often fail simply because the participants and physicians cannot be blinded to the test conditions.)

Phytomedicines merit special interest in comparison with other "complementary" medical therapies because rational phytotherapy is inherently in tune with scientific thinking. For many physicians, this academic stature is an essential prerequisite for their own acceptance of phytomedicine within modern clinical practice and thus for its successful utilization in patients.

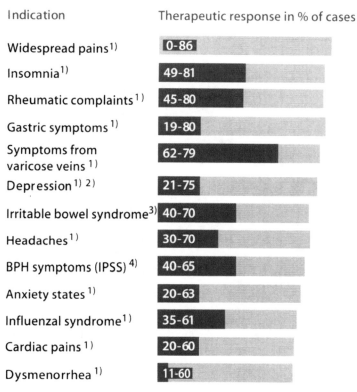

Indication | Therapeutic response in % of cases

Widespread pains[1]) **0-86**

Insomnia[1]) **49-81**

Rheumatic complaints[1]) **45-80**

Gastric symptoms[1]) **19-80**

Symptoms from varicose veins[1]) **62-79**

Depression[1]) [2]) **21-75**

Irritable bowel syndrome[3]) **40-70**

Headaches[1]) **30-70**

BPH symptoms (IPSS)[4]) **40-65**

Anxiety states[1]) **20-63**

Influenzal syndrome[1]) **35-61**

Cardiac pains[1]) **20-60**

Dysmenorrhea[1]) **11-60**

1) Gauler and Weihrauch, 1997
2) Kirsch and Sapirstein, 1998
3) Maxwell et al., 1997
4) Metzker et al., 1996; Nickel et al., 1996 and 1998

Figure 1.6. ▲ Cure rates related to psychodynamic (placebo) effects in mild and moderately severe disorders treated by family physicians (after Schulz, 2000).

1.5.4 Costs and Benefits

The number of drug prescriptions covered by statutory health insurance in Germany declined by 30 % from 1992 to 2001. The costs per prescription during the same period rose by 78 %. The sharp drop in prescriptions mainly affected phytomedicines (see Table A1 in the Appendix). Initially, it was hoped that these containment measures would save money, but this has not been the case. On the contrary, the overall drug costs between 1993 and 2001 rose more sharply than during the comparable period from 1981 to 1990 (Fig. 1.7). The authors of the *German Drug Prescription Report* (Schwabe and Paffrath, 2000, 2001) justified the drastic curtailment of prescription numbers in recent years by calling it a "comprehensive modernization of drug therapy." The decline in pre-

Millions of Rx

Billions of euros

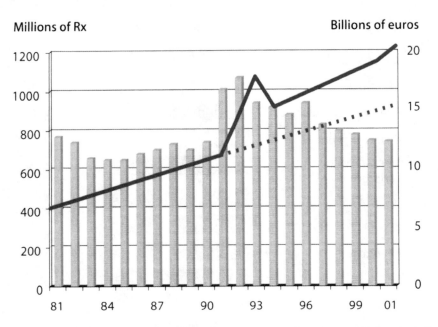

Figure 1.7. ▲ Drugs covered by national health insurance in Germany from 1981 to 2001, by sales (yellow line) and number of prescriptions (columns). Former East German states are included starting in 1991 (after Schwabe and Paffrath, 2000–2002).

scriptions, according to the 1999 and 2000 editions of the *Report*, has freed up the financial resources necessary for sharp sales increases in innovative classes of drugs, such as the 30 % marketing gain that was recorded for selective serotonin reuptake inhibitors (SSRIs) in the years 1999 and 2000.

One year later, however (Schwabe and Paffrath, 2002), the SSRIs were being re-evaluated. In Chapter 1 of the 2002 *Drug Prescription Report*, the section previously titled "Modernization of Drug Therapy" had been replaced by a "Pharmacotherapeutic Analysis of the Cost Increase." The SSRIs were no longer discussed under the heading of "Innovative Drugs" but under "Analog Products." In Chapter 43 by Lohse et al., it was noted that broad advances in the treatment of depression would no longer be achieved with new antidepressant drugs in the coming years but through measures such as "rational augmentation strategies." The authors did not elaborate on the meaning of this new term. Other press reports (Heim, 2002) make it clear, however, that this concept includes an adjustment of decades of misinterpretations regarding the efficacy of antidepressant medications (see Sect. 1.5.3, paragraph 3, and Sect. 2.2.9 of this book).

To be sure, the trend toward re-evaluating physician services in the setting of antidepressant pharmacotherapy is a welcome development. But in looking to the future, we should not ignore the costs that have been associated with these pharmacologic blind alleys in the past, because the freedom of physicians to prescribe medical therapies is partly a matter of economics. Every effort must be made to determine the direction in which research funds for new therapies should be applied and where it would be

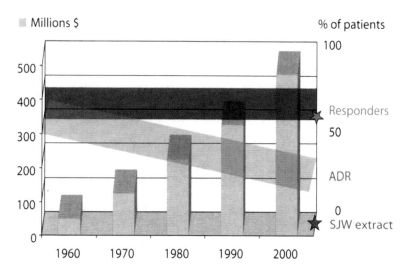

Figure 1.8. ▲ More than 30 new antidepressants have been introduced worldwide since 1960. The development costs per drug (columns) have risen 10-fold during this period. The efficacy rate (responders: horizontal bar for synthetic drugs, upper star for St. John's wort [SJW]) remained unchanged at 40–70 % of patients. The rate of adverse drug reactions (ADR: slanted bar for synthetic drugs, lower star for SJW) has fallen from approximately 50 % to 20 % of patients for synthetic drugs. The rate for SJW is approximately 2 %!

(or would have been) better to save those funds. Figure 1.8 traces the development of antidepressants since the late 1950s up to the present day. There is a consensus that drug efficacy, generally measured in terms of response rates by the Hamilton scale, was nearly constant throughout this period and that approximately 40–70 % of patients treated manifest a positive response, regardless of the product used. The incidence of adverse drug effects has declined during the past 40 years from an initial rate of approximately 50 % (tricyclic antidepressants) to a current rate of about 20 % (SSRIs) of the patients treated. In the case of St. John's wort preparations, this figure has remained a consistent 1–3 % over the years (Schulz, 2001, 2002 a).

More than 30 new drugs had to be placed on the market in order to achieve a relatively modest overall tolerance gain for synthetic antidepressants. The worldwide development costs alone that patients must pay for each of these new drugs have increased 10-fold from an estimated $50 million in the early 1960s to almost $500 million today. Comparing the above figures with St. John's wort extracts, we find that St. John's wort has roughly the same efficacy as synthetic antidepressant (see Sect. 2.2.7.3 of this book) its general tolerance is equal to the extrapolated tolerance that the synthetics will reach by the year 2030, but its development costs are roughly equal to the 1960 development costs for the synthetic drugs. This latter cost difference is reflected in per-day treatment costs, which range from approximately 40 cents (St. John's wort and amitriptyline) to $2 (alpha-2-antagonists and SSRIs). The health insurance funds in Germany spent almost $500 million for synthetic antidepressants alone in 2001. This is more money than was spent for *all* phytomedicines that were prescribed during the same year (Schwabe and Paffrath, 2002).

Unfortunately, antidepressants are not an isolated case. As we shall see in Sect. 2.1.8, the Drug Commission of the Association of German Physicians (AkdA), the American Academy of Neurology, and the British National Institute for Chemical Excellence have recently advocated the use of cholinesterase inhibitors (ChE inhibitors) in place of Ginkgo biloba extract (EGb) in patients with Alzheimer-type dementia (AkdA, 2001; Doody et al., 2001; O'Brian and Ballard, 2001). Although direct comparative studies have not been done, long-term studies covering periods of 24 to 56 weeks have been conducted separately for ChE inhibitors and EGb to determine efficacy in accordance with current EU guidelines. To date, only one psychometric scale has been widely used for assessing outcomes: the cognitive portion of the Alzheimer's Disease Assessment Scale (ADAS-Cog), which is scored from 1 to 70 (lower = better). The initial scores in the studies ranged from 20 to 30. The scores improved by approximately 2 points after 6 months' treatment with EGb and by 2–4 points with ChE inhibitors. With the ChE inhibitors, however, the relatively small differences are called into question by the occurrence of drug-specific side effects. In contrast to treatment with EGb, up to 90 % of the patients treated with ChE inhibitors experienced nausea and vomiting, raising suspicion that the apparent gain in antidepressant efficacy with the synthetic comparators was actually a methodologic effect relating to unblinding of the test groups. When treatment was discontinued, there was a more rapid reversal of therapeutic response with ChE inhibitors than with EGb. Adverse drug effects are more than 10 times more common with ChE inhibitors than EGb, and treatment costs are approximately 5 times higher (Schulz, 2003a). In absolute terms, this represents an added yearly cost of approximately $1000 per patient, with a total additional drug cost of approximately $1 billion per year in Germany alone. This burden is unacceptable given the relatively small potency advantage of ChE inhibitors, which, as just shown, may be due to the methodology of the trials, with little clinically significant benefit.

When prescribed by physicians, then, phytomedicines can be an effective counterpart to costly but dubious drugs like the examples above when used in the treatment of mild to moderate forms of depression or dementia. In passing the German Drug Law of 1976, lawmakers were on solid medical and economic ground when they elected to retain herbal medicines and confer the necessary legal status upon the plurality of pharmacologic (drug) therapies that had long existed in practice. If the modernization of synthetic drugs proceeds at a reasonable pace, it should be possible to make available to private practitioners in Germany and other European countries suitable herbal medicines for the treatment of relatively mild diseases and health problems and to continue prescribing these medications with coverage by statutory health insurance (Schulz, 2003 b). However, the prospects for such inclusion of herbal therapies in clinical practice in the U.S. are less clear, owing to the lack of an effective regulatory process to officially recognize the clinically documented benefits of numerous properly manufactured herbal and phytomedicinal preparations. In Canada, on the other hand, a new regulatory system in which so-called "Natural Health Products" or NHPs are being regulated separately from conventional foods and drugs, with the prospect that some reasonably appropriate claims may be made for some of these products leading to their presumably increased acceptance in clinical practice (Taller, 2003).

1.6   Medicinal Teas Today

Persons who prefer their daily coffee, cocoa or tea to caffeine tablets are unknowingly accepting and enjoying the pleasures of gentle-acting phytomedicines.

1.6.1   Origin of the Word "Tea." Medicinal and Nonmedicinal Teas

The word "tea" is of relatively recent origin. In 1601 a captain with the Dutch East India Company took several sacks of tea on board from a Chinese junk in Java and brought them to Holland, also bringing the name of the product, *t'e*, as it was called in the Amoy dialect of southern China. When Chinese tea found its way into other countries via Dutch and then British seaports, it retained the southern Chinese name that is familiar to us. Countries that first imported the herb by the land route through Russia adopted the name *chai*. Tea first reached Russia with a tea caravan in 1638 as *ch'a*, the name by which the herb is called in the Cantonese and Mandarin dialects of Chinese. The meaning of the term *tea* gradually broadened in the English language, first referring to the dried tea leaf, then to the beverage brewed from it, and soon it was applied to all herbs from which potable infusions can be made. The meaning of the word in any given case is determined by the context or by explanatory modifiers such as black tea, linden blossom tea, or herbal breakfast tea.

A basic distinction is drawn between:

- nonmedicinal teas that are consumed for pleasure, such as black tea and its blends, flavored teas, and tea-like products;
- medicinal teas that are used either as single teas or, more commonly, as tea mixtures (i.e., a mixture of various plant species).

For a product to be called a *tea* or *tea mixture* according to German food laws, it must consist of the leaf buds, young leaves and shoots of the tea shrub, *Camellia sinensis*, that have been prepared by methods normally used in the countries of origin (see also Sect. 5.5.1.1). Earl Gray, for example, is a mixture of teas originating from Ceylon, China, and India, to which bergamot oil is added.

Tea-like products are defined by German food laws as nonmedicinal tea substitutes made from the tops, lowers, or fruits of plants. They may bear the name *tea* only in conjunction with the name of the plant from which they are derived, e. g., apple peel tea, blackberry leaf tea, fennel tea, and rooibos tea. The latter tea, called also red bush tea, is the national drink of South Africa and has long been marketed and consumed in Europe. Rooibos tea consists of the dried leaves and branch tips of *Aspalathus linearis*, a bushy plant from the legume family distantly related to Europe's *Lupinus* species. In Germany the following herbs are offered singly or in mixtures as nonmedicinal teas: apple peels, blackberry leaves, rose hips, hibiscus flowers, raspberry leaves, life everlasting, mallow leaves, mallow flowers, peppermint leaves, sunflower blossoms, and calendula flowers. Obviously, it is sometimes difficult to draw a strict dividing line between a tea-like product and a medicinal tea. Even the pharmacodynamic action of a product does not provide a differentiating feature. For example, the effects of a cup of real tea are easier to demonstrate than the effects of a cup of linden blossom tea owing to the caffeine content of the regular tea. Thus, it is not surprising that shrewd businessmen occasionally try to represent a tea as medicinal while circumventing the German Drug Law. The basic determinants of whether a tea is a medicine or a food in any given case are the designated purpose of the product and consumer expectations. In Germany, the labels of tea-like products are not allowed to mention physiological actions or medicinal uses – a provision that can be formally circumvented by using magazine ads or printed information pamphlets to modify consumer expectations. In the U.S., medicinal teas may make relatively mild claims for their actions and benefits when they are sold as "dietary supplements" in accordance with the the Dietary Supplement Health and Education Act of 1994 (DSHEA) (Blumenthal and Israelsen, 2000). In Canada, as note above, medicinal teas can be regulated as Natural Health Products and contain on their labels government-recognized claims and benefits.

1.6.2   Medicinal Teas and Their Actions

Tea infusions can be prepared from single herbs or from herb mixtures. About 1000 single-herb teas and blends have been approved in Germany (Hiller, 1995). Common medicinal tea herbs and their indications are listed in Table 1.3 and 1.4. Exotic single-herb teas like those from the traditional medicine of India, China, or South American countries should not be prescribed if at all possible, i.e., at least in Germany. The pharmacist may be able to procure such exotic herbs, but by German law he or she can dispense the tea only if he or she can guarantee the pharmaceutical quality of the product. Usually these products have not been properly tested, so they cannot be legally dispensed (see also Sect. 1.6.8).

A typical medicinal tea consists of several herbs; thus, it represents the prototype of what is termed in Germany a fixed drug combination. In European phytotherapy the general rule is that it is considered sound pharmaceutical practice to have no more than 4–7 herbs in a blended tea (Wichtl, 1989). (This policy obviously contrasts with the practice in Asian systems of traditional medicine in which numerous herbs – often more than 7 and as many as 12 or more – are employed according to an empirical system that is based on the cosmological and philosophical tenets of the particular culture.))

Examples of tea mixtures acceptable in German phytotherapy can be found in pharmacopeias and in the standard approval criteria established by German health authorities. The compositions and formulations of these tea mixtures are given in the special section of this book dealing with specific indications. There have been only a few controlled clinical studies on the efficacy of medicinal teas published in the medical literature. (Lindemuth, 2000; Brinckmann et al., 2003)

Table 1.3.

Indications for the use of medicinal teas.

A. **Psychosomatic disorders**
   A1   Anxiety and restlessness
   A2   Nervous sleep disorders
   A3   Functional cardiac complaints

B. **Colds and congestion**
   B1   For phlegm congestion (expectorant teas)
   B2   For dry cough
   B3   To induce sweating
   B4   For fever

C. **Gastrointestinal disorders**
   C1   Digestive problems (flatulence, bloating)
   C2   Loss of appetite
   C3   Digestive problems associated with biliary tract dyskinesia
   C4   Mild inflammations of the gastric mucosa
   C5   Motion sickness

D. **Urinary tract disorders**
   D1   To promote diuresis
   D2   To disinfect the urine
   D3   To prevent stone disease (urolithiasis)

E. **Diarrhetic conditions**
   E1   Nonspecific, mild, transient forms

F. **Constipation**
   F1   To promote gentle bowel movements with soft stools, e.g., in patients with anal fissures or
   hemorrhoids or following anorectal surgery.
   F2   Chronic constipation, irritable colon.

G. **Local use as mouthwash or gargle**
   G1   Inflammations of the oropharyngeal mucosa
   G2   Oral hygiene

H. **Correctives**
   H1   To improve the odor or flavor of a tea mixture
   H2   To improve the appearance of a tea mixture

I. **Less common uses**
   I1   Adjuvant for excessive menstrual bleeding and other menstrual complaints
   I2   Physical and mental fatigue
   I3   Adjuvant for rheumatism

One reason for this is the challenge of adequately blinding the study participants to the extent that they can in a study of solid herbal preparations, so it is extremely difficult to establish a placebo control.

In some cases the efficacy of a medicinal tea is obvious. Anthranoid-containing herbs have a definite laxative action, teas with aromatic bitters stimulate the appetite, and nothing is usually better for an upset stomach than fasting and peppermint tea. The medicinal value of teas is based largely on empirical evidence. The contribution of the placebo effect to efficacy is probably large. The slogan, "Drink tea, wait and see," can be interpreted as a temporizing measure during the expectant phase of a still-undiagnosed illness that can calm emotions (anxiety) and reduce stress. Similar reasoning applies to patients who live in constant fear of becoming sick: "Health is just undetected disease."

The regimen that surrounds the use of a medicinal tea can positively influence the patient's subjective experience of his or her situation. The process of preparing the infusion and sipping the tea at intervals throughout the day can become a kind of relaxation exercise. A tea infusion differs from a solid dosage form of the same composition in that its sensory effects – smell, taste, and pleasant warming sensation behind the sternum – are fully appreciated. Thus, medicinal teas continue to be an effective, recommended therapy as long as they are made from herbs that are relatively free of toxicologic risk.

1.6.3 Various Forms of Medicinal Teas

Three kinds of tea are distinguished according to their external form:

▶ blended teas (containing more than one plant species),
▶ tea-bag teas,
▶ soluble teas.

All three forms are commercially produced and sold as ready-to-use products. Coarse-cut teas and tea-bag teas (filter bags) can also be made and stored in pharmacies. Most of these teas are prepared according to the specifications stated in pharmacopeias or other legal standards. Finally, the pharmacist can compound teas as prescribed by a physician, generally preparing the tea as a mixture of cut herbs.

1.6.3.1 Mixtures of Cut and Dried Herbs

Until a few decades ago, this was the only type of tea that was widely available. An example is the "sedative tea" listed in the German Pharmacopeia, 6th ed. It is prepared from:

▶ coarsely cut bogbean   4 parts
▶ coarsely cut peppermint   3 parts
▶ coarsely cut valerian   3 parts.

One advantage of such products is that the user can check the quality of the mixture by inspecting it for pest infestation, a high content of powdered herb (tea dust), etc.

Tea mixtures composed of various herbs should be shaken vigorously or stirred with a spoon before use. This ensures that small, light components that have settled during storage will not distort the ration of the ingredients.

1.6.3.3 Soluble Teas

Real tea (*Camellia sinensis*) was the first tea to be packaged in filter bags, and 80 % of it is currently sold in this form (Katalyse Environmental Group, 1981). Tea bags are advantageous in that they simplify dosing and are convenient to use. Their disadvantages relate to the finely chopped condition of the herbal material. This provides a large surface area that is accessible to air, promoting oxidative changes and the evaporation of aromatics and volatile oils. Another disadvantage is that the quality of a powdered herb is more difficult to assess by simple inspection. For example, chamomile flowers may contain excessive amounts of stem pieces (Schilcher, 1982; Bauer et al. 1989).

1.6.3.2 Tea-bag Teas

Powdered and instant teas are not teas in the strict sense. They consist of particles of a carrier substance such as lactose or maltodextrin that have been coated with a dry herbal extract. The quality of these products is variable. The filler content ranges from 50 % to 92 %, so the actual content of herbal extract is only 8–50 %. Sucrose is the vehicle used in most instant teas, and the product may contain up to 97 % sugar – a fact that should be noted by diabetics.

1.6.4 Standard Approval for Tea Mixtures

Tea mixtures that are prepared in quantity and stored in pharmaceutical laboratories, public pharmacies, and hospital pharmacies are exempt from individual approval according to the German Drug Law, as long as the tea formula is in compliance with official standards. These formulas are constantly modified as new discoveries are made and new knowledge is gained. The physician who prescribes standard teas can be certain that the herbs prescribed do not pose a toxicologic risk.

1.6.5 Teas Compounded as Prescribed by a Physician

Common abbreviations: cort. (cortex, bark); fol. (folium or folia, leaf or leaves); frct. (fructus, fruits); pericarp. (pericarpium, peel); rad. (radix, root); rhiz. (rhizome); sem. (semen or semina, seed); stip. (stipes or stipites, stem); summ. (summitates, branch tips); tub. (tuber or tubera).

Historically, the prescription written by a physician consists of six parts (Bader et al., 1985).

1. The **heading** contains the name and academic degree of the prescriber, the prescriber's address, telephone number and professional title (e. g., general practitioner), and the date on which the prescription is written.

2. The **superscription**, written Rx, is the symbol for the Latin word *recipe* (take) and directs the pharmacist to prepare the medication.

3. The **prescription** (or **inscription**) lists the ingredients and states their individual quantities relatively (in parts) or absolutely (in grams). Usually the total quantity of the prescription is 100 g. The various ingredients of the prescription have different functions and may consist of four distinct parts.

   ▶ The **base**, or chief active ingredient, such as a bitter herb in an appetite-stimulating stomach tea.

   ▶ The **adjuvant**, or supportive medicine, that acts in the same manner as the base, such as an aromatic bitter in a stomach tea.

   ▶ The **corrective**, or substance added to improve fragrance, flavor, or appearance. For example, calendula flowers, hibiscus flowers, or life everlasting flowers may be added as correctives to carminative teas (Pahlow, 1985).

   ▶ The **vehicle** or excipient, such as stabilizing or filling herbs that are added to a tea mixture to give it a suitable form or consistency. Stabilizing herbs keep the tea mixture homogeneous and, with lengthy storage, ensure that the lower third of the package has the same composition as the upper third. For example, hairy leaves can be added to help stabilize plants parts that have a smooth surface. Stabilizing herbs should be pharmacologically and toxicologically inert; an example is raspberry leaves. Coltsfoot leaves were once a popular stabilizing agent but are no longer used today due to their content of potentially hepatotoxic pyrrolizidine alkaloids.

4. The **subscription** directs the pharmacist to prepare and dispense the drug in a form suitable for use by the patient. For example, the direction "m. f. spec." stands for "*misce fiat species*," or "mix to yield a tea."

5. The **transcription** gives the necessary directions to the patient. "Take as directed" is satisfactory in most cases. The transcription may indicate when and how many times a day the tea should be consumed (see p. 35). If necessary, the physician or pharmacist should also give oral instructions on how the tea is to be prepared (see Sect. 1.6.6).

6. The **signature** appears at the bottom of the prescription blank and should be handwritten by the prescribing physician.

Formulas for Tea Mixtures

Tea formulas may be found in textbooks of phytotherapy (e. g., Weiss, 1982), books on medicinal plants (e. g., Braun and Frohne, 1987; Lindemann, 1979; Pahlow, 1979), and handbooks (e. g., Wurm, 1990). The standard approval criteria for medicinal teas (Braun, 1987) provide a reliable information source in Germany, listing tea mixtures that have a prescribed qualitative composition but a variable quantitative composition. The following guidelines are imposed:

▶ The quantitative composition of the active ingredients can be freely selected within certain ranges;

▶ free qualitative and quantitative selections can be made from a corresponding list of "other ingredients," as long as the content of these ingredients does not exceed 30 % of the tea by weight;

▶ no single "other ingredient" may exceed 5 percent of the tea mixture by weight.

The standard approval criteria refer to herbs by their common names as listed in Table 1.4. The standard tea mixture designated "cough and bronchial tea I" illustrates how the standard criteria can be used to formulate an individual prescription.

▶ Active ingredients in percentages by weight: fennel seeds 10.0–25.0, English plantain 25.0–40.0, licorice root 25.0–35.0, thyme 10.0–40.0.

▶ Other ingredients: marshmallow leaves, rose-hip pulp, Iceland moss, cornflower blossoms, lungwort leaves, mallow leaves, cowslip flowers, pansy.

▶ *Step 1*
Choose a composition that is within the ranges specified in the standard monograph, e. g.
Active ingredients

Fennel seed	10.0 g
English plantain	40.0 g
Licorice root	25.0 g
Thyme	10.0 g

Other ingredients

Mallow flowers	5.0 g
Wild thyme	5.0 g

▶ *Step 2*
If necessary, Latinize the common names, using the synonym list of pharmacopeial names in Table 1.4:

Foeniculi fruct.	10.0 g
Plantaginis lanceolatae herb.	40.0 g
Liquiritiae rad.	25.0 g
Thymi herb.	10.0 g
Malvae flos	5.0 g
Serpylli herb	5.0 g

▶ *Step 3*
List the ingredients on the prescription blank in quantitative order (if desired) and state the directions for the patient:

Rx	Date
English plantain	40.0 g
Licorice root	25.0 g
Fennel seed	10.0 g
Thyme	10.0 g
Mallow flowers	5.0 g
Wild thyme	5.0 g
Pectoral tea	
for Mrs. ...	
Drink 1 cup in the morning and in the evening.	

Oral instructions from the physician, physician's assistant, or pharmacist
Pour boiling water (150 ml = about 1 large cupful) over 1 tablespoon of tea, cover and steep for about 10 minutes, then pour through a tea strainer. Prepare each cup freshly just before use.

1.6.6 Guidelines for Tea Preparation

There are basically three ways to prepare tea:

- Infusion: Pour boiling water over the amount of herb indicated on the prescription or package (e. g., 1 teaspoon). Cover the vessel, steep for 5–10 minutes, and strain through a sieve.
- Decoction: Cover the designated amount of tea mixture with cold water and bring to a boil. Simmer for 5–10 minutes, then strain.
- Cold maceration: Cover the tea mixture with tap water, let stand for 6–8 hours at room temperature, then strain.

Cold maceration is usually recommended for herbs with a high mucilage content such as marshmallow root, psyllium, linseed, or Iceland moss (*Cetraria*) for fear that heat might reduce the viscosity of the mucilage.

A cold maceration does pose potential hygienic problems, however. The raw materials for medicinal teas may be heavily contaminated by microorganisms. There are herbs on the market that were harvested and processed under poor hygienic conditions. They may harbor large numbers of bacteria such as *Escherichia coli, Salmonella* spp., *Pseudomonas aeruginosa*, and *Staphylococcus aureus* (Hefendehl, 1984). Exposing the herb to boiling water will typically reduce the bacterial count by about 90 % (Härtling, 1983; Leimbeck, 1987). In fact, some herbal wholesale firms and suppliers have advised their clients to provide written instructions that consumers always use boiling water when preparing the teas (Wichtl, 1989).

Table 1.4.

Herbs used in medicinal teas, and their indications.*

Herb	Pharmacopeial Name	Indication (Table 1.3)
Agrimony	Agrimoniae herba	E 1, G 1
Angelica root	Angelicae rad.	C 1, C 2
Aniseed	Anisi fruct.	B 1, C 1
Avens root	Gei urbani rhizoma	C 1, E 1
Basil	Basilici herb.	C 1
Bearberry leaf	Uvae ursi fol.	D 2
Bilberry	Myrtilli fruct.	E 1, G 1
Birch leaf	Betulae folium	D 1
Bitter orange peel	Aurantii pericarp.	C 1, C 2, H 1
Black currant leaf	Ribis nigri fol.	D 1
Blackberry leaf	Rubi frutic. fol.	E 1
Blessed thistle	Cnici benedicti herb.	A 1, A 2
Blonde psyllium	Plantaginis ovatae sem.	F 2
Broom	Sarothamni scop. herb.	A 3
Buckthorn bark	Frangulae cort.	F 1
Buckthorn berries	Rhamni cathartici fruct.	F 2
Burnet-saxifrage root	Pimpinellae rad.	B 1
Calendula flowers	Calendulae flos	G 1, G 2, H 2
Caraway	Carvi fruct.	C 1, C 2
Cascara bark	Rhamni purshiani cort.	F 1
Chamomile	Matricariae flos	C 1, C 4
Chamomile, Roman	Chamomillae romanae flos	C 1, I 1
Cinchona bark	Cinchonae cort.	C 1, C 2
Cinnamon	Cinnamomi cort.	C 1, C 2, H 1
Cocoa shells	Cacao testis	H 1
Coriander seed	Coriandri fruct.	C 1, C 2
Cornflower	Cyani flos	H 2
Dandelion root and leaf	Taraxaci rad. cum herb.	C 1, C 2
Devil's claw	Harpagophyti rad.	C 1, C 2
Early goldenrod	Solidaginis gig. herb.	D 1, D 3
Elder flowers	Sambuci flos	B 3
Eucalyptus leaf	Eucalypti fol.	B 1
European aspen bark	Populi cort.	I 3
European aspen leaf	Populi fol.	I 3
Fennelseed	Foeniculi fruct.	C 1
Fumitory	Fumariae herb.	C 3
Gentian	Gentianae rad.	C 1, C 2
Ginger	Zingiberis rhizoma	C 1, C 2, C 5
Goldenrod	Virgaureae herb.	D 1, D 3
Hawthorn leaf and flowers	Crataegi fol. cum flore	A 3
Hibiscus flowers	Hibisci flos	H 1, H 2

Table 1.4.

Herbs used in medicinal teas, and their indications (*cont.*).*

Herb	Pharmacopeial Name	Indication (Table 1.3)
Hops	Lupuli strob.	A 1, A 2
Horsetail	Equiseti herb.	D 1, D 3
Iceland moss	Cetrariae lichen	B 2, C 2
Immortelle flowers	Stoechados flos	H 2
Juniper berries	Juniperi fruct.	C 1, C 2
Kidney bean pods	Phaseoli pericarpium	D 1, D 3
Knotgrass	Polygoni avicularis herb.	B 1, B 2, G 1
Lady's-mantle	Alchemillae herb.	E 1
Lavender flowers	Lavendulae flos	A 1, A 2, C 1
Lemon balm	Melissae fol.	A 2, C 1, C 2
Lesser centaury	Centaurii herb.	C 1, C 2
Licorice	Liquiritiae rad.	B 2, H 1
Linden flowers	Tiliae flos	B 2, B 3
Linseed	Lini sem.	C 4, F 1
Lovage root	Levistici rad.	D 1, D 3
Mallow flowers	Malvae flos	B 2, H 2
Mallow leaf	Malvae fol.	B 2
Marshmallow leaf	Althaeae fol.	B 2
Marshmallow root	Althaeae rad.	B 2, C 4
Maté	Mate folium	I 2
Meadowsweet flowers	Spiraeae flos	B 3
Milk thistle fruit	Cardui mariae fruct.	C 1, C 2
Mullein flowers	Verbasci flos	B 1, B 2
Nettle leaf	Urticae herba	D 1
Oak bark	Quercus cort.	E 1, G 1
Orange blossoms	Aurantii flos	A 2, H 1
Orange flowers	Aurantii flos	A 1, H 1
Orthosiphon leaf	Orthosiphonis fol.	D 1
Passion flower	Passiflorae herb.	A 1
Peppermint	Menthae pip. fol.	C 1, C 3
Plantain	Plantaginis lanceol. herb.	B 1, G 1
Primula flowers	Primulae flos	B 1
Primula root	Primulae rad.	B 1
Psyllium seed	Psyllii sem.	F 2
Raspberry leaf	Rubi idaei fol.	H 1
Raspberry root	Ononidis rad.	D 1, D 3
Rhubarb	Rhei rad.	F 1
Rose hips	Rosae pseudofructus cum fructibus	H 1
Rosemary	Rosmarini fol.	C 1
Sage	Salviae fol.	C 1, G 1, G 2
Senega snakeroot	Senegae rad.	B 1

Table 1.4.
Herbs used in medicinal teas, and their indications (*cont.*).*

Herb	Pharmacopeial Name	Indication (Table 1.3)
Senna leaves	Sennae fol.	F 1
Senna pods	Sennae fruct.	F 1
Shepherd's purse	Bursae pastoris herb.	I 1
Silverweed	Anserinae herb.	E 1, G 1
Sloe berries	Pruni spinosae fruct.	G 1
Sloe blossoms	Pruni spinosae flos	H 2
St. John's wort	Hyperici herb.	A 1
Thyme	Thymi herb.	B 2
Tormentil rhizome	Tormentilliae rhizoma	E 1, G 1
Triticum rhizome	Graminis rhiz.	D 1
Turmeric	Curcumae longae rhiz.	C 1, C 2
Valerian	Valerianae rad.	A 1, A 2
Violet rhizome	Violae rhizoma	B 1, B 2
White deadnettle	Lamii albi herb.	B 1, G 1
White deadnettle flowers	Lamii albi flos	B 1
Wild thyme	Serpylli herb.	B 1
Willow bark	Salicis cort.	B 4
Witch hazel bark	Hamamelidis cort.	E 1
Witch hazel leaf	Hamamelidis fol.	G 1
Wormwood	Absinthii herb.	A 1, A 2, A 3
Yarrow	Millefolii herb.	C 1, C 2

* The levels of evidence vary to support the potential administration for the herb for the proposed indication. The indications are listed in this table as a guide for clinicians and are based on a variety of evidence, including results from controlled clinical trials and approvals for official use by the German Commission E (Blumenthal et al., 1998; Braun et al., 1996; Meyer-Buchtela, 1999).

With regard to dosing schedule, the old rule of drinking 1 cup of tea 3 times daily is generally valid (before breakfast, at about 5:00 p. m., and before bedtime), but the following exceptions should be noted:

- Tea used as a laxative or sleep aid should be taken at night.
- Peppermint and chamomile tea for an upset stomach should be taken at the patient's usual meal times or as needed.
- Linden blossom tea and elder flower tea should be consumed hot while the patient is in bed, because much of their diaphoretic effect is based on physical warming. The sensitivity to heat stimuli shows a diurnal pattern; diaphoretic tea has no effect in the morning, but when taken in the afternoon as the body temperature is rising, it promptly induces profuse sweating (Hildebrandt et al., 1954).
- Diuretic tea is taken at breakfast time; 1 liter should be consumed in one sitting if possible.

▶ Appetite-stimulant teas are taken about 30 min. before meals. Note: Liver diseases are often associated with anorexia. Teas for the liver and gallbladder generally contain bitter-tasting herbs, so it may be advisable to take them 30 min before meals as well.

Some authors recommend medicinal teas as an adjunctive therapy in the management of chronic illnesses (Weiss, 1982), with patients drinking 2 or 3 cups daily for a period of 3–4 weeks. Long-term use is not advised due to a lack of experimental studies on the potential long-term toxicity of the herbs used in medicinal teas (see Sect. 1.6.8).

1.6.7 Teas for Infants and Children

A distinction is drawn between teas used for medicinal purposes and teas that are included in the nutritional regimen of infants and children. In practice, there is considerable overlap between the two types; for example, fennel tea can be used medicinally and as a nutritional supplement. A healthy breast-fed of bottle-fed infant normally does not require extra fluids. Potable water may be given as a thirst quencher under hot conditions (summer) or in low-humidity environments (houses with central heating). Fever and diarrhea are exceptional situations. The Nutritional Committee of the German Society of Pediatrics (1988) has published the following recommendation. If tea is given to infants between 10 days and 6 months of age, it should contain no more than 4 % carbohydrates, preferably in the form of maltodextrin. Teas for infants over 4 months old who have started teething should not contain carbohydrates. There is no objection to using protein as a vehicle in this age group. Vehicles in the form of hydrolyzed proteins (e. g., from collagen) have a molecular weight less than 5000 D in about 70 % of cases, in the range of 5000–10,000 D in 23 %, and 10,000–20,000 D in 8 %. The glycine content must be less than 25 %. If the tea is prepared as directed, using 0.5 g of tea powder per 100 mL of ready-to-drink liquid, there should be a negligible risk of hyperglycinemia (Marfort and Schmidt, 1989). Pediatric teas based on protein hydrolysates should be used only if other foreign proteins are also to be used for infant nutrition, generally after 4 months of age. This is a sound precaution when one considers the high of sensitization to foreign protein during the first months of life.

Instead of instant products, teas can be used in the form of coarsely cut leaves or teabag teas. It is always best to use teas from reputable manufacturers whose products are constantly tested for compliance with legally prescribed standards.

Given the past history of popular interest in teas for infants and children, particularly in Germany, remarkably little reliable information is available on the safety and efficacy of these products.

1.6.8 Adverse Effects and Risks

There have been no reports of objectionable side effects for the majority of medicinal teas used in Germany (Table 1.4). Arnica flowers, European mistletoe, and psyllium can trigger allergic reactions. Herbs with a high tannin content such as uva ursi leaves, lady's mantle, and tormentil rhizome can cause stomach discomfort in sensitive individuals, as can herbs with a high content of bitters such as gentian root, dandelion, and wormwood (overacidification of the stomach). The long-term use of anthranoid-containing laxative teas made from buckthorn bark, rhubarb root, senna leaves, or senna pods can lead to electrolyte losses, most notably potassium deficiency. Because the long-term use of laxatives is a form of product abuse, the resulting effects actually constitute a toxic reaction.

Pharmaceutical incompatibilities and pharmacodynamic interactions are important issues due to the common practice of prescribing teas as an adjunct to essential medications. Unfortunately, almost no clinical studies have been done in this area, so we must base our considerations on plausibility. It is conceivable, for example, that tannin-containing teas might delay the absorption of sedatives, hypnotics, antidepressants, and tranquilizers (Ludewig, 1992) and reduce the efficacy of the antidiabetic drug metformin. Tannins would presumably decrease the absorption of products containing iron, calcium, and magnesium.

Proven medicinal teas that have been used in Germany for many years are known to be free of acute toxicity over al large range of doses. Less is known about their possible chronic toxic effects except in the case of herbs that contain pyrrolizidine alkaloids, such as coltsfoot leaves. Pyrrolizidine alkaloids (PA's) are a group of about 200 structurally related compounds that have been found in some 350 plant species including medicinal plants such as *Cynoglossum* species (hound's tongue), *Petasites* species (petasites), *Tussilago farfara* (coltsfoot leaves and flowers), *Senecio* species (ragwort, liferoot), and *Symphytum* species (comfrey) (Westendorf, 1992). Toxicity to humans has been particularly well documented for the PA's occurring in *Crotolaria* species (bush tea). A latent period of weeks or months after exposure is followed by the appearance of nonspecific symptoms such as anorexia, lethargy, and abdominal pain. Further progression is characterized by emaciation, swelling of the abdomen, and liver changes that take the form of acute, subacute, and chronic veno-occlusive lesions. PA's of the type with the 1,2-unsaturated necine ring act on the centrilobular hepatocytes of the liver, destroying them in large numbers, and they damage small branches of the hepatic vein, causing endothelial disruption and predisposing to thrombosis.

Coltsfoot leaves contain relatively large amounts of hepatotoxic and hepatocarcinogenic PA's (average concentration 4.3 ppm) and most of these chemicals are released into solution when the tea is prepared (Wiedenfeld et al., 1995). In Austria and other countries, the commercial sale of coltsfoot leaves has been banned since 1994. In Germany, a maximum limit has been imposed that prohibits the consumption of more than 1µg of pyrrolizidine alkaloids per day (Bundesanzeiger No. III, Vol. 17.6, 1992). Apparently, it is assumed that there is a limit for carcinogenic compounds below which the herb can be safely used, but this assumption is controversial. In any case, coltsfoot tea is an expendable commodity that is easily replaced by other mucilaginous herbs such as marshmallow leaves and mallow leaves; hence we would recommend discontinuing any further use of coltsfoot in Germany or elsewhere.

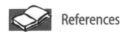 References

AkdÄ (Arzneimittelkommission der deutschen Ärzteschaft) (2002) Evidenzbasierte Therapie-Leitlinien – Demenz. Deutscher Ärzte-Verlag, Cologne, 2002, pp. 137–153.

Bak AAA, Grobbee DE (1989) The effect on serum cholesterol levels of coffee brewed by filtering or boiling. N Engl J Med 321: 142–147.

Bauer KH, Frömming KH, Führer C (1989) Pharmazeutische Technologie. 2nd edition. Thieme Verlag, Stuttgart New York: 450.

Benedum J (1998) Phytotherapie der Antike. In: Loew D, Rietbrock N (eds) Phytopharmaka IV, Forschung und klinische Anwendung. Dr. D. Steinkopff Verlag, Darmstadt: 3–11.

Blumenthal M, Busse WR, Goldberg A, Gruenwald J, Hall T, Riggins CW, Rister RS (eds.). Klein S, Rister RS (trans). (1998) The Complete German Commission E Monographs – Therapeutic Guide to Herbal Medicines. American Botanical Council, Austin, Texas. *www.herbalgram.org.*

Blumenthal M, Israelsen LD. FDA Issues Final Rules for Structure/Function Claims for Dietary Supplements Under DSHEA. *HerbalGram* 2000;48:32–8.

Braun H, Frohne D (1987) Heilpflanzenlexikon für Ärzte und Apotheker, 5th edition. Fischer Verlag, Stuttgart.

Braun R, Surmann R, Wendt R, Wichtl M, Ziegenmeyer J (eds.). Standardzulassungen für Fertig-arzneimittel: Text und Kommentar, 11. Ergänzungslieferung. Stuttgart, Germany: Deutscher Apotheker Verlag. February 1996;1499.99.99.

Brinckmann et al. (2003) Safety and Efficacy of a Traditional Herbal Medicine (Throat Coat®) in Symptomatic Temporary Relief of Pain in Patients with Acute Pharyngitis: A Multicenter, Prospective, Randomized, Double-Blinded, Placebo-Controlled Study. J Altern Comp Med 9: 285–98.

Cordell GA, Quinn-Beattie ML, Farnsworth NR (2001) The potential of alkaloids in drug discovery. Phytother Res 15: 183–205.

Doody RS, Stevens JC, Beck C, et al.: Practice parameter: Management of dementia (an evidence-based review). Neurology 2001; 56: 1154–66.

EG Kommission (2002) Richtlinie des Europäischen Parlamentes und des Rates zur Änderung der Richtlinie 2001/83/EG im Hinblick auf traditionelle pflanzliche Arzneimittel.

Eisenberg DM, Davis RB, Ettner SL et al. (1998) Trends in alternative medicine use in the United States, 1990-1997. JAMA 280:1569–75.

Ernst E, Pittler MH, Stevinson C, White A (2001) The Desktop Guide to Complementary and Alternative Medicine, an Evidence-Based Approach. Mosby, Edinburgh London New York 2001.

ESCOP (2003) Monographs on the medicinal uses of plant drugs. Thieme Stuttgart New York, 2003

Europäisches Arzneibuch, Amtliche Deutsche Ausgabe 1997. Deutscher Apotheker Verlag – Govi Verlag, Stuttgart – Eschborn, 1997.

European Pharmacopeia (2002) Extracts. 4th edition. Suppl 4.3 : 2937–8.

Gaedcke F, Steinhoff B (2000) Phytopharmaka – Wissenschaftliche und rechtliche Grundlagen für die Entwicklung, Standardisierung und Zulassung in Deutschland und Europa. Wissenschaft-liche Verlagsgesellschaft, Stuttgart 2000.

Gauler TC, Weihrauch TR (eds) (1997) Placebo: Ein wirksames und ungefährliches Medikament? Urban & Schwarzenberg, p. 31.

Haas H (1956) Spiegel der Arznei. Ursprung, Geschichte und Idee der Heilmittelkunde. Springer, Berlin Göttingen Heidelberg, 176.

Harnack GA (1980) Kinderheilkunde. Springer Verlag, Berlin Heidelberg New York.

Härtling Ch (1983) Beitrag zur Frage des mikrobiellen Zustandes pflanzlicher Drogen. Fakten und Folgerungen. Pharm Z 132: 643–644.

Hefendehl FW (1984) Anforderungen an die Qualität pflanzlicher Arzneimittel. In: Eberwein B, Helmstaedter G, Reimann J et al. (eds) Pharmazeutische Qualität von Phytopharmaka. Deutscher Apotheker Verlag, Stuttgart, 25–34.

Heim T (2002) Therapie depressiver Erkrankungen: Weg von rein medikamentösen Ansätzen. Deutsches Ärzteblatt 99: 2428.

Hildebrandt G, Engelbertz P, Hildebrandt-Evers G (1954) Physiologische Grundlagen für eine tageszeitliche Ordnung der Schwitzprozeduren. Z Klin Med 152: 446-468.

Hiller K (1995) Pharmazeutische Bewertung ausgewählter Teedrogen. Dtsch Apoth Z 135: 1425-1440.

Hypericum Depression Trial Study Group: effect of Hypericum perforatum (St. John's wort) in major depressive disorder. A randomized controlled trial. JAMA 287: 1807-14, 2002.

IfD-Umfrage 1016 (2002) Institut für Demoskopie, Allensbach/Germany, Allensbacher Archiv.

Jüttner G (1983) Therapeutische Konzepte und soziales Anliegen in der frühen Kräuterheilkunde. In: Imhof AE (ed.) Der Mensch und sein Körper. Beck, Munich, 118-130.

Keller K (1996) Herbal medicinal products in Germany and Europe: experiences with national and European assessment. Drug Inform J 30: 933-948.

Kirsch I, Sapirstein G (1998) Listening to Prozac but hearing placebo: A meta-analysis of antidepressant medication. Prevention & Treatment, 1, Article 0002a. Available on the World Wide Web: http://journals.apa.org/prevention/volume1/pre0010002a.html.

Leimbeck R (1987) Teedrogen: Wie steht es mit der mikrobiologischen Qualität? Dtsch Apoth Z 127: 1221-1224.

Lindemann G (1979) Teerezepte. Verlag Tibor Marczell, München.

Lindemuth G, Lindemuth E (2000) The efficacy of Echinacea compound herbal tea preparation on the severity and duration of upper respiratory and flu symptoms: a randomized, double-blind placebo-controlled study. J Altern Comp Med 6: 327-34.

Linden M, Osterheider M, Schaaf B, Fleckenstein G, Weber HJ (1992) Fluoxetin in der Anwendung durch niedergelassene Nervenärzte. Münch Med Wschr 134: 836-840.

Ludewig R (1989) Schulmedizin und Naturmedizin im Meinungsstreit um Arzneimittel. Plädoyer für einen Modus vivendi. Natur- und Ganzheitsmedizin 2: 40-47.

Ludewig R (1992) Tee als Genuß-, Vorbeugungs- und Heilmittel. Ein alltägliches Beispiel für die schulmedizinisch begründete Phytotherapie. Natur- und Ganzheitsmedizin 5: 185-192.

Mader FH, Weißgerber H (eds) (2003) Allgemeinmedizin und Praxis. 5th edition. Springer Verlag, Berlin Heidelberg.

Meyer-Buchtela E. Tee-Rezepturen: Ein Handbuch für Apotheker und Ärzte. Stuttgart, Germany: Deutscher Apotheker Verlag. 1999.

Montgomery SA (1999 a) Alternatives to placebo-controlled trials in psychiatry. European Neuropsychopharmacology 9 (3): 265-269.

Montgomery SA (1999 b) The failure of placebo-controlled studies. European Neuropsychopharmacology 9 (3): 271-276.

Mulrow C.D., Williams J.W., Trivendi M.: Treatment of depression: newer pharmacotherapies. AHCPR publication no. 99-E014. , 1999.

Nickel, IC (1998) Placebo therapy of benign prostatic hyperplasia: a 25-month study. Brit J Urol 81: 383-7.

Note for Guidance: Quality of Herbal Medicinal Products. European Agency for the Evaluation of Medicinal Products (EMEA). EMEA/adhoc HMPWG/114/98 (July 1998).

O'Brien JT, Ballard CG: Drugs for Alzheimer's disease. Cholinesterase inhibitors have passed NICE's hurdle. BMJ 2001; 325: 123-124.

Pahlow M (1985) Heilpflanzen in der Apotheke. Informationen und Tips aus der Praxis. Dtsch Apoth Z 125: 2663-2664.

Rees L (2001) Integrated medicine. Imbues orthodox medicine with the values of complementary medicine. BMJ 322: 119-20.

Schilcher H (1982) Gesund durch Kräuter-Tees. Möglichkeiten und Probleme der Arzneikräuter-Teezubereitungen. Apotheker-Journal, Heft 7: 36-39.

Schulz V (2000) The psychodynamic and pharmacodynamic effects of drugs: A differentiated evaluation of the efficacy of phytotherapy. Phytomed 7: 73-81.

Schulz V (2001) Incidence and clinical relevance of the interactions and side effects of Hypericum preparations. Phytomed 8:152-160.

Schulz V (2002a) Clinical trials with Hypericum extracts in patients with depression - Results, comparisons, conclusions for therapy with antidepressant drugs. Phytomed 9: 468-474.

Schulz V (2002b) Therapie depressiver Störungen: Die Polit-Pharmakologen. Der Allgemeinarzt 2002: 1363.

Schulz V (2003 a) Ginkgo extrakt or cholinesterase inhibitors in patients with dementia: What clinical trials and guidelines fail to consider. Phytomed 10 Suppl IV: 74–79.

Schulz V (2003 b) Pflanzliche Arzneimittel und Evidenz basierte Medizin: Thesen zur Rationalität der Phytotherapie. Bundesgesundheitsbl Gesundheitsforsch Gesundheitsschutz 46: 1080–85

Schwabe U, Paffrath D (eds) Arzneiverordnungsreport 2000. Springer, Berlin-Heidelberg-New York, pp 1-4; 714–742.

Schwabe U, Paffrath D (eds) Arzneiverordnungsreport 2001. Springer, Berlin-Heidelberg-New York, pp 1-4; 754–767.

Schwabe U, Paffrath D (eds) Arzneiverordnungsreport 2002. Springer, Berlin-Heidelberg-New York, pp 1-18; 652–659.

Taller JB (2003) Canada issues final Natural Health Products regulations. *HerbalGram* 60: 62–5.

Timothy B., Seidman S.N., Sysko R., Gould M. (2002): Placebo response in studies of major depression – variable, substantial, and growing. JAMA 287: 1840–47.

Weihrauch TR, Gauler TC (1999) Placebo – Efficacy and adverse effects in controlled clinical trials. Arzneim-Forsch/Drug Res 49: 385–393.

Weiss RF (1991) Lehrbuch der Phytotherapie, 7th edition, Hippokrates, Stuttgart.

Westendorf J (1992) Pyrrolizidin Alakloids – General Discussion. In: De Smet PAGM, Keller K, Hänsel R, Chandler RF (eds) Adverse effects of herbal drugs. Volume l, Springer Verlag, Berlin Heidelberg New York, 193–214.4.

Wichtl M (Hrsg) (1989) Teedrogen. 2nd edition. Wissenschaftliche Verlagsgesellschaft, Stuttgart, 10 and 26.

Wiedenfeld H, Lebada R, Kopp B (1995) Pyrrolizidinalkaloide im Huflattich. Dtsch Apoth Z 135: 1037–1046.

Withering W (1885) An Account of the Foxglove and Some of Its Medicinal Uses: with Practical Remarks on Dropsy and other Diseases. C. G. J. + J. Robinson, London, 1785. Reprinted in Med Class 2 (1937): 305–443.

2 Central Nervous System

The plant kingdom is replete with compounds and mixtures of compounds that have a stimulating or calmative effect on the central nervous system (CNS). In cases where this action is due to a single high-potency compound that can be chemically isolated, such as morphine, cocaine, or atropine, the plant and its preparations are usually considered to be outside the realm of phytotherapy (see Sect. 1.2). Herbs that contain caffeine are discussed in Sect. 3.2.1.1. Most other herbs affecting the CNS fall under the broad heading of plant sedatives. However, recent controlled therapeutic studies have identified fairly specific indications for three of the psychotropic medicinal plants and their phytomedicinal preparations. Thus, ginkgo biloba extract is considered a nootropic agent that is effective in the symptomatic treatment of cognitive deficiencies (Hartmann and Schulz, 1991; Schulz et al. 1997; Le Bars et al., 1997; Ernst and Pittler, 1999; ESCOP, 2003). Extracts from St. John's wort have proven highly effective in the treatment of mild to moderate depression and have even shown value in severe depressive disorders (Linde et al., 1996; Wong et al. 1998; Kasper, 2001; Schulz, 2002), and extracts from the kava root (*Piper methysticum* rhizome) have shown efficacy as anxiolytic drugs (Volz and Hänsel, 1994; Volz, 1997; Pittler and Ernst, 2000).

Except for ginkgo and kava, the findings on psychotropic plant drugs were compiled by Commission E in 1984 and 1985. Based on information available at that time, the Commission cited similar indications for the majority of these herbs, mentioning the symptom of unrest in nearly all its monographs (Blumenthal et al., 1998). Consequently, the indications stated for John's wort in Table 2.1 are somewhat outdated. None of the controlled studies listed in Tables 2.5 and 2.6 have confirmed sedative effects useful in treating nervous unrest with alcoholic extracts of St. John's wort, but this therapy has proven effective for various depressive mood disorders including moderate and severe depression. Since 1997, the Federal Institute for Drugs and Medical Devices in Germany has recognized "mild depression" as the only indication for most new products made from St. John's wort while recognizing that some specific products with documented efficacy are appropriate for "mild to moderate depressive episodes." Commission E

Table 2.1.
Indications for herbal remedies with psychotropic actions based on the monographs of Commission E, with the year of publication in the *Bundesanzeiger* (*German Federal Gazette*).

Herb	Year	Indication
Hops	1984	Mood disorders such as anxiety and restlessness, sleep disturbances
Kava	1990	Nervous anxiety, tension and restlessness
Lavender	1984	Mood disorders such as restlessness, insomnia, functional upper abdominal complaints
Lemon balm	1984	Nervous insomnia, functional gastrointestinal complaints
Passion Flower	1985	Nervous unrest, mild sleeplessness, nervous gastrointestinal complaints
St. John's wort	1984	Psychoautonomic disturbances, depression, anxiety, and/or nervous unrest
Valerian	1985	Restlessness, nervous insomnia

Source: Blumenthal et al.

published its monographs on gingko extracts in the summer of 1994. The therapeutic indications are reviewed in Sect. 2.1 below.

2.1 Ginkgo in the Treatment of Cognitive Deficiency

2.1.1 Introduction

The first green growth to appear at the center of Hiroshima in 1946 was the sprout of a ginkgo tree. Like all other flora and fauna in the city, the ginkgo tree originally there was incinerated when the atomic bomb was dropped on august 6, 1945. The new plant showed all the usual traits of its species and grew into a normal, full-size tree.

Extreme hardiness seems to be a characteristic of ginkgo trees, which have lived on earth for approximately 300 million years. They are as resistant to harmful insects and microorganisms as they are to the environmental toxins of modern civilization. They are commonly planted as ornamental trees along the heavily trafficked streets of major cities like Tokyo and New York. Their genetic resistance to mutagenic influences may relate to the ability of some ginkgo constituents to act as free-radical scavengers. This, in turn, may have bearing on the pharmacologic and therapeutic properties of ginkgo extracts.

The ginkgo tree died out in Europe during the Ice Age. The German physician and botanist Engelbert Kaempfer first described the tree in his book *Amoenitatum Exoticarum* (Kaempfer, 1712) following a visit to Japan. The first European ginkgo tree was planted in Utrecht, Holland, in 1730, and by 1800 the gingko had become naturalized throughout Europe. The oldest ginkgo tree in Germany (about 200 years) is believed to stand on the grounds of Wilhelmshöhe Castle near the town of Kassel. Goethe wrote a poem *Ginkgo biloba* about the bilobed ginkgo leaf in 1815 after walking the grounds of Heidelberg Castle, and he had several ginkgo trees planted near his summerhouse in Weimar.

Ginkgo biloba has no tradition as a medicinal plant in Europe. Therapeutic uses of the ginkgo seed have been described in China and other parts of eastern Asia for 2000 years and the therapeutic use of ginkgo *leaves* in traditional Chinese medicine for pulmonary complaints dates to the Ming dynasty in 1436 [Ref: Foster S. Ginkgo, *Ginkgo biloba*. Botanical Booklet Series No. 304. Austin, TX: American Botanical Council, 1996.]. A major traditional Chinese use of ginkgo is in the treatment of bronchial asthma, presumably owing to its PAF-inhibiting properties (Schmid and Schmoll, 1994). Present-day Chinese medicine uses extracts from ginkgo leaves in wound dressings. The vasoactive properties of ginkgo principles may play a role in this application.

2.1.2 Botanical Description

Ginkgo biloba (Fig. 2.1) is a dioecious plant, with male and female flowers occurring on different trees. The trees do not blossom until they are 20–30 years old. Young trees are narrow and pear-shaped, later developing a broad crown and eventually reaching a height of up to 40 m. Ginkgo trees more than 1000 years old and measuring 10–20 m in circumference have been described in China, Korea, and Japan.

The last surviving member of the family Ginkgoaceae, *Ginkgo biloba* is unrelated to any other plant species alive today. The foliage of the ginkgo tree more closely resembles that of certain ferns than that of deciduous trees, its fan-shaped leaves lacking the central rib and cross venation seen in broad-leaf trees.

2.1.3 Crude Drug and Extract

The dried green leaves of the ginkgo tree provide the crude drug from which ginkgo extracts are obtained. Leaves may be gathered from cultivated trees or from the wild. Most of the bulk herb comes from China, Japan, North and South Korea, and from plantations in Europe (southern France) and North America. The content of flavonoid glycosides is highest in fresh ginkgo leaves that are harvested in May shortly after the appearance of new foliage, while the leaves are still a pure green color (Sticher, 1993). The leaves may be gathered by climbing and picking, or they may be stripped from branches that have been cut from the tree. On plantations, leaves are machine-harvested from trees that are pruned to the size and shape of large shrubs. When dried, the leaves lose about three-fourths of their fresh weight. The dried leaves are compacted into large bales to help keep them dry and prevent moisture-related fermentation.

Ginkgo extracts are produced in standard fashion by extracting the milled leaves with polar solvents. These primary extracts, which have about a 4:1 ratio of crude herb to extract, and the dried leaves themselves are no longer marketed in Germany, but preparations containing dried leaf material (e.g., teas, capsules, etc.) and simple

Fig. 2.1. ▶ Branch of *Ginkgo biloba.*

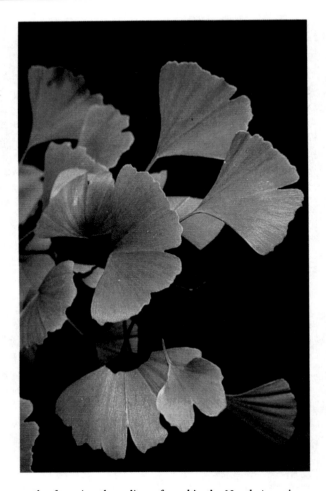

extracts (e.g., tinctures at a strength of 1:10 in ethanol) are found in the North American market. None of these products are phytoequivalent to the concentrated and standardized preparations used in published clinical trials. The monograph published by Commission E in August of 1994 (*Bundesanzeiger* No. 133) states that the only acceptable extracts are those with an herb-to-extract ratio in the range of 35:1 to 67:1 (average: 50:1) that have been extracted with an acetone-water mixture and then further purified without adding concentrates or isolated constituents (Blumenthal et al,, 1998). This standardized process eliminates unwanted components, including those that make the product less stable or pose an excessive toxicologic risk – fats, waxes, tannins, proanthocyanidins, biflavonoids, ginkgol, ginkgolic acids, proteins, and mineral components. In particular, it has been shown that ginkgolic acids incite allergic responses and other toxic reactions (Becker and Skipworth, 1995; Hausen, 1998; Jaggy and Koch, 1997). The extracts suitable for use in drug manufacture are nearly free of ginkgolic acids (< 5 ppm) as required by the Commission E (Blumenthal et al., 1998) and a recent monograph in the *German Pharmacopeia* (DAB 2000). The two leading extracts meeting these criteria are designated in the technical literature as EGb 761 and LI 1370.

2.1.4 Key Constituents, Analysis, Pharmacokinetics

The monograph published by Commission E lists the following characteristics of medicinal ginkgo extracts: 22–27 % flavonoid glycosides, determined by high-performance liquid chromatography (HPLC) as quercetin, kaempferol, and isorhamnetin and calculated as acylflavonoids with the molecular weight $M_r = 756.7$ (quercetin glycosides) and $M_r = 740.7$ (kaempferol glycosides); 5–7 % terpene lactones, consisting of about 2.8–3.4 % ginkgolides A, B, and C and 2.6–3.2 % bilobalide; and less than 5 ppm ginkgolic acids. Analytic and production-related variations are included in the ranges indicated (Blumenthal et al., 1998).

Other chemicals present in the extracts include hydroxykynurenic acid, shikimic acid, protocatechuic acid, vanillic acid, and p-hydroxybenzoic acid. For quantitative analysis, the key constituents are separated from the extract by HPLC. Additionally, gas chromatographic techniques are used for analysis of the ginkgolides and bilobalide. The flavonoid glycosides are hydrolyzed with methanol and hydrochloric acid prior to chromatographic separation. Safe upper limits have been established for the concentration of ginkgolic acids, which are considered toxic and allergenic.

The pharmacokinetics of ginkgo extracts have been studied in experimental animals and in humans. Experiments with the radiolabeled extract EGb 761 in rats showed a 60 % absorption rate. Human studies with EGb 761 indicated an absolute bioavailability of 98–100 % for ginkgolide A, 79–93 % for ginkgolide B, and at least 70 % for bilobalide (Hänsel et al., 1993; DeFeudis, 1998). Ginkgolides A and B and bilobalide were absorbed in a dose-linear fashion when administered orally to rats (30, 55, and 100 mg/kg). The maximum plasma levels (approximately 100–400 ng/mL) were reached at 0.5–1 h, and the plasma half-life was 1.7–3 h (Biber and Koch, 1999). The pharmacokinetics of ginkgolides A and B and of bilobalide were tested in 12 healthy subjects following the oral and parenteral administration of EGb 761. The bioavailability of ginkgolide A and B after oral administration was 80 % and 88 %, respectively, while that of bilobalide was only about 1 %. The plasma half-life was approximately 10 h for ginkgolide A and 4 h for the other two substances. The 48-h urinary excretion was 72 % for ginkgolide A and 30–40 % for the other two substances (Fourtillan et al., 1997). In studies with the extract LI 1370, the plasma flavonoid levels in healthy subjects showed a dose-dependent rise after the ingestion of 50 mg, 100 mg, and 300 mg and were maximal at 2–3 hours (Nieder, 1991).

2.1.5 Animal Pharmacology, Human Pharmacology, and Toxicology

Some 300 original papers have been published on the pharmacologic actions of ginkgo extracts (surveys in: Oberpichler and Krieglstein, 1992; Hänsel et al., 1993; Rupalla et al., 1995; DeFeudis, 1998). Most of the studies were performed with the extract EGb 761. The 1994 Commission E monograph summarizes the experimentally documented pharmacologic actions of EGb 761 as follows:

▶ increases tolerance to hypoxia, especially in brain tissue;
▶ inhibits the development of post-traumatic or toxin-induced brain edema and hastens its resolution;
▶ reduces retinal edema and retinal lesions;
▶ inhibits the age-related decline of muscarinic choline receptors and α_2-adrenergic receptors; promotes choline uptake in the hippocampus;
▶ improves memory and learning capacity and aids in the compensation of disturbed equilibrium, acting particularly at the level of the microcirculation;
▶ improves the rheologic properties of the blood;
▶ scavenges toxic oxygen-derived free radicals;
▶ inhibits platelet activation factor (PAF) and exerts an neuroprotective effect (Blumenthal et al., 1998)

As with other phytomedicines, all the primary constituents of ginkgo extracts are assumed to contribute in their totality to the therapeutic effect. But some pharmacologic actions can be related to specific groups of compounds. For example, the ginkgo flavonoids (mostly rutin derivatives) are efficient free-radical scavengers We know from experimental studies in animals and humans that rutin raises the threshold for the seepage of blood from capillary vessels, an effect generally described as decreased capillary fragility.

The ginkgolides inhibit platelet activating factor (PAF). A bioregulator synthesized in mammalian cell membranes in response to various stimuli, PAF mediates various physiologic responses and, when excessive, can initiate pathophysiologic processes. It induces platelet aggregation in the blood and functions as a key mediator in allergic inflammatory processes. PAF receptors have been detected in various tissues including the brain. PAF-induced platelet aggregation is known to occur in zones of incomplete ischemia, e. g., at the periphery of an infarcted area. The ginkgolides and bilobalide, whose chemical structures are unique in nature, have also demonstrated characteristic neuroprotective properties in various pharmacologic models (Braquet, 1988, 1989; Krieglstein et al., 1995).

Studies in experimental models have been supplemented by a number of pharmacologic studies in humans. In an open trial, Itil et al. (1998) compared the effect of a single test dose of 40 mg of tacrine with that of 240 mg of ginkgo extract in 18 patients with Alzheimer dementia based on computer-analyzed EEGs (CEEGs). The authors found that the ginkgo extract had "typical cognitive CEEG activator profiles" in more of the subjects (8 of 18) than tacrine (3 of 18). Rigney et al. (1999) conducted a double-blind study with a multiple crossover design in which they tested the effect of 120–300 mg of ginkgo extract on cognitive performance in healthy subjects with psychomotor tests. The authors found a dose-dependent positive response, especially in memory performance, that was more pronounced in the subjects 50–59 years of age than in younger subjects. Mix and Crews (2000) conducted a placebo-controlled study in 40 healthy subjects 55–86 years of age. The ginkgo-treated group received 180 mg/d of ginkgo extract (EGb 761) for 6 weeks. Three neuropsychological tests demonstrated positive effects on cognitive functioning. A followup randomized double-blind, placebo-controlled trial by the same authors (Mix & Crews, 2002) demonstrated benefits of a daily dose of 180 mg ginkgo extract (EGb 761) on routine memory tasks.

In contrast to the four previous studies, one randomized placebo-controlled study in 230 elderly subjects (average 69 years) treated for 6 weeks with 120 mg/d of the ginkgo extract EGb 761 showed no significant improvements in cognitive function compared with placebo. However, the blinding in this study was imperfect since the test medication in the ginkgo-treated group consisted of coated tablets while the placebo was administered in gelatin capsules (Solomon et al., 2002). Another open, randomized study was conducted in a population of 5028 healthy elderly subjects (average age 69 years), 1000 of whom received 120 mg of ginkgo extract (LI 1370) daily for 4 months while the remaining 4028 (control group) received no anti-dementia medication. The subjects were surveyed at 0, 1, 3, and 4 months with validated self-rated scales on activities of daily living. After 4 months of treatment, statistically significant differences were found in the ability of the group treated with ginkgo extract to cope with their daily activities (Cockle et al., 2000).

The toxicity of therapeutically applied ginkgo extracts is very low. Tests in mice showed an LD_{50} of 7725 mg/kg on oral administration and 1100 mg/kg) on intravenous administration. An acute LD_{50} could not be determined in rats. Tests for mutagenic, carcinogenic, and genotoxic effects were negative (Hänsel et al., 1993; Alaoni-Yonsseti, 1999; DeFeudis, 1998; Alaoui-Youssefi, 1999).

2.1.6 Clinical Efficacy in Patients with Cognitive Deficiency

The symptomatic treatment of cognitive deficits due to organic brain disease is considered the primary indication for ginkgo extracts. There is no single definition for the term cognitive deficits. In medical parlance it has been largely synonymous with cerebral insufficiency, an older term reflecting the etiologic hypothesis that stenotic vascular changes with aging cause a progressive decrease in cerebral blood flow, leading to a decline in mental and physical functioning. The clinical manifestations include impairment of memory and other cognitive functions, affective symptoms such as anxiety and depression, and physical complaints such as tinnitus, vertigo, and headache (Fig. 2.2). The older etiologic concept of cerebrovascular insufficiency has been largely abandoned since it was shown that neuronal degeneration like that occurring in Alzheimer's disease is a more frequent cause of impaired mental functioning in elderly patients. At present, a deficiency of the neurotransmitter acetylcholine in the cerebral cortex is considered a very consistent neurobiological finding in patients with Alzheimer-type dementia.

The clinical features of these central nervous system disorders correspond to the syndrome of dementia, which is characterized by disturbances of memory, cognition, and emotional control. Both the broadened classification of mental disorders in the DSM-IV (American Psychiatric Association, 1995) and the 10th revision of the international disease classification of the WHO (ICD 10, German Institute for Medical Documentation and Information, 1994) define dementia as a pattern of disturbance in which multiple higher mental functions are simultaneously affected. The cardinal symptoms are impairment of memory, abstract thinking, and psychomotor functions such as speech. Changes in mood, social functioning, and personality may also be pres-

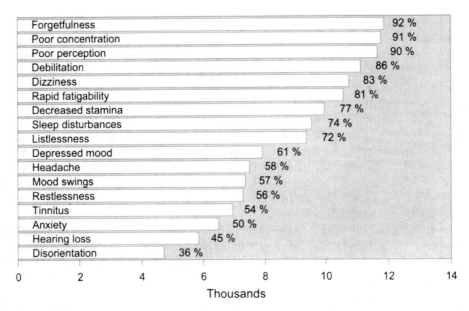

Symptom	Percentage
Forgetfulness	92 %
Poor concentration	91 %
Poor perception	90 %
Debilitation	86 %
Dizziness	83 %
Rapid fatigability	81 %
Decreased stamina	77 %
Sleep disturbances	74 %
Listlessness	72 %
Depressed mood	61 %
Headache	58 %
Mood swings	57 %
Restlessness	56 %
Tinnitus	54 %
Anxiety	50 %
Hearing loss	45 %
Disorientation	36 %

Thousands

Fig. 2.2. ▲ Frequency distribution of typical symptoms in 13,565 patients diagnosed with dementia (multi-infarct dementia, Alzheimer's dementia, mixed type). Results based on a survey of 1357 private physicians (Burkard and Lehrl, 1991).

ent. The main criterion for diagnosing dementia as defined by ICD 10 is the presence of cognitive intellectual impairment that affects multiple areas and has reached a degree of severity that significantly interferes with activities of daily living (Dilling et al., 1993).

Based on its pharmacologic actions and clinical effects, ginkgo extract since 2000 is listed in the ATC-classification under *anti-dementia-drugs* (ATC-code N06DX02), i. e., agents that act on the central nervous system and tend to improve cognitive performance. A definite mechanism of action has not yet been established for nootropic drugs. It is generally thought that nootropic drugs act by their ability to stimulate populations of nerve cells that are still functional (stabilization of adapter capacity) or protect them from pathologic influences (neuroprotective effects). Our understanding of the mechanism of action of *anti-dementia-drugs* is based largely on studies in experimental animals since it us rarely possible to conduct this type of biochemical and pharmacodynamic research in human subjects (Kanowski, 1991; Oberpichler and Krieglstein, 1992; Itil et al., 1996).

The therapeutic efficacy of nootropic drugs can be meaningfully tested only in human subjects, the best subjects being patients with dementia. By the late 1980's, no definite guidelines had yet been established for testing drugs that improve cognitive functions. At the same time, most of the 39 controlled clinical studies on the use of ginkgo special extracts in patients with cognitive deficits (Table 2.2) were conducted in the 1980's (surveys in: Kleijnen and Knipschild, 1992a, b; Hopfenmüller, 1994; Volz and Hänsel, 1994; Oken et al., 1998, Ernst and Pittler, 1999; ESCOP, 2003). The criteria used to assess efficacy in these studies were improvements in typical symptoms and complaints (Fig. 2.3) and improved performance in psychometric tests.

Table 2.2.
The results of 40 controlled clinical studies in dementia patients.

Year	Author	Design	Subjects	Daily Dosage (mg)	Duration (weeks)	Preparation
1975	Moreau	PDB	60	120	12	EGb 761
1976	Augustin	PDB	168	120	24	EGb 761
1977	Israel	POS	48	240	8	EGb 761
1978	Leroy	VDB	60	120	8	EGb 761
1981	Dieli	PDB	40	120	8	EGb 761
1982	Eckmann	PDB	50	120	4	EGb 761
1982	Haan	VOS	60	87.5	2	EGb 761
1982	Krauskopf	VDB	20	120	8	EGb 761
1983	Pidoux	PDB	12	160	12	EGb 761
1985	Geßner	VDB	60	120	12	EGb 761
1986	Hindmarch	PDB	8	120–160	single dose	EGb 761
1986	Arrigo	PDB	80	120	6	EGb 761
1986	Weitbrecht	PDB	40	120	12	EGb 761
1987	Israel	PDB	80	160	12	EGb 761
1987	Wesnes	PDB	54	120	12	EGb 761
1988	Halama	PDB	40	120	12	EGb 761
1989	Hofferberth	PDB	36	120	8	EGb 761
1989	Vorberg	PDB	100	112	12	LI 1370
1990	Eckmann	PDB	58	160	6	LI 1370
1990	Gerhardt	VDB	80	120	6	EGb 761
1990	Schulz	PDB	77	150	12	LI 1370
1990	Rabinovici	PDB	99	150	12	LI 1370
1991	Brüchert	PDB	209	150	12	LI 1370
1991	Schmidt	PDB	99	150	12	LI 1370
1991	Halama	PDB	50	150	12	LI 1370
1991	Hartmann	PDB	45	150	12	LI 1370
1991	Hofferberth	PDB	50	150	6	LI 1370
1991	Maier-Hauff	PDB	50	150	6	LI 1370
1991	Rai	PDB	27	120	24	EGb 761
1992	Gräßel	PDB	72	160	24	EGb 761
1992	Hörr	PDB	40	200	4	EGb 761
1992	Ihl	PDB	20	240	12	EGb 761
1992	Hofferberth	PDB	40	240	12	EGb 761
1992	Michaelis	PDB	52	120	8	EGb 761
1994	Vesper	PDB	86	150	12	LI 1370
1996	Kanowski	PDB	216	240	24	EGb 761
1996	Haase	PDB	40	240 (i.V.)	4	EGb 761
1997	Maurer	PDB	20	240	12	EGb 761
1997	LeBars	PDB	309	120	52	EGb 761
2000	van Dongen	PDB	214	160–240	24	Egb 761

NOTE: The extract EGb 761 was used in 29 of these studies, the extract LI 1370 in 11. A total of 2909 patients was included in the studies. The dose generally ranged from 120 to 240 mg/day, and treatment was generally continued for 8-12 weeks (reviews and original quotes from the studies may be found in Kleijnen and Knipschild, 1992; Volz and Hänsel, 1994; Hopfenmüller, 1994; Kanowski, 1996; and LeBars, 1997, Ernst and Pittler, 1999; ESCOP, 2003). **Abbreviations: PDB** = placebo-controlled double-blind study; **POS** = placebo-controlled open study; **VDB** = double-blind study comparing ginkgo extract with synthetic nootropic drugs; **VOS** = open study comparing ginkgo extract with synthetic nootropic drugs.

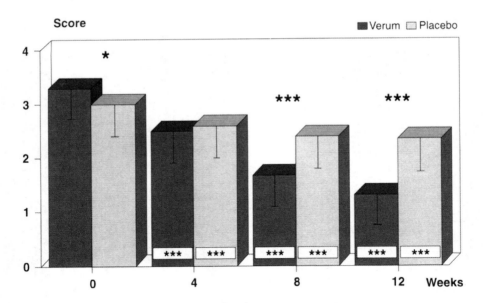

Fig. 2.3. ▲ Typical rating of individual symptoms like that used in older studies. Severity of the symptom of "dizziness." Eight to 12 weeks' therapy was needed before the ginkgo-treated patients showed significant improvement (*** = p < 0.001) relative to the placebo (Vorberg et al., 1989).

Psychometric assessment of cognitive abilities (memory, concentration, speech, construction, motor function) Standard: *Alzheimer's Disease Assessment Scale (ADAS-cog)* Observers: psychologists, office personnel, physicians

Activities of daily living, social behavior, care needs (personal care, dressing, shopping, eating, self-direction, mobility) Sample test: *Geriatric Evaluation by Relatives Rating Instrument (GERRI scale)* Observers: family members and caregivers

Global assessment of the patient by the physician (cognitive abilities, behavior, activities of daily living) Sample test: *Clinical Global Impression of Change (CGI-C)* Observer: physician interviewing the patient and caregivers

Fig. 2.4. ▲ Demonstrating the efficacy of antidementia drugs in accordance with the CPMP guidelines of July, 1997 (Lovestone et al., 1997).

In 1991, the German Federal Health Agency established new criteria for testing the efficacy of nootropic drugs (German Federal Health Agency, 1991). In July of 1997, the Committee for Proprietary Medicinal Products (CPMP) adopted these criteria in its "Note for Guidance on Medicinal Products in the Treatment of Alzheimer's Disease" (Lovestone et al., 1997). Besides the primary goal of improving dementia symptoms or delaying their progression, the new guidelines require that nootropic therapy also improve functioning in daily activities and reduce the patient's care needs. The guidelines limit clinical testing to patients with primary degenerative dementias of the Alzheimer type, vascular dementias, and mixed forms of both. They also require that efficacy be demonstrated on three mutually independent levels of observation (Fig. 2.4).

To demonstrate efficacy in the pharmacotherapy of dementia, it is necessary to show improvement on at least two or the three test levels with regard to cognition, activities of daily living, and overall clinical impression. A number of psychometric test procedures have been developed and applied for each of the three levels. Only one scale has been widely utilized as an outcome measure in recent studies: the cognitive portion of the Alzheimer's Disease Assessment Scale (ADAS-Cog) (Ihl und Weyer, 1993; Ihl, 2002). This scale is scored from 1 to 70 points (lower = better). The yearly progression in untreated Alzheimer patients is 2–10 points. The patients in the studies had a baseline score between 20 and 30 points. In a number of studies, patients were classified as "responders" if their score improved by 4 or more points during at least 24 weeks of therapy.

Two of the studies listed in Table 2.2 (Kanowski et al., 1996; Le Bars et al., 1997) satisfy these new guidelines for nootropic drugs from a methodologic standpoint. For example, the study by Le Bars et al. (1997) was a multicenter placebo-controlled double-blind study of 236 patients with mild to moderate Alzheimer-type dementia and 73 patients with vascular dementia conforming to ICD-10 diagnostic criteria. All 309 patients were treated for a period of 52 weeks, during which time the ginkgo-treated group received a daily dose of 120 mg of the extract EGb 761. Three validated scales corresponding to the observation levels in Fig. 2.4 were used to evaluate the outcomes: Geriatric Evaluation by Relative's Rating Instrument (GERRI) for daily activities, the Alzheimer's Disease Assessment Scale-Cognitive Subscale (ADAS-Cog) for psychometric testing, and Clinical Global Impression of Change (CGIC) to evaluate psychopathology.

The outcome evaluations at 26 weeks and especially at 52 weeks showed statistically significant gains in the patients treated with gingko extract. Significant improvements were found in competence with daily activities (GERRI, Fig. 2.6) and in cognitive functioning (ADAS-Cog, Fig. 2.5). Psychopathologic evaluation (CGIC) showed no significant difference between the EGb and placebo groups. The same was true of adverse side effects, although the patients taking EGb had a somewhat higher incidence of gastrointestinal complaints than the placebo group. The patients with Alzheimer-type dementia showed greater improvement in GERRI and ADAS-Cog than the patients with multi-infarct dementia. The degree of improvement in ADAS-Cog scores was comparable to the results of an earlier study that had a similar design but used the synthetic nootropic drug tacrine (Le Bars et al., 1997).

The results of Kanowski et al. (1996) and Le Bars et al. (1997, 2000) have been called into question by the results of another study (van Dongen et al., 2000). The design of this study did not conform to the CPMP testing guidelines for anti-dementia drugs, however (Fig. 2.4). The study, which began in 1994, was conducted in 214 patients who were residents of retirement and nursing homes. They were treated with 240 mg or 160 mg of ginkgo extract daily or with placebo tablets, which contained 2 mg of quinine for

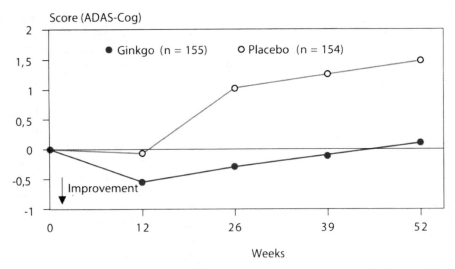

Fig. 2.5. ▲ Results of a study patterned after the guidelines in Fig. 2.4, comparing the Alzheimer's Disease Assessment Scale-Cognitive Subscale (ADAS-Cog) scores of the gingko-treated and placebo groups. While the patients treated with ginkgo extract maintained a constant level of cognitive performance over the 52-week study period, the placebo group showed a degree of decline (rising ADAS-Cog score) that would be expected to occur as a result of progression. The intergroup difference at 52 weeks was statistically significant (p < 0.01) (Le Bars, 1997).

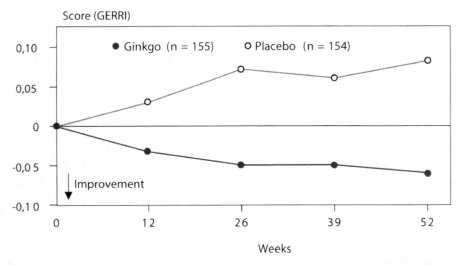

Fig. 2.6. ▲ Same study as in Fig. 2.5. Geriatric Evaluation by Relative's Rating Instrument (GERRI) was used to evaluate competence with daily activities. The GERRI score improved in patients treated with ginkgo extract but worsened in the placebo group. The intergroup differences at 26 and 52 weeks were statistically significant (p < 0.05 and p < 0.01) (Le Bars, 1997).

flavor (Knipschild et al., 1998). Two randomizations were done at 4 and 12 weeks, and by the end of the 24-week study period only 123 patients (79 ginkgo, 44 placebo) were available for final evaluation. The study population included patients with mild to moderate dementia not further specified as well as patients with age-associated memory disorders. The testing procedures did not include the ADAS-Cog scale. No significant differences were found between any of the treatment groups or treatment levels. The results are very difficult to interpret, however, due to problems of methodology (Le Bars, 2002).

Thus, more rigorous study designs have documented the therapeutic efficacy of ginkgo extract in the treatment of dementia. This does not diminish the importance of the positive results of many earlier studies, however (Table 2.2). Testing according to the new CPMP guidelines for nootropic drugs has certain drawbacks compared with the simpler protocols used in earlier studies. For example, psychometric tests corresponding to the cognitive level in Fig. 2.4 require a minimal degree of cooperation and therefore can be used only in patients with mild rather than severe cognitive deficits. But treatment with a nootropic drug is the only therapeutic option for patients with severe cognitive impairment, who cannot cooperate sufficiently to benefit from cognitive training. Older studies using gingko extracts could be performed even in patients with severe cognitive deficits. Since the majority of these studies showed benefits from ginkgo use, there should be no objection to trying ginkgo extract in severe forms of dementia rather than limiting its use to mild or moderate cases.

2.1.7 Indications, Dosages, Risks, and Contraindications

The 1994 Commission E monograph recognizes the following indications for the special ginkgo extracts defined in Sect. 2.1.3 and 2.1.4 above.

▶ Symptomatic treatment of deficits due to organic brain disease as part of a comprehensive therapy program in demential syndromes with these principal features: memory impairment, concentration difficulties, depression, vertigo, tinnitus, and headache.
  The primary target group includes demential syndromes in patients with primary degenerative dementia, vascular dementia, and mixed forms of both.
  Note: Before treatment with ginkgo extracts is started, it should be determined whether the patient's symptoms are caused by an underlying disease that would require specific treatment.
▶ Improvement of pain-free walking distance in patients with Fontaine Stage IIa or IIb peripheral arterial occlusive disease (PAOD, aka intermittent claudication) as an adjunct to physical therapy, particularly ambulatory exercise.
▶ Vertigo or tinnitus of vascular or involutional origin (Blumenthal et al., 1998).

The use of ginkgo extract for arterial occlusive disease is discussed more fully in Sect. 3.3.2. Its efficacy in the treatment of vertigo and tinnitus not associated with dementia (Fig. 2.2) was tested in eight older studies, with mostly positive results (survey in Hänsel et al., 1993, and DeFeudis, 1998). Of special interest is the potential value of gingko in the treatment of tinnitus, which occurs occasionally in about 10 % of the population and significantly affects the quality of life in approximately 1 %. A recent placebo-controlled double-blind study in 99 outpatients confirmed the therapeutic efficacy of ginkgo extract for this indication (Morgenstern and Biermann, 1997). Another study conducted in 978 patients did not, however (Drews und Davies, 2001). A meta-analysis of five randomized studies confirmed the efficacy of ginkgo extract in the treatment of tinnitus, but the value of the analysis appears limited due to methodologic errors (Ernst and Stevinson, 1999). It bears emphasis that the Commission E approval for ginkgo for tinnitus is limited to tinnitus of vascular and involutional etiology.

The indications and dosages stated in the European ESCOP monograph (ESCOP, 2003) are largely identical to those indicated by Commission E. The total daily dose in both monographs is 120–240 mg of crude dry extract is taken in 2 or 3 separate doses. Most of the clinical studies demonstrating efficacy (Table 2.2) employed doses in the range of 120–160 mg/day. A minimal 8-week course of treatment is recommended in patients with dementia (see Fe. 2.3), and the patient should be reevaluated at 3 months to determine whether it is appropriate to continue therapy. The only contraindication to ginkgo is a hypersensitivity to *Ginkgo biloba* preparations. Side effects are very rare and consist of mild gastric upset, headache, or allergic skin reactions (Table 2.3). There are no known interactions with other drugs.

The only contraindication noted in the monographs is hypersensitivity to gingko extract preparations. Side effects consist of very rare instances of mild gastrointestinal discomfort, headache, or allergic skin reactions. Seven cases of hemorrhage in patients taking ginkgo-containing products have been reported in the literature (Rowin and Lewis, 1996; Rosenblatt und Mindel, 1997; Vale, 1998; Fessenden et al., 2001). The antagonism of ginkgolides to platelet-activating factor (Braquet et al., 1988, 1989) has been cited as a possible cause. There has been no case in which a definite causal link could be established between hemorrhage and ginkgo use. Despite some theoretical concerns about the potential for interaction with blood-thinning drugs, several interaction stud-

Table 2.3.
Frequency of side effects during 3 months' treatment with the ginkgo extract LI 1370 (10,815 patients) and with various synthetic nootropic drugs (2141 patients) (Burkard and Lehrl, 1991).

Patients, side effects	Number (%) with LI 1370	Number (%) with other nootropic drugs
Total number of patients	10,815 (100 %)	2141 (100 %)
– with no side effects	10,632 (98.31 %)	2025 (94.58 %)
– with side effects	183 (1.69 %)	116 (5.42 %)
Nausea	37 (0.34 %)	16 (0.75 %)
Headache	24 (0.22 %)	5 (0.23 %)
Stomach problems	15 (0.14 %)	15 (0.70 %)
Diarrhea	15 (0.14 %)	1 (0.05 %)
Allergy	10 (0.09 %)	2 (0.09 %)
Anxiety, restlessness	8 (0.07 %)	19 (0.89 %)
Sleep disturbances	6 (0.06 %)	11 (0.51 %)
Other	68 (0.63 %)	47 (2.20 %)

ies in humans have shown no evidence of interactions with aspirin or with phenpro-coumon-type anticoagulants (Juretzek et al., 2002).

2.1.8 Therapeutic Significance

Today there are approximately 1 million people in Germany who suffer from some form of dementia requiring treatment. Projections indicate that this number will double to approximately 2 million by the year 2030 (Bickel, 1997). In the United States, it is estimated that 9 million persons will have Alzheimer dementia by that time (Doody et al., 2001). Nonpharmacologic treatment options are basically limited to positive reinforcement and the counseling of patients and their caregivers. Cognitive training programs actually do more harm than good in many of these patients (Small et al., 1997). Both the American Academy of Neurology and the British National Institute for Clinical Excellence have recently advocated the use of cholinesterase inhibitors in patients with Alzheimer dementia (Doody et al., 2001; O'Brian und Ballard, 2001). In the opinion of the Drug Commission of the Association of German Physicians (AkdA), the pharmacotherapy of dementia "has not yet reached a desirable level of efficacy." But the AkdA goes on to state the following in its therapeutic guidelines for dementia: "In dementia as in other serious diseases for which satisfactory treatment options are not yet available, the physician should strive to achieve small improvements and relief whenever possible, especially since it cannot be predicted whether and to what degree the patient will respond to an anti-dementia drug" (AkdA, 2001).

A number of drugs have been tested and used in the treatment of dementia during the past 30 years. The different categories of drugs reflect the ever-changing views on the pathogenesis of dementia (decreased blood flow, impaired neuronal glucose utilization or calcium homeostasis, glutamate excess or acetylcholine deficiency in central synapses). During the past decade, the hypothesis that Alzheimer-type dementia is based on a "cholinergic deficit" in central synapses has led to the development of a new class of drug, the cholinesterase (ChE) inhibitors. Today the ChE inhibitors tacrine, donepezil, rivastigmine, and galantamine are available as synthetic counterparts to ginkgo extract (EGb). As the newest link in the chain of anti-dementia drugs, the ChE inhibitors have a distinct advantage over the older nootropic drugs, including EGb, in that they have been investigated in accordance with the most up-to-date testing guidelines (CPMP, 1997). This does not mean, however, that the results of all earlier clinical studies (see Table 2.2) are worthless. Moreover, the advantage of up-to-date efficacy tests must be weighed against the disadvantage of a shorter period of clinical experience with ChE inhibitors. It is also important to consider other criteria for the therapeutic use of these drugs, such as tolerance, patient acceptance, and treatment costs.

Official recommendations on the treatment of dementia (AdkA, 2001; Doody et al., 2001; O'Brian and Ballard, 2001) are based almost entirely on statistical efficacy data from controlled studies in recent years. The Drug Commission of the Association of German Physicians made the following statement in its recommendations on the treatment of dementia: "Of the anti-dementia drugs presented here, the acetylcholinesterase inhibitors should definitely be considered the agents of first choice for Alzheimer dementia from the standpoint of proven efficacy. There is very little evidence from clinical studies to support the alternative use of other groups of drugs. Official approval, individual response, and tolerance should be considered as additional criteria" (AkdA, 2001). The AkdA notes that their recommendations were made strictly "from the standpoint of proven efficacy." This proof is suspect, however, because of the difficulties in blinding studies on ChE inhibitors due to the frequency of gastrointestinal side effects such as nausea and vomiting (Schulz, 2003; see also Sect. 1.5.4, paragraph 5). Also, the discontinuation of ChE inhibitors is followed swiftly by cognitive relapse. This has been observed to a much lesser degree after the discontinuation of traditional nootropic agents, especially ginkgo extract (Rainer et al., 2001). This could have major practical relevance when we consider that, in many cases, treatment with anti-dementia drugs cannot be continued to the end of the patient's life even in primary responders.

The anti-dementia agents that have been most widely prescribed in Germany thus far are standardized gingko extracts. These products have been prescribed by doctors for more than 30 years, and they continue to enjoy a high acceptance rate among patients. The incidence of adverse side effects is a few percent (Table 2.3). By contrast, typical side effects were observed in 20–70 % of all patients treated with ChE inhibitors, with allowance for nocebo effects (Schulz, 2003). Percentages this high mean that in the day-to-day use of these agents, the patients or their family members, if not the physician him or herself, will tend to reduce the dosage to a more tolerable level, which may be below the therapeutic range.

Another problem is treatment costs. ChE inhibitors cost 3–6 times more than clinically documented ginkgo extracts. In absolute terms, the change to ChE inhibitors represent an added yearly cost of approximately $1000 per patient, assuming an optimum dosage. Applied to a population of 1 million patients requiring treatment, the total additional drug cost in Germany alone would be approximately $1 billion per year. This financial burden is unacceptable when we consider the relatively small efficacy advantage of ChE inhibitors, which may be due to a methodologic cause, and the distinct possibility that the placebo effect may be more important for this indication than the nature of the drug itself.

Drug Products

The *Rote Liste 1998* (Red List – the German equivalent of *Physicians' Desk Reference*) contains a total of 16 conventional pharmaceutical ginkgo preparations, which is twice the number stated in the 1998 edition of *Rational Phytotherapy*. All of these products meet the specifications of the 1994 Commission E monographs in their active constituents. Five gingko products are currently included in the list of the 100 most commonly prescribed phytomedicines in Germany (Appendix).

References

AkdÄ – Arzneimittelkommission der deutschen Ärzteschaft (2002) Evidenzbasierte Therapie-Leitlinien – Demenz. Arzneimittelkommission der deutschen Ärzteschaft, Deutscher Ärzteverlag, Cologne, pp 137–151.
Alaoui-Youssefi A (1999) Antineoclastic effects of Ginkgo biloba extract (EGB 761) and some of its constituents in irradiated rats. Mutation Res 445: 99–104.

Becker LE, Skipworth GB (1975) Ginkgo-tree dermatitis, stomatitis and proctitis. JAMA 231: 1162-1163.

Biber A, Koch E (1999) Bioavailability of ginkgolides and bilobalide from extracts of Ginkgo biloba using GC/MP. Planta Med 65: 192-193.

Bickel H: Allgemeine Gerontopsychiatrie; Grundlagen des normalen und pathologischen Alterns. In Förstl H (eds.): Lehrbuch der Gerontopsychiatrie. Ferdinand Enke Verlag, Stuttgart 1997: 1-15.

Blumenthal M, Busse WR, Goldberg A, Gruenwald J, Hall T, Riggins CW, Rister RS (eds.). Klein S, Rister RS (trans). (1998) The Complete German Commission E Monographs – Therapeutic Guide to Herbal Medicines. American Botanical Council, Austin, Texas. *www.herbalgram.org.*

Braquet P (ed) (1988) Ginkgolides. Chemistry, Biology, Pharmacology and Clinical Perspectives. Vol l. JR Prous Science, Barcelona.

Braquet P (ed) (1989) Ginkgolides. Chemistry, Biology, Pharmacology and Clinical Perspectives. Vol II. JR Prous Science, Barcelona.

Brüchert E, Heinrich SE, Ruf-Kohler P (1991) Wirksamkeit von LI 1370 bei älteren Patienten mit Hirnleistungsschwäche. Münch Med Wschr 133 (Suppl 1): 9-14.

Bundesgesundheitsamt (1991) Empfehlungen zum Wirksamkeitsnachweis von Nootropika im Indikationsbereich "Demenz" (Phase III). Bundesgesundheitsblatt 7: 342-350.

Burkard G, Lehrl S (1991) Verhältnis von Demenzen vom Multiinfarkt- und vom Alzheimertyp in ärztlichen Praxen. Münch Med Wschr 133 (Suppl. 1): 38-43.

Cockle SM, Kimber S, Hindmarch I (2000) The effects of *Ginkgo biloba* extract (LI1370) supplementation on activities of daily living in free-living older volunteers: a questionnaire survey. Hum Psychopharmacol Clin Exp 15: 227-235.

CPMP – Committee for Proprietary Medicinal Products (1997) Note for Guidance on Medicinal Products in the Treatment of Alzheimer's Disease. London, September 1997, CPMP/EWP/553/95.

DAB. *Deutsches Arzneibuch* (DAB Ergänzungslieferung 2000). Stuttgart, Germany: Deutscher Apotheker Verlag. 2000.

DeFeudis FV (1998) Ginkgo Biloba Extract (EGb 761): From Chemistry to the Clinic. Ullstein Medical, Wiesbaden.

Deutsches Institut für medizinische Dokumentation und Information (ed) (1994) ICD-10. Internationale und statistische Klassifikation der Krankheiten und verwandter Gesundheitsprobleme. 10. Revision. Bd 1. Urban + Schwarzenberg, Munich Vienna Baltimore.

Dilling H, Mombour W, Schmidt MH: ICD-10; Internationale Klassifikation psychischer Störungen. Verlag Hans Huber, Bern, 1993.

Doody RS, Stevens JC, Beck C, et al.: Practice parameter: Management of dementia (an evidence-based review). Neurology 2001; 56: 1154-66.

Drews S, Davies E (2001) Effectiveness of *Ginkgo biloba* in treating tinnitus: double blind, placebo controlled trial. BMJ 322: 73-75.

Dutta-Roy AK (1999) Inhibitory effect of Ginkgo biloba extract on human platelet aggregation. Platelets 10: 298-305

Ernst E, Pittler MH (1999) Ginkgo biloba for dementia. A systematic reviews of double-blind, placebo-controlled trials. Clin Drug Invest 17: 301-308.

Ernst E, Stevinson C (1999) *Ginkgo biloba* for tinnitus: a review. Clin Otolaryngol 24: 164-7.

ESCOP (2003) Monographs on the medicinal uses of plant drugs. Folium ginkgo – Ginkgo leaf. Thieme Stuttgart New York, 2003.

Fessenden JM, Wittenborn W, Clarke L (2001) Ginkgo biloba: A case report of herbal medicine and bleeding postoperatively from a laparascopic cholecystectomy. Am Surg 67: 33-35.

Fourtillan JB, Brisson AM, Girault J et al. (1997) Proprietes pharmacocinetiques du Bilobalide et des Ginkgolides A et B chez le sujet sain apres administrations intraveineuses et orales d'extrait de Ginkgo biloba (EGb 761). Therapie 50:137.

Haase A, Halama P, Hörr R (1996) Wirksamkeit kurzdauernder Infusionsbehandlungen mit Ginkgo biloba-Spezialextakt EGb 761 bei Demenz vom vaskulären und Alzheimer-Typ. Z Gerontol Geriat 29: 302-309.

Hänsel R, Keller K, Rimpler H, Schneider G (eds) (1993) Hagers Handbuch der Pharmazeutischen

Praxis, 5th edition, Drogen E-O. Springer Verlag, Berlin Heidelberg New York: 268-292.

Hartmann A, Schulz V (Hrsg) (1991) Ginkgo biloba: Aktuelle Forschungsergebnisse 1990/91. Münch Med Wschr 133: S1-S64.

Hausen BM (1998) The sensitizing capacity of ginkgolic acids in guinea pigs. American Journal of Contact Dermatitis 9: 146-148.

Hopfenmüller W (1994) Nachweis der therapeutischen Wirksamkeit eines Ginkgo biloba-Spezial-extraktes. Metaanalyse von 11 klinischen Studien bei Patienten mit Hirnleistungsstörungen im Alter. Arzneim Forsch/Drug Res 44: 1005-1013.

Ihl R, Weyer G: Die Alzheimer`s Disease Assessment Scale (ADAS). Weinheim: Beltz Test, 1993.

Ihl R: Demenzerkrankungen - Was bringen die neuen Antidementiva? MMW - Fortschr Med 2002; 144: 424-429.

Itil TM, Eralp E, Ahmed I, Kunitz A and Itil KZ (1998) The pharmacological effects of ginkgo biloba, a plant extract, on the brain of dementia patients in comparison with tacrine. Psychopharmacol Bull 34:391-7.

Itil TM, Eralp E, Tsambis E, Itil K, Stein U (1996) Central nervous system effects of Ginkgo biloba, a plant extract. Am J Therap 3: 63-73.

Jaggy H, Koch E (1997) Chemistry and biology of alkylphenols from Ginkgo biloba L. Pharmazie 52: 735-738.

Juretzek W, Kaddour HH, Habs M (2002) Blutungsgefahr unter Ginkgo? Der Hausarzt 39/19: 76-78.

Kanowski S (1991) Klinischer Wirksamkeitsnachweis bei Nootropika. Münch Med Wschr 133: S5-S8.

Kanowski S, Herrmann WM, Stephan K, Wierich W, Hörr R (1996) Proof of efficacy of the ginkgo biloba special extract EGb 761 in outpatients suffering from mild to moderate primary degenerative dementia of the Alzheimer type and multi-infarct dementia. Pharmacopsychiatry 4: 149-158.

Kasper S (2001) *Hypericum perforatum* - a review of clinical studies. Pharmacopsychiatry 34 Suppl 1. S51-S55.

Kaempfer E (1712) Amoenitarum Exoticarum. Fasciculi V, Rerum Persicarum Ulterioris Asiae. Henrici Wilhelmini Mayeri, Aulae Lippiacae Typographi, 1712.

Kleijnen J, Knipschild P (1992 a) Ginkgo biloba for cerebral insufficiency. Br J Clin Pharmac 34: 352-358.

Kleijnen J, Knipschild P (1992 b) Ginkgo biloba. Lancet: 1136-1139.

Krieglstein J, Ausmeier F, El-Abhar H, Lippert K, Welsch M, Rupalla K, Henrich-Noack P (1995) Eur J Pharm Sci 3: 39-48.

Le Bars PL (2002) Conflicting results on ginkgo research. Forsch Komplementärmed Klass Naturheilkd 9: 19-20.

Le Bars PL, Kieser M, Itil KZ (2000) A 26-week analysis of a double-blind, placebo-controlled trial of the Ginkgo biloba extract EGb 761 in dementia. Dement Geriatr Cogn Disord 11: 230-237.

LeBars PL, Katz MM, Berman N, Itil TM, Freedman AM, Schatzberg AF (1997) A placebo-controlled, double-blind, randomized trial of an extract of Ginkgo biloba for dementia. JAMA 278: 1327-1332.

Linde K, Ramirez G, Mulrow CD, Pauls M, Weidenhammer W, Melchart D (1996) St. John's wort for depression - an overview and meta-analysis of randomized clinical trials. Br Med J 313: 253-258.8.

Lovestone S, Graham N, Howard R (1997) Guidelines on drug treatment for Alzheimer's disease. Lancet 350: 232-233.

Maurer K, Ihl R, Dierks T, Frölich L (1997) Clinical efficacy of Ginkgo biloba special extract EGb 761 in dementia of the Alzheimer type. J Psychiat Res 31: 645-655.

Mix JA, Crews WD (2000) An examination of the efficacy of *Ginkgo biloba* extract EGb 761 on the neurophysiologic functioning of cognitively intact older adults. J Alternative Complementary Medicine 6: 219-229.

Mix JA, Crews WD (2002) A double-blind, placebo-controlled, randomized trial of *Ginkgo biloba* extract EGb 761® in a sample of cognitively intact older adults: neuropsychological findings. Hum Psychopharmacol Clin Exp 17:267-77.

Morgenstern C, Biermann E (1997) Ginkgo-Spezialextrakt EGb 761 in der Behandlung des Tinnitus aurium. Fortschritte der Medizin 115: 7–11.

Müller WE, Kasper S (ed) (1997) Hypericum extract (LI 160) as an herbal antidepressant. Pharmacopsychiat 30 (suppl II): 71–134.

Nieder M (1991) Pharmakokinetik der Ginkgo-Flavonole im Plasma. Münch Med Wschr 133: S61–S62.

O'Brien JT, Ballard CG: Drugs for Alzheimer's disease. Chilinesterase inhibitors have passed NICE's hurdle. BMJ 2001; 325: 123–124.

Oberpichler-Schwenk H, Krieglstein J (1992) Pharmakologische Wirkungen von Ginkgo-biloba-Extrakt und -Inhaltsstoffen. Pharmazie in unserer Zeit 21: 224–235.

Oken BS, Storzbach DM, Kaye JA (1998) The efficacy of Ginkgo boloba on cognitive function in Alzheimer's disease. Arch Neurol 55: 1409–15.

Pittler MH, Ernst, E (2000) Efficacy of kava extract for treating anxiety: systematic review and meta-analysis. J Clin Pharmacol 20: 84–89.

Rainer M, Mucke HAM, Krüger-Rainer C, Kraxberger E, Haushofer M, Jellinger KA: Cognitive relapse after discontinuation of drug therapy in Alzheimer's disease: cholinersterase inhibitors versus nootropics. J Neural Transm 2001; 108: 1327–33.

Rigney U, Kimber s, Hindmarch I(1999) The effects of acute doses of standardized ginkgo boloba extract on memory and psychomotor performance in volunteers. Pytotherapy Res 13: 408–415

Rosenblatt M, Mindel J (1997) Spontaneous hyphema associated with ingestion of Ginkgo biloba extract. N Engl J Med 336: 1108.

Rowin J, Lewis SL (1996) Spontaneous bilateral subdural hematomas associated with chronic Ginkgo biloba ingestion. Neurology 46: 1775–1776.

Rupalla K, Oberpichler-Schwenk H, Krieglstein J (1995) Neuroprotektive Wirkungen des Ginkgo-biloba-Extrakts und seiner Inhaltsstoffe. In: Loew D, Rietbrock N (eds) Phytopharmaka in Forschung und klinischer Anwendung. Steinkopff Verlag, Darmstadt: 17–27.

Schmid M, Schmoll H (Hrsg) (1994) Ginkgo. Wissenschaftliche Verlagsgesellschaft mbH Stuttgart.

Schulz V (2002) Clinical trials with Hypericum extracts in patients with depression – Results, comparisons, conclusions for therapy with antidepressant drugs. Phytomed 9: 468–474.

Schulz V (2003) Ginkgo extract or cholinesterase inhibitors in patients with dementia: what clinical trials and guidelines fail to consider. Phytomedicine 10 Suppl IV: 74–79.

Schulz V, Hübner WD, Ploch M (1997) Clinical trials with phyto-psychopharmacological agents. Phytomedicine 4: 379–387.

Small GW, Rabins PV, Barry PP et al.: Diagnosis and treatment of Alzheimer's disease and related disorders. Consensus statement of the American Association for Geriatric Psychiatry, the Alzheimer's Association, and the American Geriatrics Society. JAMA 1997; 278: 1363–71.

Solomon PR, Adams F, Silver A, Zimmer J, DeVeaux R (2002) Ginkgo for memory enhancement: a randomized controlled trial. JAMA 288: 835–840.

Sticher O (1993) Ginkgo biloba – Ein modernes pflanzliches Arzneimittel. Vierteljahresschrift der Naturforschenden Gesellschaft in Zürich 138/3: 125–168.8.

Vale S (1998) Subarachnoid haemorrhage associated with Ginkgo biloba. Lancet 352: 36.

Vesper J, Hänsgen KD (1994) Efficacy of Ginkgo Biloba in 90 Outpatients with Cerebral Insufficiency Caused by Old Age. Phytomedicine 1: 9–16.

Volz HP (1997) Kava-Kava und Kavain: Pflanzliches Anxiolytikum, Eine kristische Analyse der klinischen Studien. Münch med Wschr 139: 42–46.

Volz HP, Hänsel R (1994) Ginkgo biloba – Grundlagen und Anwendung in der Psychiatrie. Psychopharmakotherapie 1: 70–76.6.

Vorberg G, Schenk N, Schmidt U (1989) Wirksamkeit eines neuen Ginkgo-biloba-Extraktes bei 100 Patienten mit zerebraler Insuffizienz. Herz + Gefäße 9: 396–401.

Wong AHC, Smith M, Boon HS (1998) Herbal remedies in psychiatric practice. Arch Gen Psychiatry 55: 1033–1044.

2.2   St. John's Wort (SJW) as an Antidepressant

2.2.1   Introduction

St. John's wort (SJW, Fig. 2.7) has been used in herbal healing for more than 2000 years. Paracelsus may have known about its use in the treatment of psychiatric disorders (Czygan, 1993). The German poet-physician Justinus Kerner (1786–1862) reported on the use of St. John's wort in the treatment of mood disorders in the early nineteenth century (Engelhardt, 1962).

With the rise of scientifically oriented medicine, SJW was all but forgotten as a psychotropic drug. A full century passed before reports were again published on the successful use of St. John's wort in the treatment of depression (Daniel, 1939).

A treatise on the St. John's wort was one of the first herbal monographs published by Commission E during its 12 years of activity in the former German Federal Health Agency. The monograph was published in the *Bundesanzeiger* on December 5, 1984, and has been translated with all other Commission E monographs by the American Botanical Council (Blumenthal et al., 1998). Based on information available at the time, the Commission cited depressed mood as the indication for SJW, making specific reference to psychoautonomic disturbances and anxiety and/or nervous unrest. During the next 10 years, definitive clinical and pharmacologic studies were conducted that enabled the indications for SJW to be defined more precisely. The original German studies were published in a number of professional journals including *Nervenheilkunde* (12/1993: pp. 268–366; 23 articles), *Geriatric Psychiatry and Neurology* (7/1994: pp. 1–68; 17 articles), and *Pharmacopsychiatry* (30/1997: pp. 71–134, 12 articles; 31/1998: pp. 1–60, 8 articles; 34/2001: pp. 1–156, 31 articles). Today, alcoholic extracts of St. John's wort are placed in the category of herbal antidepressants.

2.2.2   Botanical Description

The genus *Hypericum* occurs throughout the world and encompasses 378 known species. The 1986 *Deutscher Arzneimittel-Codex* (German Drug Codex) identifies *Hypericum perforatum* as the species from which the crude drug is obtained. St. John's wort is an herbaceous plant that grows to a height of about 60 cm. It has yellow, star-shaped flowers with numerous long stamens and opposing leaves studded with translucent glandular dots. The stem bears two characteristic longitudinal ridges that distinguish the plant from other species of *Hypericum*. SJW grows wild throughout much of Europe, Asia, North America, and South America, showing a preference for dry, sunny locations. It is found on roadsides, railway embankments, and in clearings. The mesophyll of the leaves contains spherical glands filled with a highly refractive volatile oil that is secreted by the plant. Holding a leaf against the light displays numerous translucent dots that give it a perforated appearance, hence the botanical name *perforatum* (Hänsel et al., 1993).

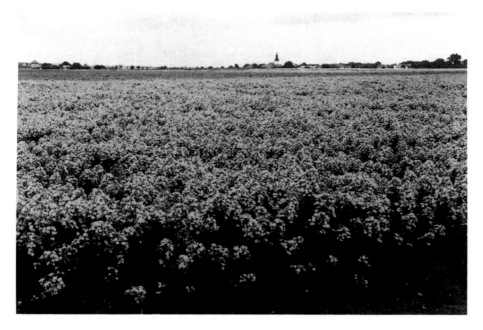

Fig. 2.7. ▲ Cultivated St. John's wort [SJW] (*Hypericum perforatum*) just before harvest.

2.2.3 Crude Drug and Extract

In years past, SJW was mainly gathered in the wild, but now most of this herb is obtained by controlled cultivation (in Germany, Poland, and South America). Herbs for medicinal use should be gathered when the flowers start to open. The harvested material should be dried rapidly but carefully to preserve the content of the secretory glands. The drying temperature should not exceed 30–40°C. The key constituents of SJW (see Sect. 2.2.4) are most concentrated in the buds, flowers, and distal leaves, so the pharmaceutical and therapeutic quality of the extracts is highly dependent on the quality of the original herbal material. Quality testing in drug manufacture is accomplished by quantitative measurement of the hypericins contained in the crude drug or extracts; poorer grades are identified and discarded.

All antidepressant medications made from SJW are based on alcoholic extracts, generally with an herb-to-extract ratio in the range of 4:1 to 7:1. So far, the only clinical proof of therapeutic efficacy for depression and other symptoms has been furnished for products that use methanol or ethanol as the solvent. Evidence to date shows that the highest yield of key constituents is obtained by extracting the dried herb with aqueous methanol containing 20–40 % water. The extraction must be performed in darkness with temperatures raised only briefly to 60–80°C (Niesel, 1992; Wagner and Bladt, 1993).

2.2.4 Key Constituents, Analysis, Pharmacokinetics

Rubbing a bud or flower from the SJW between the fingers immediately creates a red-to-purple stain caused by certain constituents of the plant: hypericin, pseudohypericin, protohypericin, protopseudohypericin, and cyclopseudohypericin, all belonging to the group of naphthodianthrones. The dried plant parts contain an average of about 0.1 % of these compounds while extracts contain approximately 0.2–0.3 %. The only analytic method that meets current qualitative and quantitative standards is HPLC (see Fig. 1.3). Animal studies suggest that the hypericin compounds contribute to the antidepressant activity of the whole extract (Butterweck et al., 1998). The hypericins are also important from a safety standpoint, as they may cause photosensitization in fair skinned individuals with overdosing (see Sect. 2.2.5).

The phloroglucinol derivative hyperforin seems to be another important antidepressant constituent of SJW. This has been demonstrated in pharmacologic models (Chatterjee et al., 1998; Müller et al., 1998; Bhattacharya, 1998; Müller et al., 2001; Cervo, 2002) and in a multicenter clinical study (Laakmann et al., 1998). The reproductive parts of H. perforatum (flowers and unripe seeds) have about a 1–4 % content of hyperforin and the related compound adhyperforin (Nahrstedt and Butterweck, 1997; Erdelmeier, 1998). Most of the ethanol and methanol extracts that are sold commercially contain approximately 2–6 % hyperforin (Melzer et al., 1998). This means that both the crude drug and its alcohol extracts contain at least 10 times more hyperforin than hypericins. Hyperforin is unstable, however, and is subject to oxidative breakdown. Apparently it is protected in the living plant by the presence of antioxidant compounds such as flavonoids. The same principle can be used in alcoholic whole extracts by adding antioxidants such as ascorbic acid to improve hyperforin stability (Erdelmeier, 1998). The therapeutic efficacy of SJW extracts cannot be attributed to hyperforin alone, however, because extracts with a very low hyperforin content have also proven effective in three clinical studies (Schrader et al., 1998, 2000; Woelk, 2000). Pharmacologic results in animal behavior models have shown that, besides hypericin and hyperforin, the efficacy of the extract depends upon the presence of other components such as rutin (Nöldner und Schötz, 2002).

Besides these species-specific components, the dried herbs and extracts also contain significant amounts of some very common plant constituents such as flavonoid derivatives (e. g., rutin and hyperoside), xanthone derivatives, biflavones (e.g. amentoflavon), procyanidines, and a volatile oil (Nahrstedt and Butterweck, 1997). The herb contains no more than about 1 % of the volatile oil, which is isolated by steam distillation. Hypericum oil is made by macerating the ground fresh flowers of SJW in olive oil (25:100 ratio). Hypericum oil is a traditional topical remedy for use on wounds and burns (see Chap. 8).

For many years, the hypericin compounds (especially hypericin and pseudohypericin) were considered the key constituents of hypericum medications. It has been shown, however, that while the hypericins contribute to the antidepressant activity of SJW, they are not the only active components present in the whole extract (Müller et al., 1998). They are responsible for the skin photosensitization that may occur in susceptible (usually light-skinned) individuals. While there have been no documented cases of serious photosensitization in patients treated with St. John's wort, three studies have been performed in a total of 76 patients to estimate the risk associated with a possible overdose (Brockmöller et al., 1997; Kerb et al., 1996). The daily doses in these studies ranged from 300 mg to 3600 mg of the St. John's wort methanol extract LI 160. The maximum plasma levels measured at 3–4 hours (pseudohypericin) and at 6–7 hours (hypericin) after drug ingestion were between 14 and 111 µg/L for hypericin and between 7 and 83 µg/L for pseudohypericin, depending on the dose. The systemic bioavailability of hypericin was calculated at 14–21 %. The elimination half-life was 24 to 48 hours for hypericin and 12 to 24 hours for pseudohypericin. This leads to a cumulative rise in plasma levels over a 14-day period of repetitive use (Fig. 2.8). Following the intravenous injection of hypericin in rhesus monkeys at a dose of 2 mg/kg (n=3) and 5 mg/kg (n=1), elimination followed a biphasic course with an initial half-life of 3 h and a terminal half-life of 26 h. Hypericin could not be detected in the cerebrospinal fluid of the animals (Fox et al., 2001). The correlation of hypericin levels with photosensitization symptoms is discussed in Sect. 2.2.6.

One study showed a dose-dependent rise of plasma hyperforin levels in rats and healthy volunteers following the oral administration of a SJW extract containing 5 % hyperforin. The maximum plasma levels in rats were reached at approximately 3 hours after dosing. Maximum plasma levels in 6 healthy volunteers, ranging from about 100 µg/L to 400 µg/L, were reached about 4 hours after the oral administration of 300 mg, 600 mg, and 1200 mg of the extract, depending on the dose. The elimination half-life in rats was approximately 3 hours in the early phase and 8–9 hours in the late phase. The elimination half-life in the healthy subjects ranged from 9 to 12 hours. A

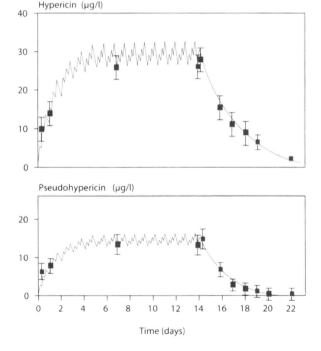

Fig. 2.8. ◀ Plasma levels of hypericin and pseudohypericin in patients taking 1800 mg SJW extract daily for 14 days. The curves represent the mean predicted plasma levels. The mean values for the measured plasma levels (n = 50) and their 95 % confidence interval are also shown (Brockmöller et al., 1997).

computer simulation showed that with a t.i.d. regimen of 300 mg of the extract, a steady-state plasma concentration of hyperforin is reached in approximately 24–26 hours (Biber et al., 1998). Another study was performed in 12 healthy subjects who took 2700 mg of the hypericum extract LI 160 daily. The plasma levels measured about 4 hours after dosing ranged from 40 to 80 µg/L for hypericin and from 1000 to 1800 µg/L for hyperforin (Franklin et al., 1999).

Comparing the data currently available for hypericins with the data available for hyperforin, we can draw the following conclusions: Hyperforin levels are at least 10 times higher than hypericin levels both in alcohol extracts and in the blood plasma after oral dosing. Hyperforin, like the hypericins, is relatively stable in the plasma, and its pharmacokinetics are proportional to the administered dose. Both hyperforin and hypericins could contribute to therapeutic efficacy based on their pharmacokinetics (Müller and Chatterjee, 1998; Singer et al., 1999).

2.2.5 Pharmacology

To appreciate the voluminous literature on studies in pharmacologic models with SJW extracts and with fractions and components isolated from them, we refer the reader to current reviews (Nathan, 1999; Greenson et al., 2001; Müller, 2002; ESCOP, 2003). Here we shall limit our discussion to studies that are useful in understanding the effects of SJW on the central nervous system. Ultimately, only treatment studies in depressed patients can prove the therapeutic efficacy of SJW as an antidepressant. But pharmacology can advance our understanding in lesser ways, e.g., by elucidating possible mechanisms of action. The cumulative results of test series, rather than of individual studies, provide the most suitable basis for evaluation. The most useful test systems are biochemical models in vitro and ex vivo and also behavioral models in live animals.

2.2.5.1 Biochemical Models

Most currently known antidepressants inhibit the active, energy-dependent reuptake of monoamines (norepinephrine, serotonin, dopamine) into the neuron from the synaptic gap. The inhibition of monoamine uptake forms the basis for the classic hypotheses on the pathophysiology of depression and the mechanism of action of antidepressant drugs, which are classified accordingly as MAO inhibitors, norepinephrine-reuptake inhibitors, selective serotonin-reuptake inhibitors. When used for a period of several days to several weeks, these drugs also induce sustained adaptive changes in certain receptor systems. These changes can be investigated experimentally in isolated synaptosomes, isolated neurons or glia cells, or by feeding experiments in animals followed by examination of the corresponding receptor systems in brain preparations (Müller et al., 1997 and 2002; Riederer et al., 1993).

Today, alcoholic extracts of St. John's wort have been tested in almost all biochemical models (reviews in Nathan, 1999; Greenson 2001; Müller et al., 1997; Müller, 2002). While these authors cannot confirm the MAO inhibition (Bladt and Wagner, 1994) they all describe a inhibitory effect on the synaptosomal uptake of serotonin, dopamine, and

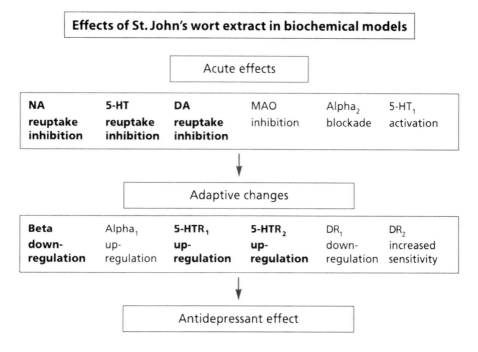

Fig. 2.9. ▲ Typical changes that can occur with antidepressants tested in biochemical models. Boldface: marked effects that have been observed in model experiments with the SJW.

Abbreviations:
NA = norepinephrine, 5-HT = 5-hydroxytryptamine, DA = dopamine, MAO = monoamine oxidase, Alpha = alpha receptors, 5-HTR = 5-hydroxytryptamine receptors, DR = dopamine receptors.

norepinephrine. The half-maximal inhibitory concentrations for these three neurotransmitters are 2 µg/mL. These concentrations are also considered therapeutically relevant in human patients (Müller et al., 1997, 1998; Beary and Bu, 1998). Studies have also shown adaptive changes in the CNS of rats after 14 days of treatment, most notably a significant increase in the density of cortical beta and an increase in cortical 5-HT$_2$ receptors (Müller et al., 1997; Gleitz and Teufel-Mayer, 1998). Hyperforin has recently been identified as an important constituent for these effects (Müller and Chatterjee, 1998). The effects of St. John's wort extract that have been documented in biochemical models thus far are reviewed in Fig. 2.9.

2.2.5.2 Behavioral Models in Animals

Experimental pharmacology includes at least 9 valid animal models in which small rodents are used to test the efficacy of antidepressants. These models are based on two fundamental principles: the principle of pharmacologic interaction (e.g., with reserpine or apomorphine) and induced behavioral change such as "learned helplessness" or

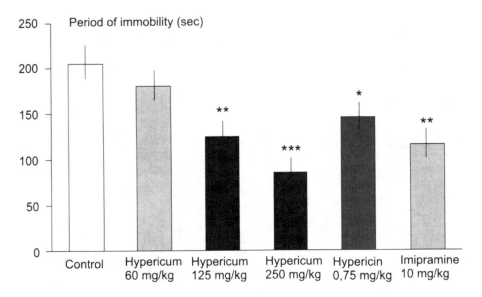

Fig. 2.10. ▲ Pharmacologic activity of a standardized St. John's wort extract (hypericum) compared with pure hypericin (0.75 mg = amount contained in 250 mg extract) and the standard antidepressant drug imipramine as measured by the Porsolt swimming test. The whole extract was significantly more active than the equivalent amount of hypericin. Imipramine was about 10 times more active than the whole extract, reflecting the approximate dose relationship of both substances when used therapeutically in human patients (Butterweck et al., 1997).

"behavioral despair" in rats (Porsolt et al., 1991). These models have already been used in several studies to test the hypericum extracts.

Tests in mice and rats have demonstrated typical effects consisting of reserpine antagonism, a shortened duration of anesthesia, and a reduction of immobility time in the Porsolt despair test (Butterweck et al., 1997, 1998; Winterhoff et al., 1993). The ratio of hypericum extract to imipramine at effective dose levels was approximately 10:1, reflecting the practice-established dose ratios used in the treatment of depressed patients (active dose of hypericum extract = 900 mg/d, for imipramine = 50–150 mg/d). Another group of authors administered two hypericum extracts intraperitoneally in same animal model, compared them with imipramine and fluoxetine, and found almost identical effective dosages in the range of 10–30 mg/kg (De Vry et al., 1999). Studies on isolated fractions and compounds have shown that several classes of compounds, including hypericins, contribute synergistically to the effect of the whole extract and that solubility-mediating substances can act as co-effectors to enhance the bioavailability of the drug (Butterweck et al., 1997, 1998). A review of the experimental pharmacology was published by Nathan (1999).

2.2.6 Toxicology, Photosensitization

The toxicologic properties of hypericum extract LI 160 have been tested both acutely and over a period of 26 weeks in mice, rats, and dogs. The maximum test dose was 5000 mg/kg. The first intolerance reactions appeared at 900 mg/kg/day, and the LD_{50} was greater than the maximum dose. None of the tests showed evidence of genotoxic or mutagenic effects (Leuschner, 1995).

Photosensitization and even phototoxic reactions (hypericism) are known to occur in grazing animals, especially sheep and cattle, that have consumed large amounts of St. John's wort (Araya and Ford, 1981; Giese, 1980). Feeding dried SJW to calves did not produce symptoms at a dose of 1 g/kg, but animals that were given doses of 3 g/kg and 5 g/kg and exposed to sunlight approximately 4 h later manifested erythema, restlessness, and diarrhea (Araya and Ford, 1981). When fresh SJW was fed to sheep in doses of 4–16 g/kg, even the lowest dose produced skin symptoms and also a rise in the plasma levels of a number of enzymes (Kako et al., 1993). The hypericin content in 5–10 g of dried herb made from flowering SJW is approximately equal to the amount contained in 1 g of a commercial SJW extract. Thus, when the experience gained from feeding experiments in calves and sheep is applied to humans, it is reasonable to assume that a serious phototoxic reaction would be likely to occur after the consumption of approximately 0.3–0.6 g/kg of extract. In a patient weighing 70 kg, this would correspond to approximately 20–40 g of extract, which is about 30 times the therapeutic daily dose. Indeed, when 30–40 mg of hypericin (equal to the amount of hypericin and pseudohypericin in about 20 g of extract) was administered intravenously in AIDS patients to test for antiviral effects, the patients developed severe phototoxic reactions that forced termination of the study (Gulick et al., 1999). It is reasonable to conclude, then, that phototoxic skin reactions can result from an overdose of SJW (e.g., in a suicide attempt), but this would not be expected to occur at therapeutic dose levels.

Studies have been done in human subjects to determine the threshold dose at which initial signs of photosensitization occur. In one placebo-controlled crossover study, 13 healthy male subjects took 900, 1800, and 3600 mg of hypericum extract once a day. The lowest dose, 900 mg/day, has been established as the effective daily dose by most clinical studies. In another study, 50 healthy subjects of both sexes took 600 mg 3 times daily (t.i.d.) for 15 days. In both tests the subjects were exposed on days 1 and 15 to ultraviolet-A (UV-A) and UV-B irradiation of standard duration and intensity 4 h after taking the morning dose. The skin reactions were assessed at 5 h, 20 h, and 7 days after the UV exposures as the minimum erythematous dose (MED) in one study and as the minimum pigmentation dose (MPD) in the other.

In hypericum-treated subjects who had been exposed to UV light, a slight decrease in the MED and a slight but statistically significant decrease in the MPD were found on day 15 of treatment. This led the authors to conclude that taking a high dose of SJW for a prolonged period of time would slightly increase the patient's tendency to tan from sun exposure. Phototoxicity symptoms, however, would not be expected to occur at the recommended therapeutic dose levels (see Sect. 2.2.8). In the event of an overdose equaling several times the recommended therapeutic dose, the patient should avoid exposure to UV light for one week due to the relatively long elimination half-life of hypericin and pseudohypericin (Brockmöller et al., 1997; Bernd et al., 1999; Golsch et al., 1997; Schempp et al., 1999).

2.2.7 Clinical Efficacy in Depressed Patients

Traditionally, SJW has been taken medicinally in the form of a tea. Such a preparation delivers a single dose equivalent to an aqueous extract of 2–3 g of the dried herb. Dividing the minimum dose of 2 g of the dried herb by 7 (based on the usual herb-to-extract ratio, see Sect. 1.3.1) gives a minimum single dose equivalent to approximately 300 mg for the dry extract. This may be considered a reasonable standard dose by the physician who relies on empirical principles in the practice of phytotherapy and believes that they will yield positive therapeutic results. The majority of the studies listed in Tables 2.4 and 2.5 conform to this requirement.

2.2.7.1 Methods in the Clinical Testing of Antidepressants

Antidepressant pharmacotherapy in the modern, efficacious sense of the word began in 1957 with the introduction of imipramine. Since then, more than 30 new drugs have been added, the most recent being the *selective serotonin-reuptake inhibitors* (SSRIs). The results of approximately 1500 controlled clinical studies on the therapeutic efficacy of antidepressants have been published thus far (Kirsch and Sapirstein, 1998). These results can be validly compared with one another, because the underlying methodology has not changed fundamentally for four decades. Most studies have used the Hamilton Depression Rating Scale (HAMD) as their main outcome measure. This observer rating scale was published in 1960, a few years after the introduction of the first tricyclic antidepressants (Hamilton, 1960). The physician assigns individual scores based on the severity of 17 or 21 items and adds them together to yield a total score expressing the severity of the illness. Scores up to about 12 are classified as normal, up to about 20 as mild depression, up to about 25 as moderate depression, and higher than 25 as severe depression. Treatment response can be assessed by the decrease in total score.

Both the FDA and European approval agencies have issued guidelines for the clinical testing of antidepressants during the past 15 years. The Committee for Proprietary Medical Products (CPMP) issued a guideline in April, 2002, to update the EU guidelines, stating that the participants recruited for clinical antidepressant trials must have a mild, moderate, or severe "major depressive disorder" as defined by the diagnostic criteria of the DSM VI or ICD 10. Efficacy for acute depressive episodes (preferably of moderate severity) must be documented in controlled studies that are conducted over a 4- to 6-week period. Besides the HAMD Scale (usually the 17-item version), the Montgomery-Asberg Depression Scale (MADRS) is also an acknowledged tool for the physician assessment of specific features. In both scales, patients whose total scores improve by at least 50 % with therapy are classified as responders (Anonymus, 2002).

Table 2.5.

Selection of 10 controlled clinical studies in depressed patients using St. John's wort preparations based on ethanol extracts.

First author, year	Cases	Daily dose (extract)	Duration (days)	Reference therapy	Responders (hypericum vs. reference therapy)
Harrer, 1991	116	3 ml (300 mg)	42	Placebo	66 % vs. 25 %
Quandt, 1993	88	4.5 mL (450 mg)	28	Placebo	71 % vs. 7 %
Schrader, 1998	159	500 mg	42	Placebo	56 % vs. 15 %
Laakmann, 1998	147	900 mg	42	Extr. 0.5% hf., Placebo	49 % vs. 39 % vs. 33 %
Philipp, 1999	263	1050 mg	56	Imipramine, placebo	76 % vs. 67 % vs. 63 %
Harrer, 1999	149	800 mg	42	Fluoxetin	71 % vs. 72 %
Lenoir, 1999	348	?	42	0.5 mg/d hypericin vs. 1 mg/d hypericin vs. 3 mg/d hypericin	62 % vs. 65 % vs. 68 %
Schrader, 2000	240	500 mg	42	Fluoxetine	60 % vs. 40 %
Woelk, 2000	324	500 mg	42	Imipramine	43 % vs. 40 %
Kalb, 2001	72	900 mg	42	Placebo	62 % vs. 43 %

NOTE: For the liquid preparations, a solids content of 10% was assumed in calculating the dose in mg. Cases were classified as responders if their total HAMD score improved by more than 50% during the course of treatment.

Table 2.4.

Selection of 12 controlled clinical studies in patients with depressive disorders treated with a St. John's wort extract produced with 80% methanol in water (v/v).

First author, year	Cases	Daily dose (extract)	Duration (days)	Reference therapy	Responders (hypericum vs. reference therapy)
Lehrl, 1993	50	450–900 mg	28	Placebo	42 % vs. 25 %
Sommer, 1994	105	450–900 mg	28	Placebo	67 % vs. 28 %
Harrer, 1994	102	900 mg	28	Maprotiline	61 % vs. 67 %
Hübner, 1994	39	900 mg	28	Placebo	70 % vs. 47 %
Vorbach, 1994	135	900 mg	42	Imipramine	64 % vs. 58 %
Hänsgen, 1996	102	900 mg	42	Placebo	70 % vs. 24 %
Wheatley, 1997	165	900 mg	42	Amitriptyline	60 % vs. 78 %
Vorbach, 1997	209	1800 mg	42	Imipramine	35 % vs. 41 %
Shelton, 2001	200	900–1200 mg	56	Placebo	33 % vs. 21 %[1]
HDT Study Group, 2002	340	900–1500 mg	56	Placebo, Sertraline	24 % vs. 32 % vs. 25 %
Lecrubier, 2002	375	900 mg	42	Placebo	53 % vs. 42 %

[1] Patients with mild to moderate depression

2.2.7.2 Studies on the Efficacy of St. John's Wort Extracts

The results of 37 controlled clinical trials with SJW extracts had been published by the end of 2002. These studies included more than 4000 patients, most suffering from mild or moderate depression. The data from 22 major studies conducted since 1990 are summarized in Tables 2.4 and 2.5. Additional information, including details on the studies cited in the two tables and in the text, can be found in the following reviews: Harrer und Schulz, 1993; Linde et al., 1996; Volz, 1997; Kasper, 2001; Schulz, 2002a; Blumenthal et al., 2003, ESCOP, 2003. The pharmacologically active components in the test preparations were either ethanol/water extracts (50 % or 60 % v/v, Table 2.4) or methanol/water extracts (80 % v/v, Table 2.5). The reference therapies consisted of placebo, synthetic antidepressants, or in two studies (Martinez et al., 1994; Wheatly, 1999) phototherapy. The main outcome measures in most of the studies were a reduction in total score or the response rate in the Hamilton Depression Scale.

Several studies from the early 1990s (involving extracts made with 50 % or 60 % ethanol in water, see Table 2.4) were conducted with liquid preparations (fresh plant tinctures). The amounts of dry extract administered in these studies could only be estimated from the published data. The estimated dosages used in the 10 studies shown in Table 2.4 ranged from 300 mg/d to 1050 mg/d of extract. Five of the 10 studies were placebo-controlled, and the SJW extracts were significantly superior to placebo in all five. Two studies each compared St. John's wort with imipramine or fluoxetine and found that hypericum was equal to or even better than the synthetic comparators. For the present, only preliminary results are available for another placebo-controlled study with an ethanol extract in 207 patients. After 6 weeks of therapy, the total average score in the placebo-treated patients fell from 22 to 14 points while the score in the hypericum-treated group fell from 22 to 11.5 points. The difference between the groups was statistically significant (Gensthaler, 2001).

The results of a total of 17 controlled studies using the 80 % methanol/water extract were published after 1990. Eight of these studies compared the hypericum extract with placebo, three with sertraline, and one each with maprotiline or amitriptyline. The dosages were in the range from 450 to 1800 mg of extract per day. Statistical analysis of the Hamilton total score showed significant differences in six of eight placebo-controlled studies in favor of SJW extract. The two studies that additionally used phototherapy (Martinez et al., 1994; Wheatley, 1999) showed no additive benefit from the concurrent use of both therapies. In seven studies comparing SJW extract with a total of four synthetic antidepressants, a significant advantage was found at the end of 6 weeks' treatment for amitriptyline (Wheatley, 1997), but no significant differences were found in comparison with sertraline (Brenner, 2000; HDT Study Group, 2002; van Gurp, 2002), imipramine (Vorbach et al., 1994, 1997), or maprotaline (Harrer et al., 1994). The data from 12 of the 17 studies using the methanol extract are summarized in Table 2.5.

The results of these studies indicate no significant differences in the efficacy of the two alcoholic extracts. Taken as a whole, all of the study results suggest that the threshold of efficacy for relieving specific symptoms and complaints in depression is approximately 300 mg of extract per day. When administered in doses of approximately 500–1000 mg of extract per day under medical supervision, the SJW preparations tended to be more effective than placebo and just as effective as the four synthetic reference products. This assessment is valid for mild to moderate depressive episodes but not for severe forms of depression, which are not an indication for SJW extracts.

Two controlled double-blind studies were conducted to determine which of the pharmacologically active ingredients (see 2.2.4) contributed most to the antidepressive

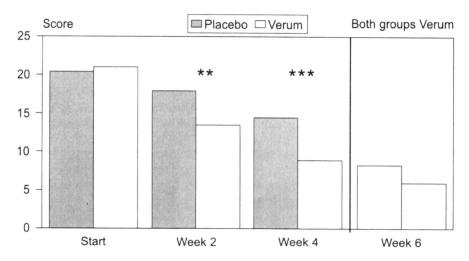

Fig. 2.11. ▲ Mean scores in the Hamilton Depression Scale (HAMD). Placebo-controlled, double-blind study in 101 depressed patients treated with 900 mg SJW extract daily compared with a placebo. A parallel group design was followed until week 4; thereafter both groups received the SJW extract. Scores recorded in weeks 2 and 4 showed statistically significant differences between SJW and placebo (*** = p < 0.001). Scores in weeks 5 and 6, when both groups received SJW showed marked improvement in the original placebo group (Hänsgen et al., 1996).

efficacy of the whole extracts in human patients. One of the studies (Lenoir et al., 1999) used three extracts containing different amounts of hypericins (equivalent to daily doses of 0.5 mg, 1 mg, or 3 mg), and the other study (Laakmann et al., 1998) used two extracts containing different amounts of hyperforin (equivalent to daily doses of 4.5 mg or 45 mg). The latter study was placebo-controlled. While increasing the hypericin dose did not produce a significant increase in efficacy (HAMD responder rates of 62 %, 65 %, and 68 %), a higher dose of hyperforin did result in in some benefit (HAMD responder rates of 39 % vs. 49 %).

As an example, Fig. 2.11 shows the results of a placebo-controlled double-blind study in 101 outpatients with moderately severe depression (meeting the criteria for major depression according to the Diagnostic and Statistical Manual [DSM] III-R). The patients received either 300 mg of hypericum extract or a placebo t.i.d. for 4 weeks. Both groups then received the hypericum extract for an additional 2 weeks. With allowance to typical placebo effects, the results at 4 weeks showed a statistically highly significant difference in favor of the group treated with the hypericum extract. As expected, a smaller difference was seen after both groups had taken the hypericum extract for an additional 2 weeks (Hänsgen et al., 1996).

Figure 2.12 shows the results of a study comparing SJW with a standard therapy in 135 depressed patients. As in the previous trial, the patients had been selected according to the criteria in the Diagnostic and Statistical Manual (DSM-III-R). For 6 weeks the patients received either 300 mg of hypericum extract t.i.d. or 25 mg of imipramine t.i.d. All drugs were administered in the form of look-alike coated tablets. Response was evaluated by the HAMD rating scale as well as two other validated observer- and self-

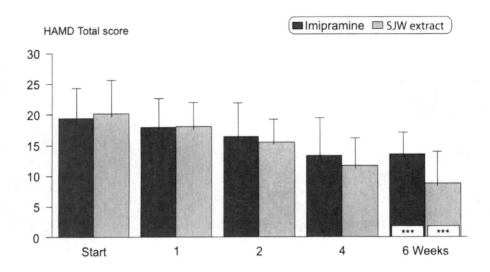

HAMD Total score

Fig. 2.12. ▲ Mean values and standard deviations of total HAMD scores recorded during 6 week's treatment with 900 mg/day SJW extract (67 patients) compared with 75 mg/day imipramine (68 patients). Statistical analysis showed that both medications were equally effective (Vorbach et al., 1994).

rating scales. The HAMD scores showed similar declines in both treatment groups, decreasing from 20.2 to 8.8 in the hypericum-treated patients and from 19.4 to 10.7 in the patients treated with imipramine (Vorbach et al., 1994).

Figure 2.13 shows the result of a double-blind study comparing the hypericum extract "STEI 300" (1050 mg/day) with imipramine (100 mg/day) and placebo. A total of 251 patients suffering a current episode of moderate depression (ICD 10: F32.1 and F33.1) were treated in 3 parallel-groups for 8 weeks. The main outcome measures were the change from baseline, in the Hamilton Depression Score (17 HAMD), Hamilton Anxiety Scale (HAMA), Clinical Global Impressions (CGI), Zung Self Rating Depression Scale (SDS) as well as Quality of Life assessment (SF-36), and adverse events profile. The hypericum extract was superior in reducing 17-HAMD scores (-15.4) compared to placebo (-12.1) and equally efficacious as imipramine (-14.2). Comparable results were found in the other scales. The rate of adverse events of hypericum (0.5 events/patient) was in the range of the placebo group (0.6) but lower than under imipramine treatment (1.2) (Philipp et al., 1999).

2.2.7.3 Pharmacotherapy of Depression: What Contributes to Efficacy?

The study described in Fig 2.13 is not alone in demonstrating a remarkably high placebo success rate. Examination of the data from the other studies in Tables 2.4 and 2.5 shows that while the relative efficacy of the placebo was not always very pronounced, it generally equalled more than 50 % of the overall effect achieved with the true drug. Moreover, the studies comparing SJW extracts with standard synthetic drugs showed no significant differences in efficacy. Meta-analyses of multiple studies have yielded

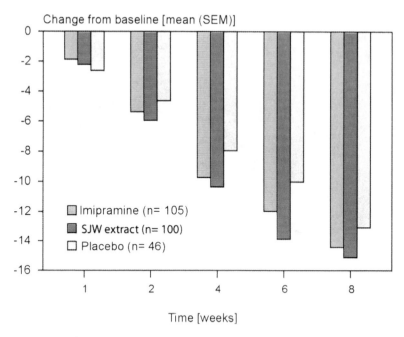

Fig. 2.13. ▲ Mean change from baseline in the 17-HAMD total score at all visits in the intention to treat analysis. 8 weeks treatment with 1050 mg SJW extract, 100 mg imipramine or placebo. Statistical analysis showed that SJW was more effective than placebo and at least as effective as imipramine (Philipp et al., 1999).

similar results (Gaster and Holroyd, 2000; Mulrow et al., 2000; Volz and Laux, 2000). The worldwide attention that has been focused on the St. John's wort phenomenon has caused many experts to reexamine the question of who and what contribute most to the effectiveness of antidepressant pharmacotherapy.

In a meta-analysis of more than 80 studies on new synthetic antidepressants, the Agency for Health Care Policy and Research in the United States found an average response rate of 32 % to placebo versus 50 % to the antidepressants (Mulrow et al., 1999). Calculations showed that in 22 major treatment studies using SJW extracts (Tables 2.4, 2.5), the response rates were 31 % on placebo (mean value of 13 studies) and 56 % on the therapeutic agents (mean value of 21 studies). Thus, the potentially decisive role of the physician in the success of antidepressant pharmacotherapy does not depend chiefly on whether an herbal or synthetic product has been prescribed. In another example, a randomized double-blind study was conducted in Norway to compare the efficacy of two "modern" antidepressants in general practice settings (NORDEP study). Sixty-one general practitioners treated 372 depressed patients for periods of 24 weeks. The success rates are shown in Fig. 2.14 Statistical analysis indicated a 47 % remission rate on placebo compared with 61 % on sertraline and 54 % on mianserin (Malt et al., 1999).

The uncritical reliance on statistical data from such studies fails to recognize, however, that the study results with synthetic antidepressants (unlike those with St. John's wort extract) are often compromised by "unblinding" of the test groups. The overrating

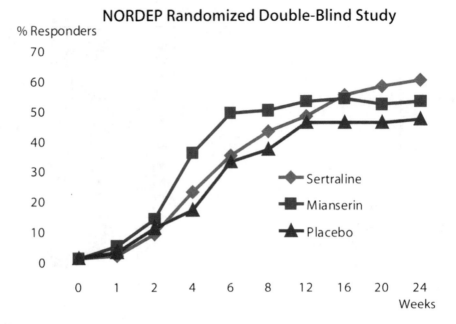

Fig. 2.14. ▲ randomized double-blind study was conducted in physicians' offices in Norway to compare the efficacy of two "modern" antidepressants (NORDEP Study). Sixty-one general practitioners treated 373 depressed patients for periods of 24 weeks. Statistical analysis indicated a 47% rate of remissions on placebo compared with 61% on sertraline and 54 % on mianserin (Malt et al., 1999).

of presumed pharmacodynamic effects in such cases is caused by side effects that are so typical of a particular drug that they give an experienced researcher early clues to the group identity in a statistically significant number of cases. The result can be false-positive findings and the misinterpretation of results (Kirsch and Sapirstein, 1998; Schulz, 1999 and 2002).

This raises a recent example: the results of a large U.S. trial to test the antidepressant efficacy of a SJW extract compared with the standard synthetic drug sertraline and a placebo were published in April of 2002 (Hypericum Depression Trial Study Group, 2002). The trial, financed with more than $5 million in public funds, indicated no significant differences among the three treatment groups in the primary outcome measure (change in the HAMD total score from baseline). Faced with this awkward situation, the authors noted that the standard drug sertraline, which has been approved as an antidepressant internationally and by the FDA, demonstrated a secondary outcome of at least a small advantage of 2 score points over SJW and the placebo. Unfortunately, this justification was based on a disregard for other data. The section of the paper titled "Assessment of Blindness to Treatment" contained the following statement: "Correct guesses for clinicians totaled 66 % for sertraline, 29 % for hypericum, and 36 % for placebo (p=0.001)." In other words, the physicians knew the correct group identity in 52 of the 79 patients who had been treated with sertraline! But the testing physicians in this study would most likely have expected sertraline to have some degree of efficacy, and this would be sufficient to account for the slight difference that was noted in favor of that drug. The same phenomenon is operative in most studies of tricyclic antidepressants, probably to an even greater degree. Drug-specific side effects occur in approximately 30–60 % of all patients treated with these agents, compared with 15–30 % of patients treated with the newer synthetic antidepressants and only 1–3 % of patients treated with St. John's wort extracts!

In summary, these facts and figures make it clear that, regardless of the synthetic or herbal origin of the agents used in antidepressant pharmacotherapy, from one-half to two-thirds of the therapeutic effect is referable to the self-healing powers of the patient and their stimulation by the treating physician, while a smaller portion is referable to the pharmacodynamic actions of the drugs. All prevailing treatment guidelines for depression disregard this scientifically confirmed reality, as they continue to overemphasize the importance of the drugs themselves and ignore the effect of the "therapeutic context." The practical application of this discovery would be of major importance in improving both the tolerance (see Sect. 2.2.9) and the economy (see Sect. 1.5.4) of antidepressant therapy.

2.2.8 Indications, Dosages, Risks, and Contraindications

The monograph on SJW published by Commission E of the German Federal Health Agency on December 5, 1984, cites the following indications for hypericum preparations: psychoautonomic (psychovegetative) disturbances, depressive mood disorders, anxiety and/or nervous unrest (Blumenthal et al., 1998). Considering that none of the numerous controlled clinical studies in Tables 2.4 and 2.5 had been published at the time this monograph was issued, we must credit the Commission with making a fairly accurate appraisal of the herb's therapeutic applications considering the somewhat relatively limited clinical data upon which their findings are based. In the light of what is known today, however, medications made from SJW should be classified strictly as antidepressants when administered in the proper form and dosage. SJW may benefit psychoautonomic disturbances and anxiety and/or nervous unrest only within the context of its overall antidepressant activity. Generally, though, marked improvement cannot be expected until the patient has taken the product for several weeks. Preparations of SJW do not produce acute effects, so they are not suitable for use as daily sedatives or sleeping aids.

In 1998 this prompted the German Federal Institute for Drugs and Medical Devices to depart from the indications stated in the Commission E monograph and use the more specific indication of "mild to moderate depressive episodes" in the new approval of products with proven efficacy. This indication corresponds to the ICD 10 diagnostic categories F32.0 and F32.1, consistent with the inclusion criteria used in the controlled studies (Tables 2.4 and 2.5). The pan-European ESCOP monograph additionally cites the ICD 10 categories F33.0 and F33.1 (ESCOP, 2003). The package insert for German consumers is required to state that the product is intended for use in "temporary mild to moderate depression."

Dosing recommendations for SJW are still based on the daily dose of 2–4 g of crude drug stated in the Commission E monograph. Stating this in terms of alcohol (methanol or ethanol) extracts, which have an herb-to-extract ratio of 4–8 in almost all commercial products, the minimum recommended dose is 300 mg of extract daily, with a normal dose range of 500–900 mg/d. As a result, the dose recommendation of "0.2–1 mg total hypericin" stated in the Commission E monograph is considered outdated and has been rescinded by the Federal Institute for Drugs and Medical Devices in Germany. Current dose recommendations are no longer based on total hypericin but strictly on the total amount of extract contained in the finished drug product. The hypericin and hyperforin content of the product is still an important consideration, however. As discussed in Sect. 2.2.4, a methanol or ethanol extract of SJW should contain approximately 0.1–0.3 % hypericins and 1–6 % hyperforin. For the reasons stated in the preceding sections, an initial daily dose of 500–1000 mg of a high-quality extract should be prescribed in depressed patients. If maintenance therapy is indicated following a positive response or if only certain symptoms require treatment in milder cases, daily doses of 300–600 mg of total extract may be sufficient.

Even the 1984 monograph mentioned photosensitization as a possible side effect of SJW therapy. As explained in Sect. 2.2.6, this reaction is caused by hypericins that are absorbed from St. John's wort preparations, but the number of reported cases of skin reactions in humans is small at the recommended therapeutic doses (1 case in 300,000 patients; Schulz, 2001). As stated in Sect. 2.2.6, however, it is likely that a single dose (20–40 g of extract) equal to approximately 30 times the recommended daily dose could cause significant phototoxic reactions in humans. If such an extreme amount were ingested, as in a suicide attempt, the patient would have to be screened from all sunlight and other UV light for one week due to the long elimination half-life of hypericins. If this important precaution is followed, even a massive overdose should not cause serious complications. It is conceivable that SJW might interact with other photosensitizing drugs, producing an additive effect, but so far there have been no reports of this.

Recent in vitro studies have raised the question of whether there may be a risk of cataract formation due to the hypericin contained in SJW (Schey et al., 2000; Sgarbossa et al., 2000). Both of these experimental studies used isolated hypericin rather than SJW preparations. In one study the hypericin was incubated with a protein isolated from calf lenses (α-crystallin) and in the other with the calf lenses themselves. The hypericin concentrations in the incubates were 50 µM (equal to about 25 mg/L) in the first case and 100 µM (equal to about 50 mg/L) in the second case. This contrasts significantly with the levels measured in pharmacokinetic studies in humans (see Sect. 2.2.4), where the average plasma concentration after 1800 mg/d (twice the normal daily dosage) of SJW extract for 14 days was approximately 30 µg/L. This is about one one-thousandth the concentrations used in the in vitro experiments cited above. Lens opacities have never been reported during or after the prolonged therapeutic use of SJW. Cataracts, moreover, are not a typical feature of the condition in veterinary medicine known as "hypericism" – the photosensitization associated with livestock that have consumed significant amounts of SJW on the open range.

There are significant risks associated with the concomitant use of SJW preparations and certain drugs, however. Numerous studies suggest that the mechanism of pharmacokinetic interactions with SJW extract involves the drug-metabolizing enzyme

CYP3A4 and the transport protein P-glycoprotein. It may be that other mechanisms are also involved in these interactions, however. So far, researchers have not been able to relate the interactions to a specific ingredient in SJW. The interactions associated with St. John's wort have been diligently recorded and researched in recent years and described in numerous publications. The reader may consult three current reviews for additional details (Ernst et al., 1998; Schulz, 2001; Johne et al., 2002). Based on current clinical and experimental data, comedication with SJW extract should be avoided in patients who are taking cyclosporin- or tacrolimus-type immunosuppressant drugs with a narrow therapeutic range, coumarin-type anticoagulants, or virostatic drugs in the form of protease inhibitors or noncompetitive reverse transcriptase inhibitors. Also, SJW extract should not be combined with other antidepressants, especially SSRIs.

Second most frequent, interactions of St. John's wort had been communicated with oral contraceptives. Women experienced breakthrough bleeding, spotting or changed menstrual patterns with concurrent use of SJW extracts suggesting a decrease in the efficacy of oral contraceptive medication. So far, unwanted pregnancies have been related to SJW co-medication in 11 women (Schwarz et al., 2003; Henderson et al., 2002). However the results of clinical studies investigating the effect of treatment with hypericum extracts on combination oral contraceptives, are contradictory. The preliminary evaluation of ethinylestradiol concentrations in 10 women did not reveal significant alterations during concomitant treatment with hypericum (Käufeler et al., 2000). In two further open studies (Hall et al., 2003; Pfrunder et al., 2003) groups of 12 and 17 young women took a combination of either 20 µg ethinylestradiol and 150 µg desogestrel or 35 µg ethinylestradiol and 1mg norethinodron over three menstrual cycles. The first menstrual cycle was regarded as control, in the second and third cycles either 600-900 mg or 900 mg hypericum dry extract was taken daily. Measurement of endogenous hormone levels (oestradiol and progesterone; primary endpoints) showed that none of the 29 subjects ovulated in the 3-month study period. There was a significant decrease of about 40 % for the AUC of desogestrel (as the metabolite 3-ketodesogestrel); blood levels of ethinylestradiol and norethinodron were not changed. An increase in breakthrough bleeding (2 to 3 times more frequently than in the control cycle) was reported in both studies. The authors thus suggest that non-compliance as a consequence of increased bleeding may cause the suspected risk for undesired pregnancies. However this hypothesis is questionable since 20–60 % of women using such contraceptives complain of interim bleeding even when no enzyme-inducing co-medication is being used (Rosenberg et al., 1996). Possibly these effects – which were purely subjectively reported by the women – were due to a nocebo-effect (subjects were informed of the possibility at the start of the study, study design was not blind).

A quite different assessment as an indicator of possible interactions is required from spontaneous reported cases of breakthrough bleeding. Between 1991 and 1999 roughly 9 million people were treated with the SJW product Jarsin. Only eight cases of breakthrough bleeding were reported in this period of time. Because about three-quarters of the Jarsin® users were women, at least four million were women of child-bearing age. That equates to one report of breakthrough bleeding per half a million treated women in this age group (Schulz and Johne, 2004). This incidence is several powers of ten lower than the spontaneous rate to be expected during the ingestion of low dose oestrogen preparations (Rosenberg et al., 1996). Therefore, it must be suspected that some of the reports of breakthrough bleedings and unwanted pregnancies may have been triggered by adverse publicity to SJW during last years.

Other rare side effects are gastrointestinal complaints, allergic skin reactions, fatigue, and unrest (Ernst et al., 1998). Due to a lack of experience and clinical data on the effect of SJW on pregnant and nursing women, the contraindication of SJW in these conditions without appropriate professional supervision would be prudent.

2.2.9 Therapeutic Significance

Depression is the most common psychiatric disorder. Epidemiologic studies indicate a 13–20 % prevalence of depressive symptoms in the population as a whole, with a 2–5 % prevalence of severe depression. Thus, adjustment disorders with depressed mood, brief depressive reactions, and mild depressive episodes are about 5–10 times more prevalent in the general population than full-blown clinical depression. The lifetime prevalence of depressive disorders requiring treatment is about 10–20 %, because depressive disorders have a high rate of recurrence and mood disturbances may progress to depression. Untreated episodes of depression usually last from 6 to 9 months; antidepressant medication prescribed by a private physician is generally continued for 1–3 months. Depression can occur at any age but shows a statistical peak around age 50 (Riederer, 1993; Smith, 1992).

Epidemiologic data show that most patients with depression are not treated by specialists in neurology or psychiatry, and very few are hospitalized for treatment. Most depressed patients are treated by their family doctors on an outpatient basis. But two criteria are particularly important for selecting an antidepressant medicine in general practice: tolerance (lack of side effects) and treatment costs.

Adverse side effects occur in approximately 30–60 % of patients treated with tricyclic antidepressants and in approximately 13–30 % of patients taking the newer antidepressants. Generally these effects occur within a few days after the drug is started, preceding the onset of a therapeutic response. Working patients in particular may find these side effects so troublesome (sedation!) that they stop taking the medication on their own, depriving themselves of any further therapeutic benefit. On the other hand, several observational studies (Albrecht et al., 1994; Woelk et al., 1994; Schakau et al., 1996) in a total of approximately 8000 patients have shown that the incidence of adverse effects with SJW extracts is only about 1–3 %, which is at least 10 times lower than with synthetic antidepressants.

Given the high development costs of new synthetic antidepressants (see Sect. 1.5), the daily treatment costs average about 40 cents for SJW preparations and for the older drug amitriptyline, which has numerous side effects. These costs average from $1.50 to $2.00 per day for alpha-2 antagonists and SSRIs. The "augmentation strategies" recommended by the authors of the *Drug Prescription Report* (Lohse et al., 2002), with doctors prescribing the medical products that are the best accepted by patients and have the fewest side effects and lowest costs, are, from both an ethical and economic standpoint, the only correct solution for the future.

2.2.10 Drug Products

The *Rote Liste 2004* identifies 34 single-herb SJW products that are marketed in Germany. All of these products contain dry extract of SJW as their pharmacologically active ingredient. Since 1998 SJW products are approved by the German Federal Institute for Drugs and Medical Devices with the indication of "mild to moderate depressive episodes".

 References

Albrecht M, Hübner WD, Podzuweit H, Schmidt U (1994) Johanniskraut-Extrakt zur Behandlung der Depression. Der Kassenarzt 41: 45–54.
Anonymus (2002) Note for guidance on clinical investigation of medicinal products in the treatment of depression. The European Agency for the Evaluation of Medicinal Products: CPMP/ EWP/518/97 rev 1. EMEA 2002.
Araya OS, Ford EJH (1981) An investigation of the type of photosensitization caused by the ingestion of St. John's wort (Hypericum perforatum) by calves. J Comp Pathol 91: 135–141.
Bergmann R, Nüßner J, Demling J (1993) Behandlung leichter bis mittelschwerer Depressionen. TW Neurol Psychiatr 7: 235–240.
Bernd A, Simon S, Ramirez Bosca A, Kippenberger S, Diaz Alperi J, Miquel J, Villalba Garcia JF, Pamies Mira D, Kaufmann R (1999) Phototoxic effects of Hypericum extract in cultures of human keratinocytes compared with those of Psoralen. Photochemistry and Photobiology 69: 218–221.
Bhattacharya SK, Chakrabarti A, Chatterjee SS (1998) Activity profiles of two hyperforin-containing hypericum extracts in behavioral models. Pharmacopsychiat 31 (Suppl): 22–29.
Biber A, Fischer H, Römer A, Chatterjee SS (1998) Oral bioavailability of hyperforin from hypericum extract in rats and human volunteers. Pharmacopsychiat 31 (Suppl): 36–43.
Bladt S, Wagner H (1994) Inhibition of MAO by fractions and constituents of hypericum extract. J Geriatr Psychiatry Neurol 7 (Suppl 1): 57–59.
Blumenthal M, Hall T, Goldberg A et al. (eds.) (2002) The ABC Clinical Guide to Herbs. Austin, TX: American Botanical Council.
Bollini P, Pampallona S, Tibaldi G, Kupelnick, B, Munizza C (1999) Effectiveness of antidepressants: meta-analysis of dose-effect relationship in randomised clinical trials. Brit J Psychiatry 174: 297–303.
Bove GM (1998) Acute neuropathy after exposure to sun in a patient treated with St. John's wort. The Lancet 352: 1121–1122.
Brenner R, Azbel V, Madhusoodanan S, Pawlowska M (2000) Comparison of extract of hypericum (LI 160) and sertraline in the treatment of depression: a double-blind, randomized pilot study. Clin Therap 22: 411–419.
Brockmöller J, Reum T, Bauer S, Kerb R, Hübner WD, Roots I (1997) Hypericin and pseudohypericin: pharmacokinetics and effects on photosensitivity in humans. Pharmacopsychiatry 30 (Suppl): 94–101.
Butterweck V, Petereit F, Winterhoff H, Nahrstedt A (1998) Solubilized hypericin and pseudohypericin from Hypericum perforatum exert antidepressant activity in the forced swimming test. Planta Med 64: 291–294.
Butterweck V, Wall A, Liefländer-Wulf U, Winterhoff H, Nahrstedt A (1997) Effects of the total extract and fractions of *Hypericum perforatum* in animal assays for antidepressant activity. Pharmacopsychiatry 30 (Suppl): 117–124.
Cervo L, Rozio M, Ekalle-Soppo CB et al. (2002) Role of hyperforin in the antidepressant-like activity of *Hypericum perforatum* extracts. Psychopharmacology 164: 423–8.

Chatterjee SS, Nöldner M, Koch E, Erdelmeier C (1998) Antidepressant activity of Hypericum perforatum and hyperforin: the neglected possibility. Pharmacopsychiat 31 (Suppl): 7-15.

Czygan FC (1993) Kulturgeschichte und Mystik des Johanniskrautes. Z Phytother 14: 276-281.

Daniel K (1939) Inhaltsstoffe und Prüfmethoden homöopathisch verwendeter Arzneipflanzen. Hippokrates lo: 5-6.

De Vry J, Maurel S, Schreiber R, de Beun R, Jentzsch KR (1999) Comparison of hypericum extracts with imipramine and fluoxetine in animal models of depression and alcoholism. European Neuropsychopharmacology 9: 461-8.

Engelhardt A (1962) Justinus Kerner und das Johanniskraut. Apotheker-Dienst Roche 3: 51-55.

Erdelmeier CAJ (1998) Hyperforin, possibly the major non-nitrogenous secondary metabolite of hypericum perforatum L. Pharmacopsychiat 31 (Suppl): 2-6.

Ernst E (1999) Second thoughts about safety of St John's wort. Lancet 354: 2014-5.

Ernst E, Rand JI, Barnes J, Stevinson C (1998) Adverse effects profile of the herbal antidepressant St. John's wort (Hypericum perforatum L.). Eur J Clin Pharmacol 54: 589-594.

ESCOP (2003) Monographs on the medicinal uses of plant drugs. Hyperici herba - St John's Wort. Thieme Stuttgart New York, 2003.

Fox E, Murphy RF, McCully CL, Adamson PC (2001) Plasma pharmacokinetics and cerebrospinal fluid penetration of hypericin in nonhuman primates. Cancer Chemother Pharmacol 47: 41-44.

Franklin M, Chi J, McGavin C, Hockney R, Reed A, Campling G, Whale RWR, Cowen PJ (1999) Neuroendocrine evidence for dopaminergic actions of hypericum extract (LI 160) in healthy volunteers. J Biol Psychiat, in press.

Gaster B, Holroyd J (2000) St John's wort for depression. A systematic review. Arch Intern Med 160: 152-156.

Gensthaler BM (2001) Johanniskraut ist Placebo überlegen. Pharm Ztg 146 Nr. 24 (Vorläufige Mitteilung vom 24.06.01).

Giese AC (1980) Hypericism. Photochem Photobiol Rev 5: 229-255.

Gobbi M (1999) Hypericum perforatum L. extract does not inhibit 5-HAT transporter in rat brain cortex. Arch Pharmacol 360: 262-269.

Golsch S, Vocks E, Rakoski J, Brockow K, Ring J (1997) Reversible Erhöhung der Photosensitivität im UV-B-Bereich durch Johanniskrautextrakt-Präparate. Der Hautarzt 48: 249-252.

Gordon J (1998) SSRIs and St John's wort: possible toxicity? Am Fam Physician 62: 31.

Greenson JM, Sanford B, Monti DA (2001) St. John's Wort (Hypericum perforatum): a review of the current pharmacolocical, toxicological and clinical literature. Psychopharmacology 153: 402-14.

Gulick RM, McAuliffe V, Holden-Wiltse J et al.: Phase I studies of hypericin, the active compound in St. John's Wort, as an antiretroviral agent in HIV-infected adults. Ann Intern Med 130: 510-514, 1999.

Halama P (1991) Wirksamkeit des Johanniskrautextraktes LI 160 bei depressiver Verstimmung. Nervenheilkunde 10: 250-253.

Hall SD, Wang Z, Huang SM, Hammann MA et al. (2003) The interaction between St John's wort and oral contraceptive. Clin Pharmacol Ther 74: 525-535.

Hamilton M (1960) A rating scale for depression. J Neurol Neurosurg Psychiatry 23: 56-61.

Hänsel R, Keller K, Rimpler H, Schneider G (eds) (1993) Hagers Handbuch der Pharmazeutischen Praxis, 5th edition, Drogen E-O. Springer Verlag, Berlin Heidelberg New York, pp. 268-292.

Hänsgen KD, Vesper J (1996) Antidepressive Wirksamkeit eines hochdosierten Hypericum-Extraktes. Münch Med Wschr 138: 29-33.

Harrer G (1999) Comparison of equivalence between the St. John's wort extract LoHyp-57 and fluoxetine. Arzneim-Forsch/Drug Res 49: 289-296.

Harrer G, Hübner WD, Podzuweit H (1994) Effectiveness and tolerance of the hypericum extract LI 160 compared to maprotiline: a multicenter double-blind study. J Geriatr Psychiatry Neurol 7 (Suppl 1): 28-28.

Harrer G, Schmidt U, Kuhn U (1991) "Alternative" Depressionsbehandlung mit einem Hypericum-Extrakt (Alternative treatment of depression with an extract of Hypericum). TW Neurol Psychiatr 5: 710-716.

Harrer G, Schulz V (1994) Clinical investigation of the antidepressant effectiveness of hypericum. J Geriatr Psychiatry Neurol 7 (Suppl 1): 6–8.

Henderson L, Yue QY, Bergquist C, Gerden B, Arlett P (2002) St John's wort (Hypericum perforatum): drug interactions and clinical outcomes. Br J Clin Pharmacol 54:349–56.

Hoffmann J, Kühl ED (1979) Therapie von depressiven Zuständen mit Hypericin (Therapy of depressive states with St. John's Wort). Z Allg Med 55: 776–782.

Hübner WD, Lande S, Podzuweit H (1994) Hypericum treatment of mild depression with somatic symptoms. J Geriatr Psychiatry Neurol 7 (Suppl 1): 12–14.

Hypericum Depression Trial Study Group: Effect of Hypericum perforatum (St. John's Wort) in major depressive disorder. A randomized controlled trial. JAMA 287: 1807–14, 2002.

Jenike MA (ed) (1994) Hypericum: a novel antidepressant. J Geriatr Psychiatry Neurol 7: Sl–S68.

Johne A, Brockmöller J, Bauer S, Maurer A, Langheinrich M and Roots I (1999) Pharmacokinetic interaction of digoxin with an herbal extract from St John's wort (Hypericum perforatum). Clin Pharmacol Ther 66: 338–345.

Johne A, Mai I, Bauer S et al. (2002) Übersicht zu Interaktionsstudien mit Johanniskrautextrakten. In: Schulz V, Rietbrock N, Roots I, Loew D (eds) Phytopharmaka VII – Forschung und klinische Anwendung. Steinkopff, Darmstadt, pp. 149–161.

Kako MDN, Al-Sultan II (1993) Studies of sheep experimentally poisoned with Hypericum perforatum. Vet Hum Toxicol 35: 298–300.

Kalb R, Trautmann-Sponsel RD, Kieser M (2001) Efficacy and tolerability of hypericum extract WS 5572 versus placebo in mildly to moderately depressed patients. Pharmacopsychiatry 34: 96–103.

Kasper S (2001) Hypericum perforatum – a review of clinical studies. Pharmacopsychiatry 34 Suppl 1: pp. 51–S55.

Käufeler R, Meier B, Brattström A (2000) Johanniskrautextrakt Ze 117 – Klinische Wirksamkeit und Verträglichkeit. In: Reitbrock N, Donath F, Loew D, Roots I, Schulz V, eds. Phytopharmaka VI Forschung und Klinische Anwendung. Darmstadt: Steinkopff; 2000:84–9.

Kerb R, Brockmöller J, Staffeldt B, Ploch M, Roots I (1996) Single-dose and steady-state pharmacokinetics of hypericin and pseudohypericin. J Clin Pharmacol Therapeutics 40: 2087–2093.

Kirsch I, Sapirstein G (1998) Listening to Prozac but hearing placebo: a meta-analysis of antidepressant medication. Prevention & Treatment, 1, Article 0002a. Available on the World Wide Web: http://journals.apa.org/prevention/volume1/pre0010002a.html.

Kugler J, Weidenhammer W, Schmidt A, Groll S (1990) Therapie depressiver Zustände (Therapy of depressive disorders). Z Allg Med 66: 21–29.

Laakmann G, Schüle C, Baghai T, Kieser M (1998) St. John's wort in mild to moderate depression: the relevance of hyperforin for clinical efficacy. Pharmacopsychiatry 31 (Suppl 1): 54–59.

Lecrubier Y, Clerc G, Didi R, Kieser M (2002) Efficacy of St. John's Wort WS 5570 in major depression: a double-blind, placebo-controlled trial. Am J Psychiatry 159: 1361–366.

Lehrl S, Willemsen A, Papp R, Woelk H (1993) Ergebnisse von Messungen der kognitiven Leistungsfähigkeit bei Patienten unter der Therapie mit Johanniskraut-Extrakt. Nervenheilkunde 12: 281–284.

Lenoir S, Degenring FH, Saller R (1999) A double-blind randomized trial to investigate three different concentrations of a standardised fresh plant extract obtained from the shoot tips of Hypericum perforatum L. Phytomedicine 6: 141–146.

Leuschner J (1995) Gutachten zur experimentellen Toxikologie von Hypericum-Extrakt Ll 160. Lichtwer Pharma GmbH, Berlin.

Linde K, Ramirez G, Mulrow CD, Pauls M, Weidenhammer W, Melchart D (1996) St. John's wort for depression–an overview and meta-analysis of randomized clinical trials. Br Med J 313: 253–258.

Lohse MJ, Lorenzen A, Möller-Oerlinghausen B (2002) Psychopharmaka. In: Schwabe U, Paffrath D (eds) Arzneiverordnungsreport 2002. Springer, Berlin-Heidelberg-New York, pp. 641–678.

Malt UF, Robak OH, Madsbu HP, Bakke O, Loeb M (1999) The Norwegian naturalistic treatment study of depression in general practice (NORDEP)-I: Randomised double blind study. BMJ 318: 1180–4.

Martinez B, Kasper S, Ruhrmann S, Möller HJ (1994) Hypericum in the treatment of seasonal affective disorders. J Geriatr Psychiatry Neurol 7 (Suppl 1): 29–33.

Melzer M, Fuhrken D, Kolkmann R (1998) Hyperforin im Johanniskraut. Deutsche Apotheker Zeitung 138: 56–62.

Müller WE (2003) Current St. John's wort reseach from mode of action to clinical efficacy. Pharmacolocical Research 47: 101–9.

Müller WE, Chatterjee SS (eds) (1998) Hyperforin and the antidepressive activity of St. John's wort. Pharmacopsychiat 31 (Suppl): 1–60.

Müller WE, Kasper S (eds) (1997) Hypericum Extract (LI 160) as an herbal antidepressant. Pharmakopsychiat 30 (Suppl II): 71–134.

Müller WE, Schäfer C, Rolli M, Wonnemann R (1997) Effects of hypericum extract LI 160 on neurotransmitter uptake systems and beta-adrenergic receptor density. Pharmacopsychiat 30 (Suppl): 102–107.

Müller WE, Singer A, Wonnemann M (2001) Hyperforin – Antidepressant activity by a novel mechanism of action. Pharmacopsychiatry 34 Suppl 1: S98–S102

Müller WE, Singer A, Wonnemann M, Hafner U, Rolli M, Schäfer C (1998 a) Hyperforin represents the neurotransmitter reuptake inhibiting constituent of hypericum extract. Pharmacopsychiat 31 (Suppl): 16–21.

Müller WE, Singer A, Wonnemann M, Rolli M, Schäfer C, Hafner U (1998 b) Wirkungen von standardisiertem Johanniskraut-Extrakt (LI 160) in biochemischen Modellen antidepressiver Wirksamkeit. Psychopharmakotherapie 5 (Suppl 8): 40–45.

Mulrow CD, Williams JW, Chiquette E et al. (2000) Efficacy of newer medications for treating depression in primary care patients. Am J Med 108: 54–64.

Mulrow CD, Williams JW, Trivendi M (1999) Treatment of depression: newer pharmacotherapies. AHCPR publication no. 99–E014.

Nahrstedt A, Butterweck V (1997) Biologically active and other chemical constituents of the herb of Hypericum perforatum L. Pharmacopsychiat 30 (Suppl): 129–134.

Nathan PJ (1999) The experimental and clinical pharmacology of St John's wort (Hypericum perforatum L.). Molecular Psychiatry 4: 333–338.

Niesel S (1992) Untersuchungen zum Freisetzungsverhalten und zur Stabilität ausgewählter wertbestimmender Pflanzeninhaltsstoffe unter besonderer Berücksichtigung moderner phytochemischer Analysenverfahren. Inaugural-Dissertation. Freie Universität Berlin.

Nöldner M, Schötz K (2002) Rutin is essential for the antidepressant activity of Hypericum perforatum extracts in the forced swimming test. Planta Med 68: 577–580.

Orth HCJ, Hauer H, Erdelmeier CAJ, Schmidt PC (1999) Orthoforin: The main degradation product of hyperforin from Hypericum perforatum L. Pharmazie 54: 76–77.

Pfrunder A, Schiesser M, Gerber S, Haschke M, Bitzer J, Drewe J (2003) Interaction of St John's wort with low-dose oral contraceptive therapy: a randomized controlled trial. Br J Cin Pharmacol 56: 683–90.

Philipp M, Kohnen R, Hiller KO (1999) Hypericum extract versus imipramine or placebo in patients with moderate depression: randomised multicentre study of treatment for eight weeks. BMJ 319: 1534–9.

Porsolt RD, Lenégre A, McArthur RA (1991) Pharmacological models of depression. In: Animal Models in Psychopharmacology – Advances in Pharmacological Sciences. Birkhäuser, Basel (Switzerland) 1991, pp. 137–159.

Quandt J, Schmidt U, Schenk N (1993) Ambulante Behandlung leichter und mittelschwerer depressiver Verstimmungen. Der Allgemeinarzt 2: 97–102.

Raffa RB (1998) Screen of receptor and uptake-site activity of hypericin component of St. John's wort reveals σ receptor binding. Life Sciences 62: 265–270.

Riederer P, Laux G, Pöldinger W (1993) Neuro-Psychopharmaka. Ein Therapie-Handbuch, Vol. 3: Antidepressiva und Phasenprophylaktika. Springer-Verlag Vienna New York, pp. 1–10.

Rosenberg MJ Waugh MS, Higgins SE (1996) The effect of desogestrel, gestadone, and other factors on spotting and bleeding. Contraception 53: 85–90.

Schakau D, Hiller KO, Schultz-Zehden W, Teschner F (1996) Nutzen/Risiko-Profil von Johanniskrautextrakt. STEI 300 bei 2404 Patienten mit psychischen Störungen unterschiedlicher Schweregrade. Psychopharmakotherapie 3: 116–122.

Schempp CM, Winghofer B, Langheinrich M, Schöpf E, Simon JC (1999) Hypericin levels in human serum and interstitial skin blister fluid after oral single-dose and steady-state administration of Hypericum perforatum extract. Skin Pharmacol Appl Skin Physiol 12: 299–304.

Schey KL, Patat S, Chignell CF, Datillo M, Wang RH, Roberts JE: Photooxidation of lens á-crystallin by hypericin (active ingredient in St. John's wort). Photochemistry and Photobiology 2000; 72: 200–203.

Schlich D, Braukmann F, Schenk N (1987) Behandlung depressiver Zustandsbilder mit Hypericum (Treatment of depressive disorders with Hypericum). Psycho 13: 440–447.

Schmidt U, Harrer G, Kuhn U, Berger-Deinert W, Luther D (1993) Wechselwirkungen von Hypericum-Extrakt mit Alkohol. Nervenheilkunde 12: 314–319.

Schmidt U, Schenk N, Schwarz I, Vorberg G (1989) Zur Therapie depressiver Verstimmungen (On the therapy of depressive disorders). Psycho 15: 665–671.

Schrader E, Meier B, Brattström A (1998) Hypericum treatment of mild to moderate depression in a placebo-controlled study. A prospective, double-blind, randomized, placebo-controlled, multicentre study. Human Psychopharmacology 13: 163–169.

Schrader E, on behalf of the Study Group (2000) Equivalence of St John's wort extract (ZE 117) and fluoxetine: a randomized, controlled study in mild to moderate depression. Int Clin Psychopharmacol 15: 61–68.

Schulz V (1999) Stellenwert von Hypericum-Extrakten in der Therapie leichter bis mittelschwerer Depressionen. In: Loew D, Blume H, Dingermann T (eds) Phytopharmaka V – Forschung und klinische Anwendung. Steinkopff-Verlag, Darmstadt, pp. 151–156.

Schulz V (2000) The psychodynamic and pharmacodynamic effects of drugs: a differenciated evaluation of the efficacy of phytotherapy. Phytomed 7: 73–81.

Schulz V (2001) Incidence and clinical relevance of the interactions and side effects of Hypericum preparations. Phytomed 8:152–160.

Schulz V (2002) Clinical trials with hypericum extracts in patients with depression – Results, comparisons, conclusions for therapy with antidepressant drugs. Phytomed 9: 468–74.

Schulz V, Johne A (2004) Side effects and drug interactions. In: Müller WE (ed) Milestones in Drug Therapy: St. John's Wort and its active principles in depression and anxiety. Birkhäuser. Basel (Switzerland) 2004.

Schwarz UL, Büschel B, Kirch W (2003) Unwanted pregnancy on self-medication with St John's wort despite hormonal contraception. Br J Clin Pharmacol 55: 112–113.

Sgarbossa A, Angelini N, Gioffre D, Youssef T, Lenci F, Roberts JE: The uptake, location and fluorescence of hypericin in bovine intact lens. Current Eye Research 2000; 21: 597–601.

Shelton CR, Keller MB, Gelenberg A et al. (2001) Effectiveness of St. John´s wort in major depression: a randomized controlled trial. JAMA 285: 1978–85.

Smith AL, Weissmann MM (1992) Epidemiology. In: Paykel ES (ed) Handbook of Affective Disorders. Churchill Livinstone, 2nd edition, pp. 111–129.

Sommer H, Harrer G (1994) Placebo-controlled double-blind study examining the effectiveness of a hypericum preparation in 105 mildly depressed patients. J Geriatr Psychiatry Neurol 7 (Suppl 1): 9–11.

Stevinson C, Ernst E (1999) Safety of hypericum in patients with depression. A comparison with conventional antidepressants. CNS Drugs 11: 125–132.

Suzuki O, Katsumata Y, Oya M, Bladt S, Wagner H (1984) Inhibition of monoamine oxidase by hypericin. Planta Med 50: 272–274.

Thiebot M, Martin P, Puech AJ (1992) Animal behavioral studies in the evaluation of antidepressant drugs. Brit J Psych 160 (Suppl. 15): 44–50.

Van Gurp G, Meterissam GB, Haiek LN, McCruscer J, Bellavance F (2002) St John's wort or sertraline? Randomized controlled trial in primary care. Canadian Family Physician 48: 905–912.

Volz HP (1997) Controlled clinical trials of hypericum extracts in depressed patients – an overview. Pharmacopsychiat 30 (Suppl): 72–76.6.

Volz HP, Hänsel R (1995) Hypericum (Johanniskraut) als pflanzliches Antidepressivum. Psychopharmakotherapie 2: 1–9.

Volz HP, Laux P (2000) Potential treatment for subthreshold and mild depression: A comparison of St. John's wort extracts and fluoxetine. Comprehensive Psychiatry 41: 133–137.

Vorbach EU, Arnoldt KH, Christl D (1997). Effectiveness and tolerance of St. John's wort extract LI

160 versus imipramine in patients with severe depressive episodes according to ICD-10. Pharmacopsychiat 30 (Suppl): 81–85.

Vorbach EU, Hübner WD, Arnoldt KH (1994) Effectiveness and tolerance of the hypericum extract LI 160 in comparison with imipramine: randomized double-blind study with 135 outpatients. J Geriat Psychiatry Neurol 7 (Suppl 1): 19–23.

Werth W (1989) Psychotonin M versus Imipramin in der Chirurgie (Psychotonin M vs. imipramine in surgery). Der Kassenarzt 15: 64–68.

Wheatley D (1997) Amitriptyline-controlled trial of hypericum extract LI 160. Pharmacopsychiat 30 (Suppl): 77–80.

Wheatley D (1999) Hypericum in seasonal affective disorder (SAD). Current Medical Research and Opinion 15: 33–37.

Winterhoff H, Hambrügge M, Vahlensieck W (1993) Testung von Hypericum perforatum L. im Tierexperiment. Nervenheilkunde 12: 341–345.

Woelk H (2000) St John's wort extract versus tricyclic antidepressant: a randomised, controlled study in mild to moderate depression. BMJ321: 536–539.

Woelk H, Burkard G, Grünwald J (1994) Benefits and risks of the hypericum extract LI 160: drug monitoring study in 3250 patients. J Geriatr Psychiatry Neurol 7 (Suppl 1): 34–38.

Yue YY, Gerden B (2000) Letter to the editor. Lancet 355: 576–7.

2.3 Kava as an Anxiolytic

2.3.1 Introduction

When Europeans discovered the island world of Oceania in the 18th century, they learned about the custom of kava drinking. Natives of Polynesia, Melanesia, and Micronesia harvested the large rhizome of the kava shrub (*Piper methysticum*), masticated it, and mixed it with water and coconut milk to make a beverage that produced a calming, relaxing effect without altering consciousness. Published reports on kava quickly led to studies aimed at isolation the psychotropic active principle and elucidating its chemical structure. It was not until 1966 that the German pharmacologist H. J. Meyer proved that the characteristic effects of the kava beverage were due to kavapyrones (kavalactones). These compounds are poorly water-soluble and, to become bioavailable, must be converted to a finely divided form. The first kava product to appear on the conventional drug market contained synthetic kawain. Most subsequent kava products have contained extracts from the kava rhizome; only the extract-based products are considered true phytomedicines. The pharmacy, pharmacology, and clinical characteristics of kava preparations are reviewed in Hänsel et al. (1999).

2.3.2 Botanical Description

The kava shrub (*Piper methysticum*) grows to a height of 2–3 m. It has large, hard-shaped leaves and bears numerous small flowers arranged in clusters shaped like ears of corn. The crude drug is obtained from the large, branched, juicy rhizome which can weigh up to 10 kg (Fig. 2.15). The actual origin of the kava plant is unknown but may have been Vanuatu (formerly New Hebrides). As Polynesians settled the surrounding

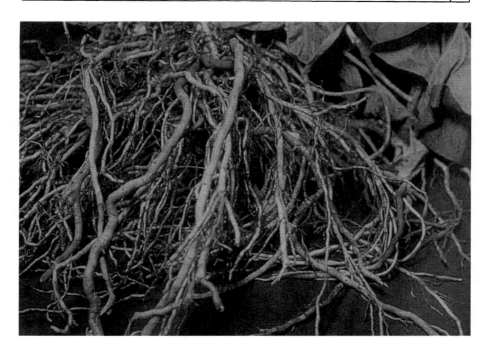

Fig. 2.15. ▲ Kava (*Piper methysticum*): roots of a young plant.

Pacific islands, the shrub became naturalized to areas as far east as Hawaii. Today kava is cultivated commercially, and no longer grows in the wild.

2.3.3 Crude Drug and Extract

The crude drug consists of the dried rhizome. It has a faintly aromatic odor and a slightly bitter, soapy, acrid taste. Chewing a piece of kava rhizome causes prolonged numbness of the tongue and stimulates salivation.

The kava beverage is made by chewing or grinding the dried rhizome, macerating it in cold water, and straining off the liquid. Medicinal extracts are prepared by extracting the dried herb with an ethanol-water mixture (for extracts containing about 30 % kavapyrones) or with an acetone-water mixture (for extracts containing about 70 % kavapyrones). The herb-to-extract ratio is about 12–20:1 in both preparations. Kavapyrones are very poorly soluble in water, so for medicinal use they must be placed in colloidal solution or at least converted to a finely divided form to promote absorption from the gastrointestinal tract.

2.3.4 Key Constituents, Analysis, Pharmacokinetics

The kava rhizome is among the few phytomedicines whose key active constituents (see Sect. 1.2) are known. They are the kavapyrones (kavalactones), including kawain (1–2 % in the crude drug), dihydrokawain (0.6–1 %), methysticin (1.2–2 %), and dihydromethysticin (0.5–0.8 %). The dried herb should contain at least 3.5 % kavapyrones, calculated as kawain. Quantitative analysis of the kawains is accomplished by photometric assay of the total fraction or of its individual components following separation by HPLC or by electrokinetic chromatography (Lechtenberg et al., 1999). Despite their low water solubility, kawain and dihydrokawain were shown to be readily absorbed from the gastrointestinal tract. In experiments with mice, plasma levels of approximately 2 µg/mL kawain were measured 30 min after the oral administration of 100 mg/kg b. w. of a kava extract containing 70 % kavapyrones. Kawain levels in the brain tissue were approximately the same and paralleled the time course of the plasma levels. The kavapyrones have a plasma half-life ranging from 90 min to several hours. Bioavailability depends strongly on the galenic formulation and can vary 10-fold among different preparations (Hänsel et al., 1999).

2.3.5 Pharmacology and Toxicology

The four pyrones of the kawain-methysticin type act centrally as muscle relaxants and anticonvulsants; their actions are comparable to those of mephenesin. They exert a strong protective effect against experimental strychnine poisoning and are superior in this regard to all previously known, non-narcotic strychnine antagonists. The kawains and methysticins reduce the excitability of the limbic system as measured by electrical stimulation of corresponding brain areas in rabbits; this is analogous to the effect produced by benzodiazepine. Methysticin and dihydromethysticin show marked neuroprotective properties in mice and rats, significantly reducing the volume of an ischemic infarction induced by ligation of the middle cerebral artery. The two methysticins have the same potency as memantine in this infarction model. Peripherally, the kawains act as local anesthetics comparable in potency to the topical anesthetics cocaine and benzocaine (Jamieson et al., 1989; Backhaus and Krieglstein, 1992). In vitro studies in a platelet model have shown that kava extract as well as kavapyrones isolated from the extract inhibit monoamine oxidase B (MAO-B). This action is considered an important mechanism for their psychotropic activity (Uebelhack et al., 1998). Another group of authors has shown that kavapyrones interact with GABA-A receptors but do not alter the levels of the neurotransmitters dopamine and serotonin in the CNS when fed to rats (Boonen and Häberlein, 1998; Boonen et al., 1998). In the light of recent extensive data on the pharmacology of kava extracts and their constituents, however, their mechanism of action most likely involves an allosteric effect on the GABA-A-receptor complex, inhibition of the voltage-gated Na-channel, and an attack on the H_3 receptor (Kretzschmar, 1995; Hänsel et al., 1999).

A kava extract containing 70 % kavapyrones was tested for toxic effects in rats and dogs over a 26-week period. The maximum dose was 320 mg/kg (rats) or 60 mg/kg (dogs). The highest doses were associated with mild histopathologic changes in liver and kidney tissues. The dogs tolerated 24 mg/kg/day and the rats 20 mg/kg/day with no adverse reactions. Testing of the same extract in corresponding in vitro models showed no evidence of mutagenic potential. Only dihydromethysticin has been tested for genotoxicity, and no teratogenic effects were observed (Kretschmar, 1995; Hänsel et al., 1999).

There have been reports from Australia and the South Sea region of toxic reactions in humans following the consumption of kava beverages. The following symptoms were observed after the ingestion of 300–400 g of dried rhizome powder per week: ataxia, skin rash, hair loss, yellowish discoloration of the skin and sclerae, yellowing of the fingernails and toenails, redness of the eyes, visual accommodation difficulties, hearing impairment, swallowing difficulties, respiratory problems, loss of appetite, and loss of body weight. It should be noted that these dose levels were at least 100 times higher than the clinically tested doses (Table 2.6) and the recommended therapeutic doses (Hänsel et al., 1999).

2.3.6 Clinical Efficacy

The therapeutic efficacy of an anxiolytic drug can be documented only by clinical trials in patients; studies in healthy subjects are of no value. Human pharmacologic studies are nevertheless useful in that they can provide evidence of possible mechanisms of action, associated effects, and side effects. A kava extract containing 70 % kavapyrones (designated in the literature as WS 1490, brand name Laitan®) was investigated in four human pharmacologic studies (Johnson et al., 1991; Emser and Bartylla, 1991; Herberg, 1991; Münte et al., 1993). The first two studies were open, and the last two were double-blinded and placebo-controlled. The key parameters were drug-induced EEG changes and psychometric tests of intellectual and motor functioning. According to the authors, the observed EEG changes and (partial) psychometric test results showed no evidence of a decline in vigilance or responsiveness in subjects who took the extract for up to 14 days at doses equivalent to 105 mg, 210 mg, or 420 mg of kavapyrones daily. The author of one study (Herberg, 1991) concluded that use of the kava extract did not impair the ability to drive a motor vehicle. In another human pharmacologic study using a crossover design, a kava extract standardized to 30 % kavapyrones (brand name Antares 120, equivalent to 120 mg/day kavalactones) was compared to a placebo over a treatment period of 7 days. The results, based on quantitative EEG studies and psychometric testing, were similar to those of the studies described above (Gessner and Cnota, 1994).

To date, a total of 12 controlled double-blind studies have been published on the therapeutic efficacy of kava kava in patients (Pittler and Ernst, 1999). Three of the studies were done with an extract standardized to 15 % kavapyrones (Bhate et al., 1989; Warnecke et al., 1990) and nine with an extract standardized to 70 % kavapyrones (WS 1490). Details on the studies are shown in Table 2.6. The results of the study by Bhate et al. are of dubious clinical relevance due to the brief duration of treatment (2 doses of 60 mg kavapyrones) and the nature of the results (nonstandard scoring scale, relatively small numerical differences between the treatment groups).

Table 2.6.
Clinical double-blind studies of kava extract preparations in patients with anxiety disorders due to various causes.

First author, year	Cases (n)	Dose (mg/dl)	Duration (days)	Indications, outcome measures, and results
Bhate, 1989	59	60	2	Surgical patients. Improvement in perioperative mood, questionable clinical relevance
Warnecke, 1990	40	30–60	56–84	Climacteric symptoms. Kuppermann index and ASI scale significant vs. placebo
Warnecke, 1991	40	210	56	Climacteric symptoms. HAMA, DSI and Kuppermann index significant vs. placebo
Kinzler, 1991	58	210	28	Anxiety syndrome. HAMA, EWL, CGI, FSUCL index significant vs. placebo
Woelk, 1993	172	210	42	Anxiety syndrome. HAMA, CGI, KEPS, and EAAS not significant vs. oxazepam and bromazepam
Volz, 1996	101	210	168	Anxiety syndrome. HAMA, CGI, and Bf-S after 7 weeks significantly better than placebo
Lehmann, 1996	58	210	28	HAMA, CGI, FSUCL significantly better than placebo
Malsch, 2000	40	105–210	35	HAMA, BF-S significantly better than placebo
Boerner, 2003	120	120	56	HAMA responders: kava 77 %, opipramol 76 %, buspirone 74 %
Lehrl, 2003	61	140	28	HAMA, CGI significantly better than placebo
Geier, 2003	50	105	28	HAMA, CGI significantly better than placebo
Gastpar, 2003	141	105	28	ASI im Trend, BS-F, CGI significantly better than placebo

NOTE: The dose figures (column 3) are based on kavapyrones. Except for Bhate (1989), Warnecke (1990), and Boerner (2000), the authors used a uniform extract with a 70 % content of kavapyrones. **Abbreviations: ASI** = Anxiety Status Inventory, **HAMA** = Hamilton Anxiety Scale, **DSI** = Depression Status Inventory, **CGI** = Clinical Global Impressions, **Bf-S** = von Zerssen mood scale, **EWL** = adjective list, **FSUCL** = Fischer Somatic Symptoms or Undesired Effects Checklist, **KEPS** = brief test for evaluating personality structure, **EAAS** = Erlanger scale for anxiety, aggression, and tension.

Warnecke et al. (1990, 1991) conducted two placebo-controlled clinical trials, each involving 40 women with menopausal symptoms. Each of the studies used different preparations and dosages (see Table 2.7). The duration of treatment was at least 56 days in both studies. In the second study, the total score on the Hamilton Anxiety Rating Scale (HAMA) was used as the confirmatory parameter, and three other scales were used as adjuncts. The total HAMA score showed significant improvement after just 1 week on the kava extract and reached a plateau after 4 weeks' therapy. Overall, the therapeutic response was highly significant in relation to the placebo (p < 0.001).

In the study of Kinzler et al. (1991), 58 patients from 18 to 60 years of age with symptoms of anxiety, tension, or agitation of nonpsychotic origin were tested against a placebo in a 4-week double-blind comparative study. Again, the confirmatory parameter was the total score on the Hamilton Anxiety Rating Scale. A comparison of the groups after 1 week's therapy already showed a significant disparity in total scores. This difference continued to increase over the next 3 weeks. The results of the adjunctive rating scales

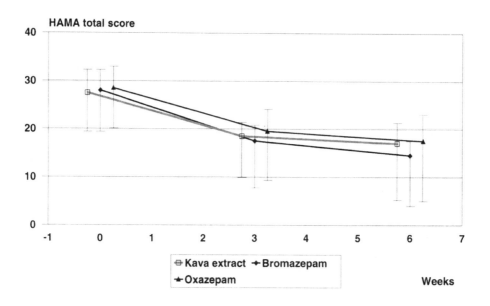

Fig. 2.16. ▲ Progression of scores of the Hamilton Anxiety Scale (HAMA) during 6 weeks' treatment with a kava extract equivalent to 210 mg/day kavapyrones compared with 15 mg/day oxazepam and 9 mg/day bromazepam. There were no statistically significant differences in the degree of improvement achieved in the three treatment groups (Woelk et al., 1993).

correlated with the HAMA scores. Surprisingly, no unpleasant or adverse side effects were observed in patients taking the medication.

In a study by Woelk et al. (1993), the effect of a daily dose equivalent to 210 mg of kavapyrones was compared with that of 15 mg/day oxazepam or 9 mg/day bromazepam in a double-blind study lasting 6 weeks. The main study criterion was a decline in total score on the HAMA rating scale. When a total of 164 treatment protocols had been completed, the improvement in symptoms was approximately the same in all three treatment groups (Fig. 16). Because the statistical analysis focused on the degree of difference rather than the demonstration of equivalence, however, we cannot conclude that the drugs are equally effective in the strict sense.

One criticism that has been leveled at all clinical studies with kava extracts is that the inclusion criteria were not sufficiently rigorous and allowed the inclusion of a heterogeneous population (depression with anxious features, panic disorders, phobias, somatoform disorders, and generalized anxiety disorders) (Volz and Hänsel, 1994; Volz, 1997).

Six randomized, placebo-controlled double-blind studies were conducted in accordance with current testing and Good Clinical Practice (GCP) guidelines. The efficacy and tolerance of the kava extract WS 1490 were tested over a 6-month period in 101 outpatients with nonpsychotic anxiety disorders according to DSM-III-R criteria (300.22–24, 329). The daily dose was 300 mg of extract, equivalent to 210 mg kavapyrones. The main criterion was the change in total HAMA scores from the start of therapy to its termination (week 24). A comparison of the change in total HAMA scores showed significant differences relative to the placebo group starting in week 8 (Fig. 2.17). The parameters of secondary interest (Clinical Global Impressions and Mood Scale) showed similar changes. Six of the kava patients reported unpleasant side effects, two involving gastric complaints that may have been related to the test medication. Nine of the placebo patients reported objectionable side effects (Volz and Kieser, 1996).

In another study, 129 outpatients diagnosed with generalized anxiety disorder (ICD-10 F 40.1) were treated alternately with 400 mg of kava LI 150, 10 mg of buspirone, or 100 mg of opipramol for 8 weeks. The main outcome measure was the rate of responders and full remissions corresponding to a 50 % reduction in symptoms or a score less than 9 in the HAMA scale. No significant differences were found in the responses of the three treatment groups. Over 75 % of the patients with moderate to severe anxiety disorder were classified as responders (Boerner et al., 2003). Further studies using the extract WS 1490 have been published (Gastpar and Klimm, 2003) or completed (Loew, 2002; Schmidt et al., 2002). In a meta-analysis of seven double-blind studies, Pittler and Ernst (2000) concluded that kava extracts were significantly superior to placebo as a symptomatic treatment for anxiety.

Besides the 6 double-blind therapeutic studies with kava extracts, a total of 9 double-blind studies have been conducted with the isolated compound dl-kawain. Two of the studies compared kawain with reference drugs and 7 compared it with a placebo. The therapeutic results achieved with doses of 200–600 mg/day in these studies were similar to the results of studies using extracts, but they were also similar with regard to deficiencies noted in the study methodologies (Volz and Hänsel, 1994; Volz, 1997). Nevertheless, the placebo-controlled studies in particular allow the application of the results obtained with extracts to pure compounds and vice-versa to a certain degree,

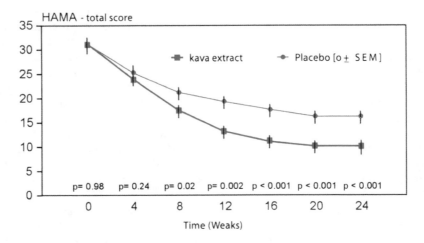

Fig. 2.17. ▲ Progression of Hamilton anxiety scores (HAMA) during 24 weeks' treatment with a kava extract equivalent to a dose of 210 mg/d kavapyrones. The graph shows the mean values SEM for 52 kava patients and 49 placebo patients with nonpsychotic anxiety disorders (Volz and Kieser, 1997).

although treatment with isolated compounds is, by definition, outside the bounds of phytotherapy (Sect. 1.2).

2.3.7   Side Effects and Risks

In an observation of 4049 patients who took 105 mg/day of an extract standardized to 70 % kavapyrones for 7 weeks, objectionable side effects were documented in 61 patients, representing an incidence of 1.5 %. The side effects were mild in nature and reversible. Most consisted of gastrointestinal complaints or allergic skin reactions. A 4-week study in 3029 patients who took 800 mg/day of an extract standardized to 30 % kavapyrones (= 240 mg kavapyrones) showed a 2.3 % incidence of unpleasant side effects. All these effects were mild, consisting of 9 cases of allergic reactions, 31 cases of gastrointestinal discomfort, and 22 cases of headache or dizziness (Hänsel et al., 1994; Hoffmann and Winter, 1993). A 47-year-old woman got a dermatomyositis-like illniss 2 weeks after ingestion of Kava Kava (no further details on the preparation; Gurn-Razuman et al., 1999).

The prolonged use of kava can cause a transient, reversible yellowish discoloration of the skin and its appendages; the product should be discontinued if this occurs. Allergic skin reactions can occur in rare cases. There have also been reports of impaired visual accommodation, pupillary dilation, and disturbances of oculomotor equilibrium. Twenty-nine of 200 chronic kava drinkers from Polynesia had pellagra-like skin changes that did not respond to 4 weeks' treatment with 100 mg niacinamide (Ruze, 1990). Chronic abuse of kava preparations has been associated with even more serious toxic effects (Siegel, 1976).

Liver damage has been recognized as a potential side effect of kava use since 1998 (Stahl et al., 1998) . A large number of authors and research groups have critically analyzed the data for kava products as well as alternative anxiolytic drugs (Pittler and Ernst, 2000; Blumenthal, 2002; Davidson et al., 2002; Ernst, 2002; Loew, 2002; Schmidt et al., 2002; Teschke et al., 2002 and 2003; Waller, 2002; Schulze et al., 2003). An analysis of known isolated cases made it clear that there were only a few cases that bore a likely causal relationship to kava use, and there was only one case that was confirmed through reexposure to kava. In all other cases, the contributions from other hepatotoxic agents such as alcohol or hepatitis infections remained unclear. A marked discrepancy is apparent between the frequency of hepatotoxic reports in Germany and Switzerland compared with those in other countries. At present there is still too little data available for distinguishing between drug idiosyncrasy and dose-dependent toxicity. Liver damage from exposure to benzodiazepines such as diazepam, oxazepam, or bromazepam is known to occur, but its incidence cannot yet be calculated with any accuracy. A semi-quantitative analysis indicates that the incidence of liver damage from benzodiazepine anxiolytics is comparable to that associated with kava-containing products. Nevertheless, the Federal Institute for Drugs and Medical Devices (BfArM) withdrew its approval for kava preparations in June of 2002 and issued a recall for all products. It justified this action by citing an adverse risk/benefit ratio and noting the availability of safer, more effective alternatives that are free of liver toxicity. This decision was not supported by most authorities and drew sharp criticism from some authors (Davidson et al., 2002; Ernst, 2002; Loew, 2002; Schmidt et al., 2002; Teschke, 2002; Teschke et al., 2003; Schulze et al., 2003).

In the United States, the issue of potential hepatotoxicity of kava preparations was first raised in a press release from the American Botanical Council (ABC) in December 2001. ABC suggested that consumers seek medical advice before taking kava if they have a history of liver disease, if they are taking hepatotoxic drugs, or if they are consuming alcohol. In addition, ABC suggested that since the adverse reports known at that time were associated with chronic use, that patients not take kava on a daily basis for more than four weeks and that consumers should discontinue use if symptoms of jaundice occur (ABC, 2001). In March 2002 the U.S. Food and Drug Administration issued a public warning that closely paralleled the recommendations of ABC (FDA, 2002). Shortly thereafter, various herbal industry associations approved warnings on labels of kava products to reflect most of the ABC and FDA recommendations. At the time of the publication of this book, kava dietary supplements were still available for retail sale in the U.S.

2.3.8 Indications and Dosages

The results of clinical studies indicate that mild anxiety states due to various causes are the primary indication for the use of kava preparations. Commission E defined the indications as "conditions of nervous anxiety, stress, and restlessness" (Blumenthal et al., 1998) in its 1990 monograph on kava rhizome. The doses of kava extracts used in clinical studies (Table 2.7) were in the range of 60–210 mg of kava pyrones daily. Generally the duration of use should not exceed three months. Due to the instances of liver toxicity, it has been suggested that the duration of treatment should generally be limited to one month and that all kava products should be made available by prescription only, thereby allowing the physician to monitor the patient's liver enzyme levels to help reduce potential chances of a toxic reaction (Teschke 2002; Teschke et al. 2003). This recommendation is moot in Germany, of course, where these products are no longer officially approved.

2.3.9 Therapeutic Significance

Kava preparations are an herbal alternative to synthetic anxiolytics and tranquilizers, particularly the benzodiazepines. Based on the study of Woelk et al. (1993), suitable kava preparations appear to have an efficacy comparable to that of benzodiazepines in the treatment of anxiety symptoms. In contrast to benzodiazepines, previous experience with the therapeutic use of kava preparations has shown no evidence that there is any potential for physical or psychological dependency (Hänsel et al., 1994 and 1999). This represents a significant advantage of kava preparations over the benzodiazepines.

2.3.10 Drug Products

The 2003 edition of the *Rote Liste* no longer includes kava preparations as a result of the German BfArM's removal of all kava-based phytomedicines from the German market in 2002 due to concerns about potential hepatotoxicity.

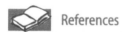 References

ABC. American Botanical Council announces new safety information on kava. Austin, TX: American Botanical Council, Dec. 20. 2001.

Backhaus C, Krieglstein J (1992) Extract of kava and its methysticin constituents protect brain tissue against ischaemic damage in rodents. J Pharmacol 215: 265–269.

Bhate H, Gerster G, Gracza E (1989) Orale Prämedikation mit Zubereitungen aus Piper methysticum bei operativen Eingriffen in Epiduralanästhesie. Erfahrungsheilkunde 6: 339–345.

Blumenthal M (2002) Kava safety questioned due to cases of possible link to liver toxicity: Expert analyses of case reports shows there is insufficient evidence to make causal connection. HerbalGram 55:26–32.

Blumenthal M, Busse WR, Goldberg A, Gruenwald J, Hall T, Riggins CW, Rister RS (eds.). Klein S, Rister RS (trans). (1998) The Complete German Commission E Monographs – Therapeutic Guide to Herbal Medicines. American Botanical Council, Austin, Texas. *www.herbalgram.org*.

Boerner RJ, Sommer H, Berger W, Kuhn U, Schmidt U, Mannel M (2003) Kava-kava extract LI 150 is as effective as opipramol and buspirone in generalized anxiety disorder – An 8-week randomised, double-blind multicenter clinical trial in 129 outpatients. Phytomedicine 10 Suppl IV: 38–49.

Boonen G, Ferger B, Kuschinsky K, Häberlein H (1998) In vivo effects of the kavapyrones (+)-dihydromethysticin and ()-kavain on dopamine, 3,4-dihydrophenylacetic acid, serotonin and 5-hydroxyindoleacetic acid levels in striatal and cortical brain regions. Planta Med 64: 507–510.

Boonen G, Häberlein H (1998) Influence of genuine kavapyrone enantiomers on the GABA_A binding site. Planta Med 64: 504–506.

Denham A, McIntyre M, Whitehouse J (2002) Kava – the unfolding story: report of a work in progress. J Altern Compl Med 8: 237–63

Emser W, Bartylla K (1991) Verbesserung der Schlafqualität. TW Neurol Psychiatr 5: 636–642.

Ernst E (2002) Marktrücknahme des pflanzlichen Anxiolyticums Kava: Nutzen unter-, Risiken überschätzt? MMW – Fortschr Med 40: 898.

FDA. Kava-containing dietary supplements may be associated with severe liver injury. (Consumer Advisory). U.S. Food and Drug Administration, Mar. 25, 2002.

Gastpar M, Klimm HD for the Kava Study Group (2003) Treatment of anxiety, tension and restlessness states with Kava special extract WS 1490 in general practice: A randomized placebo-controlled double-blind multicenter study. Phytomedicine 10: 631–9.

Geier FP, Konstantiniwicz T (2004) Kava treatment in patients with anxiety. Phytother Res 18: 297–300.

Geßner B, Cnota P (1994) Untersuchung der Vigilanz nach Applikation von Kava-Kava-Extrakt, Diazepam oder Placebo. Z Phytother 15: 30–37.

Guro-Razuman S, Anand P, Hu Q, Mir R (1999) Dermatomyositis-like illness following Kava-kava ingestion. J Clin Reumatol 5: 342–345.

Hänsel R (1996) Kava-Kava (Piper methysticum G. Forster) in der modernen Arzneimittelforschung. Protrait einer Arzneipflanze. Zeitschrift für Phytotherapie 17: 180–195.

Hänsel R, Keller K, Rimpler H, Schneider G (Hrsg) (1994) Hagers Handbuch der Pharmazeutischen Praxis, 6th edition, Drogen E – O. Springer Verlag, Berlin Heidelberg New York: 201–221.

Hänsel R, Woelk H, Volz HP, Faust V (eds) (1999) Therapie mit Kava-Kava. Aesopus-Verlag, Stuttgart: 1–80.

Herberg KW (1991) Fahrtüchtigkeit nach Einnahme von Kava-Spezial-Extrakt WS 1490. Z Allg Med 67: 842–846.

Hofmann R, Winter U (1993) Therapeutische Möglichkeiten mit einem hochdosierten standardisierten Kava-Kava-Präparat (Antares 120) bei Angsterkrankungen. V. Phytotherapiekongress; Bonn 3.–5. Nov.

Jamieson DD, Duffield PH, Cheng D, Duffield AM (1989) Comparison of the central nervous system activity of the aqueous and lipid extrakt of kava (Piper methysticum). Arch Int Pharmacodyn 301: 66–80.

Johnson E, Frauendorf A, Stecker K, Stein U (1991) Neurophysiologisches Wirkprofil und Verträglichkeit von Kava-Extrakt WS 1490. TW Neurol Psychiatr 5: 349–354.

Kinzler E, Krömer J, Lehmann (1991) Wirksamkeit eines Kava-Spezial-Extraktes bei Patienten mit Angst-, Spannungs- und Erregungszuständen nicht-psychotischer Genese. Arzneim Forsch /Drug Res 41: 584–588.

Kretzschmar R (1995) Pharmagologische Untersuchungen zur zentralnervösen Wirkung und zum Wirkungsmechanismus der Kava-Droge (Piper methysticum Forst) und ihrer kristallinen Inhaltsstoffe. In: Loew D, Rietbrock H (eds) Phytopharmaka in Forschung und klinischer Anwendung Band I, Steinkopff-Verlag, Darmstadt: 30–38.

Lechtenberg M, Quandt B, Kohlenberg FJ, Nahrstedt A (1999) Qualitative and quantitative micellar electrokinetic chromatography of kavalactones from dry extracts of Piper methysticum Forst. and commercial drugs. J Chromatogr A 848: 457–464.

Lehmann E, Kinzler E, Friedemann J (1996) Efficacy of a special kava extract (Piper methysticum) in patients with states of anxiety, tension and excitedness of non-mental origin – A double-blind placebo-controlled study of four weeks treatment. Phytomedicine 3: 113–119.9.

Lehrl S (2004) Clinical efficacy of Kava extract WS 1490 in sleep disturbances associated with anxiety disorders. J Affective Disord 78: 101–110.

Loew D (2002) Kava-Kava-Extrakt. Deutsche Apotheker Zeitung 141: 1012–20.

Malch U, Kieser M (2001) Efficacy of Kava-kava in the treatment of nonpsychotic anxiety, following pretreatment with benzodiazepines. Psyhopharmacology 157: 277–283.

Münte TF, Heinze HJ, Matzke M, Steitz J (1993) Effects of oxacepam and an extract of kava roots (Piper methysticum) on event-related potentials in a word recognition task. Neuropsychobiology 27: 46–53.

Pittler MH, Ernst E (2000) Efficacy of kava extract for treating anxiety: systematic review and meta-analysis. J Clin Pharmacol 20: 84–89.

Ruze P (1990) Kava-induced dermopathy: a niacin deficiency? Lancet: 1442–1445.

Schmidt M, Nahrstedt A, Lüpke NP (2002) Piper methysticum (Kava) in der Diskussion: Betrachtungen zur Qualität, Wirksamkeit und Unbedenklichkeit. Wien Med Wschr 152: 382–8.

Siegel RK (1976) Herbal intoxication. Psychoactive effects from herbal cigarettes, tea and capsules. JAMA 236:473–476.

Schulze J, Raasch W, Siegers CP (2003) Toxicity of kava pyrones, drug safety and precautions – a case study. Phytomedicine 10 Suppl IV: 68–73.

Strahl S, Ehret V, Dahm HH, Maier KP (1998) Nekrotisierende Hepatitis nach Einnahme pflanzlicher Heilmittel. Dtsch Med Wochenschr 123: 1410–1414.

Stevinson C, Huntley A, Ernst E (2002) A systematic review of the safety of kava extract in the treatment of anxiety. Drug Safety 25: 251–261.

Teschke R (2002) Hepatotoxizität durch Kava-Kava. Risikofaktoren und Prävention. Deutsches Ärzteblatt 99: 2671–7.

Teschke R, Gaus W, Loew D (2003) Kava extracts: Safety and risks including rare hepaticotoxology. Phytomed 10: 440–46.

Uebelhack R, Franke L, Schewe HJ (1998) Inhibition of platelet MAO-B by kava pyrone-enriched extract from Piper methysticum forster (Kava-Kava). Pharmacopsychiat 31: 187–192.

Volz HP, Hänsel R (1994) Kava-Kava und Kavain in der Psychopharmakotherapie. Psychopharmakotherapie 1: 33–39.

Volz HP, Kieser M (1997) Kava-kava extract WS 1490 versus placebo in anxiety disorders – a randomized placebo-controlled 25-week outpatient trial. Pharmacopsychiat 30: 1–5.

Waller DP. Report on Kava and Liver Damage. Silver Spring, MD: American Herbal Products Assn. 2002.

Warnecke G (1991) Psychosomatische Dysfunktionen im weiblichen Klimakterium. Klinische Wirksamkeit und Verträglichkeit von Kava-Extrakt WS 1490. Fortschr Med 109: 119–122.

Warnecke G, Pfaender H, Gerster G, Gracza E (1990) Wirksamkeit von Kawa-Kawa-Extrakt beim klimakterischen Syndrom. Z Phytother 11: 81–86.

Woelk H, Kapoula O, Lehrl S, Schröter K, Weinholz P (1993) Behandlung von Angst-Patienten. Z Allg Med 69: 271–277.

2.4 Restlessness and Sleep Disturbances

States of nervous unrest and sleep disturbances are considered traditional indications for the use of preparations made from valerian, lavender, hops, lemon balm, and passion flower. These are gentle herbs that do not produce strong sedative or hypnotic effects. Although valepotriates and valerenic acids isolated from valerian, demonstrate sedative effects in some experimental settings, the final concentrations of these compounds in medicinal preparations are so relatively low that they could hardly account for the observed sedative or tranquilizing effects in humans.

Valerian and lavender are somewhat unique in that their actions and efficacy have been better documented (for selected valerian extracts) than for the other three herbs mentioned above. Moreover, valerian is a widely known herb both in Germany and abroad, so a separate section will be devoted to its discussion.

2.4.1 Valerian

2.4.1.1 Medicinal Plant

The medicinal valerian used in northern latitudes (*Valeriana officinalis*, Fig. 2.18) is but one of approximately 250 valerian species that occur worldwide. Native to Europe and the temperate zones of Asia, it is an erect perennial that reaches a height of about 50–150 cm. It prefers damp, swampy areas and blooms from June to August, developing tiny white to pink flowers that grow in terminal cymes. Valerian for medicinal use is cultivated and harvested from September to October. Besides the official medicinal species, there are other valerian species (*V. edulis, V. japonica, V. indica*) whose therapeutic uses are not based on the tradition and experience of European medicine. Indian valerian and especially the Mexican species (*V. edulis*) are associated with a potentially higher therapeutic risk due to their high content of valepotriates (up to 8 %).

Fig. 2.18. ► European valerian (*Valeriana officinalis*).

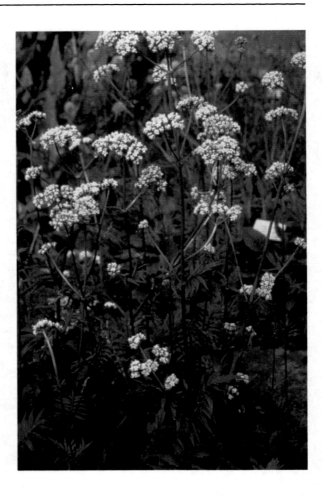

2.4.1.2 Crude Drug and Extract

Only the root of European valerian (*Valeriana officinalis*) is used as an official drug. The characteristic unpleasant odor of valerian, strongly reminiscent of isovaleric (isovalerenic) acid and camphor, appears only after the root has been cut and dried. The cut, dried root is used in tea preparations. Pharmaceutical products are mainly produced from aqueous or aqueous-alcoholic extracts (70 % ethanol, herb-to-extract ratio 4–7:1). The aqueous and ethanol extracts of valerian root are by no means equivalent in the quality of their actions, however, and they are used in different dosages. The dose for aqueous extracts is based on the traditional tea application, which uses a minimum dose of 2 g of dried herb (root) and a herb-to-extract ratio of 5:1 to yield a single dose of approximately 400 mg. The dose for alcoholic dry extracts is not easily derived from traditional applications, and clinical studies with specific extracts are needed to gain better information on proper dosing.

2.4.1.3 Key Compounds, Analysis, and Pharmacokinetics

The dried root contains, on average, 0.5–2 % volatile oil. The characteristic odor is caused by small amounts of isovaleric acid, which is formed by the breakdown of valepotriates. The concentrations of these constituents are subject to seasonal variations (Bos et al., 1998). More than 100 constituents have been identified to date, but it is unknown which of them is responsible for the characteristic medicinal actions of the root. Medicinal valerian contains 0.3–0.8 % of the two sesquiterpenes valerenic acid and acetoxyvalerenic acid. These characteristic constituents do not occur in species that grow outside Europe. Thus, both compounds make suitable marker compounds for testing the pharmaceutical quality of valerian extracts.

The carefully dried root also contains up to 1 % valepotriates (up to 8 % in Mexican valerian). Chemically, these compounds are esters of lower fatty acids, i. e., of acetic acid, isovaleric acid, and β-acetoxyisovaleric acid, with a trivalent alcohol. The alcohol component displays the C_{10} carbon skeleton of monoterpenes and contains an epoxy ring, which is mainly responsible for the instability and mutagenic potential of valerian extracts (see Sect. 2.4.1.4). Because the valepotriates are unstable in an acid or alkaline environment and at higher temperatures, they can be administered only in solid dosage forms (preferably enteric-coated tablets), not in liquid preparations (tinctures).

Three studies have been published on the absorption, distribution, and elimination of the components of valerian extracts in humans. Two of the studies report results with ^{14}C-labeled isovaltrate (Fink, 1982) and dihydrovaltrate (Wagner et al., 1980). But isovaltrate and dihydrovaltrate are compounds from the class of valepotriates, and extracts from European valerian root contain only trace amounts of them. Another study in mice was performed with ^{14}C-labeled baldrianal/homobaldrianal, which apparently is absorbed well but is subject to a strong first-pass effect in the liver (Dieckmann, 1988).

2.4.1.4 Pharmacology and Toxicology

About 20 original studies have been published on the experimental pharmacology of valerian root preparations and substances produced from them. Surveys of these studies may be found in Hänsel et al. (1994), and ESCOP (1997). Pharmacologic studies have focused on various constituents of the valerian root. Attention was first directed to the volatile oils because it was thought that the action of valerian was mediated by olfactory receptors (Hazelhoff et a., 1984). The volatile oil of valerian consists mainly of valeric acid and isovaleric acid. Other authors tested the valepotriates as possible active principles. Behavioral tests in cats given 10 mg of valepotriates mixture/kg by stomach tube showed a calmative effect manifested by a decrease in restless, fearful, and aggressive behaviors (Eickstedt, 1969). Later studies in rats showed that valepotriates exerted no central nervous system effects in either low or high doses (up to 50 mg/kg) (Grusla, 1987; Krieglstein, 1988).

Experimental studies of valerenic acids in laboratory animals demonstrated sedative and anticonvulsant activity (Hendriks et al., 1985). Riedel, Hänsel, and Ehrke (1982) performed in vitro studies showing that valerenic acid decreased the degradation rate of γ-aminobutyric acid (GABA). The most recent studies (Santos et al., 1994) showed an increased concentration of GABA in the synaptic cleft after the administration of valerian. These authors used a valerian extract rather than isolated valerenic acid. They found that this extract increased the secretion of GABA from the synaptosomes and inhibited its reuptake. Ortiz (1999) found additional effects of valerian extracts on flunitrazepam binding. He concluded that valerian extracts have effects on GABA (A) receptors, but can also interact at other presynaptic components of GABAergic neurons. GABA is considered an important inhibitory neurotransmitter that plays a key role in stress and anxiety. Cavadas et al. (1995) have noted, however, that the effects on GABA-A receptors observed in vitro can hardly account for the in-vivo sedative effect because of the low concentration of valerenic acid. Other animal studies have shown that the whole extract has calmative effects on the CNS that are not referable to valerenic acids, valepotriates, or the volatile oil fraction (Krieglstein, 1988).

Two valerian root extracts were tested for their behavioral effects in mice and rat models. An ethanol extract was administered in mice by a single intraperitoneal injection in doses up to 100 mg/kg. While definite sedative effects were not observed, the extract did show anticonvulsant activity against picrotoxin and significantly prolonged the duration of thiopental-induced anesthesia (Hiller et al., 1996). In another study, an aqueous valerian root extract caused significant sedation in mice when administered orally in doses of 20 and 200 mg/kg. Spontaneous motility 120 min after dosing was reduced by 25 % and 36 %, respectively. Diazepam administered at doses of 5 and 25 mg/kg caused a 77 % and 90 % motility reduction in the same experiment. The valerian extract also prolonged thiopental-induced sleeping time by a factor of 7.6 when administered at 200 mg/kg, and it demonstrated anticonvulsant properties (Leuschner et al., 1993).

No studies have yet been published on the acute toxicity of whole valerian extracts, only of fractions or single constituents. Von Skramlik (1959) tested the volatile oil of valerian root, and Rücker et al. (1978) and Hendriks et al. (1985) performed studies with valeranone and valerenic acid. Cytotoxic effects of potential therapeutic relevance were found with valepotriates and baldrinals and with chemical derivatives of both compounds, but these effects were not observed with valerenic acids or tinctures poor in valepotriates (Bos et al., 1998). Because of their chemical instability, however, the valepotriates are apparently cytotoxic only in vitro. Even high doses (1350 mg/kg) produced no detectable cytotoxic effects in rats (Tufik, 1985). A mixture of three valepotriates was administered orally in pregnant rats for 3 weeks, with groups of 10 rats each receiving a dose of 0, 6, 12, or 24 mg/kg. Five animals from each group were killed at the end of the 3-week period. Neither the mothers nor the fetuses showed pathologic changes on external examination. Internal examination of the fetuses showed an increased incidence of delayed ossification at doses of 12 and 24 mg/kg. Effects on neonatal rat development were investigated in the remaining 20 animals. No differences were found between the control group and the three groups that received different valepotriate dosages. The authors concluded that valepotriates had no deleterious effects on the mothers or their offspring at the tested dose levels (Tufik et al., 1985). In another study, an alcoholic extract of valerian root was administered to rats by intraperitoneal injection at doses of 400–600 mg/kg for a period of 45 days. No significant body-weight changes or blood changes were observed in comparison with control animals (Rosecrans et al., 1961). A similar extract was administered orally in rats at doses of 300–600 mg/kg for 30 days. Again, no significant differences were found in growth, organ weight, or hematologic and biochemical parameters at the end of the observation period (Fehri et al., 1991).

Studies on mutagenic potential have dealt exclusively with constituents isolated from the crude drug, i.e., valepotriates and baldrinals. Studies on bacterial mutagenicity were done using strains of *Salmonella typhimurium* and *Escherichia coli*. The test substances consisted of a valtrate/isovaltrate mixture (60:40) as well as dihydrovaltrate, baldrinal, and homobaldrinal. The studies were done with and without metabolic activation. While the valepotriates showed mutagenic effects only with metabolic activation at concentrations higher than 1.0 μmol/plate, the baldrinals were mutagenic both with and without metabolic activation at concentrations of just 0.1–0.3 μmol/plate (von der Hude et al., 1985, 1986). The effects of baldrinal and homobaldrinal on the clonogenic in-vitro growth of various hematopoietic cells were tested at concentrations of 10^{-8} to 10^{-4} M. A concentration of 10^{-4} M was necessary to significantly inhibit the growth of mouse hematopoietic stem cells and of colonies of human T-lymphocytes, leading the authors to conclude that the amounts of baldrinal contained in commercial preparations do not have significant cytotoxic effects (Braun et al., 1986). This does not mean, however, that the baldrinals are entirely without genotoxicity. The target organ for mutagenic risk after oral administration would be the liver, because while baldrinals are well absorbed, they are subject to a strong first-pass effect and are eliminated by the liver. As a result, only valerian preparations that are low in valepotriates, and thus in baldrinals, can be recommended for use in human patients (Dieckmann, 1988).

2.4.1.5 Pharmacologic Effects in Humans and Clinical Efficacy in Patients

Tables 2.7 and 2.8 review a total of 14 controlled studies dealing with valerian preparations containing no other herbal extracts, including 9 clinical pharmacologic studies in healthy volunteers and 5 studies in patients with sleep disorders. The dosage figures shown in column 3 refer to different extract preparations, however. Six studies (Schulz et al., 1994, 1998; Kuhlmann et al., 1999; Donath et al., 2000; Vorbach et al., 1995; Dorn, 2000) employed a standardized ethanol extract (70 % v/v, herb:extract ratio 4–7:1, valerenic acid content 0.4–0.6 %), and four studies (Leathwood and Chauffard, 1983, 1985; Kamm-Kohl et al., 1984; Balderer and Borbely, 1985) used freeze-dried aqueous extracts (herb:extract ratio 3–6:1). The remaining studies either used extracts with defined amounts of valepotriates (Gessner und Klasser, 1984), unspecified extracts (Jansen, 1977; Kohnen and Oswald, 1988), or the pulverized herb (Francis, 2002). Due to the inconsistencies in the preparations used and in the studies themselves, the clinical evidence for valerian as a treatment for insomnia was described as inconclusive in a meta-analysis (Stevinson und Ernst, 2000).

Leathwood reported in 1983 and 1984 on the results of studies in three groups of healthy subjects. In each case the test dose was taken only once. Two groups consisting of 128 and 8 subjects evaluated their subjective sleep parameters by filling out a self-rating scale the morning after taking the medication. Both studies by Leathwood showed a significant reduction in latency to sleep onset compared with a placebo. The quality of sleep was also improved in one of the three studies. Comparison of the response to 450 mg and 900 mg showed no sign that the measured effects were dose-dependent. In

Table 2.7.
Placebo-controlled double-blind studies of valerian extract pharmacology in volunteers.

First author, year	Cases (N)	Dose (mg/d)	Duration (d)	Methods	Results
Studies with a defined valerian extract produced with 70% ethanol in water					
Schulz, 1994, crossover design	14	405	17	Sleep EEG, self-rating scale	Increase in long-wave sleep and K-complex density; reduction of sleep stage 1. No significant change in sleep latency, waking time, or quality of sleep.
Schulz, 1998	12	1200	1	Pharmaco-EEG, Flicker fusion frequency (CFF)	EEG: characteristic waveform changes compared with placebo and diazepam. CFF: no decrease in vigilance
Kuhlmann, 1999	102	600	114	VDD, Cognitrone, TT	No impairment of respon siveness or driving ability
Donath, 2000, Crossover design	16	600	114	Pharmaco-EEG Polysomnograph Mood questionnaire	No intergroup differences after 1 day; at 14 days: SWSL*, SWS%-TIB*. 3 AEs with valerian, 18 AEs with placebo!
Studies with other single-herb valerian preparations					
Leathwood, 1983, PDB, aqueous extract	128 / 29	400 / 400	11	Self-rating scale, sleep EEG	Sleep latency shortened* Sleep quality improved* Sleep EEG n.s.
Leathwood, 1985, aqueous extract	8	450 / 900	1	Self-rating scale	Sleep latency shortened** No dose-response relationship
Gessner, 1984, crossover design, extract of Mexican valerian standardized to 20 % valepotriates	11 / 9	60 / 120	1 / 1	EOG, EMG of nuchal muscles, EKG, bilateral centro-occipital and frontocentral, EEG, mood	Greater reduction of sleep stage 4, slight reduction of REM activity, slight increase in stages of awake, sleep 1, and sleep 2. Dose-depend-ent change in beta activity. No unpleasant aftereffects from the medication
Balderer, 1985, PDB crossover, aqueous extract	10 / 8	450 / 900 / 450	1 / 1	Self-rating scale, sleep EEG	Dose-dependent shortening of sleep latency ** and time awake * Sleep EEG n.s.

Table 2.7.
(cont.)

First author, year	Cases (N)	Dose (mg/d)	Duration (d)	Methods	Results
Kohnen, 1988, PDB with undefined valerian extract vs. propranolol vs. propranolol + valerian extract	40	100 20 20+ 100	1 1	Pulse rate, alertness test (solving math problems), mood	No effect of valerian extract on physiologic activation. No differences between medication and placebo in solving addition problems

Abbreviations: EEG = electroencephalogram, **EMG** = electromyogram, **EOG** = electro-oculogram, **SWSL** = slow-wave sleep (deep sleep) latency, **SWS%-TIB** = slow-wave sleep % of time in bed; **VDD**= Vienna determination device, **TT** = tracking test. Significance: n.s. = not significant, * = p < 0.05, ** = p < 0.01, *** = p < 0.001. **AEs** = adverse events.

a separate group of 29 subjects, EEG traces recorded in a sleep laboratory showed no significant differences in comparison to placebo.

Balderer and Borbely (1985) reported similar results in a study of healthy subjects. A self-rating scale in 10 subjects indicated a significant decrease in latency to sleep onset and nocturnal awakening, but the sleep EEG's showed no objective evidence of significant effects.

Two other pharmacodynamic studies (Schulz et al., 1994; Schulz and Jobert, 1998) dealt with the effects of ethanol extracts in patients with sleep disorders. The second study (1995) used a randomized crossover design to compare valerian extract (1200 mg) with diazepam (10 mg), lavender extract (1200 mg), passion flower extract (1200 mg), kava extract (600 mg), and a placebo. All these substances were associated with distinctive patterns of quantitative EEG responses. The herbal extracts, unlike diazepam, caused a relative increase of amplitudes in the theta band of EEG frequencies. The herbs also differed from diazepam in that none of the extracts caused a relative amplitude increase in the beta frequency band. Instead, they tended to cause a reduction in this range that was especially marked with valerian and lavender. The herbal extracts showed varying patterns of effects in the long-wave delta frequency range. Marked increases were observed with lavender extract, moderate increases with valerian and passion flower extract, and decreases with kava extract.

Donath et al. (2000) found no improvement over placebo in 14 patients with insomnia (ICSD code 1.A.1) who were treated with a single dose of 600 mg of valerian extract. After 14 days' treatment with 600 mg/d, they measured a significant increase in the duration of deep sleep relative to total time in bed. Remarkably, the patients treated with valerian in this study reported significantly fewer "adverse events" than in the placebo group (3 vs. 18).

Kuhlmann et al. (1999) conducted a study in 102 volunteers to determine the effect of valerian on the ability to drive a car or operate machinery safely. The authors found that neither a single dose of 600 mg of valerian extract or repeated evening doses over a 14-day period had adverse effects on reaction time, alertness, or concentration.

Pharmacodynamic studies in humans, especially when limited to measurable changes in the pharmaco-EEG, are not sufficient in themselves to prove therapeutic

Table 2.8.
Controlled double-blind studies of valerian preparations in patients with sleep disorders.

First author, year, design, extract	Cases (N)	Dose (mg/d)	Duration (d)	Methods	Results
Studies with a defined valerian extract produced with 70% ethanol in water					
Vorbach, 1996, comparison with placebo	121	600	28	SQ-B, CGI, Bf-S, SRA	SQ*, FOR*, CIW**, SOD**, TE***, CS**, SRA*
Dorn, 2000, comparison with oxazepam, 70 % ethanol	75	600	28	SQ-B, CGI, Bf-S, SRA, HAMA	Comparable efficacy of valerian extract and oxazepam
Studies with other single-herb valerian preparations					
Jansen, 1977, undefined extract, comparison with placebo	150	300	30	Observer rating scale (10 items psychic, 8 somatic)	Progressive reduction of nearly all symptoms over a 30-day period in patients with sleep disorders at a geriatric hospital; no statistical analysis.
Kamm-Kohl, 1984, Aqueous extract, comparison with placebo	80	270	14	von Zerssen Bf-S, NOSIE scale, sleep score	Significant improvements in mood (Bf-S**), behavioral deficits (NOSIE**), and difficulties falling and staying asleep in patients at a geriatric hospital.
Francis, 2002, powdered crude drug from V. edulis, crossover vs. placebo	5	500 1500	14	Sleep EEG, SL, NTA, TST, SQ	Children with intelligence deficit and insomnia. SL*; NTA*; TST**; SQ**

Abbreviations: **EEG** = electroencephalogram, **Bf-S** = von Zerssen Mood Scale, **NOSIE** = Nurses Observation Scale for Inpatient Evaluation, **HAMA** = Hamilton Anxiety Scale, **CGI** = Clinical Global Impressions, **SF-B** = Görtelmeyer Sleep Questionnaire, **SQ-B** = Görtelmeyer Sleep Questionnaire Type B, **SRA** = sleep rating by the physician, **SL** = sleep latency; **NTA** = noctural time awake; **SQ** = sleep quality, **SOD** = severity of disease, **FOR** = feeling of refreshment after sleep, **CIW**= changes in well-being, **SOD** = severity of desease, **TE** = therapeutic efficacy, **TST** = total sleep time; **CS** = clinical status; statistical significance: **n.s.** = not significant, * = p < 0.05, ** = p < 0.01, *** = p < 0.001.

efficacy. This can be done only by conducting controlled treatment studies in suitable patient groups. Only five such studies are currently available, one of which (Jansen, 1977) should be disregarded due to a lack of statistical validity by present-day standards. Of the remaining four studies, one used powdered dried herb (Grancis, 2002), one used an aqueous extract (Kamm-Kohl et al., 1984), and the other two used the ethanol extract described above.

Kamm-Kohl et al. (1984) studied the effects of valerian in sleep-disturbed patients from geriatric hospitals. The study involved 150 patients treated for 30 days and 80 patients treated for 14 days, using two standard observer rating scales and a scoring system for rating difficulties falling asleep and staying asleep. The results after 14 days'

SF-B - Feeling rested after sleep

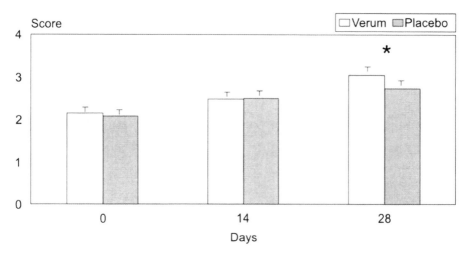

Fig. 2.19. ▲ Effect of 4 weeks' treatment with an ethanol valerian extract (600 mg/day) compared with a placebo. The results were assessed by the Görtelmayer sleep questionnaire (SF-B) and statistically evaluated. A significant difference between valerian and placebo is seen only after a 4-week course of treatment (Vorbach et al., 1996).

treatment showed statistically significant improvements in mood (von Zerssen mood scale), behavioral disturbance (NOSIE), and difficulties falling and staying asleep (sleep score).

The results of a placebo-controlled double-blind study by Vorbach et al. (1996) are even more impressive. This study involved 121 patients who had experienced significant sleep disturbance for a period of at least 4 weeks. Patients with depression (HAMD > 16) and patients who were taking or had taken medication that could affect sleep were excluded from the study. Therapeutic efficacy was evaluated by four standard rating scales: a physician-rated sleep scale (SRA), the Görtelmayer sleep questionnaire (SF-B), the von Zerssen mood scale (Bf-S), and the Clinical Global Impressions (CGI) scale. All rating scales were administered before the start of treatment, at 14 days, and at 28 days.

The results of this study are shown graphically in Figs. 2.19–2.21. It is noteworthy that the patients observed virtually no acute effects during the initial days of treatment. All the rating scales showed marked placebo effects over the 4-week course of treatment, with the result that the physician-rated sleep scale (SRA) showed no statistically significant differences between the valerian extract and the placebo. The Görtelmayer sleep questionnaire (SF-B) showed no difference at 14 days, but by 28 days there was a significant difference favoring the valerian-treated group (Fig. 2.19). The von Zerssen mood scale (Bf-S) also showed significant intergroup differences after 28 days of treatment (Fig. 2.20). The most pronounced differences were seen with the Clinical Global Impressions (CGI) scale. Ratings by both patient and physician showed very marked

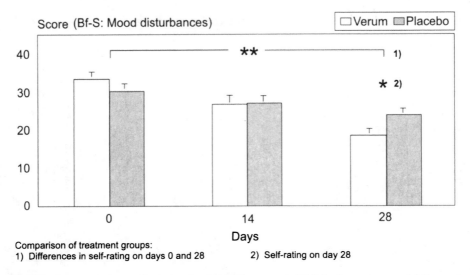

Comparison of treatment groups:
1) Differences in self-rating on days 0 and 28   2) Self-rating on day 28

Fig. 2.20. ▲ Same study as in Fig. 2.19, using the von Zerssen scale (Bf-S) for the assessment of daily mood. The valerian and placebo groups show no significant difference after 2 weeks' treatment, but by 4 weeks there is significant improvement with the valerian preparation compared with the placebo.

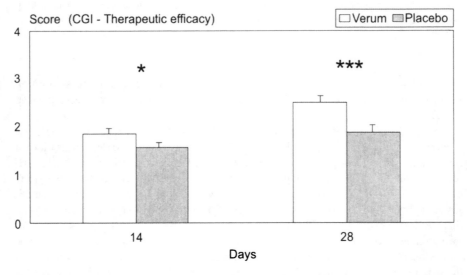

Fig. 2.21. ▲ Same study as in Fig. 2.19. Evaluation and statistical analysis of efficacy after 4 weeks' treatment, scored by the physician and patient using Clinical Global Impression (CGI) criteria. Marked intergroup differences are seen at 4 weeks compared with 2 weeks.

differences in favor of the valerian extract, with statistical analysis indicating a significant difference at 14 days ($p < 0.05$) and a highly significant difference at 28 days ($p < 0.001$; Fig. 2.21).

The results of this study suggest that valerian preparations probably do not produce immediate effects like those of a typical sleep aid, and that 2–4 weeks' therapy is needed to achieve significant improvements, especially in daily mood. The lack of an acute response need not be a disadvantage in sleep-disturbed patients, however, because acute effects can promote dependency and can interfere with necessary psychotherapeutic measures. The delayed onset of action particularly distinguishes valerian preparations from the benzodiazepines, although the sleep-inducing effect of valerian after 4 weeks' use was comparable to that of oxazepam (Dorn, 2000). Patients should clearly understand that the onset of action is delayed so that they will not stop taking the medication prematurely. Sleep aids and sedatives are generally associated with immediate effects, which valerian apparently does not possess.

In addition to studies dealing with valerian therapy alone, there are several studies dealing with the combined use of valerian extract and other herbal calmatives. The results obtained with single-herb valerian products are supported by results with two fixed combination products in which valerian is combined with lemon balm extract (Albrecht et al., 1995; Dressing et al., 1992, 1996) and with hops (Gebhardt et al., 1996; Vonderheid-Guth et al., 2000). In a placebo-controlled double-blind study, the therapeutic efficacy of a valerian-lemon balm combination was tested in 68 patients with insomnia who took a daily dose of 630 mg of valerian extract plus 320 mg of lemon balm extract for 14 days. A multiparameter rating scale showed that the combination product was significantly more effective than the placebo (Dressing et al., 1996). The same product was tested in a placebo-controlled study in 54 subjects for its effect on driving ability in comparison with flunitrazepam and a placebo. It was found that objectively measurable impairment of performance in vigilance and reaction tests occurred only in the group that received flunitrazepam (Gebhardt et al., 1996). A recent summary of 29 clinical trials conducted on preparations made with valerian only as well as valerian combined with other herbs is found in Blumenthal et al. (2003).

2.4.1.6 Indications, Dosages, Risks, and Contraindications

The monograph on valerian root published by the Commission E in 1985 cites "restlessness, sleeping disorders based on nervous conditions" as the indications for use (Blumenthal et al., 1998). The results of subsequent clinical studies (Table 2.8) essentially confirm the indications stated in the monograph. However, the results of Vorbach et al. (1996) suggest that it would be better to replace the word "insomnia" (i.e., difficulty falling asleep) with "sleep disturbances." As for dosage, the monograph recommends taking 2–3 g of the dried herb one or more times daily. Based on the study by Vorbach et al. (1996), the ethanol extract tested in the study should be taken in a dose of about 600 mg 2 h before bedtime.

No contraindications, side effects, or drug interactions are mentioned in the Commission E monograph. As a precaution, the ESCOP monograph (2003) recommends that valerian not be used during pregnancy, lactation, or in children younger than 3 years of age. Only a few adverse reactions have been reported in the few controlled treatment studies that have been performed to date. Vorbach et al. (1996) noted three adverse reactions in 61 patients of the valerian group: two cases of headache and one case of morning grogginess. To date, only one spontaneous ADR has been reported for the most commonly prescribed single-herb valerian product in Germany(brand name Sedonium®). Two hours after taking the product, a 57-year-old woman had a paradoxical reaction consisting of restlessness, nervousness, and difficulty falling asleep. So far there has been only one reported case of a patient attempting suicide by taking a valerian overdose. An 18-year-old girl swallowed approximately 20 g (40-50 capsules at 470 mg each) of powdered valerian root obtained as a retail product. Three hours later she was admitted to a hospital ICU with complaints of weakness, abdominal pain and cramping, tightness in the chest, tremors in the hands and feet, and grogginess. Her respiration and circulation were stable. Body temperature and other physical findings were normal except for mydriasis, and she had a normal ECG and blood chemistry. All of her symptoms resolved spontaneously within 24 h. The authors concluded that a valerian overdose equal to approximately 20 times the recommended therapeutic dose appears to be benign (Willey et al., 1995).

2.4.1.7 Therapeutic Significance

Nervousness and sleeping difficulties (insomnia) affect approximately one-fifth of the population and are very common indications for valerian use. Complaints of sleeping problems increase with aging, and women are affected more often than men. Untreated or inadequately treated insomnia is associated with an increased risk of various physical and mental disorders, including depression. Insomnia therefore requires therapeutic intervention. Nonpharmacologic measures should be tried before resorting to pharmacologic therapy. Sensitive counseling by the physician can be very beneficial in cases of this kind. For example, Gauler and Weihrauch (1997) noted clinically significant placebo effects in approximately 40–80 % of sleep-disturbed patients within the framework of controlled double-blind studies. It should be added, however, that a significant portion of this "psychodynamic" effect (Schulz, 2000) is linked to the ritual of taking the medication. There are no objective figures available on the exclusive use of behavioral or physical therapeutic measures. The current pharmacologic treatment of nervousness and insomnia relies mainly on benzodiazepines and has a number of serious risks such as sedation hangover, impaired responses, rebound insomnia, respiratory depression, and drug dependency. Given these hazards, the risk-to-benefit ratio of benzodiazepines is probably questionable in a majority of patients. Valerian products that conform to pharmaceutical specifications provide a low-risk alternative for the pharmacologic treatment of nervousness and insomnia. Despite centuries of medical experience with valerian root preparations, there is no evidence that the herb promotes dependency. Because valerian root acts gradually and is not useful for the acute treatment of insomnia, suitable counseling and physical therapeutic measures are necessary during the initial weeks of use to ensure compliance, especially in patients already accustomed to using benzodiazepines or other synthetic drugs. Based on the information available from scientific studies, the pharmacodynamic effect of valerian helps to promote and restore natural sleep after at least 2–4 weeks of use.

2.4.2 Lavender Flowers

2.4.2.1 Medicinal Plant, Crude Drug, and Lavender Oil

Lavender flowers consist of the dried blossoms of the true lavender plant (*Lavendula angustifolia*), which are gathered just before they are fully open (Fig. 2.22). The plant is a small, branched shrub that grows up to 60 cm high and is native to the Mediterranean region. Lavender flowers have at least a 1.5 % content of essential oil. Their main constituents are linalyl acetate, linalool, campher, beta-ocimene, and cineol. The herb also contains up to 12 % tannins. True lavender oil, which is extracted from the fresh flowering tops by steam distillation, contains linalyl acetate and linalool as its main constituents. True lavender oil is distinguished from "spike lavender oil," which is derived from a broad-leafed variety of lavender (*L. latifolia*) and contains up to 35 % cineol. Additional pharmaceutical information can be found in Hänsel et al. (1993) and Lis Balchin (2002).

2.4.2.2 Pharmacology and Toxicology

Preparations made from lavender flowers, chiefly from lavender oil, are believed to have a calmative effect on the central nervous system as well as neuroprotective, anticonvulsant, antimicrobial, and various other pharmacologic properties. Reviews of the extensive literature can be found in Fröhlich (1968), Hänsel et al. (1993), Buchbauer (1996), Blumenthal et al. (2000), Cavanagh and Wilkinson (2002), und Lis Balchin (2002). Our present discussion will be limited to the cerebral effects of lavender.

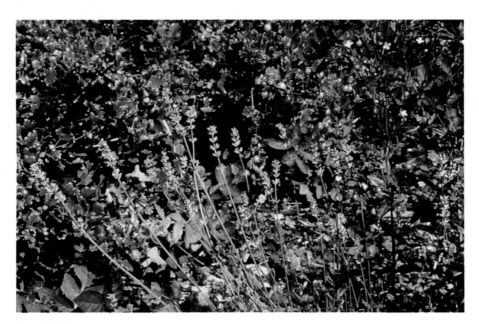

Fig. 2.22. ▲ Lavender (*Lavandula angustifolia*).

An experiment was conducted on GABA-A receptors obtained from the rat brain to measure their effect on specific membrane potentials. Various preparations of lavender oil potentiated the effect of GABA-A. The authors concluded that low concentrations of lavender oil increase the affinity of GABA for the receptors, acting in a manner similar to known sedatives such as benzodiazepine and barbiturates (Aoshima und Hamamoto, 1999).

To date, lavender oil is the only lavender preparation for which pharmacologic studies in animals and humans have been reported (Lis-Balchin, 1999). Intraperitoneal doses of approximately 100–200 mg/kg lavender oil in mice and rats showed anticonvulsant effects against electric shock, inhibitory effects on spontaneous motor activity, and additive effects when combined with several narcotics (Atanassova-Shopova, 1970). Multiple oral doses of 0.4 mg/kg lavender oil in mice followed by the intraperitoneal injection of 40 mg/kg pentobarbital significantly reduced the time of sleep onset and prolonged the duration of sleep relative to a control group (Guillemain, 1989). A significant depression of motor activity was observed in mice exposed to a lavender atmosphere in a dark cage after 30, 60, and 90 min. Linalool and linalyl acetate alone showed similar effects. The plasma levels of linalool rose in proportion to the length of exposure. Lavender oil completely inhibited stimulation by caffeine, and linalool and linalyl acetate inhibited caffeine stimulation by about 50 % (Buchbauer et al., 1991). In another series of tests, the inhalation of lavender oil vapor caused a dose-dependent suppression of convulsions induced in mice by pentylenetetrazole, nicotine, and electric shock (Yamada et al., 1994).

In a controlled experiment, the behavior of 2 × 20 pigs was observed at 10-minute intervals during 2 hours of road travel. The cortisol concentrations in saliva samples were also analyzed as a measure of stress. On day 1, the bedding in the transport vehicle consisted of plain straw. On day 2, the straw was impregnated with lavender oil. The animals were more active on the lavender straw (the incidence of animals lying down was 7 % with lavender vs. 34 % without lavender). Symptoms of travel sickness (foaming at the mouth, retching and vomiting) were significantly less common in the lavender condition than in the control group (total of 3/20 with lavender vs. 9/20 without). The cortisol concentration in the saliva, as a measure of stress, showed no significant differences between the two groups (Bradshaw et al., 1998).

The LD-50 values associated with a single oral dose of lavender oil in rats or with dermal application in rabbits were 5 mL/kg or higher (Buchbauer et al., 1991; Hänsel et al., 1993). No other results on the toxicology of lavender have been reported. More comprehensive studies on acute and subacute toxicity and teratogenicity have been reported for spike oil (oleum spicae, derived from *L. latifolia*), which differs in its quantitative but not its qualitative composition from the typical ingredients in lavender oil. The acute LD-30 for spike oil administered subcutaneously in mice was 40 mL/kg. In guinea pigs, on the other hand, an oral dose of only 3.2 mL/kg was lethal. Oral doses of 0.4 mL/kg administered to guinea pigs daily for 12 weeks had no apparent toxic effects on the animals or their organs except for significant enlargement of the adrenal glands (with no change in organ structure). The results of studies on reproductive toxicity in a total of 357 mice from 30 litters were classified as "nonteratogenic" (Fröhlich, 1968).

2.4.2.3 Pharmacokinetics

No studies have been published on the pharmacokinetics of constituents derived from lavender oil following oral administration. In inhalation experiments in mice, a direct correlation was found between inhalation time and the plasma levels of linalool. Levels of 3 ng/mL linalool and 11 ng/mL linalyl acetate were measured following 1-hour exposure to a lavender atmosphere (Jirovetz et al., 1990). Linalool was partially bound to glucuronic acid. After 15 minutes of inhalation, the constituents were found not only in the blood but also in the brain (Buchbauer et al., 1991, 1996). Linalool and linalyl acetate were detectable in the blood of volunteers following the dermal application of lavender oil (Jäger et al., 1992).

Based on a systematic review of the bioavailability and pharmacokinetics of natural volatile terpenes in animals and humans, Kohlert et al. (2000) conclude that these compounds are probably eliminated from the body with a half-life of approximately 1 hour, so that there is no risk of accumulation. The available data also suggest that the terpene components of the essential oils are rapidly absorbed following oral, dermal, or inhalational administration. A small portion is exhaled through the lungs unchanged. Most is broken down metabolically to carbon dioxide or excreted by the kidneys in conjugated form (Kohlert et al., 2000).

2.4.2.4 Clinical Pharmacology

Studies on the pharmacodynamic effects of *L. officinalis* preparations in healthy volunteers have, with one exception (Schulz et al., 1998), administered the preparations by inhalation in the form of aromatherapy. The outcome measures in these studies were the effects of the lavender preparations on the electrophysiologic activity of the CNS, moods and emotions, cognitive functions, and on physiologic circulatory parameters.

The study by Schulz et al. (1998) was a double-blind multi-crossover study in 12 female volunteers to test the effect of an ethanol extract of lavender flowers (single oral dose of 1200 mg) on the EEG and on alertness measured with a visual analog scale (VAS) in comparison with a placebo, diazepam, and seven other plant extracts. The EEG and VAS were obtained just before, 120 min after, and 180 min after ingestion of the test substance. The results of the self-rated VAS indicated that diazepam, valerian extract, and lavender extract caused pronounced sedation, while the extracts of St. John's wort, lemon balm, and California poppy (*Eschscholzia californica*) did not differ significantly from placebo. The quantitative EEG also showed definite changes with the three sedative agents, but the change profile with diazepam differed markedly from that associated with valerian and lavender (Schulz et al., 1998).

In another study, seven human subjects who had inhaled lavender oil showed a significant decline in selective EEG potentials (contingent negative variation, CNV), that correlate with vigilance, expectancy, and alertness. Lavender oil was considered to have a sedating and relaxing effect when compared with various other substances. Unlike nitrazepam, however, lavender oil had no effect on heart rate or reaction time (Torii et al., 1991).

In another study the administration of lavender oil vapor by surgical mask in 10 subjects significantly prolonged decision-making time in a computer-controlled reaction test, but movement time was unaffected. The authors interpreted this as evidence of central sedation with no effect on motor function. In a second experiment, the same group of authors tested the reaction time of 24 subjects in a vigilance task. Again, the lavender oil caused a significant increase in reaction time while jasmine vapor caused a significant reduction (Karamat et al., 1992).

Sugawara et al. (1998 and 2000) conducted a controlled experiment to study the effects of optically active linalools administered with an inhalator in healthy subjects. The effects were assessed by quantitative EEG analysis and by an original self-rated scale to evaluate 13 odor qualities. The authors found that the two enantiomers produced different effects in the quantitative EEG and in terms of odor perception compared with the racemate.

Diego et al. (1998) had 40 healthy adults inhale lavender or rosemary aromas and assessed the effect by quantitative EEG analysis, a self-rated mood scale (profile of mood states = POMS), and a cognitive performance test (math computations). The lavender group showed increased beta power in the EEG, had a more relaxed and less depressed mood in the POMS, and performed the math computations faster and more accurately. The rosemary group showed decreased beta power in the EEG, and they were only faster but not more accurate in completing the math computations.

In a study conducted by Vernet-Maury et al. (1999), 15 male and female subjects 22–28 years of age inhaled five different odorants in random order with a face mask. The subjects filled out an 11-point hedonic scale to rate the "pleasantness" or "unpleasantness" of each odorant. Six autonomic nervous system (ANS) responses were simultaneously recorded: skin potential (mV), skin resistance (kOhm), skin temperature, skin blood flow, heart rate, and respiratory rate. Based on prior methodologic studies, a decision tree was used to relate each of the six ANS parameters to a basic emotional state: happiness, surprise, sadness, fear, anger, and disgust. Typical and reproducible correlations were found between the hedonic evaluation and the reaction profile for the ANS parameters. Comparison of the effects of the five odorants showed that lavender elicited the most "happiness," followed by ethyl acetate. Camphor induced either "happiness," "surprise," or "sadness" (depending on the subjects' past histories), while acetic and butyric acid mainly induced "anger" and "disgust".

Degel und Köster (1999) conducted a prospective randomized study in a total of 108 women and men (average age 30 years) who completed a fixed series of cognitive performance tests (creative, narrative, and mathematical) in three different rooms weakly scented with lavender, jasmine, or placebo. The mood of each subject was rated at the end of the tests. On statistical average, mood was rated better after exposure to lavender than jasmine. In the cognitive tests as well, lavender generally had a more positive effect while jasmine had a more negative effect.

Saeki (2000) performed a crossover study in 10 women 19–21 years of age to test the effect of soaking the feet in a hot water bath with or without lavender oil (4 drops in 4 L of water at an initial temperature of 40 °C) on five autonomic nervous system functions (EKG, heart rate, respiratory rate, heart rate variability, and fingertip blood flow). It was found that the lavender foot bath produced a significant increase in blood flow but did not alter the other parameters.

Romine et al. (1999) conducted a controlled experiment in which two groups of 10 men each performed physical exercise (level walking at a fast pace) for 2 min. Afterward they rested in a room for 10 min, during which the experimental group was exposed to lavender aromatherapy while the control group was not exposed to an odor. Recovery was assessed by measuring blood pressure and pulse rate immediately after the exercise and at the end of rest period. The recovery measures showed the same progression with and without lavender. Due to the mild level of exercise, however (mean immediate postexercise values were 132/79 mm Hg and 85 bpm!), the outcome of this experiment was fairly predictable.

Motomura et al. (1998) performed a randomized study in which 42 healthy students were exposed to a defined psychological stress in a room that had been treated with 3 mL of lavender oil or with no odorant. A psychological checklist for stress and tension showed significant stress reduction with lavender oil with no adverse effects on heart rate, blood pressure, or the ability to perform memory tasks.

Two additional studies dealt with measuring the olfactory effects of lavender oil on the brain. Brand et al. (1999) measured bilateral electrodermal potentials in 20 women and 10 men following unilateral exposure to lavender oil (one nostril). They found that the perception of the odor stimulus was localized to the individually determined cerebral hemisphere regardless of the side of exposure. Di Nardo et al. (2000) measured the perfusion of specific brain areas by single photon emission computed tomography (SPECT) in 9 men and 6 women before and after specifically defined olfactory interval stimulation with lavender water in both nostrils. The perfusion of certain brain areas increased significantly during the 10-min exposure period (e.g., +25 % in the gyrus rectus).

2.4.2.5 Treatment Studies (Aromatherapy)

While numerous studies have been conducted on the clinical pharmacology of lavender, so far only five controlled clinical studies have been published on the efficacy of lavender preparations in patients. Three of the studies involved the inhalation of lavender oil vapor in a room, and two involved the use of lavender oil in massage therapy.

Hardy et al. (1995) reported on a pilot study in four geriatric patients who suffered from insomnia. Patient 1 had been on 10 mg of temazepam for 1 year, patient 2 on 25 mg of promazine hydrochloride for 3 years, patient 3 had been taking 1 capsule of chlormethiazole for 7 months, and patient 4 had no prior medications. The sleep time of the four patients was measured for 6 weeks according to a fixed scheme: 2 weeks with premedication, 2 weeks without premedication, and 2 weeks with nighttime use of a lavender oil vaporizer. The sleep times of the four patients were significantly shorted by an average of 1 h during the 2 weeks without medication, but after the lavender therapy was started they returned to the values prior to discontinuation of the psychotropic drugs.

Dale und Cornwell (1994) reported on a controlled study in a total of 635 women during the postpartum period. For 10 days after childbirth, the patients received a faily full bath (initially at the hospital, later at home under the supervision of a midwife) with 6 drops of a volatile oil added to the bath water. To determine the effect on postpartum well-being, the women were randomly assigned to three groups of approximately equal size. The first group received natural lavender oil, the second a synthetic mixture of lavender-like odorants, the third an oil with a pure, volatile chemical compound. Two visual analog scales for the self-rating of daily discomfort and mood were used as a confirmatory parameter evaluating well-being. The results on day 5 with lavender oil were somewhat better than with the two synthetic oils, although the difference was not statistically significant. The results on the other days showed no intergroup differences in terms of well-being and mood.

A recent open study demonstrated more positive results of aromatherapy in women following childbirth. Over an 8-year period, a total of 8058 patients at a large obstetric hospital in England received combined aromatherapy in which lavender oil was only one of 10 essential oils that were used. Fifty percent of all the women in this study rated the aromatherapy as helpful, while 14 % rated it as unhelpful. A total of 100 women (1.2 %) reported adverse events (60 nausea, 15 itching, 13 headache, 9 precipitous labor) but did not believe that they were related to the aromatherapy (Burns et al., 2000).

Two randomized studies were done to investigate the effect of lavender oil massages in reducing levels of stress and anxiety in 12 patients (Buckle et al., 1993) and in 43 patients (Dunn et al., 1995). In the latter study, treatment with lavender oil resulted in significantly greater improvement than massage alone.

2.4.3.6 Indications, Dosage, and Risks

In its monograph on lavender flowers, Commission E described the indications for internal use as "mood disturbances such as restlessness or insomnia, functional abdominal complaints (nervous stomach irritations, Roehmheld syndrome, meteorism, nervous intestinal discomfort" (Blumenthal et al., 1998) recommending 1–2 teaspoons of dried herb per cup of tea or 1–4 drops of lavender oil (about 20–80 mg) taken with a sugar cube. An extract prepared from 100 g of dried flowers in 2 liters of hot water can be added to bath water for external use.

None of the clinical or clinical-pharmacologic studies cited here contain reports of adverse events that the investigators could relate to the lavender preparations. In the topical application of cosmetic preparations whose ingredients included lavender oil, three women aged 28, 71, and 76 years experienced a contact allergic reaction with dermatitis or mucosal inflammation. The inflammation cleared completely after the product was discontinued (Coulson and Khan, 1999; Varma et al., 2000). Available monographs and reviews on this subject (Anonymus, 1984; Hänsel et al., 1993; De Smet et al., 1993; Wolf, 1999; Blumenthal et al., 2000) conclude that lavender oil is safe to use. The U.S. Food and Drug Administration has classified *L. officinalis* as safe, including it in the list of substances "Generally Recognized as Safe" (GRAS) (Anonymus, 1975) and in the database of "Everything Added to Food in the United States" (EAFUS) (Anonymus, 2001).

2.4.2.7 Therapeutic Role

Both empirical medicine and the experimental and clinical studies cited above lend credence to the sedative and relaxing effects of lavender flowers and the lavender oil derived from them. Although it is reasonable to suppose that these effects are mediated by the olfactory receptors, the results of animal studies and the good lipid solubility of the lavender oil ingredients suggests that lavender may act directly on the central nervous system, even after oral administration. Corresponding studies have not yet been done in humans and should be conducted as soon as possible, especially since the efficacy of aromatherapy is difficult to evaluate due to methodologic problems. The studies to date suggest, however, that lavender oil may be effective in patients with anxiety disorders (Cooke und Ernst, 2000) and that lavender oil preparations could become a potential substitute for kava products, which are no longer available in Germany and several other countries.

2.4.3 Hops, Lemon Balm, Passion Flower

Monographs published by Commission E cite restlessness and sleep disturbances as the indications for treatment with hop strobiles, lemon balm leaves, passion flower, and lavender flowers (Blumenthal et al., 1998) (see Table 2.1). These indications are based on herbal tradition and empirical medicine. There have been no controlled clinical studies that can demonstrate efficacy in accordance with current standards. Available pharmacologic data are fragmentary and do not permit a definitive evaluation. Virtually no single-herb products are available for the indications stated above, although the four herbs and their extracts do occur as ingredients in numerous combination products.

2.4.3.1 Hop Strobiles and Hop Glands

While hops have been used in traditional European medicine as a tonic, diuretic, and aromatic bitter, the use of hops as a calmative is a more recent development. The fatigue- and sleep-promoting effects of hops were discovered when it was noticed that hop pickers tired easily, apparently due to the transfer of hop resin from their hands to their mouths (Tyler, 1987). But the assumption that hop resin has a sedative action when administered orally could not be confirmed by experimental studies (Hänsel and Wagener, 1967; Stocker, 1967). Hop-picker fatigue might be caused by inhaling the volatile oil of the hop plant, but ordinary extraction eliminates the volatile oil from the finished product.

Hop strobiles are the female flowers of the cultivated hop plant (*Humulus lupulus*, Fig. 2.23). They contain bitter principles including humulone and lupulone. These principles combine to form hop resin which occurs in 15–30 % concentration in the strobiles and 50–80 % in the hop glands (lupulin). The strobiles also contain up to 1 % volatile oil and up to 4 % tannins. Only the fresh dried herb contains these substances in full concentration. The bitter principles in particular beak down rapidly during storage, their concentration decreasing by 50–70 % in 6 months (Hänsel and Schulz, 1986).

Stored hops contain up to 0.15 % methylbutenol, which is too volatile to persist in hop extracts but may form there from bitter acids. In experiments with mice and rats, methylbutenol was found to have sedative properties when administered in high doses (Wohlfarth et al., 1983). Due to the volatility of methylbutenol, the only preparation that can contain active amounts of this principle is the hops pillow used in traditional folk medicine. Its concentration in extracts is probably much too low to be effective (Wohlfarth, 1983).

Fig. 2.23. ▶ Hops (*Humulus lupulus*).

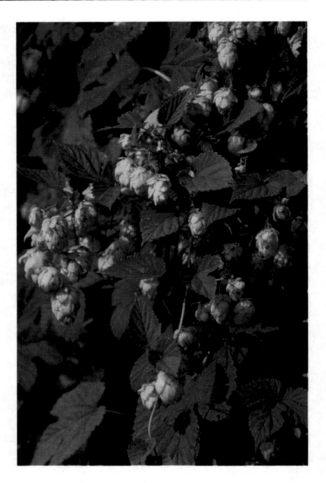

When lupulone and ethanol hop extract were tested in four pharmacologic models in mice (motor activity in an exercise wheel, locomotor activity in an exercise box, barbiturate-potentiating effects, tests on a rotating cylinder), oral doses of 10–500 mg/kg were found to have no demonstrable sedative effects (Hänsel and Wagener, 1967). Similar studies in 15 human subjects treated with 250 mg of a lipophilic hop concentrate for 5 days showed no sleep-inducing effects in any of the subjects tested (Stoker, 1967) (see Sect. 7.3).

Based on information currently available, there is no toxicologic risk associated with hops. The LD_{50} for orally administered hop extract or lupulones in mice is in the range of 500–3500 mg/kg (Hänsel et a., 1993).

The Commission E monograph of December 5, 1984, cites "discomfort due to restlessness or anxiety and sleep disturbances " as the indications for hops. The recommended dose is 0.5 g of the dried herb, or its equivalent in extract-based products, taken one to several times daily.

2.4.3.2 Lemon Balm Leaves

This herb consists of the dried leaves of the lemon balm plant (*Melissa officinalis*), which today is cultivated commercially. The leaves emit a fragrant lemony odor when bruised. They contain at least 0.05 % of a volatile oil whose main components are citronellal, geranial, and neral. Lemon balm leaves also contain phenol carboxylic acids, including about 4 % rosmarinic acid. Lemon balm oil is produced by steam distillation from fresh or dried herb gathered at the start of or during the flowering period. Citronellal, geranial, and neral together constitute about 50–75 % of lemon balm oil (Schultze et al., 1995). In the only experimental study to date on possible sedative effects, lemon balm oil was administered in doses of 3–100 mg/kg. Some effects were demonstrated (Wagner and Sprinkmeyer, 1973), but the absence of a dose-dependent response suggests that the effects were nonspecific.

The Commission E monograph of December 5, 1984, cites "nervous sleeping disorders and functional gastrointestinal complaints" as the indications for balm leaves and preparations made from them (Blumenthal et al., 1998. The recommended single dose is 1.5–4.5 g of the dried herb.

2.4.3.3 Passion Flower

Passion flower consists of the dried, leafy aerial parts, which may include the flowers and young fruits, of *Passiflora incarnata*, a tropical climbing vine native to southern North America. The main constituents of passiflora are flavonoids (up to 2.5 %), coumarin, and umbeliferone. The occurrence of harmala alkaloids, once considered responsible for the effects of the herb, has been disputed (Koch and Steinegger, 1980).

Extracts of passion flower were found to reduce spontaneous locomotor activity in mice and prolong their sleep when administered by the oral and intraperitoneal routes (Speroni and Minghetti, 1988). In one study, an aqueous extract from *P. edulis* produced a hypnotic sedative effect in human subjects but also showed signs of hepatotoxicity and pancreatotoxicity (Maluf et al., 1991). There have been no controlled therapeutic studies with single-herb preparations based on extracts from P. Mayer (1995) reviewed the pharmaceutical quality, constituents, and pharmacologic testing of this herb.

Commission E, in its monograph of November 30, 1985, described the indications for passion flower as states of nervous unrest and recommended an average daily dose of 4–8 g of dried herb or its equivalent in passiflora preparations (Blumenthal et al., 1998).

2.4.4 Sedative Teas

Sedative teas, known also as nerve teas or slumber teas, are most commonly prepared from valerian root, hop strobiles, or balm leaves. Herbs containing volatile oils are frequently used as additives, e. g., chamomile flowers, lavender flowers, orange blossoms, peppermint leaves, and bitter orange peel. Chamomile is widely regarded as a mild calmative and sleep-aid in England and the U. S., where it enjoys almost the same status as valerian does in Germany.

The tea formula listed in the *German Pharmacopeia* 6th edition contains the bitter leaf bogbean (*Menyanthes trifoliata*) as a major ingredient (40 %). It might be asked how an appetite-stimulating bitter herb could contribute to the efficacy of a sedative tea. For centuries, Europeans have considered bitter-tasting herbs to have general beneficial effects on health, almost equating the efficacy of a medicine with its bitterness. This deeply rooted cultural attitude may have heightened the psychological readiness of the user to believe in the hypnogenic potency of the tea. Of course, the possibility that future clinical trials may determine that bitter herbs have a sedative action on the central nervous system cannot be ruled out; However, such a general statement may be a bit simplistic, as bitter principles in various herbs may be combined with compounds with a CNS stimulating or a CNS sedating activities.

A handbook issued by the Drug Approval and Pharmacopeia, Commission in France lists the following herbs used in the treatment of nervousness and mild sleep disturbances: valerian root, black horehound (*Ballota foetida*), hop strobiles, corn poppy flowers, lavender flowers, linden flowers, balm leaves, passion flower, bitter orange leaves, bitter orange flowers, woodruff, hawthorn flowers, and lemon verbena leaves (*Aloysia triphylla*).

Tea Formulations

Indications: nervousness, difficulty falling asleep.

Preparation and dosing guidelines: Pour boiling water (about 150 mL) over 1 tablespoon of tea, cover and steep for about 10 min, then pass through a tea strainer. Drink 1 cup of freshly made tea 2 or 3 times during the day and before bedtime.

Directions to patient: One heaping tablespoon per cup (about 150 mL) of tea 2 or 3 times daily and before going t bed.

Nerve tea formula in German Pharmacopeia 6		
Rx	Bogbean leaves	40.0
	Peppermint leaves	30.0
	Valerian root	30.0
	Prepare tea	
	Directions to patient (see above)	

Nerve tea formula in Swiss Pharmacopeia 6		
Rx	Valerian root	25.0
	Orange blossoms	20.0
	Passion flower	20.0
	Crushed aniseed	15.0
	Balm leaves	10.0
	Peppermint leaves	10.0

Nerve tea formula in German Pharmacopeia 7

Rx	Valerian root	50.0
	Balm leaves	25.0
	Peppermint leaves	25.0

Nerve tea formula in Austrian Pharmacopeia 9

RX	Valerian root	60.0
	Balm leaves	10.0
	Peppermint leaves	10.0
	Orange blossoms	10.0
	Bitter orange peel	10.0

2.4.5 Drug Products

The *Rote Liste 2003* lists under the heading of "Sedatives and Hypnotics" 15 single-herb valerian products, one product each based on balm and passion flower, 16 two-herb products containing valerian and hops, and 42 multiherb combinations that contain valerian along with at least two other medicinal herbs.

Based on currently available information, *Valeriana officinalis* is the only species that should be used in official valerian preparations. These products should be produced according to approved standards, and their efficacy should be tested by therapeutic studies. They should contain an adequate amount of the active principle (see Sect. 2.4.1.6). Products with a high content of valepotriates should no longer be used because of their potential toxicity (see Sect. 2.4.1.4).

 References

Albrecht M, Berger W, Laux P; Schmidt U, Martin C (1995) Psychopharmaka und Verkehrssicherheit. Der Einfluß von Euvegalforte auf die Fahrtüchtigkeit und Kombinationswirkungen mit Alkohol. Z Allg Med 71: 1215-1225.

Anonymus (1975) Safe and unsafe herbs in herbal teas. Department of Health Education and Welfare. Public Health Service. FDA, Wasington DC.

Anonymus (1984) Monographie *Lavandulae flos* (Lavendelblüten) Banz 228 vom 5.12.1984.

Anonymus (2001) FDA/CFSAN/OPA: EAFUS List. *http://vm.cfsan.fda.gov/dms/eafus.html*.

Aoshima H, Hamamoto K (1999) Potentiation of GABA-A receptors expressed in *Xenopus* oocytes by perfume and phytoncid. Biosci Biotechnol Biochem 63: 743-748.

Atanassova-Shopova S, Roussinov KS (1970) On certain central neurotropic effects of lavender essential oil. Bull Inst Physiol 8: 69-76.

Balderer G, Borbély AA (1985) Effect of valerian on human sleep. Psychopharmacol 87: 406-409.

Blumenthal M, Hall T, Goldberg A et al. The ABC Clinical Guide to Herbs. Austin, TX: American Botanical Council, 2003.

Blumenthal M, Goldberg A, Brinckmann J (2000) Herbal Medicine. Expanded Commission E Monographs. American Botanical Council, Austin, USA, pp. 226-229.

Blumenthal M, Busse WR, Goldberg A, Gruenwald J, Hall T, Riggins CW, Rister RS (eds.). Klein S,

Rister RS (trans). (1998) The Complete German Commission E Monographs – Therapeutic Guide to Herbal Medicines. American Botanical Council, Austin, Texas. *www.herbalgram.org.*

Bos R, Hendriks H, Scheffer JJC, Woerdenbag HJ (1998) Cytotoxic potential of valerian constituents and valerian tinctures. Phytomedicine 5 (3): 219–225.

Bos R, Woerdenbag HJ, van Putten FMS, Hendriks H, Scheffer JJC (1998) Seasonal variation of the essential oil, valerenic acid and derivatives, and valepotriates in *Valeriana officinalis* roots and rhizomes, and the selection of plants suitable for phytomedicines. Planta Med 64: 143–147.

Bounthanh C, Bergmann C, Beck JP, Haag-Berrurier M, Anton R (1981) Valepotriates, a new class of cytotoxic and antitumor agents. Planta Med 41: 21–28.

Bradshaw RH, Marchant JN, Meredith MJ, Broom DM (1998) Effects of lavender straw on stress and travel sickness in pigs. Journal of Alternative and Complementary Medicine 4: 271–275.

Brand G, Millot JL, Henquell D (1999) Olfaction and hemispheric asymmetry: unilateral stimulation and bilateral electrodermal recordings. Neuropsychobiology 39: 160–164.

Braun R, Dieckmann H, Machut M, Echarti C, Maurer HR (1986) Untersuchungen zum Einfluß von Baldrianalen auf hämatopoetische Zellen in vitro, auf die metabolische Aktivität der Leber in vivo sowie zum Gehalt in Fertigarzneimitteln. Planta Med: 446–450.

Braun R, Dittmar W, Machut M, Weickmann S (1982) Valepotriate mit Epoxidstruktur – beachtliche Alkylantien. Dtsch Apoth Z 122:1109–1113.3.

Braun R, Dittmar W, von der Hude W, Scheutwinkel-Reich M (1985) Bacterial mutagenicity of the tranquilizing constituents of valerianaceae roots. Naunyn- Schmiedeberg's Arch Pharmacol Suppl 329: R 28.

Buchbauer G (1996) Aromatherapie: Methoden der Erforschung. Deutsche Apotheker Zeitung 136: 2939–2944.

Buchbauer G, Jirovet L, Jäger W, Dietrich H, Plank C, Karamat E (1991) Aromatherapy: evidence for sedative effects of the essential oil of lavender after inhalation. Z Naturforsch 46 c: 1067–1072.

Buckle J (1993) Aromatherapy: does it matter which lavender EO is used? Nurs Times 89: 32–35.

Burns EE, Blamey C, Ersser SJ, Barnetson L, Lloyd AJ (2000) An investigation into the use of aromatherapy in intrapartum midwifery practice. Journal of Alternative and Complementary Medicine 6: 141–147.

Cavadas C, Araujo I, Cotrim MD, Amarai T, Cunha AP, Macedo T, Fontes Ribeiro C (1995) In vitro study on the interaction of Valeriana officinalis L. extracts and their amino acids on GABAA receptor in rat brain. Arzneim.-Forsch/Drug Res 45 (II): 753–755.

Cavanagh HMA, Wilkinson JM (2002) Biological activities of lavender essential oil. Phytother Res 16: 301–308.

Cooke B, Ernst E (2000) Aromatherapy: a systematic review. Brit J General Practice 50: 493–496.

Coulson ICH, Khan ASA (1999) Facial "pillow" dermatitis due to lavender oil allergy. Contact Dermatitis 41: 111.

Dale A, Cornwell S (1994) The role of lavender oil in relieving perineal discomfort following childbirth: a blind randomized clinical trial. J Adv Nurs 19: 89–96.

De Smet PAGM, Keller K, Hänsel R, Chandler RF (1993) Adverse effects of herbal drugs. Springer, Berlin Heidelberg New York, pp. 8–12.

Degel J, Köster EP (1999) Odors: implicit memory and performance effects. Chem Senses 24: 317–325.

Di Nardo W, Di Girolamo S, Galli A et al. (2000) Olfactory function evaluated by SPECT. Am J Rhinol 14: 57–61

Dieckmann H (1988) Untersuchungen zur Pharmakokinetik, Metabolismus und Toxikologie von Baldrianalen. Inauguraldissertation, Freie Universität Berlin.

Diego MA, Jones NA, Field T et al. (1998) Aromatherapy positively affects mood, EEG patterns of alertness, and math computations. Int J Neuro Sci 96: 217–234.

Donath F, Quispe S, Diefenbach K, Maurer A, Fietze I, Roots I (2000) Critical evaluation of the effect of valerian extract on sleep structure and sleep quality. Pharmacopsychiat 33: 47–53.

Dorn M (2000) Wirksamkeit und Verträglichkeit von Baldrian versus Oxazepam bei nichtorganischen und nichtpsychiatrischen Insomnien: Eine randomisierte, doppelblinde, klinische Vergleichsstudie. Forsch Komplementärmed Klass Naturheilkd 7: 79–84.

Dreßing H, Köhler S, Müller WE (1996) Verbesserung der Schlafqualität mit einem hochdosierten Baldrian-Melisse-Präparat. Eine placebokontrollierte Doppelblindstudie. Psychopharmakotherapie 3: 124-130.

Dreßing H, Riemann D, Löw H, Schredl M, Reh C, Laux P, Müller WE (1992) Bei Schlafstörungen gleichwertig? Baldrian-Melisse-Kombination versus Benzodiazepin. Therapiewoche 42: 726-736.

Dunn C, Sleep J, Collett D (1995) Sensing an improvement: an experimental study to evaluate the use of aromatherapy, massage and periods of rest in an intensive care unit. J Adv Nursing 21: 34-40.

Eickstedt KW v, Rahmann R (1969) Psychopharmakologische Wirkungen von Valepotriaten. Arzneim-Forsch 19: 316-319.

ESCOP (2003) Monographs on the medicinal uses of plant drugs, Valerianae radix. Thieme Stuttgart New York, 2003.

Fehri B, Aiache JM, Boukef K, Memmi A, Hizaoui B (1991) Valeriana officinalis et Crataegus oxyacantha: Toxicité par administrations réitérées et investigations pharmacologiques. J Pharm Bel 46: 165-176.

Fink C (1982) Analytik, Pharmakokinetik und pharmakologische Wirkung der Valepotriate unter besonderer Berücksichtigung des Valtrats. Dissertation, Universität Marburg.

Francis AJP, Dempster RJW (2002) Effect of valerian, Valeriana edulis, on sleep difficulties in children with intellectual deficits: randomized trial. Phytomedicine 9: 273-9.

Fröhlich E (1968) Lavendelöl: Übersicht der klinischen, pharmakologischen und bakteriologischen Studien. Wien Med Wochenschr 118: 345-350.

Gauler TC, Weihrauch TR (1997) Placebo – Ein wirksames und ungefährliches Medikament? Urban + Schwarzenberg, Munich, Vienna, Baltimore.

Gerhard U, Ninnenbrink N, Georghiadou Ch, Hobi V (1996) Effects of two plant-based sleep remedies on Vigilance. Schweiz Rsch Med 85: 473-481.

Geßner B, Klasser, M (1984) Untersuchung der Wirkung von Harmonicum Much® auf den Schlaf mit Hilfe polygraphischer EEG-Aufzeichnungen. Z EEG-EMG 15: 45-51.

Grusla D (1987) Nachweis der Wirkung eines Baldrianextraktes im Rattenhirn mit der 14C-2-Desoxyglucose-Technik. Dissertation, Phillipps-Universität, Marburg.

Guillemain J, Rousseau A, Delaveau P (1989) Effets neurodépresseurs de l'huile essentielle de Lavandula angustifolia Mill. Ann Pharmaceutique Francaises 47: 337-343.

Hänsel R (1984) Bewertung von Baldrian-Präparaten: Differenzierung wesentlich. Dtsch Apoth Z 124: 2085.

Hänsel R, Keller K, Rimpler H, Schneider G (1993) Hagers Handbuch der Pharmazeutischen Praxis. Drogen E-O, 5th edition. Springer Verlag Berlin Heidelberg: 455.

Hänsel R, Keller K, Rimpler H, Schneider G (1993) Hagers Handbuch der Pharmazeutischen Praxis. Drogen E-O, 5th edition. Springer Verlag Berlin Heidelberg; pp. 630-644.

Hänsel R, Keller K, Rimpler H, Schneider G (1994) Hagers Handbuch der Pharmazeutischen Praxis. Drogen P-Z, 5th edition. Springer Verlag Berlin Heidelberg: 1067-1095.

Hänsel R, Schulz J (1982) Valerensäuren und Valerenal als Leitstoffe des offizinellen Baldrians. Dtsch Apoth Z 122: 215-219.

Hänsel R, Wagener HH (1967) Versuche, sedativ-hypnotische Wirkstoffe im Hopfen nachzuweisen. Arzneim Forsch/Drug Res 17: 79-81.

Hardy M, Kirk-Smith MD, Stretch DD (1995) Replacement of drug treatment for insomnia by ambient odour. Lancet 346: 701.

Hazelhoff B (1984) Phytochemical and Pharmacological Aspects of Valeriana compounds. Dissertation, Universität Groningen.

Hendriks H, Bos R, Woerdenbag HJ, Koster AS (1985) Central nervous depressant activity of valerenic acid in the mouse. Planta Med 51: 28-31.

Hiller KO, Zetler G (1996) Neuropharmacological studies on ethanol extracts of Valeriana officinalis L.: behavioural and anticonvulsant properties. Phytother Res 10: 145-151.

Jager W, Buchbauer G, Jirovetz L, Fritzer M (1992) Percutaneous absorption of lavender oil from a massage oil. J Soc Cosmet Chem 43: 49-54.

Jansen W (1977) Doppelblindstudie mit Baldrisedon. Therapiewoche 27: 2779-2786.

Jirovetz L, Buchbauer G, Jäger W et al. (1990) Determination of lavender oil fragrance compounds in blood samples. Fresenius Z Anal Chem 338: 922–923.

Kamm-Kohl AV, Jansen W, Brockmann P (1984) Moderne Baldriantherapie gegen nervöse Störungen im Senium. Med Welt 35: 1450–1454.

Karamat E, Ilmberger J, Buchbauer C, Rößlhuber K, Rupp C (1992) Excitatory and sedative effects of essential oils on the human reaction time performance. Chemical Senses 17: 847.

Koch H, Steinegger E (1980) Untersuchungen zur Alkaloid- und Flavonoidführung von Passiflora-Arten. Vortrag, gehalten auf dem Intern Research Congress on Natural Products, Straßburg 1980. Publiziert in den Abstracts of Posters.

Kohlert C, Rensen IV, März R, Schindler G, Graefe EU, Veit M (2000) Bioavailability and pharmacokinetics of natural volatile terpenes in animals and humans. Planta Med 66: 495–505.

Kohnen R, Oswald WD (1988) The effects of valerian, Propranolol, and their combination on activation, performance, and mood of healthy volunteers under social stress conditions. Pharmacopsychiatry 21: 447–448.

Krieglstein J, Grusla D (1988) Zentraldämpfende Inhaltsstoffe im Baldrian. Dtsch Apoth Z 128: 2041–2046.

Kuhlmann J, Berger W, Podzuweit H, Schmidt U (1999) The influence of valerian treatment on reaction time, alertness and concentration in volunteers. Pharmacopsychiat 32: 235–241.

Leathwood PD, Chauffard F (1983) Quantifying the effects of mild sedatives. J Psychiat Res 17: 115–122.

Leathwood PD, Chauffard F (1985) Aqueous extract of valerian reduces latency to fall asleep in man. Planta Med 51: 144–148.

Leuschner J, Müller J, Rudmann M (1993) Characterisation of the Central Nervous Depressant Activity of a Commercially Available Valerian Root Extract. Arzneim-Forsch/Drug Res 43 (I): 638–641.

Lis Balchin M (Ed.) (2002) Lavender – The genus Lavandula. Taylor & Francis, London and New York, 2002.

Lis-Balchin M, Deans S, Eaglesham E (1998) Relationship between bioactivity and chemical composition of commercial essential oil. Flavour Fragr J 13: 98–104.

Lis-Balchin M, Hart S (1999) Studies on the mode of action of essential oil lavender (Lavandula angustifolia P. Miller). Phytother Res 13:540–2.

Maluf E, Barros HMT, Frochtengarten ML, Benti R, Leite JR (1991) Assessment of the hypnotic/sedative effects and toxicity of Passiflora edulis aqueous extract in rodents and humans. Phytother Res 5: 262–266.

Meier B (1995) Passiflorae herba – pharmazeutische Qualität. Z Phytother 16: 90–99.9.

Motomura N, Sakurai A, Yotsuya Y (1998) A psychophysiological study of lavender odorant. Memoirs of Osaka Kyoiku University III/47: 281–287.

Ortiz JG (1999) Effects of Valeriana officinalis extracts on sup(3)H)flunitrazepam binding, synaptosomal sup(3)H)GABA uptake, and hippocampal sup(3)H)GABA release. Neurochem Res 24: 1373–8.

Riedel E, Hänsel R, Ehrke G (1982) Hemmung des Gamma-Aminobuttersäureabbaus durch Valerensäurederivate. Planta Med 46: 219–220.

Romine IJ, Bush AM, Geist CR (1999) Lavender aromatherapy in recovery from exercise. Perceptual and Motor Skills 88: 756–758.

Rosecrans JA, Defeo JJ, Youngken HWjr (1961) Pharmacological investigation of certain Valeriana officinalis L. extracts. J Pharm Sci 50: 240–244.

Rücker G, Tautges J, Sieek A, Wenzel H, Graf E (978) Untersuchungen zur Isolierung und pharmakodynamischen Aktivität des Sesquiterpens Valeranon aus Nardostrachys jatamansi DC. Arzneim-Forsch/Drug Res 28: 7.

Saeki Y (2000) The effect of foot-bath with or without lavender essential oil on the autonomic nervous system: a randomized trial. Complementary Therapies in Medicine 8: 2–7.

Santos MS, Ferreira F, Cunha AP et al. (1994) An aqueous extract of valerian influences the transport of GABA in synaptosomes. Planta Med. 60: 278–279.

Schultze W, König WA, Hilkert A, Richter R (1995) Melissenöle. Dtsch Apoth Z 135: 557–577.

Schulz H, Jobert M, Hübner WD (1998) The quantitative EEG as a screening instrument to identify sedative effects of single doses of plant extracts in comparison with diazepam.

Phytomedicine 5: 449–458.

Schulz H, Stolz C, Müller J (1994) The effect of a valerian extract on sleep polygraphy in poor sleepers. A pilot study. Pharmacopsychiat 27: 147–151.

Schulz V (2000) The psychodynamic and pharmacodynamic effects of drugs: A differentiated evaluation of the efficacy of phytotherapy. Phytomedicine 7: 73–81.

Speroni E, Minghetti A (1988) Neuropharmacological activity of extracts from Passiflora incarnata. Planta Med: 488–491.

Stevinson C, Ernst E (2000) Valerian for insomnia: a systematic review of randomized clinical trials. Sleep Medicine 1: 91–99.

Stocker HR (1967) Sedative und hypnogene Wirkung des Hopfens. Schweizer Brauerei Rundschau 78: 80–89.

Sugawara Y, Hara C, Aoki T, Sugimoto N, Masujima T (2000) Odor distinctiveness between enantiomers of linalool: difference in perception and responses elicited by sensory test and forehead surface potential wave measurement. Chem Senses 25: 77–84.

Sugawara Y, Hara C, Tamura K et al. (1998) Sedative effect on humans of inhalation of essential oil of linalool: sensory evaluation and physiological measurements using optically active linalools. Analytica Chimica Acta 365: 293–299.

Torii S, Fukuda H, Kanemoto H, Miyanchi R, Hamauzu Y, Kawasaki M (1988) Contingent negative variation (CNV) and the psychological effects of odour. In: Van Toller St, Dodd GH (eds) Perfumery, The Psychology and Biology of Fragrance. Chapman and Hall, London New York: 107–146.

Tufik S (1985) Effects of prolonged administration of valepotriates in rats on the mothers and their offspring. J Ethnopharmacol 87: 39–44.

Tyler VE (1987) The New Honest Herbal. A Sensible Guide to Herbs and Related Remedies. 2nd ed Stickley Co., Philadelphia: 125–126.

Varma S, Blackford S, Statham BN, Blackwell A (2000) Combined contact allergy to tea tree oil and lavender oil complicating chronic vulvovaginitis. Contact Dermatitis 42: 309.

Vernet-Maury E, Alaoui-Ismaili Q, Dittmar A, Delhomme G, Chanel J (1999) Basic emotions induced by odorants: a new approach based on autonomic pattern results. J Autonomic Nervous System 75: 176–183.

Von der Hude W, Scheutwinkel-Reich M, Braun R (1986) Bacterial mutagenicity of the tranquilizing constituents of Valerianaceae roots. Mutation Res 169: 23–27.

von Skramlik E (1959) Über die Giftigkeit und Verträglichkeit von ätherischen Ölen. Pharmazie 14: 435–445.

Vonderheid-Guth B, Todorova A, Brattström A, Dimpfel W (2000) Pharmacodynamic effects of valerian and hops extract combination (ZE 91019) on the quantitative-topographical EEG in healthy volunteers. Eur J Med Res 5: 139–144.

Vorbach EU, Görtelmeyer R, Brüning J (1996) Therapie von Insomnien: Wirksamkeit und Verträglichkeit eines Baldrian-Präparates. Psychopharmakotherapie 3: 109–115.

Wagner H, Jurcic K (1980 b) In vitro- und in vivo-Metabolismus von 14C-Didrovaltrat. Planta Med 38: 366–376.

Wagner H, Sprinkmeyer L (1973) Dtsch Apoth Z 113: 1159. Zitiert nach: Koch- Heitzmann I, Schültze W (1984) Melissa officinalis. Eine alte Arzneipflanze mit neuen therapeutischen Wirkungen. Dtsch Apoth Z 124: 2137–2145.

Willey LB, Mady SP, Cobaugh DJ, Wax PM (1995) Valerian overdose: a case report. Vet Human Toxicol 37, 364–365.

Wohlfart R, Hänsel R, Schmidt H (1983) Nachweis sedativ-hypnotischer Wirkstoffe im Hopfen. 4. Mittlg. Die Pharmakologie des Hopfeninhaltsstoffes 2-Methyl-3-buten-2-ol. Planta Med 48: 120–123.

Wohlfart R, Wurm G, Hänsel R, Schmidt H (1983) Der Abbau der Bittersäuren zum 2-Methyl-3-buten-2-ol, einem Hopfeninhaltsstoff mit sedativ-hypnotischer Wirkung. Arch Pharmaz 315: 132–137.

Wolf A (1999) Essential oil poisoning. Clinical Toxicology 37: 721–727.

Yamada K, Mimaki Y, Sashida Y (1994) Anticonvulsive effects of inhaling lavender oil vapour. Biol Pharm Bull 17: 359–360.

3 Cardiovascular System

Phytomedicines play a significant role in the treatment of mild forms of heart failure and coronary insufficiency, in the prevention and treatment of atherosclerosis and its sequelae, and in the symptomatic treatment of chronic venous insufficiency. There are only a few herbal preparations, however, for which safety and efficacy have been adequately proven: hawthorn leaf and flower extract (heart failure and coronary insufficiency), garlic (atherosclerosis), ginkgo extract (peripheral arterial occlusive disease), and horse chestnut extract (chronic venous insufficiency). Therefore, the bulk of this chapter is devoted to these four herbs and their preparations. The closing sections deal briefly with other preparations, including herbs that contain cardioactive digitaloids and herbal remedies for angina pectoris, cardiac arrhythmias, and hypertension and hypotension.

3.1 Heart Failure and Coronary Insufficiency

The classic remedies used to treat myocardial insufficiency are the cardiac glycosides derived from purple and Grecian foxglove (*Digitalis* spp.). These compounds are colorless, bitter-tasting substances that cause local irritation. Their chemical compositions are known, and they can be synthetically produced, but for economic reasons the 14 pure glycosides or their precursors are still obtained by extraction from digitalis leaf. Because the cardiac glycosides are specific, identifiable chemical compounds that have a narrow therapeutic dose range (see Sect.1.5.5), they are not considered phytotherapeutic agents and are outside the realm of herbal medicine. Galenic preparations made from digitalis leaves are obsolete in modern pharmacotherapy. Details on the pure glycosides and their actions can be found in textbooks of pharmacology.

3.1.1 Hawthorn

3.1.1.1 Introduction

Hawthorn (*Crataegus* spp., Fig. 3.1) is a proven, established remedy for heart ailments and circulatory disorders. Apparently, the animal kingdom also benefits from the hawthorn, as illustrated by the following anecdote. In 1966, Klatt (quoted in Weiss, 1991) reported his observations on gypsy moths. For purposes of genetic research, Klatt had been inbreeding the moths for some time while feeding them their usual diet of alder leaves. Within a few years the insects showed retarded development, aged prematurely, and laid fewer eggs. The death of the entire colony seemed likely as a result of degeneration due to inbreeding. By chance, Klatt met a butterfly breeder who recommended feeding the insects hawthorn leaves instead of alder leaves. The colony recovered. The moths became larger and stronger and resumed normal egg-laying within a few months.

Weiss (1991), in a commentary on this study, emphasized that a positive response appeared only after the whole herb (leaf) had been fed continuously for a period of several weeks. As swimming tests in rats have shown, a single dose of hawthorn does not have immediate discernible effects. A similar link between therapeutic efficacy and duration of use appears to exist in cardiac patients. The only acute effects seen after a single hawthorn dose in humans were changes in parameters having little clinical relevance (Fischer et al., 1994). A 4- to 8-week course of treatment is necessary to provide

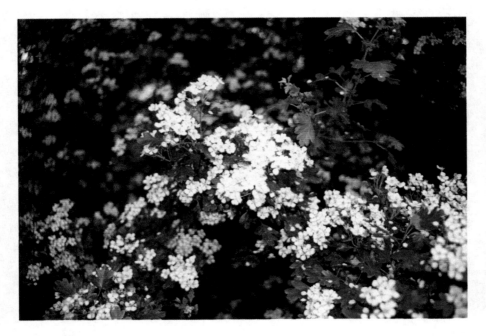

Fig. 3.1. ▲ Flowering branch of hawthorn (*Crataegus* species).

significant improvement in subjective complaints and exercise tolerance (Tauchert and Loew, 1995).

3.1.1.2 Medicinal Plant

Hawthorn is a member of the family Rosaceae, but the unpleasant aroma of its blossoms attracts only flies. The tall shrubs are distributed throughout Europe and America, growing at elevations up to 1600 m above sea level. They prefer hillsides and sunny slopes. The name of the plant derives from its fruits, or haws, and its sharp thorns. Only the white-blooming hawthorn is used therapeutically; the red-blooming garden variety of hawthorn has no recognized medicinal uses.

3.1.1.3 Crude Drug and Extract

Herbs of the species *Crataegus monogyna* and *C. oxyacantha* are used in the production of hawthorn-based medicines. Therapeutic efficacy has been most reliably documented for hawthorn leaves and flowers. The *German Pharmacopeia* (DAB 1996) describes the crude drug as consisting of the dried tops (about 7 cm long) of the flowering shrub. The dried herb has a faint, distinctive fragrance and a slightly bitter or astringent taste. A fixed combination of hawthorn flowers, leaves, and fruits has also been recognized as having therapeutic efficacy. By themselves, the dried berry-like fruits (haws) have a sweet mealy or mucilaginous taste.

The revised 1994 Commission E monograph on the hawthorn recognizes two water-and-alcohol extracts of dried hawthorn leaves with flowers (herb-to-extract ratio 4–7:1) and the fixed combination mentioned above as having therapeutic efficacy (Blumenthal et al., 1998). Efficacy is presumed likely for other preparations, especially the liquid extract described in DAB 1996 and alcoholic extracts made from leaves or flowers alone, but this has not yet been firmly established by double-blind clinical studies.

3.1.1.4 Key Constituents, Analysis, Pharmacokinetics

The main constituents that have been isolated from hawthorn are flavonoids, procyanidins, catechins, triterpenoids, aromatic carboxylic acids, amino and purine derivatives, and various other compounds (Hänsel et al., 1992). The key constituents for testing pharmaceutical quality are the flavonoids, calculated as hyperoside according to DAB 1996, and the oligomeric procyanidins, calculated as epicatechin. At present there are standard analytic methods for determining the flavonoids in hawthorn but not the oligomeric procyanidins (Sticher et al., 1994). The flavonoids content of the crude drug is approximately 1 % for the leaves and flowers but only about 0.1 % for the berries. The content of oligomeric procyanidins in the leaves and flowers is believed to be approximately 1–3 % (Kreimeyer, 1997). The Commission E monograph recommends a daily dose of 160–900 mg hawthorn extract with a designated content of flavonoids (4–30 mg) or oligomeric procyanidins (30–160 mg) (Blumenthal et al., 1998). Kaul (1998) has reviewed more than 250 references in the scientific literature, giving particular attention to studies dealing with the pharmaceutical quality and pharmacology of hawthorn preparations. A further review was published by the *American Herbal Pharmacopoeia*

(Upton, 1999). The pharmacokinetics and bioavailability of the flavonol quercetin was reviewed and studied in humans by Graefe et al. (1999).

3.1.1.5 Pharmacology

The cardiovascular effects of hawthorn have been described in a number of original works. Most studies have dealt with aqueous and alcoholic extracts as well as various fractions and constituents. The older studies were summarized in three survey works (Ammon and Händel, 1981 a–c). Summaries of more recent pharmacologic studies on hawthorn may be found in Siegel and Casper (1995) and in Kaul (1998).

In vitro studies of hawthorn effects on myocardial contractility have been done in isolated frog heart, isolated guinea pig heart (Langendorff preparation), and isolated atria, and in vivo studies have been done in anesthetized cats and dogs. All studies showed an increased amplitude of myocardial contractions and an increase in stroke volume. An increase in coronary blood flow was also demonstrated in isolated guinea pig heart. Studies in various anesthetized species have consistently shown a decrease in heart rate, although an increase was observed in isolated guinea pig heart.

Important results are available from studies on models of myocardial ischemia in rats (Krzeminski and Chatterjee, 1993), isolated rat myocardial cells (Pöpping et al., 1995), human coronary arteries (Siegel et al., 1994), and isolated perfused guinea pig heart (Joseph et al., 1995; Al Makdessi et al., 1996 and 1999).

The antiarrhythmic effects of an extract made from hawthorn leaves and flowers were tested in an ischemic model in rats (left coronary artery ischemia for 7 min, then reperfusion for 15 min). Reperfusion-induced ventricular fibrillation occurred in 88 % of the animals in the control group but in less than 20 % of the animals that had received 0.5 mg/kg or 5 mg/kg of the hawthorn extract. Significant reductions were also seen in the duration of fibrillations and the occurrence of tachycardia. The same model was used to study the effect of 100 mg/kg of the extract, administered orally for 6 days, on lethality, fibrillations, tachycardia, and CPK elevation. Reperfusion in the control group was followed by a precipitous fall in blood pressure; only 8 of the 16 animals survived, and all survivors had ventricular fibrillations. The animals treated with hawthorn had no hypotensive crises, and all survived with no episodes of ventricular fibrillation. The differences were statistically significant (Kurcok, 1992; Krzeminski and Chatterjee, 1993).

An isolated rat heart model was used to investigate the effects of 3 months' preliminary treatment with a hawthorn extract (2 % in standard feed) on the release of lactate dehydrogenase (LDH) during coronary ischemia and subsequent reperfusion. The rise in LDH levels during the reperfusion phase was significantly lower in the hawthorn group (p<0.01) than in the control group. The authors interpreted this as a cardioprotective effect with the stabilization of membrane structures (Makdessi et al., 1996). The results of Chatterjee et al. (1997) indicate that oligomeric procyanidins, as orally active constituents of hawthorn extract, may play a significant role in the cardioprotective effect of hawthorn.

One group was unable to confirm the preventive effect of hawthorn extract on ischemia- and reperfusion-induced arrhythmia in studies of rat hearts in situ and in Langendorff preparations. Seventeen rats were fed with 0.5 g/kg hawthorn extract daily for 8 weeks. The left anterior descending coronary artery was ligated for 20 min and subsequently reperfused. The hawthorn extract did not affect either the latent period to the onset of arrhythmias or the intensity of the arrhythmias compared with the untreated control group (Rothfuss et al., 2001).

In one study, hawthorn extract increased the amplitude and duration of isolated rat myocardial cell contractions within a few minutes after exposure. The effect began at extract concentrations of 30 g/mL and rose steadily as the concentration was increased to about 120 g/mL (Fig. 3.2). Calculations show that achieving this effect in an adult patient would require a daily dose of 600–900 mg, based on the assumption that the active principle is distributed in an extracellular volume of approximately 15–20 L (Pöpping et al., 1995). At concentrations of 90–180 µg/mL, the extract significantly lengthened the apparent refractory period from 144 min to 420 min (Fig. 3.3). This effect, which occurred even after prior stimulation of the cells with isoproterenol, is opposite to that of cardiac glycosides which shorten the refractory period. This difference is particularly striking when it is noted that agents with a positive inotropic action are generally arrhythmogenic while antiarrhythmic agents are negatively inotropic. Hawthorn extract is unique in that it is positively inotropic but appears to stabilize the heart rhythm (Pöpping et al., 1995).

The known ability of hawthorn to increase coronary blood flow was tested in isolated human coronary arteries. Wall forces and membrane potentials were measured in normal vascular segments and in atherosclerotic segments taken from heart transplants. Both parameters changed roughly in proportion to the concentration of the

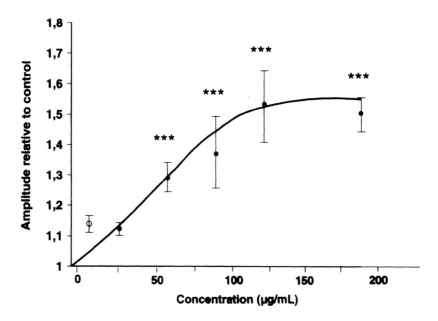

Fig. 3.2. ▲ Concentration-dependent effect of hawthorn extract on the amplitude of the contraction of isolated heart cells. The error bars indicate standard deviation from the mean (*** = p < 0.001; t-test for independent random samples) (Pöpping et al, 1995).

active principle. The degree of vascular relaxation was 14 % of the resting tonus in the normal arteries and 8 % in the arteries with atherosclerotic lesions (Siegel et al., 1994; Siegel and Casper, 1995; Siegel et al., 1996). In experiments on isolated Langendorff rat hearts perfused at a constant pressure, the hawthorn extract WS 1442 (1 to 10 µg/mL) produced a dose-dependent increase in coronary blood flow by up to 100 %. The flow increase was maximal at approximately 2 min, and the flow rate was still elevated at 60 min. Studies indicate an endothelium-dependent relaxation of the coronary vessels due to the stimulation of endothelial NO (nitric oxide) release and the inhibition of NO breakdown by the extract (Koch 2000).

Comparative studies were conducted in isolated perfused guinea pig hearts (Langendorff preparations) to study the effects of various inotropic agents – epinephrine (EPI), amrinone (AM), milrinone (MIL), digoxin (DIG), and hawthorn leaf and flower extract (CRA) – on selected functional parameters. Simultaneous recording of contractile force, spontaneous heart rate, AV conduction time, coronary flow, and effective refractory period made it possible to establish cardioactive profiles for each of the agents tested. All the agents except CRA caused a concentration-dependent shortening of the effective refractory period in addition to their known inotropic effects (max. shortening: 38 % with 1×10^{-5} mol/L EPI, 26 % with 7×10^{-7} mol/L DIG, 13 % with 1–10^{-4} mol/L MIL, and 1.6 % with 5×10^{-4} mol/L AM). In terms of positive inotropism, the shortening of the refractory period was most pronounced with MIL (1.32 ms/mN). By contrast, CRA markedly prolonged the effective refractory period, increasing it by a

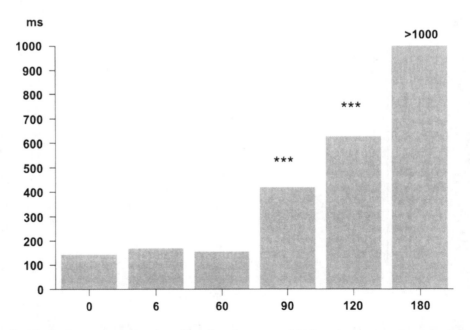

Fig. 3.3. ▲ Concentration-dependent effect of hawthorn extract (LI132) on the apparent refractory period (*** = p < 0.001; t-test for independent random samples) (Pöpping et al., 1995).

maximum of 10 %, i.e., by 2.54 ms/mN. Thus, CRA differs fundamentally from the reference drugs in that its inotropic action is associated with a lengthened refractory period, indicating that it may have less arrhythmogenic potential (Fig.3.4; Joseph et al., 1995; Müller et al., 1996). On the molecular level of action, hawthorn extract has been classified as a phytopharmacologic potassium-channel activator based on measurements in rabbit heart papillary muscle and in human coronary arteries (Siegel et al., 1996).

The inotropic effect of hawthorn extract WS 1442 was tested ex vivo in myocardial tissue removed surgically from 8 patients with NYHA (New York Heart Association) stage IV heart failure and from 8 nonfailing controls. The extract displaced radiolabeled strophanthin from its receptors but did not affect adenylate cyclase activity. In isolated left ventricular papillary muscle, WS 1442 significantly increased the force of contraction and improved frequency-dependent force generation. The authors conclude that the pharmacologic mechanism of hawthorn extract is similar to the positive inotropic action of cardiac glycosides, but with a more favorable force-frequency relationship (Schwinger et al., 2000).

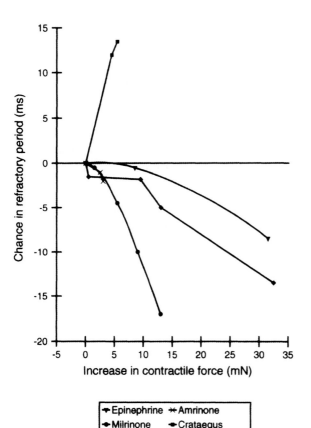

⬥ Epinephrine	⟶ Amrinone
⬥ Milrinone	⬥ Crataegus
⬥ Digoxin	

Fig. 3.4. ◀ Correlation between the change in the effective refractory period of the ventricular myocardium and the increase in force of ventricular contraction. The graph shows the mean values of the changes relative to the initial value (Joseph et al., 1995).

3.1.1.6 Toxicology

Acute toxicity studies have been performed in mice and rats using a water-and-ethanol extract designated WS 1442 (45 % ethanol m/m, herb-to-extract ratio 4–7:1). No deaths occurred following oral doses as high as 3000 mg/kg body weight. With intraperitoneal administration, the LD_{50} was 1170 mg/kg for mice and 750 mg/kg for rats. Associated toxic symptoms were sedation, dyspnea, and tremor. No toxic effects were observed in rats and dogs following the oral administration of 30, 90, and 300 mg of the same extract per kg body weight for 26 weeks. The Ames test, chromosome aberration test, mouse lymphoma test, and micronucleus test indicated no genotoxic or mutagenic effects from the extract. Oral doses up to 1.6 g/kg b.w. in rats and rabbits produced no teratogenic effects. In rats, moreover, the extract did not affect prenatal or postnatal development, nor did it alter the fertility of treated male and female rats or their F1 offspring (Schlegelmilch and Heywood, 1994; ESCOP 1999).

3.1.1.7 Clinical Efficacy

The results of 17 clinical studies in a total of 926 patients were published between 1981 and 2002 on the therapeutic efficacy of hawthorn extract (Table 3.1; reviews of the literature may be found in Tauchert, Siegel and Schulz, 1994; Loew, 1994; Tauchert and Loew, 1995, Blumenthal et al., 2003; Upton, 1999). Eleven of these studies were performed in 779 patients using alcoholic extracts of hawthorn leaves and flowers (Eichstädt et al., 1989; Weikl u. Noh, 1992; Leuchtgens, 1993; Bödigheimer u. Chase, 1994; Schmidt et al., 1994; Tauchert et al., 1994; Förster et al., 1994; Weikl et al., 1996; Eichstädt et al., 2001; Zapfe, 2001; Tauchert, 2002). The majority of patients enrolled in the studies had been diagnosed with NYHA stage II heart failure. The best outcome measures for evaluating efficacy were found to be exercise tolerance measured by standard bicycle ergometry, anaerobic threshold measured by spiroergometry, ejection fraction measured by radionuclide ventriculography or magnetic resonance imaging (Eichstädt et al., 1989, 2001; Weikl and Noh, 1992), as well as subjective complaints rated by a simple scoring system or the von Zerssen Symptom List. The clinical presentation, electrocardiogram, and chest films were less useful indicators of therapeutic response. Based on ergometric performance parameters, a minimum daily dose of 160 mg extract represents the threshold of efficacy. Whether a daily dose of 900 mg extract would provide optimum efficacy remains an open question.

Almost all the studies showed improvements in clinical symptoms, even at doses less than 300 mg/day. Given the subjective nature of the complaints, however, it is reasonable to assume that significant placebo effects influenced the evaluations. As an example, Fig. 3.5 shows the frequency of symptoms and complaints in 78 patients who had been treated with either 3x200 mg hawthorn extract or a placebo for 8 weeks as part of a double-blind study. Despite marked placebo effects, the graph shows that significantly more patients became free of complaints while on treatment with the hawthorn extract. The semiquantitative scoring scale showed improvement from 0.90 to 0.28 in the hawthorn-treated group versus 0.92 to 0.69 in the placebo group. The difference between the groups was statistically highly significant (Schmidt et al., 1994).

Table 3.1.
Controlled clinical studies using alcohol hawthorn extracts at doses of 160--900 mg taken for periods of 21-112 days published between 1981 and 2002.

Year	First author	Cases	Dose (mg/day)	Days	Key parameters
1981	Iwamoto	80	180	42	B, DFP
1982	Kümmell	19	180	42	SZI
1983	Hanak	60	180	21	AT
1986	Pozenel	22	180	28	DFP
1986	O'Connolly	36	180	42	DFP
1987	O'Connolly	31	180	42	DFP
1989	Eichstädt	20	480	28	EF, AT
1992	Weikl u. Noh	7	240	28	EF
1993	Leuchtgens	30	160	56	B, DFP
1994	Bödigheimer	85	300	28	AT
1994	Schmidt	78	600	56	AT, B
1994	Tauchert	132	900	56	AT
1994	Förster	72	900	56	AS
1996	Weikl	136	160	56	DFP, B
2001	Eichstädt	40	480	28	EF
2001	Zapfe	40	240	84	AT, DFP
2002	Tauchert	209	900–1800	112	AT, B

NOTE: 16 out of 17 of these studies used objective criteria such as exercise tolerance on a bicycle ergometer, the pressure-rate product, noninvasive measurements of the ejection fraction, and t he anaerobic threshold measured by spiroergometry (surrey in Tauchert et al., 1994, and Loew, 1997). **B** = Subjective complaints/mood; **DFP** = pressure-frequence-product; **SZI** = systolic interval; **AT** = bicycle ergometer exercise tolerance; **EF** = ejection fraction; **AS** = anaerobic threshold measured by spiroergometry.

Objective improvement in cardiac performance was demonstrated most clearly in six double-blind clinical studies using bicycle ergometry (Leuchtgens, 1993; Schmidt et al., 1994; Tauchert et al., 1994; Weikl et al., 1996; Tauchert, 2002) or spiroergometry (Förster et al., 1994). Five of the studies tested hawthorn against a placebo, and one study with 132 patients compared the efficacy of hawthorn with that of captopril.

The effect of hawthorn on average exercise tolerance over a 56-day treatment period is compared with a placebo in Fig. 3.6. In the placebo-controlled study, the average ergometric exercise tolerance rose from 79 to 107 watts in the patients treated with hawthorn extract but rose only from 71 to 76 watts in the placebo-treated group. This indicates a highly significant superiority of the hawthorn extract over the placebo. The improvement is particularly marked at moderate levels of exertion in the range of 100–125 watts (Schmidt et al., 1994). In the study comparing hawthorn with captopril, equivalent average tolerance increases were observed in both groups: from 83 to 97 watts with hawthorn extract and from 83 to 99 watts with captopril. Thus, the hawthorn preparation offers better tolerance than the ACE inhibitor captopril while providing equal therapeutic efficacy (Tauchert et al., 1994).

Spiroergometric studies also showed statistically significant advantages of hawthorn over a placebo. One advantage was the favorable effect of hawthorn on the time of onset of the anaerobic threshold. Hawthorn therapy did not alter the resting heart rate and

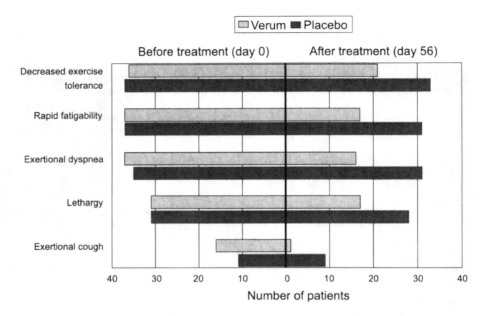

Fig. 3.5. ▲ Frequency of key symptoms before and after treatment with 600 mg/day hawthorn extract. At 56 days, patients on the drug showed significantly greater symptom reductions than patients on the placebo (Schmidt et al., 1994).

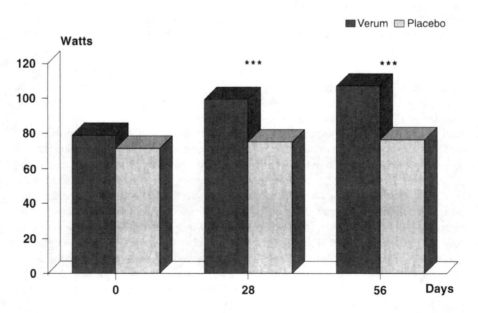

Fig. 3.6. ▲ Mean values of bicycle ergometric exercise tolerance during 56 days' treatment with 600 mg/day hawthorn extract. A statistically significant increase in exercise tolerance was noted in the hawthorn-treated group relative to the placebo (*** = p < 0.001) (Schmidt et al., 1994).

blood pressure, and during maximum exercise the blood pressure and heart rate increased less with hawthorn than with the placebo, leading to significant differences in the pressure-rate product (Förster et al., 1994).

As for side effects, a review of controlled clinical studies in a total of 367 patients treated with hawthorn showed two cases each of nausea and headache and one case each of palpitations, soft stool, and migraine headache. In all cases the physicians conducting the studies questioned the relation of the complaints to the test medication. The patient and physicians consistently rated the tolerance of the medication as "good" or "excellent".

In a multicenter double-blind study, 209 patients diagnosed with NYHA stage III heart failure were randomly assigned to groups that received a placebo (n=70), 900 mg/d of the hawthorn extract WS 1442 (n=69), or 1800 mg/d of the hawthorn extract (n=70) for 16 weeks in addition to basic diuretic therapy with 25 mg and 50 mg triamterene. Exercise tolerance at bicycle ergometry increased significantly relative to placebo only in the group that received 1800 mg of the hawthorn extract daily. Both of the groups treated with the extract showed significant improvements over the placebo group in both general and disease-specific complaints (Zerssen Symptom List) (Fig. 3.7). The group treated with 1800 mg/d reported the lowest incidence of adverse effects, consisting mainly of dizziness (1.4 % vs. 10 % in the placebo group). The author attributed this to a gain in cardiac performance (Tauchert, 2002).

A randomized, placebo-controlled double-blind study of the hawthorn extract WS 1442 (the SPICE study) is currently in progress. The study will evaluate patients treated with 900 mg of the extract daily over a 2-year period for the progression of cardiac

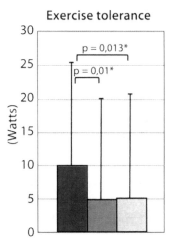
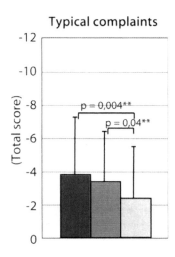

Fig. 3.7. ▲ A multicenter double-blind study was performed in 209 patients with advanced heart failure (NYHA stage III) over a 16-week period. The patients were randomly assigned to two groups in which basic diuretic therapy was supplemented by either hawthorn extract (900 or 1800 mg/day) or a placebo. Exercise tolerance rose significantly relative to placebo only in the patients who received 1800 mg/day. With regard to subjective improvement, both doses of the hawthorn extract were significantly superior to placebo (after Tauchert, 2002).

morbidity and mortality (primary outcome measures) as well as exercise tolerance, echocardiography, and quality of life (secondary outcome measures). The study, covering approximately 2400 patients with NYHA stage II or III heart failure from 140 centers in Europe, began in 1998 and is scheduled to end in 2004 (Holubarsch et al., 2000).

In the controlled clinical studies that have been performed to date in a total of 506 patients who received the hawthorn extract, there have been five reports of back pain and four reports each of dizziness, bronchitis, or head cold. Two patients each experienced nausea, gastroenteritis, headache, or angina, and one each complained of palpitations, "soft stool," flatulence, arthritis, or migraines. In all cases the physicians felt that the relationship of these adverse events to the test medication was absent or questionable. The incidence of similar events in placebo-treated patients was the same or higher.

As part of an observational study, 940 physicians in private practice tested the tolerance and efficacy of a hawthorn product in 3664 patients with NYHA stage I or stage II heart failure. The product was taken in a dose of 300 mg t.i.d. Forty-eight of the patients (1.3 %) reported 72 adverse reactions, most notably gastrointestinal complaints (24 cases), palpitations (10), vertigo (7), headache (7), and flushing (3). The physicians confirmed a link to medication use for just 7 of the gastrointestinal cases, 3 of the palpitation cases, 2 cases of headache or vertigo, and 1 case each of circulatory problems, sleeplessness, and apprehension. An analysis of statistical subgroups was particularly noteworthy in connection with the use of hawthorn products in patients susceptible to bradycardiac or hypotensive circulatory problems. This analysis showed that a fall in blood pressure during hawthorn treatment occurred in initially hypertensive patients but not in patients who were normotensive or hypotensive at the start of therapy. It was also found that a decrease in heart rate occurred only in tachycardiac patients and not in patients with initially normal or bradycardiac rates (Schmidt et al., 1998).

In a study conducted among 221 practitioners, 1011 patients with NYHA stage II heart failure were observed during and after a 24-week regimen of 900 mg of WS 1442 daily. During the course of the therapy, the physicians noted improvements in fatigue, exercise tolerance, palpitations, and exertional dyspnea. In 83 % of the patients, preexisting ankle edema was relieved at the end of the 24 weeks. Almost half the patients experienced relief of nocturia that had been present at baseline. Heart rate decreased by an average of 3.4 bpm. The resting systolic blood pressure fell by an average of 5.9 mm Hg and the diastolic pressure by 2.2 mm Hg. Maximum exercise tolerance rose from an initial 88.75 W (for 7.1 min of exercise) to 102.5 W (for 8.2 min of exercise). The ejection fraction determined by M-mode echocardiography rose from an average of 47.9 % to 51.1 %. A total of 14 adverse events were recorded. In two of these cases (epigastric fullness, right-sided facial pain accompanied by tachycardia and vomiting), the attending physicians suspected that there may have been a link to the hawthorn therapy but considered this unlikely. Most of the physicians rated the tolerance as excellent (71.2 %) or good (27.5 %) (Tauchert et al., 1999).

3.1.1.8 Indications, Dosages, Risks, and Contraindications

The updated 1994 Commission E monograph of hawthorn leaves and flowers states that the extract is indicated for "decreasing cardiac output as described in functional Stage

II of NYHA" (Blumenthal et al., 1998). The recommended dosage is 160–900 mg/day of the crude water-and-alcohol extract with a designated content of flavonoids (4–20 mg) or oligomeric procyanidins (30–160 mg). Based on the results of the treatment studies that used objective criteria, however (Table 3.1), the recommended dose should be toward the upper end of the relatively broad range stated in the monograph, i.e., 600–900 mg (as high as 1800 mg/d initially; see Fig. 3.7) of extract per day. Hawthorn preparations should be taken orally and should be continued for at least 6 weeks. There are no known risks, contraindications, or herb-drug interactions.

3.1.1.9 Therapeutic Significance

The therapeutic significance of hawthorn preparations compared with other cardioactive drugs is based on the relationship of efficacy and tolerance and the severity of the patient's illness. Heart failure is defined as an inability of the diseased heart to maintain an adequate supply of oxygen and nutrients to the peripheral tissues. Mainstays in the pharmacologic treatment of heart failure include ACE (angiotensin-converting enzyme) inhibitors, diuretics, and positive inotropic agents, especially the cardiac glycosides. The efficacy of digitalis was recently tested in a double-blind study in which 3397 patients were treated with digoxin and 3402 patients with a placebo for periods averaging 37 months (The Digitalis Investigation Group, 1997). A total of 1263 deaths occurred in the placebo group and 1274 in the digoxin group. While the digoxin patients had fewer deaths due to the progression of heart failure (hospital admissions were 19 % lower in the digoxin group), they showed a higher incidence of fatal arrhythmias. This provides a rationale for avoiding the use of cardiac glycosides in milder forms of heart failure (NYHA II) in favor of treatment with hawthorn extract. The positive inotropic effect of hawthorn, unlike that of the cardiac glycosides, is associated with a lengthening rather than shortening of the refractory period. While a shortened refractory period predisposes to arrhythmias, the lengthening effect of hawthorn extract helps to stabilize the cardiac rhythm. The incidence of adverse drug reactions in the controlled studies with hawthorn extract was about 6 %, and it was only 1.3 % in the observational study (Schmidt et al., 1998). Table 3.2 underscores the low risk of this therapy. To date there have been no reports of life-threatening cardiac arrhythmias, which are considered a limiting factor in the use of cardiac glycosides.

Therapeutic risk	Crataegus	Digitalis
Therapeutic range	Very large	Very small
Dosage errors	No danger	High risk
Arrhythmogenic potential	None	Relatively large
Renal function impairment	Not a problem	Danger of intoxication
Diuretics, laxatives	Can be safely used	Require potassium monitoring
Tolerance to oxygen deficit	Increased	Reduced

Table 3.2.
Comparison of the therapeutic risks of hawthorn extract and cardiac glycosides.

3.1.1.10 Drug Products

The *Red List 2003* lists a total of 57 single-herb hawthorn products under the heading of Herbal Heart Remedies and another 16 combination products that contain hawthorn.

3.1.2 Herbs Containing Digitaloids

Digitaloids are cardioactive glycosides that exert a digoxin-like action but are not derived from *Digitalis* species. The digitaloids include, most notably, convallatoxin, cymarin, oleandrin, G- and K-strophanthin, and proscillaridin. The principal sources of digitaloids are false hellebore, lily-of-the-valley, squill bulbs, and oleander leaves. Extracts from digitaloid herbs each contain more than one cardioactive glycoside. Up to 40 structurally related glycosides may be present along with a quantitatively dominant principal glycoside (Table 3.3). Various other compounds are extracted along with the cardiac glycosides, so digitaloid extracts can have a very complex composition. As a result, the monitoring and control of active levels is a formidable task, comparable to therapy with digitalis glycosides; this is a serious drawback given the narrow therapeutic range of cardiac glycosides (Loew, 1997).

There are no qualitative differences between the digitaloids and the classic cardiac glycosides digoxin and digitoxin in terms of their pharmacologic mechanism of action and cardiac efficacy. All these compounds are positively inotropic, negatively chronotropic, negatively dromotropic, and positively bathmotropic. Digitaloids and digitalis glycosides differ in their pharmacokinetics, however, particularly in their rates of absorption and clearance. The shorter duration of action cited by advocates as a major advantage of digitaloid preparations correlates with lower absorption rates. As a result, treatment with digitaloid herbs carries a higher overall risk than treatment with isolated cardiac glycosides. Another difficulty is that digitaloid extracts do not meet phytotherapeutic requirements for a broad therapeutic range (see Sect. 1.5.2). Thus, physicians who have no personal experience with these products should use them only with great caution.

3.1.2.1 False hellebore

The crude drug is prepared by drying the aerial parts of *Adonis vernalis* gathered while the plant is in bloom. Most of the bulk herb is imported from Hungary, Bulgaria, and Russia. Standardized hellebore powder consists of pulverized crude drug whose activity in guinea pig heart corresponds to a content of 0.2 % cymarin. The *German Pharmacopeia* (DAB 1996) describes the powdered drug as containing approximately 0.25 % cardiac glycosides, representing a complex mixture of about 20 components. These glycosides are similar to K-strophanthin in their chemical structure and pharmacokinetic properties. The 1988 Commission E monograph states that false hellebore is indicated for "mild heart failure, especially when accompanied by nervous symptoms." The contraindications, side effects, and risks are the same as for cardiac glyco-

Table 3.3.
Pharmacokinetic parameters of digitaloid glycosides compared with digitoxin and digoxin (after Loew, 1997).

	(Digitoxin)	(Digoxin)				
Number of glycosides considered	1	1	ca. 27	ca. 40	ca. 25	ca. 30
Principal glycoside	Digitoxin	Digoxin	Cymarin	Convalla-toxin	Oleandrin	Proscilla-ridin A
Absorption (%)	95–100	60–80	15–37	10	65–86	20–30
Half-life $t_{1/2}$ (h)	ca. 200	ca. 40	13–23	–	–	23–49
Daily activity loss (%) Verlust (%)	7–10	20–25	28–39	40–50	41	30–50
Duration of action (d)	10–21	4–8	2,8	–	2,65	2–3
Protein binding (%)	90–97	20	–	16	50	85
Excretion	Renal, biliary	Mainly renal	Mainly renal	Renal, biliary	Renal, biliary	Mainly renal

sides. No single-herb products based on false hellebore are available commercially in Germany, but there are products that combine the herb with other digitaloids (e.g., Corguttin, Miroton).

3.1.2.2 Lily-of-the-Valley

The crude drug is prepared by drying the aerial parts of *Convallaria majalis* gathered during the flowering period. The standardized powdered drug has a 0.2–0.3 % content of cardioactive glycosides, which number more than 30. The principal glycosides are convallatoxin and convallatoxol. Convallatoxin has an absorption rate of about 10 % and 24-h clearance rate of about 50 %. The maintenance dose is 0.2–0.3 mg intravenously and 2–3 mg orally. The indications stated in the Commission E monograph of 1987 are "mild exertional failure, age-related cardiac complaints, and chronic cor pulmonale." The contraindications, side effects, and risks are the same as for cardiac glycosides. A single-herb product based on lily-of-the-valley is marketed in Germany under the brand name Convacard. Also, there are a number of combination products containing other digitaloids and other active ingredients.

3.1.2.3 Squill Powder

The crude drug is prepared by gathering the inner scales of the squill bulb (*Urginea maritima*) after the flowering season, cutting them into transverse and longitudinal strips, and drying and pulverizing them. Depending on its origin, squill powder contains 0.15–2 % cardioactive glycosides. The principal glycosides are scillaren A and proscillaridin, which comprise about two-thirds of the total glycoside fraction; the other third consists of at least 25 other constituents. According to DAB 1996, squill powder is adjusted to an activity corresponding to 0.2 % proscillaridin.

The gastrointestinal absorption rate is about 15 % for scillaren and 20–30 % for proscillaridin. The half-life of proscillaridin is approximately 24h. The daily dose ranges from 0.1 to 0.5 g of the standardized squill powder.

The 1985 Commission E monograph states that the indications for squill powder are "mild forms of heart failure, even in patients with impaired renal function." The contraindications, side effects, and interactions are the same as for digitalis glycosides. Single-herb products based on powdered squill are marketed in Germany under the brand names Digitalysat N Bürger and Scillamiron. There are also a number of combination products that contain other digitaloids.

3.1.2.4 Oleander Leaves

The crude drug consists of the dried leaves of *Nerium oleander*. Native to the Mediterranean, oleander derives its species name from the similarity of the shape of leaves to those of the olive tree. The cardioactive glycoside fraction of oleander leaves is dominated by oleandrin, whose aglycone is closely related to the gitoxin of the purple foxglove. Only fragmentary data are available on the pharmacokinetics of oleandrin. Commission E in its 1988 monograph did not recommend oleander extract as a medicinal agent, but in 1993 the Commission did ascribe therapeutic value to a fixed combination of false hellebore liquid extract, lily-of-the-valley powdered extract, squill powdered extract, and oleander-leaf powdered extract based on clinical studies of the commercial product (Miroton). The indication was described as "mild forms of heart failure with circulatory lability." The following contraindications were noted: NYHA stage III or IV heart failure, treatment with digitalis glycosides, digitalis intoxication, hypercalcemia, potassium deficiency states, bradycardia, and ventricular tachycardia.

3.1.2.5 Drug Products

The *Rote Liste 1998* lists four single-herb digitaloid products. Additionally, there is a digitaloid combination product that is among the 100 most frequently prescribed phytomedicines in Germany (Table A3).

3.1.3 Other Cardioactive Plant Drugs

Extract from *Ammi visnaga* fruits and the compounds isolated from them, khellin and visnagin, improve myocardial perfusion by increasing blood flow through the coronary vessels. These actions form the basis for the use of visnaga extract in relieving angina due to coronary heart disease. Reports of adverse effects (isolated cases of pseudoallergic reactions, reversible cholestatic jaundice, elevated hepatic transaminase levels) prompted Commission E in 1993 to withdraw its 1986 claim that ammi visnaga extract was appropriate for the treatment of "mild angina pectoris."

Antiarrhythmic agents of plant origin include the drugs ajmaline (alkaloid obtained from the root of *Rauwolfia* species), quinidine (alkaloid obtained from the bark of *Cinchona* species), and sparteine (alkaloid obtained from the broom shrub). The treatment risks associated with these compounds are similar to those of synthetic antiarrhythmic drugs. Hence it is better to use the substances in pure, isolated form rather than in the form of herbal extract-based preparations. Further information on the medicinal uses of ajmaline, quinidine, and sparteine as isolated compounds can be found in textbooks of pharmacology.

Extracts from the perennial herb motherwort (*Leonurus cardiaca*) are recommended for the treatment of nervous heart conditions. The 1986 Commission E monograph recommends an average daily dose of 4.5 g of the crude drug. The cut and dried aerial parts of motherwort occur as ingredients in "cardiovascular teas" (from Kneipp and other manufacturers), and motherwort extract is an ingredient of several combination products (e.g., Crataezyma, Oxacant).

Mixtures of herbal cardiotonics and volatile oils containing 3–12 ingredients are available for local external application. There is some rationale for products that contain ingredients with local irritating properties. Products such as Cor-Selekt ointment or Kneipp Heart Ointment are rubbed into the dermatome that is associated with the heart (an area on the left side of the chest extending down to the costal arch, and an area on the left side of the back extending roughly from the base of the neck to the inferior angle of the scapula).

3.2 Hypotension and Hypertension

Hypotension and hypertension are not considered primary indications for phythotherapy. Nevertheless, some herbal medications are suitable for short-term use in the symptomatic treatment of orthostatic complaints associated with low blood pressure and for longer-term use as a supportive therapy in patients with high blood pressure.

3.2.1 Phythotherapy of Hypotension

Hypotension ordinarily refers to blood pressure less than 100 mm Hg systolic and 60 mm Hg diastolic. Low blood pressure has no pathologic significance in itself and is even beneficial in inhibiting atherosclerotic disease. Hypotension requires treatment only if it is associated with orthostatic symptoms such as dizziness, grogginess, headache, and fatigue. Physical therapy (e.g., physical training, Kneipp regimens) and dietary measures (increased fluid and salt intake) are the mainstays of treatment, and medications are used only temporarily in a supportive role. Dihydroergotamine, a hydrogenation product of the alkaloid ergotamine, is believed to increase the tonus of capacitance vessels by the stimulation of α-adrenergic receptors, resulting in increased venous return and a rise in blood pressure. However, dihydroergotamine is a modified pure plant constituent and, as such, is not considered a phytotherapeutic agent. Pharmacology textbooks may be consulted for more details on this compound.

On the other hand, preparations made from caffeine-containing herbs and certain aromatic herbs containing volatile oils are correctly classified as herbal antihypotensives.

Extracts from the broom shrub (Scotch broom; *Cytisus scoparius*) can no longer be recommended for antihypotensive therapy. Commission E approved this herb for "functional cardiovascular complaints" in its 1991 monograph, but the main alkaloid constituent of broom, sparteine, has shown a narrow range of therapeutic utility. Also, sparteine is poorly metabolized in a significant percentage of the population who have a congenital enzyme defect, delaying the excretion of this compound by a factor of 1000 so that even low doses can pose a significant health risk. A final problem with broom extract is that its therapeutic efficacy has not been adequately documented (Eichelbaum, 1986).

3.2.1.1 Caffeine-Containing Herbs and Beverages

Caffeine and caffeine-containing beverages are agents with unpredictable antihypotensive effects. It is a common experience, however, for people with low blood pressure to feel better after drinking their morning coffee or tea. Caffeine and other methylxanthines act directly on the pressor centers of the circulatory system; they also exert mild positive inotropic and chronotropic effects on the heart. Their duration of action is approximately 1–3 h.

A morning coffee infusion is prepared with 5–8 g of roasted coffee per cup (150 mL). Roasted coffee has a caffeine content of about 1–2 %, so a total of about 100 mg of caffeine is ingested in one cup of coffee.

Dried tea leaves contain 2–5 % caffeine. But given the smaller amount of herb that is used, and the method of extraction (infusion) one cup of black tea contains only about 30–50 mg of caffeine. Other caffeine-containing herbs are guarana seeds (*Paullinia cupana*), cola seeds (*Cola nitida, C. acuminate*), maté leaves (*Ilex paraguariensis*), and cocoa beans (*Theobroma cacao*). The amounts of methylxanthines contained in these herbs are shown in Table 3.4. Extracts from guarana and cola seeds are sold over the counter in the form of chewable tablets or drink mixtures. Due to the unpredictable risks, especially to children and adolescents (lethal caffeine dose between 3 and 10 g!), efforts are being made in Germany to limit the sales of some guarana products containing a significant amount of caffeine.

Caffeine is lipid-soluble, so it is readily absorbed from the gastrointestinal tract. The monographs state that caffeine and caffeine-containing herbs are useful for the short-

Table 3.4.
Percentage content of methylxanthines in dried herbs. n.d. = not detectable (Ploss, 1994).

Herbal drug	Caffeine	Theobromine	Theophylline
Coffee	0,9–2,6	0,002	0,0005
Cola nut	2,00	0,05	n.d.
Tea leaf	2,5–5,5	0,07–0,17	0,002–0,013
Cocoa bean	0,2	1,2	n.d.
Maté	0,5–1,5	n.d.	n.d.
Guarana	2,95–5,8	0,03–0,17	0,02–0,06

n.d. = not detectable

term relief of symptoms due to mental or physical fatigue. None of the monographs address the treatment of hypotension or orthostatic complaints, but it is well known from experience that many hypotensive patients respond positively to caffeine and caffeine-containing herbs. The possible side effects of caffeine-containing herbs include stomach upset, nervousness, and sleeplessness.

3.2.1.2 Essential Oils

Analeptic is an older term denoting a restorative remedy for states of weakness that are frequently accompanied by dizziness and fainting (Aschner, 1986). Traditional formulas for analeptic preparations contained aromatic substances that stimulated the olfactory nerve and the sensory trigeminal nerve endings, causing a reflex stimulation of respiration and circulation. Among these substances were essential oils derived from aromatic herbs (plants containing volatile oils). The Commission E monographs recommend rosemary leaves (*Rosmarinus officinalis*, indicated for circulatory problems) and lavender leaves (*Lavandula officinalis*, indicated for functional circulatory disorders) as aromatic herbs for external use in balneology. Rosemary leaves contain at least 1.2 % volatile oil. A hot infusion is prepared from about 50 g of the crude drug and is added to the bath. Lavender leaves also contain at least 1.5 % volatile oil. About 100 g of lavender leaves are used to prepare a hot infusion for adding to bathwater.

Pharmacologic and clinical data that go beyond traditional empirical knowledge are available for camphor. For 2000 years, natural camphor has been extracted from the wood of the Eastern Asian camphor tree (*Cinnamomum camphora*) by steam distillation, yielding a product with at least a 96 % content of 2-bornanone. The Commission E monograph on camphor states that it is used internally in in a daily dose of 30–300 mg for the treatment of "Hypotonic circulatory regulation disorders" (Blumenthal et al., 1998). When taken in higher doses, camphor produces toxic symptoms such as muscle pain, intoxication, and generalized spasms. Single oral doses up to approximately 50 mg are reportedly safe in adults and schoolchildren (Franz and Hempel, 2000; Hempel, 2000). Acute blood pressure elevation by camphor has been documented in a placebo-controlled double-blind study in 48 patients with orthostatic hypotension. This study used a combination product, however, that contained a hawthorn berry extract in addition to camphor. One to 5 minutes after the patients took a liquid preparation containing 0 mg of camphor (placebo), 5 mg, 20 mg, or 80 mg, a statistically significant rise in systolic and diastolic blood pressure was measured at the two higher doses (Belz and Loew, 2002).

It is likely that these aromatic herbs are effective only when the molecules of their volatile oils come in contact with the nasal mucosa through inhalation. The classic prototype is smelling salts, a preparation that is no longer manufactured today. But a homemade version can be prepared by placing 1–4 drops of essential oil on a sugar cube that is then slowly dissolved in the mouth. Rubbing the oil into the temples can also be beneficial. Essential oils should not be used in infants and small children due to the danger of reflex respiratory arrest. Further clinical studies are needed to determine whether the long-term oral use of camphor-containing products can aid in the prevention of orthostatic complaints.

3.2.2 Phytotherapy of Hypertension

According to the WHO definition, hypertension is present when the blood pressure exceeds 160 mm Hg systolic and 95 mm Hg diastolic. Blood pressures in the range of 140–160 systolic and 90–95 diastolic are classified as borderline hypertension, which is usually managed by nonpharmacologic means (weight loss, low-salt diet, exercise). An herbal remedy that has been used in the treatment of mild to moderate hypertension is the whole extract made from the dried roots of Indian snakeroot (*Rauvolfia serpentina*), an evergreen shrub native to tropical Asia. The extract contains more than 50 different alkaloids, including the sympatholytic agent reserpine. Reserpine is not only one of the oldest antihypertensive agents, it is still one of the most economical. Because of its association with objectionable side effects, particularly at doses higher than 0.2 mg/day (depression, fatigue, impotence, nasal stuffiness), the use of reserpine has declined in industrialized countries, but it is still included as a standard antihypertensive agent in the WHO list of essential drugs. Because reserpine is an isolated compound with a known chemical composition, it is considered a conventional drug, not a phytotherapeutic agent.

The whole extract derived from Indian snakeroot has the same actions and side effects as reserpine when properly standardized and administered in the proper dose. Because of its narrow therapeutic range, however, rauwolfia extract does not meet the safety criteria of an acceptable phytomedicine (see Sect. 1.5.1.1., 1.5.4, and 1.5.5). Besides two combination products that cannot be recommended, the *Rote Liste 1994* cites only one standardized rauwolfia-extract-based product (Arte Rautin forte M drops) that is still marketed in Germany. The product is standardized to 7 % total alkaloids. It has no apparent advantage over reserpine therapy which is easier to control.

Several older antihypertensives that have de facto approval in Germany contain preparations made from European mistletoe (*Viscum album*), olive leaves (*Olea europaea*), and rhododendron leaves (*Rhododendron* spp.) as their active ingredients. The parenteral use of mistletoe preparations may cause a transient fall in blood pressure, but this is due to an allergic response based on the release of biogenic amines and may not signify real therapeutic benefit for hypertension. The antihypertensive effect of orally administered mistletoe preparations has not been adequately documented. Palliative use of parenteral mistletoe preparations in cancer patients is discussed in Chap. 9.

The dried leaves of the olive tree are used in Italian folk medicine as a remedy for high blood pressure, but clinical studies have not furnished definite proof of their therapeutic efficacy in hypertension.

Rhododendron leaves contain grayanotoxins, which lower blood pressure. But these compounds are highly toxic, causing nausea, vomiting, diarrhea and, at higher doses, muscular and respiratory paralysis. Consequently, rhododendron leaf extract is not considered an acceptable herbal antihypertensive.

It has been shown that spontaneously hypertensive rats can be made normotensive by adding garlic powder to their feed (Jacob et al., 1991). In a meta-analysis of eight clinical studies with coated garlic powder tablet, three of which specifically included hypertensive patients, four of the studies showed a significant reduction in diastolic blood pressures while three showed a significant reduction in systolic pressures (Silagy and

Neil, 1994). In an observational study of some 2000 patients taking 300 mg of garlic powder three times daily, 1.3 % of the patients, developed new orthostatic symptoms while on that therapy (Beck and Grünwald, 1993). In summary, it may be concluded that garlic powder preparations taken in an adequate dose (600–1200 mg/day of active ingredient) have mild antihypertensive effects that are significant both therapeutically and with regard to possible side effects and drug-drug interactions (additive effects with other antihypertensives). Based on information currently available, garlic powder preparations are the only phytomedicines that can be recommended as adjuncts in the treatment of hypertensive patients. The vasoactive properties of garlic are discussed more fully in Sect.3.3 below.

 References (for 3.1 and 3.2)

Al Makdessi S, Sweidan H, Dietz K, Jacob R (1999) Protective effect of Crataegus oxyacantha against reperfusion arrhythmias after global no-flow ischemia in the rat heart. Basic Res Cardiol 94: 71-6.
Al Makdessi S, Sweidan H, Müllner S, Jacob R (1996) Myocardial protection by pretreatment with Crataegus oxyacantha. Arzneim Forsch/Drug Res 46 (I): 25–27.
American Herbal Pharmacopoeia (1999) Hawthorn leaf with flower. American Herbal Pharmacopoeia, Santa Cruz, USA.
Ammon HPT, Händel M (1981) Crataegus, Toxikologie und Pharmakologie. Teil l: Toxizität. Planta Med 43: 105–120.
Anonymus (1984) Camphora (Campher) Bundesanzeiger 228 vom 5.12.1984.
Beck E, Grünwald J (1993) Allium sativum in der Stufentherapie der Hyperlipidämie. Med Welt 44: 516–520.
Belz GG, Butzer R, Gaus W, Loew D (2002) Camphor-Crataegus berry extract combination dose-dependently reduces tilt induced fall in blood pressure in orthostatic hypotension. Phytomedicine 9: 581-8.
Belz GG, Loew D (2003) Dose-response related efficacy in orthostatic hypotension of a fixed combination of D-camphor and fresh Crataegus berries and the contribution of the single components. Phytomedicine 10 Suppl IV: 61-67.
Belz GG, Loew D (2003) Dose-response related efficacy in orthostatic hypotension of a fixed combination of D-camphor and a fresh Crataegus Berries and the contribution of the single components. Phytomedicine 10 Suppl IV: 61-67.
Blumenthal M, Busse WR, Goldberg A et al. (1998) The Complete German Commission E Monographs - Therapeutic Guide to Herbal Medicines. American Botanical Council, Austin, Texas, 1998. www.herbalgram.org. Chatterjee SS, Koch E, Jaggy H, Krzeminski T (1997) In-vitro- und In-vivo-Untersuchungen zur kardioprotektiven Wirkung von oligomeren Procyanidinen in einem Crataegus-Extrakt aus Blättern und Blüten. Arzneim Forsch/Drug Res 47 (I): 821–825.
Blumenthal M, Hall T, Goldberg A et al. (2003) The ABC Clinical Guide to Herbs. Austin, TX: American Botanical Council.
Bödigheimer K, Chase D (1994) Wirksamkeit von Weißdorn-Extrakt in der Dosierung 3mal 100 mg täglich. Münch Med Wochenschr 136, Suppl. 1: 7-11.
Chatterjee SS, Koch E, Jaggy H, Krzeminski T (1997) In-vitro- und In-vivo-Untersuchungen zur kardioprotektiven Wirkung von oligomeren Procyanidinen in einem Crataegus-Extrakt aus Blättern und Blüten. Arzneim Forsch/Drug Res 47 (I): 821–825.
Eichelbaum M (1986) Pharmakogenetische Aspekte der Arzneimitteltherapie. In: Dölle W, Müller-Oerlinghausen B, Schwabe U (eds) Grundlagen der Arzneimitteltherapie. Wissenschaftsverlag BI, Mannheim Vienna Zurich, pp. 438–448.

Eichstädt H, Bäder M, Danne O, Kaiser W, Stein U, Felix R (1989) Crataegus-Extrakt hilft dem Patienten mit NYHA II-Herzinsuffizienz. Therapiewoche 39: 3288-3296.

Eichstädt H, Störk T, Möckel M, Danne O, Funk P, Köhler S (2001) Wirksamkeit und Verträglichkeit von Crataegus-Extrakt WS® 1442 bei herzinsuffizienten Patienten mit eingeschränkter linksventrikulärer Funktion. Perfusion 14: 212-217.

ESCOP (1999) Crataegi folium cum flore. Monographs on the medicinal uses of plant drugs, Fascicule 6, Exeter, UK.

Fischer K, Jung F, Koscielny J, Kiesewetter H (1994) Crataegus-Extrakt vs. Methyldigoxin. Einfluß auf Rheologie und Mikrozirkulation bei 12 gesunden Probanden. Münch Med Wschr 136 (Suppl 1): 35-38.

Förster A, Förster K, Bühring M, Wolfstädter HD (1994) Crataegus bei mäßig reduzierter linksventrikulärer Auswurffraktion. Ergospirometrische Verlaufsuntersuchung bei 72 Patienten in doppelblindem Vergleich mit Plazebo. Münch Med Wschr 136 (Suppl 1): 21-26.

Franz G, Hempel B (2000) Natürlicher D-Campher. Deutsche Apotheker Zeitung 140: 1050-56.

Hänsel R, Keller K, Rimpler H, Schneider G (Hrsg) (1992) Hagers Handbuch der Pharmazeutischen Praxis. Vol. 4, Drogen A-D. 5th Ed. Springer Verlag, Berlin Heidelberg: 1040-1056.

Hempel B (2000) Toxikologie von D-Campher. In: Rietbrock N (ed) Phytopharmaka VI - Foerschung und Praxis. Steinkopff, Darmstadt, pp.29-37.

Holubarsch CJF, Colucci WS, Meinertz T, et al. (2000) Survival and prognosis: investigation of crattaegus extract WS 1442 in congestive heart failure (SPICE) - rationale, study design and study protocol. Eur J Heart Failure 2: 431-7.

Jacob R, Ehrsam M, Ohkubo T, Rupp H (1991) Antihypertensive und kardioprotektive Effekte von Knoblauchpulver (Allium sativum). Med Welt (Suppl 7 a): 39-41.

Joseph G, Zhao Y, Klaus W (1995) Pharmakologisches Wirkprofil von Crataegus-Extrakt im Vergleich zu Epinephrin, Amrinon, Milrinon und Digoxin am isoliert perfundierten Meerschweinchenherzen. Arzneim Forsch/Drug Res 45: 1261-1265.

Kaul R (ed) (1998) Der Weißdorn. Wissenschaftliche Verlagsges. MbH, Stuttgart.

Koch E, Chatterjee SS (2000) Crataegus extract WS-1442 enhances coronary flow in the isolated rat heart by endothelial release of nitric oxide. Naunyn-Schmiedeberg's Arch Pharmacol 361 Suppl., R48, Abstr. 180.

Kreimeyer J (1997) Beiträge zur Analytik von Flavon-3-olen und oligomeren Proanthocyanidinen sowie Untersuchungen zur Pharmakologie von Wirkstoff-Fraktionen und einzelnen Procyanidinen aus einem Weißdorn-Trockenextrakt. Inaugural Dissertation, Universität Münster.

Krzeminski T, Chatterjee SS (1993) Ischemia and early reperfusion induced arrhythmias: beneficial effects of an extract of Crataegus oxyacantha L. Pharm Pharmacol Lett 3: 45-48.

Kurcok A (1992) Ischemia- and reperfusion-induced cardiac inury; effects of two flavonoids containing plant extracts possessing radical scavenging properties. Naunyn-Schmiedebergs's Arch Pharmacol 345 (Suppl RB 81) Abstr 322.

Leuchtgens H (1993) Crataegus-Spezialextrakt WS 1442 bei Herzinsuffizienz NYHA II. Fortschr Med 111: 352-354.

Loew D (1994) Crataegus-Spezialextrakte bei Herzinsuffizienz. Kassenarzt 15: 43-52.

Loew D (1997) Phytotherapy in heart failure. Phytomedicine 4: 267-271.

Müller A, Linke W, Zhao Y, Klaus W (1996) Crataegus extract prolongs action potential duration in guinea-pig papillary muscle. Phytomedicine 3: 257-261.

Pöpping S, Rose H, Ionescu I, Fischer Y, Kammermeier H (1995) Effect of a hawthorn extract on contraction and energy turnover of isolated rat cardiomyocytes. Arzneim Forsch/ Drug Res 45: 1157-1161.

Rotfuß MA, Pascht U, Kissling G (2001) Effect of long-term application of Crataegus oxyacanta on ischemia and reperfusion induced arrhythmias in rats. Arzneim-Forsch/Drug Res 51: 24-28.

Rothfuss MA, Pascht U, Kissling G (2001) Effect of long-term application of Crataegus oxyacanta on ischemia and reperfusion induced arrhythmias in rats. Arzneim-Forsch/Drug Res 51: 24-28.

Schlegelmilch R, Heywood R (1994) Toxicity of crataegus (hawthorn) extract (WS 1442). J Am Coll Toxicol 13: 103-111.

Schmidt U, Albrecht M, Podzuweit H, Ploch M, Maisenbacher J (1998) Hochdosierte Crataegus-Therapie bei herzinsuffizienten Patienten NYHA-Stadium I und II. Z Phytother 19: 22-30.

Schmidt U, Kuhn U, Ploch M, Hübner WD (1994) Wirksamkeit des Extraktes LI 132 (600 mg/Tag) bei 8wöchiger Therapie. Plazebokontrollierte Doppelblindstudie mit Weißdorn an 78 herzinsuffizienten Patienten im Stadium II nach NYHA. Münch Med Wschr 136 (Suppl 1): 13–20.

Schwinger RHG; Pietsch M, Frank K, et al. (2000) Crataegus special extract WS 1442 increases force of contraction in human myocardium cAMP-independently. J Cardiovasc Pharmacol 35: 700-7.

Siegel G, Casper U (1996) Crataegi folium cum flore. In: Loew D, Rietbrock N (eds) Phytopharmaka in Forschung und klinischer Anwendung. Steinkopff Verlag, Darmstadt: 1–14.

Siegel G, Casper U, Schnalke F (1996) Molecular physiological effector mechanisms of hawthorn extract in cardiac papillary muscle and coronary vascular smooth muscle. Phytotherapie Res 10: S195-S198.

Siegel G, Casper U, Walter H, Hetzer R (1994) Weißdorn-Extrakt LI 132. Dosis-Wirkungs-Studie zum Membranpotential und Tonus menschlicher Koronararterien und des Hundepapillarmuskels. Münch med Wschr 136 (Suppl 1): 47–56.

Silagy C, Neil A (1994) A meta-analysis of the effect of garlic on blood pressure. J Hypertension 12: 463–468.

Sticher O, Rehwald A, Meier B (1994) Kriterien der pharmazeutischen Qualität von Crataegus-Extrakten. Münch Med Wschr 136 (Suppl 1): 69–73.

Tauchert M (2002) Efficacy and safety of crataegus extract WS 1442 in comparison with placebo in patients with chronic stable New York Heart Association class-III heart failure. Am Heart J 143: 910-5.

Tauchert M, Gildor A, Lipinski J 1999) Einsatz des hochdosierten Crataegusextraktes WS 1442 in der Therapie der Herzinsuffizienz Stadium NYHA II. Herz 24: 465-474.

Tauchert M, Loew D (1995) Crataegi folium cum flore bei Herzinsuffizienz. In: Loew D, Rietbrock N (eds) Phytopharmaka in Forschung und klinischer Anwendung. Steinkopff Verlag, Darmstadt: 137–144.

Tauchert M, Ploch M, Hübner WD (1994) Wirksamkeit des Weißdorn-Extraktes LI 132 im Vergleich mit Captopril. Multizentrische Doppelblindstudie bei 132 Patienten mit Herzinsuffizienz im Stadium II nach NYHA. Münch Med Wschr 136 (Suppl 1): 27–34.

Tauchert M, Siegel G, Schulz V (1994) Weißdorn-Extrakt als pflanzliches Cardiacum (Vorwort). Neubewertung der therapeutischen Wirksamkeit. Münch Med Wschr 136 (Suppl 1): 3–5.

The Digitalis Investigation Group (1997) The effect of digoxin on mortality and morbidity in patients with heart failure. N Eng J Med 336 (8): 525–533.

Upton R (ed.) (1999) Hawthorn leaf with flower. American Herbal Pharmacopoeia, Santa Cruz, CA, USA.

Weikl A, Assmus KD, Neukum-Schmidt A, Schmitz J, Zapfe G, Noh HS, Siegrist J (1996) Crataegus-Spezialextrakt WS 1442. Fortschr Med 114(24):291–296.

Weikl A, Noh HS (1992) Der Einfluß von Crataegus bei globaler Herzinsuffizienz. Herz + Gefäße 11: 516-524.

Weiss RF (Hrsg) (1991) Lehrbuch der Phytotherapie. 7th Edition, Hippokrates Verlag Stuttgart: 223.

Zapfe G (2001) Clinical efficacy of Crataegus extract WS® 1442 in congestive heart failure NYHA class II. Phytomedicine 8: 262-266.

3.3   Atherosclerosis and Arterial Occlusive Disease

Some phytomedicines are useful in the prevention or symptomatic treatment of atherosclerosis and its sequelae. Particular value is ascribed to certain *Allium* species (garlic, onion, ramson) in the prevention of atherosclerosis, and the effects of garlic have been extensively documented by pharmacologic and clinical research. The antiatherosclerotic effects of garlic are based mainly on its vasodilating, rheologic, and lipid-reducing actions. It has been discovered that garlic lowers blood lipids by inhibiting cholesterol synthesis. Other lipid-reducing plant constituents for the secondary prophylaxis of atherosclerosis are phospholipids derived from soybeans, oat bran, and guar gum.

Special extracts from gingko (*Gingko biloba*) leaves have value in the symptomatic treatment of peripheral arterial occlusive disease. Another major application of these ginkgo extracts is in the symptomatic treatment of cognitive deficits secondary to organic brain disease (see Sect. 2.1).

3.3.1   Garlic

3.3.1.1   Historical Background

Garlic is a traditional herb. Some of the earliest references to this medicinal and culinary plant are found on Sumerian clay tablets dating from 2600–2100 BCE. Garlic was an important medicine to the ancient Egyptians, appearing in 22 of the more than 800 remedies listed in the famous Ebers papyrus (ca. 1550 BCE). The Greek historian Herodotus, who traveled through Egypt in about 450 BCE, reported that the workers who built the pyramids were given large rations of onions, radishes, and garlic. A sum of 1600 silver talents (equivalent to about US$ 10 million) was spent over a 20-year period to supply some 360,000 workers with these provisions. Herodotus went on to explain that large amounts of garlic were necessary to protect the pyramid builders from febrile illnesses.

The Israelites learned about garlic from the Egyptians. After the Hebrew slaves had been led out of Egypt, they bemoaned the loss of this valuable medicine and spice with these words:
"We remember the fish we ate in Egypt for nothing, the cucumbers, the melons, the leeks, the onions, and the garlic; but now our strength is dried up, and there is nothing at all..."
(*Numbers 11: 5-6*) (Ferne, 2004).

Garlic has been known in Europe as a healing herb since the Middle Ages. It owed much of its popularity to the Benedictine monks who grew garlic in their monastery gardens. Garlic was thought to be a valuable remedy for communicable diseases, and many references are found to its use in plagues. When Basel was struck by the plague, the Jewish population who consumed garlic regularly, reportedly fared much better than other citizens. In 1721 the plague was rampant in Marseilles. During this time a band of thieves looted the city, robbing the sick and dead alike, without contracting the disease themselves. When one of the thieves was caught, he explained that his band had regularly consumed garlic soaked in wine and vinegar.

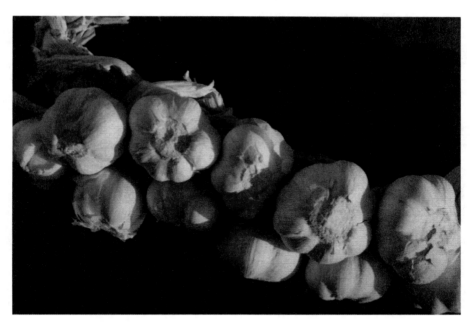

Fig. 3.8. ▲ Garlic (*Allium sativum*).

Besides its antimicrobial properties, garlic was prized by the peoples of Europe and the Orient for its effects on the heart and circulation. For example, garlic was commonly recommended as a remedy for "dropsy" (cardiac insufficiency). The lipid-reducing and antiatherosclerotic effects of garlic – a focal point of current interest – were unknown in ancient and medieval medicine because atherosclerosis was not recognized as an important disease entity until the Industrial Age. Koch et al. (1996) published a detailed account of the history of the medicinal uses of garlic.

3.3.1.2 Botanical Description

A member of the lily family, garlic (*Allium sativum*, Fig. 3.8) traces its origins to Central Asia. Today it is known only in its cultivated form. The subterranean garlic bulb is not laminar like an onion but is a composite structure consisting of 4–20 cloves, each enclosed within a dry, white leaf skin. The weight of one clove is highly variable, averaging about 1 g. Rising from the cloves are unbranched, quill-like stalks about 30–90 cm high topped by flowers arranged in a loose, globular cluster. This flower head is surrounded by a cylindrical, sharply tapered leaf, or spathe, resembling a pointed cap. The cluster is an umbel composed of about 5–7 pale flowers that bloom from June to August. Among the flowers are about 20–30 bulbils or "brood bulbs" up to 1 cm in size. Because the flowers are almost always sterile, the bulbils perform an important reproductive function.

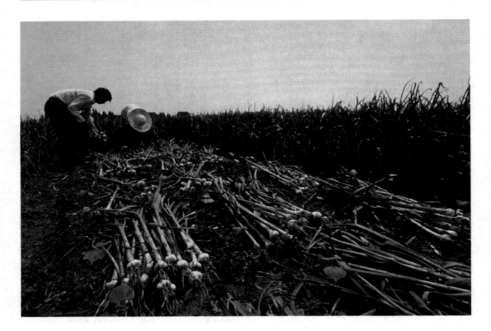

Fig. 3.9. ▲ All garlic for commercial use is cultivated.

3.3.1.3 Crude Drug

Only the garlic bulb has culinary and medicinal applications. Today it is entirely a prod-uct of commercial cultivation (Fig. 3.9). World production is approximately 2 million tons annually, with about 60 % grown in Asia (mostly China), 20 % in Europe, and 10 % each in North America and Africa (Fenwick and Hanley, 1985).

Most garlic is processed into a powdered form immediately after harvesting. Garlic powder is produced by peeling the cloves, cutting them into slices, and drying them for 3–4 days at a maximum temperature of 500C to a residual moisture content of less than 5 %. During this process the garlic loses about two-thirds of its fresh weight (Heikal et al., 1972). Drying destroys very little of the sulfur-containing constituents or the enzyme alliinase that causes their breakdown (see Sect.3.3.1.4); but the residual moisture in the garlic powder leads to a gradual but constant enzymatic decomposition and subsequent volatilization of the sulfur-containing compounds that contribute to garlic's medicinal effects. This process limits the shelf life of fresh garlic and of garlic-based medications.

Besides the powdered herb, there are other preparations that are used in medicinal garlic products. In terms of practical significance, the most important are garlic oil macerations (cold oil infusions) using fatty oils. In this process the garlic cloves are ground, covered with a vegetable oil such as corn oil or wheat germ oil, and allowed to stand so that lipophilic compounds can dissolve into the oil. A press is then used to sep-arate the oil from the solid residues. These preparations do not contain the water-solu-ble constituents of garlic.

Another process uses steam distillation to obtain essential garlic oil from freshly ground garlic. Garlic bulbs have about a 0.1–0.5 % content of water-soluble compounds.

Analogous to cold oil infusions, the compounds present in essential garlic oil no longer correspond to the original plant constituents as enzymatic and thermal breakdown transform alliin and other thiosulfinates (see Sect.3.3.1.4) into sulfur-containing products. While garlic-oil preparations are known to have certain therapeutic effects, they are not nearly as effective as garlic powder and other medicinal garlic preparations.

Garlic fermentation products (aged garlics) have been available on the pharmaceutical market for several years now. These odor-free products are fermented for several months in the presence of moisture and atmospheric oxygen, resulting in the conversion of all reactive garlic constituents into more or less inert degradation products. One would not expect these fermented products to have significant medicinal actions, nor have such actions been demonstrated in pharmacologic or clinical studies.

3.3.1.4 Key Constituents, Analysis, Pharmacokinetics

The constituents of garlic are ordinarily divided into two groups: sulfur-containing compounds and non-sulfur-containing compounds. Most of the medicinal effects of garlic are referable to the sulfur compounds and the alliin-splitting enzyme alliinase. Thus, commercial garlic preparations are often adjusted or standardized to sulfur-containing ingredients, particularly to the amino acid alliin contained in garlic powder.

Garlic cloves typically contain about 0.35 % total sulfur (about 1 % of dry weight) and about 1 % total nitrogen. The organic sulfur compounds in garlic are derived from the amino acid cysteine or its derivatives and can be subdivided into S-allylcysteine sulfoxide and γ-glutamyl-S-allylcysteines. Apparently the cysteine sulfoxides are stored in the form of γ-glutamylcysteines, which undergo a gradual hydrolytic cleavage during germination of the garlic bulb and in products that are stored. Thus, freshly harvested garlic differs markedly from stored garlic, especially in its content of γ-glutamylcysteines.

Fresh garlic contains about 0.5–1 % cysteine sulfoxides, mostly alliin, and an equal amount of γ-glutamylcysteines. Garlic powder that has been carefully dried may contain up to twice the concentrations of these constituents. Garlic powder products manufactured in Europe and in the U.S. are usually standardized to a specified content of alliin or of the allicin that is released from alliin by the action of the enzyme alliinase (Fig. 3.10). (The leading garlic product from Japan is prepared and standardized by a different criteria, where S-acetyl-cysteine, a product of the garlic decomposition cascade, is the standardized marker compound.)Alliin is separated from alliinase while it is still in the cells of an intact garlic bulb. But when the bulb is chopped or crushed, damage to the cells allows the alliin to come into contact with alliinase, and within minutes the enzyme converts the alliin into the volatile compound allicin. Allicin has an aromatic odor but is unstable in aqueous and oily solution, and within a few hours it degrades into vinyldithiins and ajoene. Cold oil infusions and distilled garlic oils contain only the products of alliin degradation.

The amount of sulfur-containing constituents in fresh garlic is highly variable (Fig. 3.11); hence the leading European garlic manufacturer has determined that it is important to standardize garlic-powder preparations to a specified concentration range of alliin. This standardization may well account for the positive, reproducible results that have been obtained in recent years with garlic-powder tablet in controlled clinical studies (see Sect.3.3.1.7).

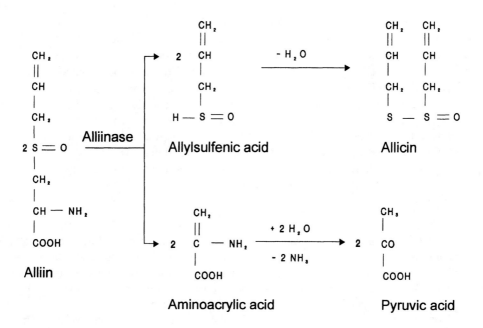

Fig. 3.10. ▲ Alliin, a natural constituent of garlic, is converted by the enzyme alliinase to allicin and pyruvic acid.

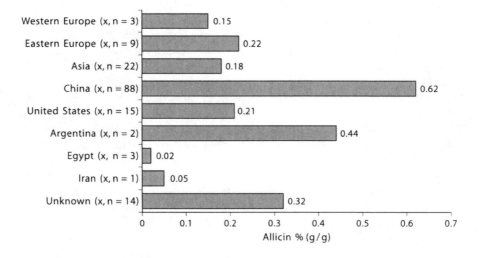

Fig. 3.11. ▲ Quantity of allicin released from garlic samples obtained from various regions of the world. The tests were performed between 1984 and 1990. Quantitative allicin release varied by up to a factor of 31 among different samples (Chinese vs. Egyptian garlic) (Pfaff, 1991).

The non-sulfur-containing constituents of garlic include alliinase and other enzymes. These enzymes appear to have significant bearing on the bioavailability of garlic principles, and the garlic should be dried in a manner that preserves the enzymes (e.g., avoiding air temperatures in excess of 50 °C). Other non-sulfur-containing garlic constituents are various amino acids, proteins, lipids, steroids, vitamins, and 12 trace elements (Block 1992; Reuter and Sendl, 1994).

Pharmacokinetics studies were performed in rats using S-labeled alliin, allicin, and vinyldithiin. Each compound was administered in a dose of 8 mg/kg, and the activity levels were determined in terms of ^{35}S-alliin. Blood levels were measured over a 72-h period along with excretion levels in the urine, feces, and expired air. Whole-animal autoradiographs were also obtained to assess organ distribution. It was found that the rates of absorption and elimination for ^{35}S-alliin were markedly higher than for the other garlic constituents. Maximum blood levels were reached within 10 min after oral administration (by stomach tube). The measured urinary levels indicated a minimum absorption rate of 65 % for allicin and 73 % for the vinyldithiins. Approximately 20 % was found in the stool, and traces were detectable in the expired air (Lachmann et al., 1994).

3.3.1.5 Experimental Pharmacology

To date, some 100 original papers have been published on the experimental pharmacology of garlic and its preparations, so it is not possible to provide here a complete listing of bibliographic references. (Surveys may be found in Reuter et al., 1994, 1995).

Most pharmacologic studies in the past 20 years have been done in animal models and have dealt mostly with the antiatherogenic, lipid-reducing, and antihypertensive effects of garlic; its inhibitory effects on cholesterol synthesis; its properties as a vasodilator and antioxidant; and its capacity to activate fibrinolysis and inhibit platelet aggregation. Older studies tended to focus on the antimicrobial properties of garlic.

Table 3.5 reviews the pharmacodynamic studies performed between 1988 and 2003 using a standardized garlic powder (approximately 1 % alliin). Taken as a whole, the results of these studies can account for the inhibitory effect of garlic on the progression of atherosclerosis (Sect. 3.3.1.7.3).

3.3.1.5.1 Effects on Atherogenesis and Lipid Metabolism

Seven groups of authors (Abramoritz, 1999; Tain, 1975; 1977; Bordia et al., 1977; Chang et al., 1980; Kamanna et al., 1984; Mand et al., 1985; Betz et al., 1989) studied the effects of the long-term (2-9 months) feeding of garlic and garlic preparations to rabbits with experimental atherosclerosis induced by a high-cholesterol diet. Most of the authors found that dietary garlic supplementation caused a statistically significant reduction of atheromatous lesions, particularly in the aorta, that averaged about 50 %. The duration of use was a highly significant factor, and a period of months was necessary to inhibit atherogenesis. Comparative studies with various garlic preparations showed that the antiatheromatous effects were due mainly to the lipophilic fractions in the garlic, with hydrophilic fractions playing a lesser role. Other authors who studied specific garlic constituents (Fujiwara et al., 1972; Itokawa et al., 1973; Zhao et al., 1983) showed that the sulfur-containing compounds have special significance in inhibiting atherogenesis. Heinle and Betz (1994) and Patumraj et al. (2000) documented antiatheromatous

Table 3.5.
Pharmacologic studies using a standardized garlic powder (with 1 % alliin). The results of these publications support for the inhibitory effect of garlic therapy on the progression of atherosclerosis.

First author, year	Study material	Effects	Inhibition of atherosclerosis
Betz, 1989	Rabbits	Antiatherogenic	++
Heinle, 1994	Rats	Antiatherogenic	++
Orekhov, 1995	Intimal cell culture	Antiatherosclerotic	++
Orekhov, 1997	Intimal cell culture	Antiatherogenic	++
Abramovitz, 1999	Mice	Antiatherogenic	++
Patumraj, 2000	Diabetic rats	Antiatherosclerotic	++
Siegel, 2003	Biosensor model	Antiatherosclerotic	++
Brosche, 1991	Rats	Inhibition of cholesterol synthesis	+
Gebhardt, 1993	Hepatocyte culture	Inhibition of cholesterol synthesis	+
Gebhardt, 1994	Hepatocyte culture	Inhibition of cholesterol synthesis	+
Gebhardt, 1995	Hepatocyte culture	Inhibition of cholesterol synthesis	+
Gebhardt, 1996	Hepatocyte culture	Inhibition of cholesterol synthesis	+
Liu, 2000	Isolated rat hepatocytes	Inhibition of cholesterol synthesis	+
Siegel, 1991	Human coronary arteries	Vasodilation	+
Jacob, 1991	Hypertensive rats	Antihypertensive	+
Das, 1995	Thrombocytes	antiplatelet effect	+
Sabban, 1997	Thrombocytes	antiplatelet effect	+
Brändle, 1997	Hypertensive rats	Life-prolonging	+
Ciplea, 1988	Rats	Cardioprotective	(+)
Ipensee, 1993	Langendorff heart (rat)	Cardioprotective	(+)
Pedraza, 1998	Rats	NO sythetase activating, Vasodilatin	+
Kourounakis, 1991	Hepatic microsomes	Antioxidative	(+)
Popov, 1994	Photochemical radicals	Antioxidative	(+)
Török, 1994	Photochemical radicals	Antioxidative	(+)
Lewin, 1994	LDL particles	Antioxidative	(+)
Siegers, 1999	Granulocytes	Antioxidative	(+)
Siegers, 1992	Colon carcinoma cells	Tumor-protective	–

effects in live rats, and Orekhow et al. (1995) observed similar effects on atherosclerotic plaque in human aortas. Jacob et al. (1993) demonstrated cardioprotective effects in rats with experimental myocardial infarction that had been fed garlic powder for 10 weeks.

Abramovitz (1999) investigated the effect of allicin as an active component of garlic on formation of fatty streaks (atherosclerosis) and lipid profile in mice. While he observed no significant differences between blood lipid profiles of groups, the microscopic evaluation of aortic sinus formation of fatty streaks showed that values for mice in the allicin-treated group were significantly lower by nearly 50 %.

The inhibitory effects of garlic on cholesterol biosynthesis were first documented by Quereshi et al. (1983) in chicken hepatocytes and monkey livers. These authors also conducted comparative studies with three extract fractions. At equivalent doses, both the whole herb and its lipophilic and hydrophilic fractions caused a 50–75 % inhibition of

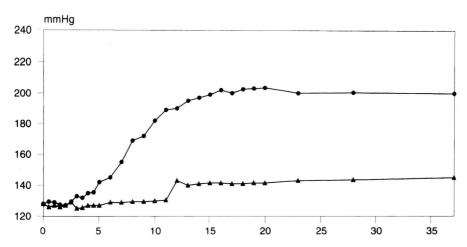

Fig. 3.12. ▲ Progression of blood pressure readings in spontaneously hypertensive rats. Time 0 corresponds to delivery of the experimental animals (at about 3 weeks of age). The animals were observed for approximately 9 months. The upper curve represents the control animals; the lower curve represents animals given an average dose of 1 g/kg b. w. garlic powder daily added to their standard feed (Jacob et al., 1991).

two key enzymes in cholesterol biosynthesis. In experiments with rat hepatocytes, Gebhardt et al. (1993, 1994) identified the steps in cholesterol biosynthesis that are influenced by garlic and its sulfur-containing constituents. The molecular mechanism of action is based on an interaction with the phosphorylation cascade of hydroxymethylglutaryl-CoA reductase (Gebhardt, 1995). Allicin inhibited the uptake of ^{14}C-acetate into neutral lipids at concentrations as low as 10 µM, making allicin the most active compound among the sulfur-containing derivatives of alliin (Gebhardt et al., 1996). These results have been confirmed by Liu and Yeh (2000) and supplemented by other systematic studies using 11 water-soluble and 6 lipid-soluble alliin derivatives.

3.3.1.5.2 Effects on Vascular Resistance, Fibrinolysis, and Platelet Aggregation
Chandorkar and Jain (1973) and Malik et al. (1981) demonstrated the ability of garlic preparations to lower blood pressure in experimental dogs.

Jacob et al. (1991) tested the effects of garlic powder added to the feed of spontaneously hypertensive rats for periods of 2 weeks to 11 months. The results of this study (Fig. 3.12) provide very impressive evidence of the antihypertensive effect of garlic, which was accompanied by a reduction in secondary myocardial injury. In a series of studies by the same group of authors in spontaneously hypertensive rats, the life span of the animals was significantly prolonged by garlic feeding (Brändle et al., 1997).

Besides the inhibition of plaque formation, the antihypertensive properties of garlic appear to be based partly on a direct vasodilating action of garlic constituents. Siegel et al. (1991, 1992) investigated these effects in isolated strips from canine carotid arteries and in isolated vascular muscle cells. They found that aqueous garlic extracts and some sulfur-containing compounds produced a strong membrane-polarizing effect, suggesting that certain garlic constituents may act as potassium channel openers. Another study showed that garlic is a potent activator of endogenous nitric oxide (NO) synthesis (Das et al., 1995). Nitric oxide is known as a powerful vasodilator whose functions include physiologic vasodilatation in response to muscular exercise (Bode-Böger et al., 1994).

The activating effect of garlic on fibrinolysis and its inhibitory effect on platelet aggregation have been demonstrated in a total of 16 experimental studies, some done in live animals and some performed in vitro. These studies and their results are reviewed in Reuter et al. (1994, 1995, 1996). Most of these studies showed that various garlic preparations as well as certain sulfur-containing metablic products of alliin act to stimulate endogenous fibrinolysis and inhibit platelet aggregation. A therapeutic trial in patients with increased platelet aggregation showed an absence of acute effects; treatment had to be continued for 2–4 weeks to achieve a significant response (Kiesewetter et al., 1993). Das et al. (1995) identified the activation of calcium-dependent nitric oxide synthetase as the mechanism by which garlic inhibits platelet aggregation.

3.3.1.5.3 Cardioprotective and Antioxidative Effects
Feeding garlic powder to rats for 11 days had a protective effect on isoproterenol-induced myocardial damage (Ciplea and Richter, 1988). In another series of tests, rats were fed a standard chow enriched with 1 % garlic powder for 10 weeks. Studies on cardioprotective effect were then performed in a Langendorff heart preparation under conditions of cardiac ischemia and reperfusion. The authors determined the time to onset of ventricular fibrillation and the size of the ischemic zone as a percentage of cardiac weight. The time to onset of arrhythmia after occlusion of the descending branch of the left coronary artery was significantly prolonged in the garlic-treated animals compared with untreated controls, and the size of the ischemic zone was significantly reduced (Isensee et al., 1993).

The formation of oxygen-derived free radicals leading to lipid peroxidation may play a key role in the pathogenesis of atherosclerosis, and therefore the antioxidative effects of garlic could contribute to its antiatherosclerotic properties. These effects have been demonstrated with garlic powder in isolated hepatic microsomes (Kourounakis et al., 1991), in isolated LDL particles (Lewin et al., 1994), and using a photochemical radical generator with chemiluminescence measurements (Popov et al., 1994; Török et al., 1994).

3.3.1.5.4 Other Actions
A number of predominantly older studies showed that garlic and its aqueous preparations had definite antibacterial and antifungal properties, with a few studies even showing evidence of antiviral activity. These studies are reviewed in Reuter et al. (1994, 1995). But while the anti-infectious effects of garlic, whose main active principle has been known since 1944 (Cavallito and Bailey, 1944), are still of interest to medical historians (see 3.3.1), they are no longer considered to have practical importance. The protective effects against *Heliobacter pylori* have prompted renewed interest in the antibacterial properties of garlic (Sivam, 2001), but so far clinical studies in human patients have been unable to confirm these effects (Graham et al., 1999; Aydin et al., 2000).

Various experimental models in rabbits, rats, and guinea pigs have demonstrated the antihypertensive properties of garlic (Mathew et al., 1973; Jain, 1977; Zacharias et al., 1980; Chang et al., 1980). The groups of Mathew and Chang concluded from their findings that garlic stimulates insulin production, but therapeutic studies have shown no evidence that garlic has antidiabetic properties in human patients.

Five studies have described antitoxic effects of garlic in cases of carbon tetrachloride, isoproteranol, and heavy metal poisoning. Garlic has exhibited tumor-inhibiting properties in 12 other studies, showing the greatest effects in sarcomas, bladder tumors, liver cell carcinomas, and isolated colon carcinoma cells (survey in Reuter and Sendl, 1994). To date there have been 20 epidemiologic studies on the effect of a garlic-rich diet on the incidence of malignant tumors in humans. The results indicate that a high dietary intake of *Allium* species has a protective effect against certain gastrointestinal tumors. Antibacterial or antimutagenic effects have been postulated as possible mechanisms (Ernst, 1997).

3.3.1.6 Toxicology

Tests of the acute toxicity of allicin in mice indicated LD_{50} values of 60 mg/kg by intravenous injection and 120 mg/kg by subcutaneous injection (Cavallito and Bailey, 1944). A more recent study on the acute toxicity of a garlic extract in rats and mice showed lethal effects following the oral, intraperitoneal, and subcutaneous administration of doses higher than 30 mL/kg (Nakagawa et al., 1984).

In another study, rats fed up to 2000 mg/kg of a garlic extract for 6 months showed no weight loss but did show a slightly reduced food intake relative to controls. There were no changes in renal function, hematologic parameters, or selected serologic parameters, and there was no evidence of any pathologic changes in organs or tissues (Sumiyoshi et al., 1984).

A study testing for genotoxicity in mouse bone marrow cells after the oral administration of garlic showed no significant changes in comparison with untreated controls (Abraham and Kesavan, 1984).

A review of other studies on the toxicology of garlic may be found in Koch (1988, 1996).

3.3.1.7 Clinical Studies

Thirty-two controlled clinical studies on garlic preparations were published from 1985 to 1999. Four of these studies were done with garlic oil or an oil maceration (Lau et al., 1987; Barrie et al., 1987; Gadkari and Joshi, 1991; Berthold et al., 1998). All the others used garlic powder preparations adjusted to an alliin content of 1.0–1.4 % (Table 3.6). Further discussions in this chapter pertain exclusively to studies that used garlic powder preparations, because the results obtained with garlic oil cannot be validly applied to powder preparations due to differences in pharmaceutical quality. Earlier studies published up until about 1994 have been reviewed in several surveys and meta-analyses (Reuter and Sendl, 1994; Reuter et al., 1995; Silagy and Neil, 1994; Warshafsky et al., 1993).

Table 3.6 lists 30 treatment studies in which garlic powder tablets were used. A total of 3689 patients was enrolled in these studies, and 2012 of the patients received garlic preparations. Four of the studies did not use control groups. Three studies compared garlic with a reference therapy, one study used matched pairs, and all the rest were double-blind studies with placebo controls. The duration of treatment ranged from 2 to 208

Table 3.6.
Review of 30 clinical studies in which standardized garlic powder tablets were used.

First author, year	Number of patients		Dose (mg/d)	Weeks	Key parameters
	Total	Taking garlic			
Ernst, 1986	20	10	600	4	CH, TG
König, 1986	53	53	600	4	CH, TG, PVD, BP
Kandziora, 1988 a	40	20	600	12	CH, TG, BP
Kandziora, 1988 b	40	20	600	12	CH, TG, BP
Harenberg, 1988	20	20	600	4	CH, TG, FL, BP
Schwartzkopff, 1988	40	20	900	12	Lipid fractions, BP
Auer, 1989	47	24	600	12	CH, TG, BP
Brosche, 1989	40	40	600	12	Lipid fractions
Vorberg, 1990	40	20	900	16	CH, TG, BP, B
Zimmermann, 1990	23	23	900	3	CH, TG
Mader, 1990	221	111	800	16	CH, TG, BP
Kiesewetter, 1991	60	30	800	5	THE, EF, PV, BP
Holzgartner, 1992	94	47	900	12	CH, TG, HDL, LDL, BP
Rotzsch, 1992	24	12	900	6	TG (postprandial)
De Santos, 1993	52	25	900	24	CH, TG, LDL, HDL, BP, B
Jain, 1993	42	20	900	12	CH, TG, BP, B
Kiesewetter, 1993 b	64	32	800	12	PVD, THA, PV, CH, BP
Saradeth, 1994	68	31	600	15	FL, PV, HKT, CH, TG, BP
Walper, 1994	1682	917	600	6	CH (vs. diet)
Simons, 1995	28	28	900	12	CH, LDL, HDL, TG, BP, LOS
De Santos, 1995	70	36	600	16	CH, LDL, HDL, BP, B
Neil, 1996	115	57	900	24	CH, LDL, HDL, TG
Orekhov, 1996	23	11	900	4	CAG, LOS, CH, TG
Adler, 1997	50	12	900	12	CH, LDL, HDL, TG
Breithaupt-Grögler, 1997	202	101	>300	>104	PWV, EVR
Isaacsohn, 1998	50	28	900	12	CH, LDL, HDL, TG
Lash, 1998	35	19	1400	12	CH, LDL, HDL, TG
McCrindle, 1998	30	15	900	8	CH, LDL, HDL
Koscielny, 1999	152	61	900	208	PQV
Superko, 2000	50	25	900	12	CH, LDL, HDL, TG

NOTE: A total of 3724 patients was enrolled, 2012 of whom were treated with garlic. The doses ranged from 300 mg to 1400 mg of garlic powder daily. The duration of treatment ranged from 2 to 208 weeks.
Abbreviations: CH = total cholesterol, LDL = LDL cholesterol, HDL = HDL cholesterol, TG = triglycerides, B = mood, PVD = walking distance and symptoms of peripheral arterial occlusive disease, BP = blood pressure reduction, FL = fibrinolysis, THA = platelet aggregation, PV = plasma viscosity, LOS = lipoprotein oxidation, CAG = cellular atherogenicity, PQV = plaque volume, PWV = pulse wave velocity, EVR = elastic vascular resistance.

weeks, depending on the goal of the study. Most of the older studies used blood lipids as confirmatory parameters, especially the total cholesterol and plasma triglycerides. One study tested the efficacy of garlic tablets by measuring the increase in walking distance in patients with peripheral arterial occlusive disease (Kiesewetter et al., 1993b).

Table 3.7.
The effect of garlic powder tablets on total serum cholesterol -- evaluated in the 21 studies listed in Table 3.6.

First author, year	Cholesterol a) before:after (mg/dL)	Difference (%) During course of treatment	Relative to placebo
Harenberg, 1988, K	278:258	-7*	-
Kandziora, 1988 b, K	314:294	-6 f	-5 ns
Schwartzkopff, 1988, R	278:274	-1 ns	-3 ns
Auer, 1989, R	268:230	-14*	-6+
Brosche, 1989	260:240	-8***	-
Vorberg, 1990, R	259:233	-21***	-17***
Mader, 1990, R	266:235	-12***	-9***
Holzgartner, 1992, K	282:210	-25***	-
Rotzsch, 1992, K	261:253	-3***	-2***
De Santos, 1993, R	267:243	-5*	-6*
Jain, 1993, R	263:247	-6**	-5**
Kiesewetter, 1993 b, R	267:234	-12***	-8*
Saradeth, 1994, R	223:214	-4*	-5*
Simons, 1995, R	(Crossover design)		ns
De Santos, 1995, K	6.47:5.76 (mmol/L)	-11*	-8 ns
Neil, 1996, R	6.96:6.91 (mmol/L)	-1 ns	-2 ns
Orekhov, 1996, R	217:201	-7 ns	-7 ns
Adler, 1997, R	6.54:5.79 (mmol/L)	-11*	-12**
Isaacsohn, 1998, R	7.1:? (mmol/L)	+2 ns	+2 ns
Lash, 1998 R	290:275	-5*	-7*
McCrindle, 1998, R	6.86:? (mmol/L)	+0.6 ns	+0.1 ns
Superko, 2000, R	245 : 243	-1 ns	-2 ns

NOTE: Column 2 shows the values before and after garlic treatment (see Table 3.6 for treatment duration and dosage). Column 3 shows the percentage changes relative to the initial value in the garlic group, and column 4 shows the difference in the percentage changes between the garlic and placebo groups at the end of treatment.

Abbreviations: * = < 0.05; ** = < 0.01; *** = < 0.001; ns = not significant; f = no information given on significance; R = double-blind placebo-controlled study; K = comparison with control group

One study tested the effect of garlic on the atherogenicity of LDL (Orekhov et al., 1996), one tested its effect on atherosclerotic plaque growth in the carotid artery (Koscielny et al., 1999), and another studied its effect on pulse wave velocity to measure the elastic properties of the aorta (Breithaupt-Grögler et al., 1997). Some studies also evaluated secondary parameters such as mood (psychometric scales), blood pressure reduction, increased fibrinolysis, and a decrease in plasma viscosity (Kiesewetter et. al., 1993c).

3.3.1.7.1 Reduction of Elevated Blood Lipids

Brosche and Platt (1990) reviewed the results of the studies from 1988 to 1990. Table 3.7 presents data from this review, supplemented by data from other studies published between 1992 and 1998. As the table indicates, 13 of the 21 studies showed significant reductions in total cholesterol during the course of treatment, and 8 studies showed significant cholesterol reductions compared with a control group. We also note, however, that significant lipid-lowering effects were found less frequently in the studies from 1995 to 1998 than in earlier studies, a circumstance that has led some authors to question the lipid-lowering effects of garlic in general (Isaacsohn et al., 1998; Berthold et al., 1998; Superko et al., 2000).

The most comprehensive placebo-controlled study on the lipid-lowering effect of garlic powder was performed by Mader et al. (1990) in 261 patients. Over a 16-week course of treatment, these authors found significant reductions in total cholesterol compared with placebo-treated controls. The most striking effects were seen in patients with initial cholesterol levels in the range of 250 to 300 mg/dL. The lipid-lowering effects of garlic powder in patients with hyperlipidemia were evaluated in two meta-analyses performed in the early 1990s. These studies concluded that, when correction is made for the placebo effect, garlic therapy can reduce total cholesterol by an average of 9 % (Warshafsky et al., 1993) or 12 % (Silagy and Neil, 1994 a) or 6 % (Stevinson et al., 2000), with a 13 % average reduction in triglycerides compared with placebo (Silagy and Neil, 1994a). These results were obtained at dose levels equivalent to 600–900 mg of garlic powder daily during treatment periods of at least 4 weeks.

3.3.1.7.2 Blood Pressure Reduction

Blood pressure changes were investigated as an associated parameter in a total of 15 studies. Table 3.8 reviews the average blood pressure measured in garlic-treated subjects at the start and conclusion of the treatment periods. The percentage differences in blood pressures measured before and after treatment are indicated. The last column in Table 3.8 shows the statistical significance relative to a placebo or controls. The table indicates that, except for two studies, all the researchers noted blood pressure reductions in the subjects who took coated garlic tablets. The reductions ranged from 2 % to 27 % of the initial values.

A meta-analysis of eight studies, including three that specifically included hypertensive patients, showed a significant reduction of diastolic blood pressure in four studies and a significant reduction of systolic blood pressure in three studies (Silagy and Neil, 1994). These authors concluded from the studies that garlic can slightly lower blood pressure when taken in doses equivalent to 600–900 mg of powder daily but that this effect is not adequate for specific antihypertensive therapy in patients with high blood pressure.

3.3.1.7.3 Inhibiting the Progression of Atherosclerosis in Humans

Given the favorable effect of garlic on typical risk factors for atherosclerosis as well as on coagulation factors and the rheologic properties of blood, it is reasonable to assume that garlic produces a net antiatherosclerotic effect (Neil and Silagy, 1994). To date, four studies have been done to test directly for this effect in humans. Two of the studies were in patients with Fontaine stage II peripheral arterial occlusive disease. König and Schneider (1986) performed an open study with 53 patients who were treated with garlic powder tablets (600 mg/d) for 12 weeks. These patients showed significant improvements in calf and toe oscillography and plethysmographic toe pressure. Kiesewetter et al. (1993b; Siegel et al., 2000) performed a placebo-controlled double-blind study in 80 patients (64 evaluable cases) who took garlic powder in a dose of 800 mg/day for 12 weeks.

Table 3.8.
Mean blood pressure readings (systolic/diastolic) before and after treatment with garlic powder tablets.

First author, year	Mean BP (mm Hg) Patients on garlic therapy			Significance Garlic vs. placebo
	Before	After	Diff.%	
König, 1986	167/107	156/97	−6/−5	−
Harenberg, 1988	137/86	126/81	−8/−9	−
Kandziora, 1988 a, R	174/99	158/83	−9/−16	−
Kandziora, 1988 b, K	178/100	167/85	−6/−15	−
Schwartzkopff, 1988, R	128/82	130/84	+2/+2	ns
Auer, 1989, R	171/101	151/90	−12/−11	*
Vorberg, 1990, R	144/90	138/87	−4/−3	*
Mader, 1990, R	151/92	143/85	−5/−8	*
Kiesewetter, 1991, R	116/73	108/67	−7/−9	*
Holzgartner, 1992, K	143/83	135/79	−6/−5	*
De Santos, 1993, R	145/90	120/80	−17/−11	*
Kiesewetter, 1993 b, R	152/85	150/82	−2/−3	*
Saradeth, 1994, R	125/80	127/83	+2/+3	ns
Simons, 1995, R	(Crossover design)			ns
De Santos, 1995, K	151/96	124/79	−27/−17	−

NOTE: The dosages and duration of treatment are shown in Table 3.6. In most of the 15 studies, BP readings were taken only as a secondary parameter. A numerical BP reduction occurred during the course of treatment in 12 of the 15 studies. Differences relative to a placebo were significant in 7 of the studies.
Abbreviations: K = comparison with a control group; R = randomized double-blind placebo-controlled study; * = statistically significant ($p < 0.05$).

The confirmatory parameter was pain-free walking distance determined by treadmill ergometry. Both the garlic and placebo groups received regular physical therapy. Walking distance in the garlic group increased by 28 % (46 meters) compared with 18 % (31 meters) in the placebo group. The difference between the two groups was significant at the 5 % level and increased steadily over the 12-week treatment period.

The same group of authors performed a prospective placebo-controlled double-blind study in a total of 280 patients from 1992 to 1998. The confirmatory parameter in this study was the change in the volume of atherosclerotic plaque in the common carotid artery, which was measured by B-mode ultrasound imaging. Of the patients initially enrolled, 152 completed the 48-month course of treatment. The increase in atherosclerotic plaque volumes was significantly reduced by 5–18 % compared with the placebo group. Age-correlated plaque growth in patients from 50 to 80 years of age decreased significantly by 6–13 % over the 4-year treatment period (Fig. 3.13). The results indicate that the antiatherosclerotic effects of garlic are both prophylactic and, in some patients, therapeutic in terms of reducing the volume of existing plaques (Koscielny et al., 1999).

Orekhov et al. (1996) performed a placebo-controlled study in a total of 23 patients with advanced coronary atherosclerosis. Eleven of the patients took a daily dose of 900 mg of garlic powder in the form of coated tablets for 4 weeks. The key parameter

Fig. 3.13. ▶ Prospective double-blind study tracing the development of atherosclerotic plaque in patients taking 900 mg of garlic powder daily for 4 years (•, n=61, regression line b) compared with a placebo (o, n=91, regression line a). Plaque growth, reflecting the progression of atherosclerosis, is significantly inhibited by garlic therapy (Koscielny et al., 1999).

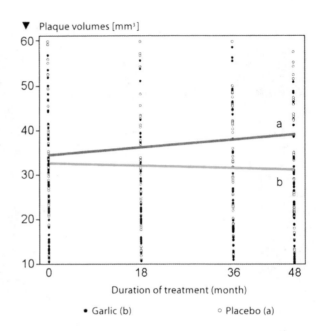

in the study was the atherogenic potential of the patients' serum and of the LDL fraction derived from it. This was measured in cultured subendothelial cells from the human aorta. The atherogenicity of the LDL fraction was significantly reduced by 38 % in the garlic-treated patients but showed no significant change following treatment with a placebo.

Breithaupt-Grögler et al. (1997) studied older, healthy adults (n=101, 50–80 years of age) who were taking more than 300 mg/day of standardized garlic powder (LI 111) for more than 2 years and compared them with an equal number of age- and sex-matched controls. The pulse wave velocity (PWV) and pressure-standardized elastic vascular resistance (EVR) were used as indices to measure the elastic properties of the aorta (Breithaupt-Grögler et al., 1992). Blood pressures and plasma lipid levels were similar in the two groups. The PWV (8.3 ± 1.46 versus 9.8 ± 2.45 m/s; p < 0.001) and EVR (0.63 ± 0.21 versus 0.9 ± 0.44 $m^2 \times s^{-2} \times mmHg^{-1}$; p < 0.001) were lower in the garlic group than in the control group. The PWV showed a significant positive correlation with age and systolic blood pressure. With any increase in age or systolic blood pressure, the PWV increased significantly less in the garlic group than in the control group (p < 0.001, Fig. 3.14). Statistical analysis showed that the effect of garlic on the PWV was independent of the cofactors of age and blood pressure. The authors concluded from these results that chronic garlic powder intake delays age-related increases in aortic stiffness.

3.3.1.7.4 Other Clinical Studies

A total of eight clinical pharmacologic studies in healthy subjects have investigated the effects of garlic on spontaneous platelet aggregation, endogenous fibrinolysis, plasma viscosity, arteriolar caliber, and blood flow velocity as determined by direct light

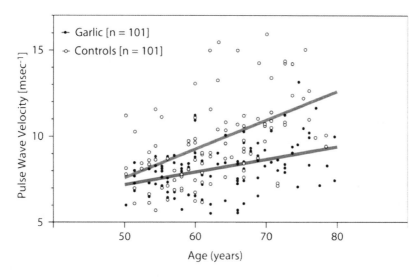

Fig. 3.14. ▲ Relationships between age and pulse wave velocity (PWV) in the garlic user (•) and control subjects (o). The slope of the lines relating age and PWV was different between the two groups (p=<0.0001). The linear regression line was less steep in the garlic group than in the control group; garlic group: PWV = 0.08 (SD, 0.017) age + 3.03 (SD, 1.081); control group: PWV = 0.18 (SD, 0.029) age - 1.25 (SD, 1.822) (Breithaupt-Grögler et al., 1997).

microscopy at the nail fold. These techniques were used to test the dose-dependence of the response to a single dose of 100–2700 mg. It was found that 300 mg of the garlic powder preparation constituted the threshold dose for significant pharmacodynamic effects. Raising the dose to 1200 mg led to proportionate increases in the demonstrable effects (Kiesewetter et al., 1993b; survey in Reuter et al., 1994). Another study was performed in 60 subjects who had an increased propensity for spontaneous platelet aggregation. These subjects took a daily dose equivalent to 800 mg of garlic powder or a placebo for four weeks in a double-blind, placebo-controlled protocol. The differences between the two treatment groups at the end of four weeks were statistically significant (Kiesewetter et al., 1993a).

3.3.1.8 Side Effects and Garlic Odor

Relatively few side effects were reported in the 30 treatment studies and 8 clinical pharmacologic studies using garlic powder preparations, although most of the older studies did not systematically investigate or document adverse reactions. Of the side effects that were reported, most were nonspecific and occurred equally in the garlic and placebo groups. Gastrointestinal discomfort and nausea were the most frequent complaints. Reports of allergic skin reactions apparently represent a more specific response. A survey by Koch (1996) showed that allergic reactions to garlic were reported in a total of 39 publications between 1938 and 1994. Most of these cases involved an allergic contact dermatitis, sometimes severe (Eming et al., 1999), which has been reported in certain occupational groups exposed to frequent contact with garlic. There have also been sporadic reports of allergic conjunctivitis, rhinitis, or bronchospasms occurring in response to garlic inhalation or ingestion (Falleroni et al., 1981; Papageorgiou et al., 1983). Other cases of severe contact dermatitis have been reported (Ehming et al, 1999).

From 1990 to 1995, a total of four studies were published on how ingested fresh garlic or garlic preparations may interact with anticoagulants or platelet aggregation inhibitors (Rose et al., 1990; Sunter, 1991; Burnham, 1995; Petry, 1995). All these studies found that garlic potentiated the anticoagulant effect, leading in one case to a life-threatening hemorrhage. Since it has been shown that garlic can increase fibrinolysis and inhibit platelet aggregation, it is reasonable to assume that these effects were indeed caused by the garlic preparations.

A more common problem associated with the use of garlic powder preparations has been the complaint of a gar-licky odor. Usually developing after several days of garlic powder ingestion, this odor is perceived on the breath and skin. A double-blind study using a 5-fold crossover design was conducted in 123 subjects to determine the incidence of garlic odor as a function of the ingested dose. The study period was divided into 2-week segments during which the participants took daily doses of 0 mg, 300 mg, 600 mg, 900 mg, and 1200 mg of garlic powder in tablet form (LI 111). All the participants kept an odor log indicating the times at which others noticed a garlic odor and classifying the severity of the odor as slight, moderate, or strong. The incidence of slight and moderate garlic odor was 10 % in the placebo group, 24 % at a dose of 300 mg/d, 36 % at 600 mg/d, 40 % at 900 mg/d, and 45 % at 1200 mg/d. Approximately 5 % of the subjects developed a strong garlic body odor only at doses of 900 and 1200 mg (Schmidt et al., 1992; Fig. 3.15).

An observational study in 1993 investigated the side effects of a regimen of 3×300 mg/day garlic powder, taken in the form of coated tablets, in a total of 1997 patients. The participants were interviewed at the start of the study and after 8 and 16 weeks of treatment. The difference between the reports on admission and the maximal reports at 8 or 12 weeks was interpreted as a specific effect of garlic use (Table 3.9). As the table indicates, garlic odor was the most frequent complaint, at 27 %, followed by gastrointestinal discomfort, orthostatic complaints, and allergic reactions. Other reported side effects included bloating, headache, dizziness, and profuse sweating (Beck and Grünwald, 1993).

3.3.1.9 Indications, Dosages, Risks, and Contraindications

The monograph on the garlic bulb published by Commission E in 1988 states that garlic preparations are indicated as "supportive to dietary measures at elevated levels of lipids in blood" and "preventative measures for age-dependent vascular changes" (Blumenthal et al., 1998). In the years since this monograph was published, the results of some 40 controlled clinical studies have become available. Initially these studies focused on secondary surrogate parameters of atherogenesis such as blood lipids, blood pressure, fibrinolysis, and platelet aggregation. But technical advances now make it possible to measure directly the progression of atherosclerosis and its response to garlic therapy in humans. Study results currently available based on primary surrogates (Breithaupt et al., 1998; Koscielny, 1999) are much closer to the pathologic substrate of atherosclerosis and therefore should form the basis for the future formulation of treat-

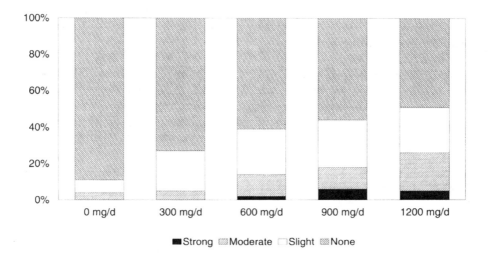

Fig. 3.15. ▲ Randomized double-blind study in 123 subjects using a 5-part crossover design; 111 of the protocols could be statistically evaluated. The subjects took o mg, 300 mg, 600 mg, 900 mg, and 1200 mg/day garlic pills for 14 days, and each participant kept an odor diary. The graph shows the percentage of subjects in the various dosage groups who perceived a garlic odor. The frequency of this complaint rises in proportion to the dosage, with about 50% of subjects reporting garlic odor at a dosage of 1200 mg/day (Schmidt et al.,1992).

Table 3.9.
Observational study on commercial garlic powder (Sapec).

Adverse side effects	Number of cases (% of 2010)		
	Admission (A)	Maximum (M)	Difference (M-A)
Nausea	149 (7 %)	262 (13 %)	113 (6 %)
Hypotension	28 (1.4 %)	54 (2.7 %)	26 (1.3 %)
Allergy	12 (0.6 %)	35 (1.7 %)	23 (1.1 %)
Other	11 (0.5 %)	27 (1.3 %)	16 (0.8 %)

NOTE: During the course of the observational study, the side effects occurring in a total of 1997 patients on treatment with the commercial product Sapec (300 mg garlic powder per coated tablet) were systematically recorded. The recommended dosage was 1 tablet taken 3 times daily. The patients were questioned on admission to the study, at 8 weeks, and at 16 weeks. The differences between statements made on admission and at 8 and 12 weeks were interpreted as possible therapy-related side effects. Gastrointestinal complaints (6 % reported nausea) and allergic reactions (1.1 %) were confirmed as known adverse effects of garlic therapy. Surprisingly, there were relatively frequent reports of orthostatic circulatory problems (1.3 % incidence of hypotension), underscoring the need to caution users about possible hypotensive effects in the prescribing literature and in package inserts for garlic medications. In the "other" category, bloating, headaches, dizziness, and out-breaks of sweating were reported somewhat more frequently during treatment than on admission (Beck and Grünwald, 1993).

ment indications. Presumably, based on these trials, the official indication for garlic therapy in Germany will be "for the prevention of general atherosclerosis (vascular thickening and hardening)."

As the great majority of studies have been done with garlic powder tablets, the approval of garlic products for atherosclerosis prevention will cover only that type of product. The dosage in most studies was 600–900 mg per day, which is roughly equivalent to ingesting 2400–3700 mg of fresh garlic. The average daily dose recommended in the Commission E monograph of July 6, 1988, is equivalent to 4 g of fresh garlic clove. This recommendation should be revised downward to approximately 900 mg of garlic powder, which is roughly equivalent to 2700 mg of fresh garlic.

The 1988 monograph characterizes the side effects of garlic preparations as "in rare instances there may be gastrointestinal symptoms, changes to the flora of the intestine, or allergic reactions" and "the odor of garlic may pervade the breath and skin" (Blumenthal et al., 1998). This list of effects is confirmed in its essence and sequence by the results of an observational study (Table 3.9), except that "hypotensive circulatory reactions," which have an incidence of more than 1 %, should be added to the list after allergic reactions. Although Commission E claimed that there were no known drug-drug interactions, based on the data available at the time the monograph was written, recent data suggest that it is possible that garlic may potentiate the effect of antihypertensive and anticoagulant medications.

3.3.1.10 Therapeutic Significance

With their overall pharmacodynamic and clinical profile, garlic powder tablets are able to slow the progression of age-related arterial changes and should therefore be classified as typical atherosclerosis remedies. While these products are not covered by health insurers under the German system (see Table 1.3), physicians are still obliged to counsel their patients on the use of garlic remedies because of their actions and potential side effects. Self-medication with garlic tablets is so widespread that its preventive value should not be underestimated, especially when one considers that these patients are leading a responsible, health-conscious lifestyle that does not burden the public health system and can very likely moderate the course and consequences of atherosclerosis.

3.3.1.11 Drug Products

The Red List 2003 includes a total of eight single-herb products, five containing garlic powder and three containing garlic oil, garlic oil maceration, or an extract as their pharmacologically active ingredients. As for the garlic powder products, controlled clinical studies have confirmed their therapeutic efficacy in the prevention of general atherosclerosis.

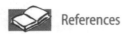 References

Abramovitz D (1999) Allicin-induced decrease in formation of fatty streaks (atherosclerosis) in mice fed a cholesterol-rich diet. Coronary Artery Disease 10: 515–519.

Adler AJ, Holub BJ (1997) Effect of garlic and fish-oil supplementation on serum lipid and lipoprotein concentrations in hypercholesterolemic men. Am J Clin Nutr 65: 445-450.

Auer W, Eiber A, Hertkorn E, Höhfeld E, Köhrle U, Lorenz A, Mader F, Merx W, Otto G, Schmid-Otto B, Taubenheim H (1989) Hypertonie und Hyperlipidämie: In leichte-ren Fällen hilft auch Knoblauch. Multizentrische placebokontrollierte Doppelblind-Studie zur lipid- und blutdrucksenkenden Wirkung eines Knoblauchpräparates. Der Allgemeinarzt 10: 205-208.

Aydin A, Ersöz G, Tekesin O, Akcicek E (2000) Garlic oil and Heliobacter pylori infection. Am J Gastroenterol 95: 563-4.

Barrie SA, Wright JV, Pizzorno JE (1987) Effects of garlic oil on platelet aggregation serum lipids and blood pressure in humans. J Orthomolec Med 2: 15-21.

Beck E, Grünwald J (1993) Allium sativum in der Stufentherapie der Hyperlipidämie. Med Welt 44: 516-520.

Berthold HK, Sudhop T, von Bergmann, K (1998) Effect of a garlic oil preparation on serum lipoproteins and cholesterol metabolism. JAMA 279: 1900-1902.

Betz E, Weidler R (1989) Die Wirkung von Knoblauchextrakt auf die Atherogenese bei Kaninchen. In: Betz E (Ed) Die Anwendung aktueller Methoden in der Arteriosklerose-Forschung, 304-311.

Blumenthal M, Busse WR, Goldberg A, Gruenwald J, Hall T, Riggins CW, Rister RS (eds.). Klein S, Rister RS (trans). (1998) The Complete German Commission E Monographs - Therapeutic Guide to Herbal Medicines. American Botanical Council, Austin, Texas. *www.herbalgram.org.*

Bode-Böger SM, Böger RH, Schröder EP, Frölich JC (1994) Exercise increases systemic nitric oxide production in men. J Cardio Risk 1: 173-178.

Bordia AK, Verma SK, Vyas AK, Khabya BL, Rathore AS, Bhu N, Bedi HK (1977) Effect of essential oil of onion and garlic on experimental atherosclerosis in rabbits. Atherosclerosis 26: 379-386.

Brändle M, Al Makdessi S, Weber RK, Dietz K, Jacob R (1997) Prolongation of life span in hypertensive rats by dietary interventions. Effect of garlic and linseed oil. Basic Res Cardiol 92: 223-232

Breithaupt-Grögler K, Ling M, Boudoulas H, Belz GG (1997) Protective Effect of Chronic Garlic Intake on Elastic Properties of Aorta in the Elderly. Circulation 96 (8): 2649-2655.

Brosche T (1989) Therapeutische Wirkungen einer Knoblauchzubereitung auf den Lipidstatus geriatrischer Probanden. Medwelt 40: 1233-1237.

Brosche T, Platt D (1990) Knoblauch als pflanzlicher Lipidsenker: Neuere Untersuchungen mit einem standardisierten Knoblauchtrockenpulver-Präparat. Fortschr Med 108: 703-706.

Brosche T, Siegers CP, Platt D (1991) Auswirkungen einer Knoblauch-Therapie auf die Cholesterin-Biosynthese sowie auf Plasma- und Membranlipide. Med Welt (Suppl 7a): 10-11.

Burnham BE (1995) Garlic as a possible risk for postoperative bleeding. Plast Recon Surg. 95: 213.

Cavallito CJ, Bailey JH (1944) Allicin, the antibacterial principle of Allium sativum. I.Isolation, physical properties and antibacterial action. J Am Chem Soc 66: 1950-1954.

Chandorkar AG, Jain PK (1973) Analysis of hypotensive action of allium sativum (garlic). Indian J Physiol Pharmacol 17: 132-133.

Chang MLW, Johnson MA (1980) Effect of garlic on carbohydrate metabolism and lipid syxnthesis in rats. J Nutr 110: 931-936.

Ciplea AG, Richter KD (1988) The Protective Effect of Allium sativum and Crataegus on Isoprenaline-induced Tissue Necrosis in Rats. Arzneim-Forsch/Drug Res 38 (II): 1583-1592.

Das I, Khan NS, Sooranna SR (1995) Potent activation of nitric oxide synthase by garlic: a basis for its therapeutic applications. Curr Med Res Opin 13: 257-263.

De Santos O, Grünwald J (1993) Effect of garlic powder tablets on blood lipids and blood pressure - a six month placebo controlled double blind study. Br J Clin Res 4: 37-44.

De Santos OS, Johns RA (1995) Effects of garlic powder and garlic oil preparations on blood lipids, blood pressure and well-being. Br J Clin Res 6: 91-100.

El-Sabban, F, Radwan GMH (1997) Influence of garlic compared to aspirin on induced photothrombosis in mouse pial microvessels, in vivo. Thrombosis Research 88: 193-203.

Eming SA, Piontek JO, Hunzelmann N, Rasokat H, Scharffetter-Kachanek K (1999) Severe toxic contact dermatitis caused by garlic. Br J Dermatol 141: 391-2.

Ernst E (1997) Can Allium vegetable can prevent cancer? Phytomedicine 4: 79-83.

Ernst E, Weihmayr T, Matrai A (1986) Knoblauch plus Diät senkt Serumlipide. Ärztliche Praxis 38:

1748–1749.

Falleroni AE, Zeiss CR, Levitz D (1981) Occupational asthma secondary to inhalation of garlic dust. J Allergy Clin Immunol 68: 156–160.

Ferne M (2004) Garlic and Onion in Classic Jewish Literature. HerbalGram 2004;61:44-47.

Fujiwara M, Itokawa Y, Uchino H, Inoue K (1972) Anti-hypercholesterolemic effect of a sulfur containing amino acid, S-methyl-L-cysteine sulfoxide, isolated from cabbage. Experientia 28: 254–255.

Gadkari JV, Joshi VD (1991) Effect of ingestion of raw garlic on serum cholesterol leve, clotting time and fibrinolytic activity in normal subjects. J Postgrad Med 37: 128–131.

Gebhardt R (1993) Multiple inhibitory effects of Garlic extracts on cholesterol biosynthesis in hepatocytes. Lipids 28 (6): 613–619.

Gebhardt R (1995) Amplification of palmitate-induced inhibition of cholesterol biosynthesis in cultured rat hepatocytes by garlic-derived organosulfur compounds. Phytomedicine 2: 29–34.

Gebhardt R, Beck H (1996) Differential Inhibitory Effects of Garlic-Derived Organosulfur Compounds on Cholesterol Biosynthesis in Primary Rat Hepatocyte Cultures. Lipids 31: 1269–1276.

Gebhardt R, Beck H, Wagner KG (1994) Inhibition of cholesterol biosynthesis by allicin and ajoene in rat hepatocytes and HepG2 cells. Biochem Biphys Acta 1213: 57–62.

Graham Y, Anderson SY, Lang T (1999) Garlic or Jalapeno pepper for treatment of Heliobacter pylori infection. Am J Gastroenterol 94: 1200-2.

Harenberg J, Giese C, Zimmermann R (1988) Effect of dried garlic on blood coagulation, fibrinolysis, platelet aggregation and cholesterol in patients with hyperlipoproteinemia. Atherosclerosis 74: 247–249.

Heikal HA, Kamel SI, Awaad KE, Khalil NF (1972) A study on the dehydration of garlic slices. Agri Res Rev 50: 243–253.

Heinle H, Betz E (1994) Effects of Dietary Garlic Supplementation in a Rat Model of Atherosclerosis. Arzneimittelforschung/Drug Res 44 (1): 614–617.

Holzgartner H, Schmidt U, Kuhn U (1992) Wirksamkeit und Verträglichkeit eines Knoblauchpulver-Präparates im Vergleich mit Bezafibrat. Arzneimittelforschung/Drug Res 42: 1473–1477.

Isaacsohn JL, Moser M, Stein EA, Dudley K, Davey JA, Liskow E, Black HR (1998) Garlic powder and plasma lipids and lipoproteins: A multicenter randomized, placebo-controlled trial. Arch Intern Med 158: 1189–1194.

Isensee H, Rietz B, Jacob R (1993) Cardioprotective Actions of Garlic (Allium sativum) Arzneim Forsch/Drug Res 43 (1): 94–98.

Itokawa Y, Inoue K, Sasagawa S, Fujiwara M (1973) Effect of S- methylcysteine sulfoxide, S-allylcysteine sulfoxide and related sulfur-containing amino acids on lipid metabolism of experimental hypercholesterolemic rats. J Nutr 103: 88–92.

Jacob R, Isensee H, Rietz B, Makdessi S, Sweidan H (1993) Cardioprotection by dietary interventions in animal experiments: Effect of garlic and various dietary oils under the conditions of experimental infarction. Pharm Pharmacol Lett 3: 131–134.

Jacob R, Rhrsam M, Ohkubo T, Rupp H (1991) Antihypertensive and kardioprotektive Effekte von Knoblauchpulver (Allium sativum). Med Welt (Suppl 7a): 39–41.

Jain AK, Vargas R, Gotzkowsky S, McMahon FG (1993) Can Garlic Reduce levels of Serum Lipids? A Controlled Clinical Study. Am J Med 94: 632–635.

Jain RC (1975) Onion and garlic in experimental cholesterol atherosclerosis in rabbits I. Effect on serum lipids and development of atherosclerosis. Atery 1: 115–125.

Jain RC (1977) Effect of garlic on serum lipids, coagulability and fibrinolytic activity of blood. Am J Clin Nutr 30: 1380–1381.

Kamanna VS, Chandrasekhara N (1984) Hypocholesteremic activity of different fractions of garlic. Indian J Med Res 79: 580–583.

Kandziora J (1988a) Blutdruck- und lipidsenkende Wirkung eines Knoblauch-Präparates in Kombination mit einem Diuretikum. Ärztliche Forschung 35 (3): 1–8.

Kandziora J (1988b) Antihypertensive Wirksamkeit und Verträglichkeit eines Knoblauch-Präparates. Ärztliche Forschung 35 (1): 1–8.

Kiesewetter H, Jung EM, Mrowietz C, Koscielny J, Wenzel E (1993a) Effect of garlic on platelet aggregation in patients with increased risk of juvenile ischaemic attack. Eur J Clin Pharmacol

45: 333–336.

Kiesewetter H, Jung F, Jung EM, Blume J, Mrowietz C, Birk A, Koscielny J, Wenzel E (1993b) Effects of garlic coated tablet in peripheral arterial occlusive desease. Clin Invest 71: 383–386.

Kiesewetter H, Jung F, Mrowietz C, Wenzel E (1993c) Wirkung von Knoblauch (Allium sativum L.), insbesondere rheologische und hämostaseologische Effekte. Hämostaseologie 13: 3–12.

Kiesewetter H, Jung F, Pindur G, Jung EM, Mrowietz C, Wenzel E (1991) Effect of garlic on thrombocyte aggregation, microcirculation, and other risk factors. Int J Clin Pharm Ther Toxicol 29: 151–155.

Koch HP, Hahn G, Lawson L, Reuter HD, Siegers CP (1996) Garlic – An Introduction to the Therapeutic Applications of Allium sativum. L. Williams & Wilkins, Baltimore.

König FK, Schneider B (1986) Knoblauch bessert Durchblutungsstörungen. Ärztliche Praxis 38: 344–345.

Koscielny J, Klüßendorf D, Latza R, Baumann-Baretti B, Mayer B Siegel G, Kiesewetter H (1999) The antiatherosclerotic effect of Allium sativum. Atherosclerosis, 144: 237–249.

Kourounakis PN, Rekka EA (1991) Effect on Active Oxygen Species of Alliin and Allium Sativum (Garlic) Powder. Res Commun Chem Pathol Pharmacol 74: 249–252.

Lachmann G, Lorenz D, Radeck W, Steiper M (1994) Untersuchungen zur Pharmakokinetik der mit 35-S markierten Knoblauchinhaltsstoffe Alliin, Allicin und Vinyldithiine. Arzneimittelforschung/Drug Res 44: 734-743.

Lash JP, Cardoso LR, Mesler PM, Walczak DA, Pollak R (1998) The effect of garlic on hypercholesterolemia in renal transplant patients. Transplantation Proceedings 30: 189–191.

Lau BHS, Lam F, Wang-Cheng R (1987) Effect of an odor-modified garlic preparation on blood lipids. Nutrition Research 7: 139–149.

Lewin G, Popov I (1994) Antioxidant Effects of Aqueous Garlic Extract 2nd Communication: Inhibition of CU^{2+}-initiated oxidation of low density lipoproteins. Arzneimittel-Forschung/Drug Research 44(1): 604–607.

Liu L, Yeh YY (2000) Inhibition of cholesterol biosynthesis by organosulfur compounds derived from garlic. Lipids 35: 197–203.

Mader FH, Auer W, Becker W, Böhm W, Brüchert E, Deutsch S (1990) Hyperlipidämie-Behandlung mit Knoblauch-Dragees. Der Allgemeinarzt 12: 435–440.

Malik ZA, Siddiqui S (1981) Hypotensive effect of freeze-dried garlic (Allium sativum) SAP in dog. JPMA 31: 12–13.

Mand JK, Gupta PP, Soni GL, Singh R (1985) Effect of garlic on experimental atherosclerosis in rabbits. Indian Heart J 37: 183–188.

Mathew PT, Augusti KT (1973) Studies of the effect of allicin (diallyl disulphide-oxide) on alloxan diabetes: Part I – Hypopglycaemic action & enhancement of serum insulin effect & glycogen synthesis. Indian J Biochem Biophys 10: 209–212.

McCrindle BW, Helden E, Conner WT (1998) Garlic extract therapy in children with hypercholesterolemia. Arch Pediatr Adolesc Med 152: 1089–1094.

Nakagawa S, Masamoto K, Sumiyoshi H, Harada H (1984) Acute toxicity test of garlic extract. J Toxicol Sci 9: 57–60.

Neil A, Silagy C (1994) Garlic: its cardio-protective properties. Curr Opinion Lipid 5: 6–10.

Neil A, Silagy C, Lancaster T, Hodgeman J, Moore JW, Jones L, Fowler GH (1996) Garlic powder in the treatment of moderate hyperlipidaemia: a controlled trial and meta-analysis. J Roy Coll Physicians London 30: 329–334.

Orekhof AN, Tertov VV (1997) In vitro effect of garlic powder extract on lipid content in normal and atherosclerotic human aortic cells. Lipids 32: 1055–60.

Orekhow AN, Pivovarova EM, Tertov VV (1996) Garlic powder tablets reduce atherogenicity of low density lipoprotein. A placebo-controlles double-blind study. Nutr Metab Cardiovasc Dis 6: 21–31.

Orekhow AN, Tertov VV, Sobenin IA, Pivovarova EM (1995) Direct Antiatherosclerosis-related Effects of Garlic. Ann Med 27: 63–65.

Papageogiou D, Corbet JP, Menezes-Brando F, Pecegueiro M, Benezra C (1983) Allergic: contact dermatitis to garlic (Allium sativum L.) identification of the allergens: the role of mono-, di- and trisulfides present in garlic. Arch Dermatol Res 275: 229–234.

Patumray S, Tewit S, Amatyakul S et al. (2000) Coparative effects of garlic and aspirin on diabetic cardiovascular complications. Drug Delivery 7: 91–96.

Pedraza-Chaverri J, Tapia E, Medina-Campos ON, de los Angeles Granados M, Franco M (1998) Garlic prevents hypertension induced by chronic inhibition of nitric oxide synthesis. Life Sciences 62: 71–77.

Petry JJ (1995) Garlic and postoperative bleeding. Plastic Recon Surg 96: 483–484.

Popov I, Blumstein A, Lewin G (1994) Antioxidant Effects of Aqueous Garlic Extract, 1st Communication: Direct detection using the photochemilumin-escence. Arzneimittel-Forschung/Drug Research 44 (1): 602–604.

Qureshi AA, Abiurmeileh N, Din ZZ, Elson CE, Burger WC (1983) Inhibition of cholesterol and fatty acid biosynthesis in liver enzymes and chicken hepatocytes by polar fractions of garlic. Lipids 18: 343–348.

Reuter HD (1995) Allium sativum und Allium ursinum: Part 2. Pharmacology and Medicinal Application. Phytomedicine 2: 73–91.

Reuter HD (1996) Therapeutic Effects and Applications of Garlic and its Preparations. In: Koch HP, Hahn G, Lawson L, Reuter HD, Siegers CP (Eds) Garlic – An Introduction to the Therapeutic Applications of Allium sativum. L. Williams & Wilkins, Baltimore.

Reuter HD, Sendl A (1994) Allium sativum und Allium ursinum: Chemistry, Pharmacology and Medical applications. Econo Med Plant Res 6: 56–108.

Rose KD, Croissant PD, Parliament CF, Levin MB (1990) Spontaneous Spinal Epidural Hematoma with Associated Platelet Dysfunction from Excessive Garlic Ingestion: A Case Report. Neurosurgery 26: 880–882.

Rotzsch W, Richter V, Rassoul F (1992) Postprandiale Lipämie unter Medikation von Allium sativum. Arzneimittel-Forschung/Drug Res 42 (II): 1223–1227.

Saradeth T, Seidl S, Resch KL, Ernst E (1994) Does garlic alter the lipid pattern in normal volunteers? Phytomedicine 1: 183–185.

Schmidt U, Schenk N (1992) Geruchsbildung bei repetierter Einnahme von standardisierten Knoblauchpulver-Dragees Kwai® (LI 111) in Abhängigkeit von der Tagesdosis. Wissenschaftlicher Bericht.

Schwartzkopff W, Bimmermann A, Schleicher J (1988) Klinische Studie mit Li 112-Knoblauchdragees. Wissenschaftlicher Bericht.

Siegel G, Emden J, Schnalke F, Walter A, Rückborn K, Wagner KG (1991) Wirkungen von Knoblauch auf die Gefäßregulation. Med Welt (Suppl 7a): 32–34.

Siegel G, Emden J, Wenzel K, Mironneau J, Stock G (1992) Potassium channel activation in vascular smooth muscle. In: Frank GB (Ed) Excitation-Contraction Coupling in Skeletal, Cardiac and Smooth Muscle, Plenum Press, New York: 53–72.

Siegel G, Klüßendorf D (2000) The anti-atherosclerotic effect of Allium sativum: Statistics re-evaluated. Atherosclerosis 150: 437–8.

Siegel G, Malmsten M, Schneider W, Michel F (2004) The effect of garlic on arteriosclerotic nanoplaque formation and size. Phytomedicine 11, in press

Siegel G, Nuck R, Schnalke F, Michel F (1998) Molecular evidence for phytopharmacological K+ channel opening by garlic in human vascular smooth muscle cell membranes. Phytotherapy Research 12: 149–151.

Siegel G, Walter A, Engel S, Walper A, Michel F (1999) Pleiotrope Wirkungen von Knoblauch. Wiener Med Wschr 149.217–224.

Siegers P, Röbke A, Pentz R (1999) Effects of garlic preparations on superoxide production by phorbol ester activated granulocytes. Phytomedicine 6: 13–16.

Silagy C, Neil A (1994) A meta-analysis of the effect of garlic on blood pressure. J Hypertension 12: 463–468.

Silagy C, Neil A (1994) Garlic as a lipid lowering agent – a meta-analysis. J R Coll Physicians 28(1): 2–8.

Simons LA, Balasubramaniam S, von Konigsmark M, Parfitt A, Simons J, Peters W (1995) On the effect of garlic on plasma lipids and lipoproteins in mild hypercholesterolaemia. Atherosclerosis 113: 219–225.

Sivam GP (2001) Protection against Heliobacter pylori and other bacterial infections by garlic. J

Nutr 131: 1106S–1108S.

Stevinson C, Pittler MH, Ernst E (2000) Garlic for treating hypercholesterolemia. Ann Intern Med 133: 420–9.

Sunter WH (1991) Warfarin and garlic. Pharm J 246: 722.

Superko R, Krauss RM (2000) Garlic powder, effect on plasma lipids, postprandial lipemia, low-density lipoprotein particle size, high-density lipoprotein subclass distribution and lipoprotein(a). JACC 35: 321–6.

Török B, Belágyi J, Rietz B, Jakob R (1994) Effectiveness of Garlic on the Radical Activity in Radical Generating Systems. Arzneimittelforschung/Drug Research 44(I): 608–611.

Vorberg G, Schneider B (1990) Therapie mit Knoblauch: Ergebnisse einer placebokontrollierten Doppelblindstudie. Natur- und Ganzheitsmedizin 3: 2–6.

Walper A, Rassoul F, Purschwitz K, Schulz V (1994) Effizienz einer Diätempfehlung und einer zusätzlichen Phytotherapie mit Allium sativum bei leichter bis mäßiger Hypercholesterinämie. Medwelt 45: 327–332.

Warshafsky S, Kamer RS, Sivak L (1993) Effect of garlic on total serum cholesterol. Ann Inter Med 119: 599–605.

Zacharias NT, Sebastian KL, Philip B, Augusti KT (1980) Hypoglycemic and Hypolipidaemic Effects of Garlic in Sucrose fed Rabbits. Ind J Physiol Pharmac 24: 151–154.

Zhao F, Chen H, Shen Y, Liu Z, Chen Y, Sun X, Cheng G, Lang L (1983) Study of synthetic allicin on the prevention and treatment of atherosclerosis. Chem Abst 98: 209.844.

Zimmermann W, Zimmermann B (1990) Senkung erhöhter Blutfette durch ein Knoblauch-Präparat: Offene Studie an stationären Patienten. Der Bayerische Internist 10: 40–43

3.3.2 Ginkgo Special Extract for Peripheral Arterial Occlusive Disease

The Commission E monograph of 1994 lists only two special extracts made from *Gingko biloba* leaves (acetone-and-water extracts with an average herb-to-extract ratio of 50:1) that are recommended for therapeutic use. The extracts are designated in the technical literature as EGb 761 (produced by Dr. Willmar Schwabe GmbH) and LI 1370 (produced by Lichtwer Pharma AG). Details on the history, pharmacy, pharmacology, and clinical aspects of these ginkgo extracts are presented in Sect. 2.1. Their use for the symptomatic treatment of peripheral arterial occlusive disease (PAOD) is considered here.

The 1994 Commission E monograph states that ginkgo special extracts are indicated in the treatment of PAOD for the "Improvement of pain-free walking distance in peripheral arterial occlusive disease in Stage II of Fontaine (intermittent claudication) in a regimen of physical therapeutic measures, in particular walking exercise" (Blumenthal et al., 1998).

Generally, patients with stage II PAOD have a pain-free walking distance in the range of 30–300 m. When this limit is reached, the oxygen deficit in the leg muscles causes the onset of pain and intermittent claudication. In cases that are not amenable to surgical correction (reopening or bypassing the stenosed segments in larger vessels), physical therapy with an emphasis on gait training is the most effective therapeutic measure. The training benefits peripheral arterial disease mainly by enlarging the caliber of the collateral arteries and increasing metabolic activities, i.e., promoting capillarization and increasing intracellular mitochondrial density to improve oxygen utilization.

Pharmacologic agents that promote blood flow act mainly by improving the rheologic properties of the blood. Gingko extracts are known to produce such an effect (see

Sect. 2.1.5). The pharmacologic action profile of ginkgo extracts implies that ginkgo should be of benefit in the symptomatic treatment of PAOD.

To date, 16 therapeutic studies have been completed dealing with the therapeutic efficacy of ginkgo special extracts in patients with Fontaine stage II peripheral arterial disease. Most of these studies had a randomized, placebo-controlled, double-blind design. The studies began with a 2- to 6-week run-in phase followed by a 3- to 6-month course of treatment with ginkgo extracts taken in daily doses of 120–160 mg. By July of 1994, most of these studies had been evaluated by Commission E and its consultants for preparation of the Commission monograph. It was concluded that in four of the placebo-controlled studies, the increase in pain-free walking distance achieved with ginkgo therapy was both statistically significant and clinically relevant. The older studies that formed that basis for the Commission E monograph have been reviewed and published in the form of two meta-analyses (Schneider, 1992; Letzel and Schoop, 1992). The features of the most important studies are summarized in Table 3.10. A typical result is shown graphically in Fig. 3.16. Most of the placebo-controlled studies showed statistically significant and therapeutically relevant gains in walking distance as a result of gingko therapy. The efficacy of the gingko special extract is comparable to that of synthetic drugs in the treatment of intermittent claudication (Letzel and Schoop, 1992). The advantage of gingko preparations over synthetic drugs is their better tolerance (see Table 2.3). Two meta-analyses of 8 ginkgo studies (Pittler und Ernst, 2000) and of 52 therapeutic trials of all agents used in the treatment of intermittent claudication (Moher et al., 2000) also confirm the superiority of ginkgo extract over placebo for the treatment of PAOD

Drug Products

See 2.1.9.

3.3.3 Other Herbs with Antiatherosclerotic Properties

The 1986 Commission E monograph states that onion (*Allium cepa*), like garlic, is useful "for the prevention of age-related vascular changes" (i.e., atherosclerosis). It must be taken in significantly higher doses than garlic, however, the Commission recommending an average daily dose of 50 g fresh onion bulb or 20 g dried herb. Onion is described as having antibacterial, lipid-reducing, antihypertensive, and platelet-aggregation-inhibiting properties.

The chemistry of the onion bulb resembles that of garlic. Instead of alliin, onion contains methyl and propyl compounds of cysteine sulfoxide. These chemicals are transformed by fermentation into the familiar eye-irritating compounds that induce lacrimation (cepaenes). In one study, the decrease in fibrinolytic activity caused by a fatty meal could be reversed by feeding the subjects onions (Menon et al., 1968). The ingestion of onion was also shown to inhibit platelet aggregation (Baghurst et al., 1977). More recent placebo-controlled studies comparable to those with garlic have not yet been conducted on the effects of onion.

Table 3.10.

Randomized placebo-controlled double-blind studies on the efficacy of gingko special extract in patients with Fontaine stage II peripheral arterial occlusive disease.

First author, year	Number of patients	Dose (mg/day)	Duration of treatment (months)	Walking distance test conditions, significance of gingko vs. placebo
Bauer, 1984	80	120	3	10% gradient, 3 km/h, **
Bulling, 1991	36	160	6	10% gradient, 3 km/h, **
Blume, 1996	60	120	6	12% gradient, 3 km/h, ***
Schoop, 1997	222	120	6	12% gradient, 3 km/h, ns/*[1]
Peters, 1998	111	120	6	12% gradient, 3 km/h, *
Blume, 1999	40	160	6	12% gradient, 3 km/h, ***

* = $p < 0.05$; ** = $p < 0.01$; *** = $p < 0.001$. [1] Significant difference in the subgroup with walking distance >75 m without a walking-through phenomenon.

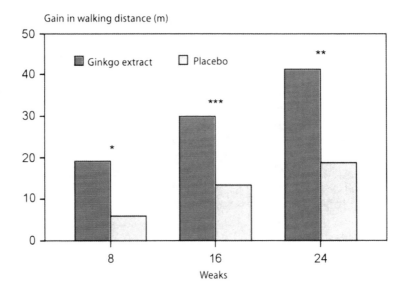

Fig. 3.16. ▲ Increase in pain-free walking distance in patients with peripheral arterial occlusive disease after 24 week's treatment with ginkgo special extract, compared with a placebo (Peters et al., 1998).

Phospholipids derived from soybeans consist of an enriched extract containing 73–79 % phosphatidylcholine. The 1994 Commission E monograph states that this phospholipid extract is useful for the treatment of mild forms of hypercholesterolemia in cases that are not adequately managed by diet and other nonpharmacologic measures (e.g., exercise and weight loss) alone. In addition, soybean phospholipids have shown hepatoprotective properties in numerous experimental models of acute toxic liver damage (e.g., caused by ethanol, carbon tetrachloride, or galactosamine). The pharmacokinetics of orally administered phospholipids have been investigated with radiolabeled agents in experimental animals. It has been shown that phospholipid is degraded to lyso-phosphatidylcholine while still in the intestine and is mainly absorbed in that form. Most phosphatidylcholine circulating in the plasma is bound to albumin. It is likely that most of the metabolites of administered soybean phospholipids are integrated into endogenous phospholipids within a few hours. Thirty-two clinical studies were evaluated in preparation for the monograph; nine were placebo-controlled studies in patients with hyperlipoproteinemia. Four of the nine placebo-controlled studies demonstrated efficacy, consisting of a reduction in total cholesterol (7–19 % of initial levels). Three studies showed significant reductions in LDL cholesterol. Triglycerides and HDL cholesterol were unaffected. The studies employed doses of 1–3 g of phospholipids per day. Lipostabil 300 forte is one example of a suitable commercial product.

Oat bran (from *Avena sativa*) was found to reduce total cholesterol by 13 % when taken in a daily dose of about 100 g for 3 weeks (Gold and Davidson, 1988). A similar study using the same daily dose administered for 14 weeks showed a 16 % total cholesterol reduction accompanied by a 21 % reduction in LDL (Fischer et al., 1991). The cholesterol-lowering effect of oat bran is apparently based on its content of gel-forming dietary fiber; wheat bran does not produce this effect.

Guar gum, a reserve polysaccharide derived from the Indian guar plant (*Cyamopsis tetragonolobus*), lowered cholesterol levels by 6–8 % and triglyceride levels by 13–17 % when taken in a dose of 15 g/day. As in the case of oat bran, this effect apparently results from the binding of primarily liver-excreted cholesterol to nonabsorbable bulk materials. Owing to their lipid-reducing effects, both of these sources of dietary fiber may be beneficial in the secondary prophylaxis of atherosclerosis (Fischer et al., 1991).

The results of a prospective epidemiologic study in 3454 Dutch citizens indicate that drinking approximately 250–400 mL of black tea daily has a protective effect against atherosclerosis and coronary heart disease. On statistical average, the adjusted risk of ischemic heart disease was reduced by 40 % compared with nondrinkers of black tea (Geleijnse et al., 1999).

3.3.3.1 Red Yeast Rice

Red yeast rice consists of the fungus *Monascus purpureus* Went grown on rice (*Oryza sativa*) and the resulting fermentation product standardized to contain 0.4 % 3-hydroxy-3-methylglutaryl coenzyme A (HMG-CoA) reductase inhibitors, principally monacolin K. The mixture also contains fatty acids, proteins, vitamins, minerals, and pigments. It was first marketed in the United States under the trade name Cholestin, but several imitative products are now also available. The use of red yeast rice in China was first recorded in 800 AD during the T'ang dynasty. In addition to being used for medicinal purposes, it was employed in making rice wine and as a taste preservative and colorant for food.

Therapeutic utility of red yeast rice in treating hyperlipoproteinemia is due primarily to monacolin K, also known as mevinolin or lovastatin, which is present in the standardized product in a concentration of 0.2 %. Eight other monacolin derivatives are also present in smaller amounts. These compounds are inhibitors of HMG-CoA reductase, the rate-limiting enzyme in endogenous cholesterol biosynthesis.

Seventeen clinical trials (8 controlled, 9 open) conducted in China support the use of red yeast rice in lowering blood lipid levels. A 1995 study on 324 hypercholesterolemic patients treated for 8 weeks with a product containing 13.5 mg of total monacolins in the 1.2 g daily dose found serum cholesterol concentrations decreased an average of 23 % and triacylglycerol levels 36.5 %. At the same time, HDL-cholesterol levels increased by 19.6 % (Wang et al., 1995).

A similar 1996 study in 101 subjects who received 10–13 mg of total monacolins daily reported total cholesterol decreases averaging 19.5 % and triacylglycerol reductions of 36.1 % in the treated group. HDL-cholesterol concentrations increased by 16.7 % (Shen et al., 1996).

Subsequently, the results of a double-blind, placebo-controlled, prospectively randomized, 12-week clinical study conducted in the United States on 83 subjects with hyperlipidemia were published (Heber et al., 1999). The subjects were instructed to consume a diet providing 30 % of energy from fat, < 10 % from saturated fat, and < 300 mg of cholesterol daily. Total cholesterol, HDL and LDL cholesterol were measured at 8, 9, 11, and 12 weeks.

In the treated group, total cholesterol concentrations decreased after 8 weeks from an average of 254 ± 36 mg/dl to 208 ± 31 mg/dl. LDL cholesterol and total triacylglycerol also decreased significantly but not HDL cholesterol. No significant changes in these parameters were noted in the placebo group. No adverse effects related to red yeast rice were reported, and no abnormal liver or renal function tests occured at any time in the subjects studied.

The effectiveness of red yeast rice in blood lipid reduction is not surprising in view of the fact that its major active constituent, monacolin K, is an approved prescription drug in the United States under the name lovastatin. Although adverse effects were not noted in the U. S. clinical trial with red yeast rice, others have reported occurence of gastritis, abdominal discomfort, and elevated levels of liver enzymes. Lovastatin has been associated with muscle pain, tenderness, and weakness, so these conditions may also occur with red yeast rice use. Red yeast rice should not be used by persons with liver disease, pregnant women, or persons under the age of eighteen.

Recommended dose of the product to maintain healthy blood lipid levels is two 600 mg capsules taken twice daily with meals. It is specifically recommended for adults with moderately high cholesterol levels ranging from 200–239 mg/dl.

Because one of the active constituents in red yeast rice, monacolin K, is chemically identical to the purified prescription drug, lovastatin, the United States Food and Drug Administration (FDA) in 1998 declared that the product was an unapproved drug and banned its import. Pharmanex, the manufacturer of the original red yeast rice preparation, Cholestin, appealed the ruling, and in June of 1998, a federal judge in the state of Utah ruled that the product was not a drug but a dietary supplement (food) as defined in the Dietary Supplement Health and Education Act of 1994 (Skinner, 1998). The FDA subsequently appealed the decision, but pending the outcome of litigation, red yeast rice is still being marketed as a dietary supplement. It is ironic that of all the botanical products sold in the United States, the FDA chose to challenge repeatedly the legality of one whose active constituents have been so thoroughly studied and demonstrated to be safe and effective.

References (for 3.3.2 and 3.3.3)

Baghurst KI, Raj MI, Truswell AS (1977) Onions and platelet aggregation. Lancet 101: 1051.

Bauer U (1984) Six-month double-blind randomised clinical trial of Ginkgo biloba extract versus placebo in two parallel groups in patients suffering from peripheral arterial insufficiency. Arzneim-Forsch/Drug Res 34: 716–720.

Blume J, Kieser M, Hölscher U (1996) Placebokontrollierte Doppelblindstudie zur Wirksamkeit von Ginkgo-biloba-Spezialextrakt EGb 761 bei austrainierten Patienten mit Claudicatio intermittens. VASA 25: 265–274.

Blume J, Kieser M, Hölscher U (1998) Randomisierte placebokontrollierte Doppelblindstudie zum Nachweis der klinischen Wirksamkeit von EGb 761 bei Patienten mit peripherer arterieller Verschlußkrankheit im Stadium IIb nach Fontaine. Fortschritte der Medizin 116: 137-43.

Blumenthal M, Busse WR, Goldberg A, Gruenwald J, Hall T, Riggins CW, Rister RS (eds.). Klein S, Rister RS (trans). (1998) The Complete German Commission E Monographs – Therapeutic Guide to Herbal Medicines. American Botanical Council, Austin, Texas. *www.herbalgram.org*.

Bulling G, von Bary S (1991) Behandlung der chronischen peripheren arteriellen Verschlußkrankheit mit physikalischem Training und Ginkgo-biloba-Extrakt 761. Med Welt 42: 702–708.

Fischer S, Berg A, Keul J, Leitzmann C (1991) Einfluß einer ballaststoffangereicherten Kost auf die Ernährungsgewohnheiten und die Blutfettwerte bei Hypercholesterinämikern. Aktuelle Ernährungsmedizin 16: 303–309.

Geleijnse JM, Launer LJ, Hoffmann A et al. (1999) Tea flavanoids may protect against atherosclerosis. The Rotterdam Study. Arch Intern Med 159: 2170-4.

Gold KK, Davidson DM (1988) Oat bran as a cholesterol-reducing dietary adjunct in an young healthy population. West J Med 148: 299–302.

Heber D, Yip I, Ashley JM, Elashoff DA, Elashoff RM, Go VLW (1999) Cholesterol-lowering effects of a proprietary Chinese red-yeast-rice dietary supplement. Am J Clin Nutr 69: 231–236.

Letzel H, Schoop E (1992) Ginkgo-biloba-Extrakt EGb 761 und Pentoxifyllin bei Claudicatio intermittens. VASA 21: 403–410.

Menon IS, Kendal RY, Dewar HA, Newell DJ (1968) Effects of onion on blood fibrinolytic activity. Brit Med J 3: 351.

Moher D, Pham B, Ausejo M, et al. (2000) Pharmacological management of intermittent claudication. A meta-analysis of randomised trials. Drugs 59: 1557-70.

Peters H, Kieser M, Hölscher U (1998) Demonstration of the efficacy of ginkgo biloba special extract EGb 761on intermittent claudication – a placebo-controlled, double-blind multicenter trial. VASA 27: 106–110.0.

Pittler MH, Ernst E (2000) *Ginkgo biloba* extract for the treatment of intermittent claudication. A metaanalysis of randomised trials. Am J Med 108: 276–81.

Schneider B (1992) Ginkgo-biloba-Extrakt bei peripheren arteriellen Verschlußkrankheiten. Arzneim Forsch/Drug Res 42: 428–436.

Schoop W (1997) Klinische Prüfung mit Ginkgo-biloba-Spezialextrakt EGb 761 bei Patienten mit peripherer arterieller Verschlußkrankheit im Stadium IIb nach Fontaine im Vergleich zu Placebo. VASA 26: 160.

Shen Z, Yu P, Su M, Chi J, Zhou Y, Zhu X, Yang C, He C (1996) A prospective study on Zhitai capsule in the treatment of primary hyperlipidemia. Nat Med J China 76: 156–157.

Skinner W (1988) Cholestin declared dietary supplement and FDA enjoined. Nat Med Law 2(1): 1,6.

Wang J, Su M, Lu Z, Kou W, Chi J, Yu P, Wang W (1995) Clinical trial of extract of *Monascus purpureus* (red yeast) in the treatment of hyperlipidemia. Clin J Exp Ther Prep Chin Med 12: 1–5.

3.4   Chronic Venous Insufficiency

Chronic venous insufficiency is the term applied to a syndrome resulting from the obstruction or persistent incompetence of deep veins or perforating veins in the lower extremities. The symptoms range from edema, cyanosis or dermatosclerosis to atrophic skin changes and crural ulceration, depending on the severity and duration of the impaired venous return and associated impairment of metabolic exchange. Chronic venous insufficiency is divided into three stages based on its degree of severity (Marshall and Loew, 1994).

Causal therapy in the form of vascular surgery is possible only in a small percentage of patients. Conservative treatment options consist of elastic compression (support stockings) and symptomatic pharmacotherapy with so-called venous remedies.

Most pharmacologic and clinical studies on herbs used in the treatment of venous disorders have dealt with horse chestnut extracts and their constituent aescins. These agents act less on the veins and venules than at the capillary level, where they exert antiexudative and antiedematous effects. Commercial products vary widely in quality, however, and only some contain active levels of antiexudative constituents. This variable quality of herbal venous remedies is a major reason why their clinical efficacy remains a controversial matter.

Proof of safety and efficacy by controlled clinical studies requires a differentiated approach to patient evaluation and follow-up. Instrumental diagnostic techniques may consist of more general procedures such as Doppler and duplex scanning, phlebodynamometry, and venous occlusion plethysmography or of more specialized procedures, such as volumetry, that can detect pharmacologic actions. Since pharmacologic therapy can influence functional vascular changes but cannot reverse pathoanatomic changes, proof of clinical efficacy must rely on techniques for determining capillary permeability, such as venous occlusion plethysmographic volumetry. Emphasis should also be placed on the follow-up of subjective complaints. Tired, heavy legs, a tense or bursting sensation, and calf pain are not mood disorders but symptoms that have major pathologic significance. If instrumental diagnostic techniques as well as clinical follow-up indicate a positive response to herbal therapy, it is reasonable to conclude that these preparations can be important in the treatment of lower-extremity venous disorders (Marshall and Loew, 1994).

3.4.1   Horse Chestnut Seed Extract

3.4.1.1   Introduction

The horse chestnut, *Aesculus hippocastanum* (family Hippocastanaceae), was introduced into northern Europe from the Near East in the sixteenth century. Extracts from horse chestnut seeds were already used therapeutically in France in the early 1800's. Several French works published between 1896 and 1909 reported successful outcomes in the treatment of hemorrhoidal ailments. Even then it was assumed that the active components belonged to the saponin class of glycosides (Hitzenberger, 1989).

3.4.1.2   Crude Drug and Extract

The German Pharmacopeia (*DAB 1996*) describes the crude drug as consisting of the dried seeds of the horse chestnut tree. (Fig. 3.17). Preparations made from other parts of the tree (leaves, bark) have also been used medicinally, but their efficacy has not been adequately proven. For simplicity, the term horse chestnut extract will hereafter refer to the extract derived from horse chestnut seeds.

The fully ripe seeds are predried by spreading them out in a thin layer in a well-ventilated area. Then they are split open and dried rapidly at a temperature of 60 °C to obtain a powdered crude drug containing 3–5 % saponins. Water-.and-alcohol mixtures are used to prepare powdered extracts, which are adjusted as needed by the addition of dextrins, to a triterpene glycoside content of 16–20 % (m/m), calculated as aescin.

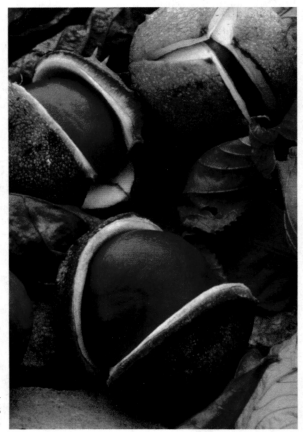

Fig. 3.17. ▶ Horse chestnut (*Aesculus hippocastanum*), opening fruits with seeds.

3.4.1.3 Chemistry and Pharmacokinetics of Aescin

Aescin is considered the main active constituent of horse chestnut extract, and isolated aescin has shown clinical efficacy on administration (Fink Serralde et al., 1975). The triterpene saponins in horse chestnut seeds form a complex mixture of saponins. The part of the mixture that tends to crystallize, called β-aescin, is itself a mixture of several glycosides. These glycosides contained in β-aescin are derived from two aglycones. Aescin is fairly soluble in water but is poorly soluble in lipid solvents. Glycoside determinations employ a method developed in 1966 and slightly modified for pharmaceutical purposes; it is based on a color reaction of triterpene glycosides with ferric chloride.

Orally administered aescin is either sparingly absorbed or undergoes a substantial first-pass effect. Its relative bioavailability compared with i.v. administration is less than 1 %. It has an absorption half-life of about 1 h and an elimination half-life of about 20 h. In subjects who took 50 mg of aescin in capsule form (brand name Venostasin retard), maximum plasma levels of approximately 20–30 ng/mL were measured 2–3 h after ingestion of the capsule (Hänsel et al., 1992).

Measurements on the bioequivalence of various galenic preparations of horse chestnut extracts were performed in 48 healthy subjects. Specific antibodies were used to measure the plasma concentrations of aescin. Maximum plasma levels of approximately 15 ng/mL were measured after the ingestion of various horse chestnut extract preparations equivalent to a single dose of 100 mg aescin. Maximum plasma levels were reached about 3 h after oral administration of the extract, and the average elimination half-life was approximately 20 h. Based on the marked variability in the plasma levels of aescin, the authors could not show bioequivalence to a reference drug in subjects who took a single dose but could do so in subjects who took the extract for 6 days (comparison of steady-state levels) (Biber et al., 1996).

3.4.1.4 Pharmacology

Studies in an animal model (rat paw edema) showed that whole horse chestnut extract was 100 times more active than the same extract with the aescin removed (Lorenz and Marek, 1960). Since then, it has been repeatedly confirmed that aescin is responsible for the antiexudative properties of horse chestnut extract, even in inflammatory and stasis-related edema (Hitzenberger, 1989).

Several authors showed that horse chestnut extract increased the tonicity of isolated veins (Annoni et al., 1979; Lock, 1974; Longiave et al., 1978). This effect was not blocked by phentolamine, proving that it is not mediated by α-adrenergic receptors. There is no evidence to date, however, that horse chestnut can significantly affect venous capacity in patients with venous insufficiency (Rudofsky et al., 1986; Bisler et al., 1986).

3.4.1.5 Toxicology

Horse chestnut extract and aescin have been tested for acute toxicity in several animal species (mouse, rat, guinea pig, rabbit, dog). The "no effect" dose is approximately 8 times higher than the dose recommended for therapeutic use in patients. Tests for chronic toxicity (34 weeks in rats and dogs) showed no cumulative toxic effects or any evidence of embryotoxic or teratogenic effects. The results of animal studies are corroborated by decades of use in patients with no reports of harmful effects due to overdosing. No studies have been published on mutagenicity or carcinogenicity (Hänsel et al., 1992).

3.4.1.6 Actions and Efficacy in Subjects and Patients

3.4.1.6.1 Studies in Healthy Subjects
Pauschinger (1987) investigated the effects of a standardized horse chestnut extract (single dose of 600 mg) on capillary filtration in a double-blind, placebo-controlled study of 12 healthy subjects. The parameters of interest were vascular capacity and the filtration coefficient as measured by venous occlusion plethysmography. While both parameters remained unchanged in the placebo-treated group, the subjects taking the extract showed a decrease in vascular capacity and filtration coefficient.

Among the clinical pharmacologic studies in healthy subjects is that of Marshall et al. (1987), who conducted a double-blind study on the development of foot and ankle edema in 19 subjects following a long-distance flight. They found that edema was significantly reduced in subjects who had taken a prophylactic dose of 600 mg horse chestnut extract prior to the flight.

3.4.1.6.2 Therapeutic Studies in Patients
Seven placebo-controlled double-blind studies were carried out with a standardized horse chestnut extract to assess its therapeutic efficacy in patients with chronic venous insufficiency. These studies, listed in Table 3.11, included a total of 558 evaluable patient treatment cycles. All the studies used daily doses of approximately 600 mg of horse chestnut extract, equivalent to 100 mg/day aescin. Most of them used a cross-over design in which each patient received both the extract and the placebo in separate treatment cycles.

The study by Alter (1973) is of limited value, despite its double-blind design, due to significant methodologic and statistical deficiencies. Subsequent studies by Neiss et al. (1976) and Friedrich et al. (1978) are of considerably greater interest. Both studies had a similar design, and both used a 0-3 point scale to rate the severity of symptoms typically associated with chronic venous insufficiency. A 4-field test was used for statistical significance. The majority of symptoms showed significantly greater improvement in the patients taking the horse chestnut extract than in patients taking a placebo.

Four additional studies were published in 1986. Steiner and Hillemanns (1986) treated 13 women diagnosed with pregnancy-related varicose veins and 7 women diagnosed with chronic venous insufficiency. Leg volumes were determined by water plethysmography, and leg circumferences were measured at three levels. Leg volumes did not change in placebo-treated patients, but treatment with horse chestnut extract led to a significant average reduction of 114 mL and 126 mL in the two patient groups. The subjective complaints and overall physician-rated efficacy were also significantly better in patients treated with the extract than in patients given a placebo.

Lohr et al. (1986) conducted a study in 74 patients with chronic venous insufficiency and proneness to lower extremity edema. Leg volumes were determined by water plethysmography and leg circumferences were directly measured before and after the

Table 3.11.

Placebo-controlled double-blind studies using a standardized horse chestnut extract (Venotasin retard).

First author, year	Number of patients	Duration (days)	Key parameters and statistical results of drug vs. placebo
Alter, 1973	96	2 × 20	Palpable findings, skin color, venous prominence, edema, dermatoses, pain, feeling of heaviness, and itching significantly improved in most patients
Neiss, 1978	212	2 × 20	Complaint scale (0–3): Edema** Calf spasms ns. Pain** Itching ns. Feeling of heaviness*
Friedrich, 1978	95	2 × 20	Complaint scale (0–3): Edema* Calf spasms** Pain** Itching ns. Feeling of heaviness*
Steiner, 1986	20	2 × 14	leg volume[1]** Subjective complaints**
Lohr, 1986	74	56	leg volume[1]** Subjective complaints**
Bisler, 1986	22	2 × 1	Filtration coefficient[2]*** (−22%) Venous capacity[2] ns. (−5%)
Rudofsky, 1986	39	28	Extravascular volume[1] [3]*** Venous capacity[2] ns. Subjective complaints*
Diehm, 1996	240	84	Leg volume[1]**

The dose in all studies was 100 mg aescin per day. Except for Lohr et al., all the authors used a crossover design for their studies. *=p<0.05; **=p<0.01; ***=p<0.001; ns. = not significant.
[1] Water plethysmography, [2] venous occlusion plethysmography, [3] measured on the foot and distal lower leg.

provocation of edema. The provocative increase in leg volume fell from 32 mL to 27 mL in the group treated with horse chestnut but rose from 27 mL to 31 mL in the placebo-treated group. Subjective symptoms were also significantly improved.

Bisler et al. (1986) and Rudofsky et al. (1986) studied the effects of horse chestnut on the intravascular volume of the lower extremity veins and on interstitial filtration (measured indirectly by venous-occlusion or water plethysmography) in patients with chronic venous insufficiency.

Bisler et al. (1986) tested the effects of a single dose of 600 mg horse chestnut extract versus a placebo. In patients taking the placebo, transcapillary filtration rose from 8.2 to 8.3 scale units over a 3-h period, but it fell from 9.4 to 7.4 units in the patients treated with horse chestnut extract. This indicated a significant 22 % reduction in the transcapillary filtration coefficient. The decrease in intravascular volume (−5 %) was not significant. This led the authors to conclude that the vein-toning action of horse chestnut extract is of far less importance than its ability to reduce capillary permeability.

Rudofsky et al. (1986) documented similar effects of horse chestnut extract over a 28-day treatment period. Whereas venous capacity before and after the therapy showed no significant differences between the extract- and placebo-treated groups, the extravascular volume changes measured in the foot and ankle at 14-28 days showed highly significant intergroup differences (Fig. 3.18). Four weeks' treatment with the horse chestnut extract also led to significant improvement in most subjective symptoms (feeling of tension, pain, leg fatigue, itching) and in the finding of leg edemas. The symptom of calf muscle spasms did not improve.

Diehm et al. (1996) carried out a study to compare the efficacy (edema reduction) and safety of compression stockings class II and dried horse chestnut seed extract (HCSE, 50 mg aescin, twice daily). Equivalence of both therapies was examined in a novel hierarchical statistical design in 240 patients with chronic venous insufficiency. Patients were treated over a period of 12 weeks in a randomized, partially blinded, placebo-controlled, parallel study design. Lower leg volume of the more severely affected limb decreased on average by 43.8 mL (n=95) with HCSE and 46.7 mL (n=99) with compression therapy for the intention-to-treat group (Fig. 3.19). Significant edema reductions were achieved by HCSE (p=0.005) and compression (p=0.002) compared to placebo, and the two therapies were shown to be equivalent (p=0.001); in this design, however, compression could not be proven as standard with regard to edema reduction

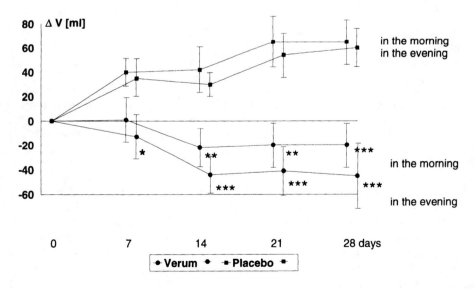

Fig. 3.18. ▲ Effect of 4 weeks' treatment with 600 mg horse chestnut extract, corresponding to 100 mg/day aescin, on volume changes in the foot and distal lower leg with a fixed, reduced blood volume (change in extravascular volume). Mean values SEM for n = 19 patients (horse chestnut extract) and n = 20 patients (placebo). * = p < 0.05; ** = p < 0.01, *** = p < 0.001 (significance comparing extracts vs. placebo) (after Rudofsky et al., 1986).

in the statistical test procedure. Both HCSE and compression therapy were well tolerated and no serious treatment-related events were reported. These results indicate that compression stocking therapy and HCSE therapy are alternative therapies for the effective treatment of patients with edema resulting from chronic venous insufficiency.

Pittler and Ernst (1998) published a meta-analysis of all controlled studies comparing horse chestnut extract with a placebo or reference therapy. The authors concluded

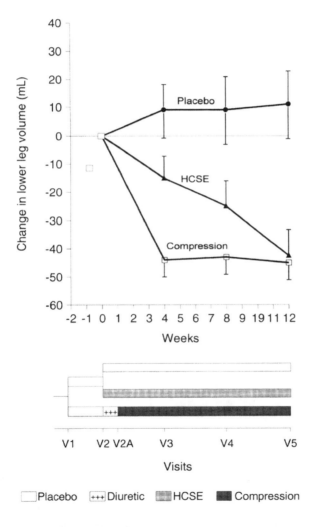

Fig. 3.19. ▲ Study design (lower) and differences (mean SEM) in lower leg volume versus baseline (upper) of the study of Siehm et al. (1996) with 240 patients. Significant reductions of lower leg volume were achieved by horse chestnut seed extract (HCSE, p = 0.005) and compression (p = 0.002) compared to placebo. The two therapies were shown to be equivalent (p = 0.001).

that all the placebo-controlled studies document the superiority of horse chestnut extract over placebo in reducing leg volume and lower leg circumference. Five studies comparing horse chestnut with rutin show equivalent effects with both medications (Pittler and Ernst, 1998).

3.4.1.7 Indications, Dosages, Risks, and Contraindications

There appears to be sufficient evidence to prove the therapeutic efficacy of horse chestnut extract in reducing leg edema and improving the typical subjective complaints associated with chronic venous insufficiency. Thus, the Commission E monograph on horse chestnut seeds published in the April 15, 1994, issue of *Bundesanzeiger* states that a standardized powdered extract of horse chestnut seeds (*DAB 1996*) adjusted to a triterpene glycoside content of 16–20 % (calculated as anhydrous aescin) is appropriate for the "treatment of complaints relating to diseases of the lower extremity veins (chronic venous insufficiency) such as pain and a feeling of heaviness in the legs, nocturnal calf muscle spasms, itching, and swelling of the legs."

The monograph further states that other noninvasive physician-prescribed measures such as elastic compression or cold water treatments should definitely be continued.

There are no known contraindications to the use of horse chestnut extract. Isolated instances of itching, nausea, and stomach discomfort have been reported as side effects.

With regard to tolerance, it should be emphasized that high tolerance has been demonstrated only for the controlled-release dosage form. The saponins contained in non-controlled-release preparations of horse chestnut extract tend to cause stomach upset when the extract is taken at therapeutic doses of 250–313 mg twice daily, equivalent to 100 mg of aescin.

3.4.1.8 Therapeutic Significance

Horse chestnut extract is the most widely prescribed oral antiedema venous remedy in Germany. Semisynthetic derivatives of plant constituents such as hydroxyethylrutin, calcium dobesilate, troxerutin, and trimethylhesperidin chalcone are also used individually or in combinations; but single-herb products, especially those based on horse chestnut seed extract, are the most commonly prescribed (Fricke, 1998).

The therapeutic efficacy of certain orally administered venous remedies has been satisfactorily established in recent treatment studies (Table 3.11), although some physicians continue to have a cautious or negative attitude (Fricke, 1998). The most important study (Diehm et al., 1996) showed a statistically significant reduction in edema by approximately 50 mL after 12 weeks' treatment with horse chestnut seed extract. Earlier studies had already demonstrated the efficacy of horse chestnut extract in the amelioration of subjective complaints (Hitzenberger, 1989). The Commission E monograph of April, 1994, pertains only to preparations that supply a daily dose of 100 mg aescin, corresponding to about 300 mg of extract in a controlled-release dosage form. Other preparations made from horse chestnut leaves, bark, and flowers have been negatively appraised and should no longer be prescribed. Extracts from other herbs (butcher's broom rhizome, sweet clover, buckwheat, grape leaves) are traditional remedies that have not been proven by up-to-date clinical studies. Caution is advised in prescribing these herbs as well as any combination products that are offered for the treatment of venous disorders.

As for chemically modified isolated plant constituents, which by definition are not phytotherapeutic agents in the strict sense (Sect.1.2 and 1.3), the compound hydroxyethylrutin has shown at least short-term efficacy in ameliorating the subjective complaints of chronic venous insufficiency. Thus it can be recommended as an alternative to horse chestnut seed extract, although there have been isolated reports of hair loss in patients using hydroxyethylrutin. One case of agranulocytosis was reported following the use of calcium dobesilate. The side effects of horse chestnut seed extract (gastrointestinal complaints, allergic skin reactions) are relatively harmless by comparison.

In contrast to herbal and semisynthetic antiedema agents, the use of diuretics is only occasionally indicated to clear venogenic edema in patients with chronic venous insufficiency. Also, a number of contraindications exist to diuretic therapy. Given the potential for hemoconcentration with impairment of venous drainage and the risk of stasis predisposing to thrombosis, diuretics are inappropriate for the long-term treatment of edema due to venous insufficiency.

3.4.2 Topical Venous Remedies

The most commonly prescribed topical venous remedies are products containing heparin. Combination products containing herbal extracts or plant constituents from the group of saponins (e.g., aescin) or flavonoids (e.g., rutin) are also used. The topical application of these agents does not produce systemic therapeutic levels of the active principle. Their therapeutic effects may be based largely on the ointment base and the tissue massage that occurs when the ointment is applied. Patients frequently experience subjective improvement in their complaints, but the benefits are not referable to specific plant constituents because all but one of the commercial preparations (Venostasin N ointment, active ingredient: horse chestnut extract) are combination products.

It is unclear whether extracts from arnica flowers are topically active and, if so, how they exert their effects. They are used as additives in the form of ethanol extracts (e.g., Arnica Kneipp Gel, Vasotonin Gel). Arnica extracts contain a volatile oil with bicyclic sesquiterpenes of the helenalin type as characteristic constituents. Helenalins cause local irritation of the skin and mucous membranes, yet they are considered to have an anti-inflammatory action. Arnica flowers induce hyperemia when applied topically to the skin in the form of a tincture or infusion.

Assessment of the efficacy of topical venous remedies is still based primarily on experience with practical use. To date there has been insufficient proof of efficacy, especially with regard to the prevention of thrombosis and the improvement of its sequelae. While local therapeutic agents are of unquestioned benefit in the treatment of chronic venous disorders, they are also associated with risks in the form of allergic sensitization and contact eczema.

3.4.3 Drug Products

The *Red List 2003* lists 30 single-herb products for internal use under the heading of Remedies for Venous Disorders. Twenty-three of these products contain horse chestnut seed extract, three contain butcher's broom rhizome extract, and one each contain sweet clover extract, buckwheat, and grapevine leaf extract as their pharmacologically active ingredients. The horse chestnut seed extracts listed below include only products that conform to the 1994 monograph and contain the active ingredient in controlled-release form with a single dose equivalent to 250–313 mg of extract, corresponding to 50 mg of aescin. All of the clinical studies cited in Table 3.11 used the product with the brand name Venostasin retard. Combination products for this indication are no longer among the 100 most frequently prescribed herbal remedies.

 References

Alter H (1973) Zur medikamentösen Therapie der Varikosis. Z Allg Med 49 (17): 1301–1304.

Annoni F, Mauri A, Marincola 17, Resele LF (1959) Venotonic activity of aescin on the human saphenous vein. Arzneim Forsch/Drug Res 29: 672.

Bisler H, Pfeifer R, Klüken N, Pauschinger P (1986) Wirkung von Roßkastaniensamenextrakt auf die transkapilläre Filtration bei chronischer venöser Insuffizienz. Dtsch Med Wschr 111: 1321–1328.

Diehm C, Trampisch HJ, Lange S, Schmidt C (1996) Comparison of leg compression stocking and oral horse-chestnut seed extract therapy in patients with chronic venous insufficiency. Lancet 347: 292–294.

Fink Serralde C, Dreyfus Cortes GO, Colo Hernandez, Marquez Zacarias LA (1975) Valoracion de la escina pura en el tratamiento del sindrome des estasis venosa cronica. Münch Med Wschr (Spanish edition) 117(1): 41–46.

Fricke U (1995) Venenmittel. In: Schwabe U, Paffrath D (eds) Arzneiverordnungs-Report '95. Gustav Fischer Verlag, Stuttgart Jena, pp 421–430.

Friedrich HC, Vogelsberg H, Neiss A (1978) Ein Beitrag zur Bewertung von intern wirksamen Venenpharmaka. Z Hautkrankheiten 53 (11): 369–374.

Hänsel R, Keller K, Rimpler H, Schneider G (1992) Hagers Handbuch der Pharmazeutischen Praxis. 5th Ed., Drogen A-D.Springer Verlag, Berlin Heidelberg New York, pp 108–122.

Hitzenberger G (1989) Die therapeutische Wirksamkeit des Roßkastaniensamenextraktes. Wien Med Wschr 139 (17): 385–389.

Locks H, Baumgartner H, Konzett H (1974) Zur Beeinflussung des Venentonus durch Roßkastanienextrakte. Arzneim Forsch 24: 1347.

Lohr E, Garanin G, Jesau P, Fischer H (1986) Ödemprotektive Therapie bei chronischer Venenin-suffizienz mit Ödemneigung. Münch Med Wschr 128: 579–581.

Longiave D, Omini C, Nicosia S, Berti F (1978) The mode of action of aescin on isolated veins: relationship with PGF_{2a}. Pharmacol Res 10: 145.

Lorenz D, Marek ML (1960) Das therapeutisch wirksame Prinzip der Roßkastanie (Aesculus hippocastanum). Arzneim Forsch 10: 263–272.

Marshall M, Loew D (1994). Diagnostische Maßnahmen zum Nachweis der Wirksamkeit von Venentherapeutika. Phlebol 23: 85–91.

Marshall M, Dormandy JA (1987) Oedema of long distant flights. Phlebol 2: 123–124.

Neiss A, Böhm C (1976) Zum Wirksamkeitsnachweis von Roßkastaniensamenextrakt beim varikösen Symptomenkomplex. Münch Med Wschr 7: 213–216.

Pauschinger P (1987) Klinisch experimentelle Untersuchungen zur Wirkung von Roßkastaniensamenextrakt auf die transkapilläre Filtration und das intravasale Volumen an Patienten mit chronisch venöser Insuffizienz. Phlebol Proktol 16: 57–61.

Pittler MH, Ernst E (1998) Horse-chestnut seed extract for chronic venous insufficiency. A criteria-based systematic review. Arch Dermatol 134: 1356–1360.

Rudofsky G, Neiß A, Otto K, Seibel K (1986) Ödemprotektive Wirkung und klinische Wirksamkeit von Roßkastaniensamenextrakt im Doppelblindversuch. Phlebol Proktol 15: 47–54.

Steiner M, Hillemanns HG (1986) Untersuchung zur ödemprotektiven Wirkung eines Venentherapeutikums. Münch Med Wschr 31: 551–552.

4 Respiratory System

For many patients, phytomedicines are the remedies of choice for the treatment of uncomplicated acute respiratory tract infections. Increasingly, these medicines, taken mainly in the form of teas and liquid preparations, are being self-prescribed by patients due to the limited insurance coverage for cold medications. One problem with this trend is that medical laypersons can rarely distinguish between a harmless course and the onset of complications that warrant prompt medical attention. But primary care physicians who understand the preference of many patients for herbal remedies (see Sect. 4.1.2) will continue to have their advice sought and can continue to provide the guidance and management that patients need.

4.1 Acute Upper Respiratory Infections

Respiratory tract infections are the most common human diseases. Adults suffer from an average of two to five respiratory infections per year, and children contract even more (AkdA, 2002). The infections may involve the upper respiratory tract (nose, paranasal sinuses, pharynx, and larynx) or the lower airways (trachea and bronchi). The upper airways constitute a mechanical barrier to inhaled microorganisms that is reinforced by the immunologic shield of the mucous membranes and the lymphoepithelial structures of the Waldeyer ring. The efficacy of certain liquid herbal preparations is linked to their ability to strengthen this immunologic barrier (see Sect. 4.7).

4.1.1 Abuse of Antibiotics

Respiratory tract infections account for two-thirds of all infections that are treated by physicians in private practice (Fig. 4.1). Most respiratory infections are caused by viruses, while bacteria are very rarely the primary cause. In theory, the viral etiology of acute bronchitis, pharyngitis, or tonsilitis allows only for symptomatic treatment to reduce irritation. In practice, however, physicians tend to be more aggressive in prescribing strong-acting medications. Up to two-thirds of patients with acute bronchitis are treated with antibiotics, even though it has been proven that these drugs do not significantly shorten the duration of illness (Altiner et al., 2001; Bent et al., 1999; Fahey et al., 2001; Little et al., 1997; Murray et al., 2000). The risks of antibiotic therapy include the potential for allergic reactions. Additionally, antibiotics alter the normal bacterial flora of the bowel and nasopharynx and promote the development of resistant bacterial strains, increasing the danger of recurrence.

This has led expert medical commissions to recommend that patients with acute respiratory infections be apprised of these risks and limitations of antibiotics and, whenever possible, receive only symptomatic treatment. Antibiotics should be reserved for selected groups of high-risk patients (e.g., those with chronic airway obstructions), even though controlled studies have not shown definite benefits even in this population. At the same time, the therapeutic guidelines concede that, contrary to the best professional advice, approximately 75 % of all antibiotic prescriptions are written for acute respiratory tract infections (AkdA, 2002). Apparently, the difficulty lies in the practical application of theoretical recommendations. Laboratory methods are not useful for the "objective" differentiation of viral and bacterial infections, mainly due to the rapid course of the disease. The predominantly clinical differentiating features (Table 4.1) are

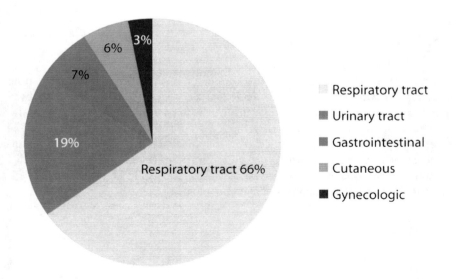

Figure 4.1. ▲ Relative frequency of infections diagnosed by office practitioners (Schwabe and Paffrath, 2001).

vague and are not useful for identifying bacterial infections that warrant antibiotic therapy.

4.1.2 The Desire of Patients to Recover

Patients who consult their physician for an acute respiratory infection mainly want one thing: to improve quickly. Some patients cannot "afford" days off from work or school, and others at least believe that they cannot. Viewed in a positive light, all of these patients want to do something on their own part to hasten their recovery. This desire of patients to recover from their illness deserves to be recognized, promoted, and encouraged. A controlled study from England documents the extent to which physicians can reinforce the self-healing powers of patients with a respiratory infection. A total of 476 patients were treated randomly with an antibiotic (n=246) or without an antibiotic (n=230). Statistical analysis of the cases showed that, except for fever, there were no statistically significant differences between the two groups in terms of complaints or duration of illness. Incidental questioning of the patients did reveal a significant difference, however. After their initial consultation, the patients were asked by a third party about their degree of satisfaction with the counseling and prescribing that their doctors had provided. Patients who were "very" satisfied improved more quickly: their average duration of illness was 4 days, compared with 6.5 days for patients who were "not at all" satisfied. This marked difference bore absolutely no relationship to whether or not antibiotics had been prescribed (Little et al., 1997).

These results show that acute respiratory tract infections are among the indications in which the "therapeutic context" and the physician (including the "herb doctor") have a greater impact on clinical response than the pharmacodynamics of the prescribed medicines (see also Sect. 1.5.3). If physicians were to rely entirely on statistically determined placebo/drug differences in making therapeutic recommendations for these indications, they run the risk of creating a side issue into the main issue and reaching a decision that is not consistent with the principles of practice-oriented, evidence-based medicine.

Table 4.1.
Differentiation of viral and bacterial respiratory tract infections (after AkdÄ, 2002).

Signs and symptoms	Suggestive of viral infection	Suggestive of bacterial infection
Onset	Gradual	Sudden
Fever	Gradual progression	Initial spike
Purulent drainage	Rare	Common
Lymph nodes	Indolent	Painful
Muscle pain	Common	Rare
Joint pain	Common	Rare
Cough	Usually dry	Purulent discharge
Auscultation	Minimal findings	Significant findings
Lung x-ray	"More than audible"	Consistent with audible findings
Leukocytosis	Moderate	Pronounced

4.2 General Phytotherapeutic Measures

When prescribed in the proper context, phytomedicines can make a useful contribution to relieving the symptoms of upper respiratory tract infections. From a pathophysiologic and pharmacologic standpoint, agents should be selected that do not further compromise the mucociliary clearance mechanism of the upper respiratory tract. Damage to this mechanism by the viral infection can pave the way for the bacterial invasion of normally germ-free sites (paranasal sinuses, inner ear, tracheal mucosa). Adequate fluid intake also helps to protect the mucous membranes and relieve irritation; medicinal teas are an excellent way to maintain this hydration.

4.2.1 Teas for Cold Relief

A proven and recommended home remedy for the initial stages of a cold (scratchy throat, malaise) consists of hot teas (usually infusions) and gradient foot baths (starting at about 33 °C and increasing the water temperature over a 20-min period according to tolerance) followed by warm bed rest to promote diaphoresis. Teas made from elder flowers, linden flowers, and meadowsweet flowers are particularly recommended for colds. Willow bark is also a component in many tea formulas (see Sect. 4.2.1.4). A strict distinction is not drawn between anti-tussive teas and bronchial teas. The efficacy of anti-tussive and bronchial teas, like that of other herbal remedies, is based only in part on specific pharmacodynamic effects. These teas are an important source of oral fluid intake as well as humidified inspiratory air, helping to reduce the viscosity of bronchial secretions and keep the mucous membranes from drying out. A daily fluid intake of approximately 2–3 liters is recommended. The use of teas is limited only in patients with cardiac or renal failure.

4.2.1.1 Elder Flowers

Elder flowers are derived from *Sambucus nigra* (Fig.4.2), a deciduous shrub that is widely distributed in Europe and central Asia. The flowering tops, which are flat compound cymes, are gathered, dried, and separated by sifting into individual flowers and peduncles and pedicels. These latter are then discarded. A crude drug of lower quality is made by drying and cutting the flowering tops, without separating the flowers from the peduncles and pedicels. Elder flowers have a faint, distinctive odor, an initially sweet taste, and an acrid aftertaste. It has not been proven that elder flowers contain diaphoretic principles despite their frequent use in formulations used to induce perspiration. Elder flower tea is prepared as follows according to the German Standard Registration: pour boiling water (150 Ml) over about 2 teaspoons (3 g) of dried elder flowers, steep for 5 min, and strain; drink 1–2 cups very hot.

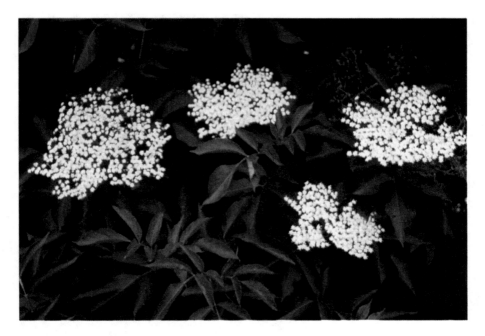

Figure 4.2. ▲ Cymes of the elder (*Sambucus nigra*).

4.2.1.2 Linden Flowers

Linden flowers are derived from two species of linden tree that are native to Europe and are often planted ornamentally along city streets: the early blooming summer linden (*Tilia platyphyllos*, Fig.4.3) and the winter linden (*T. cordata*), which blooms about 2 weeks later. The crude drug from both species is made by gathering and drying the fully developed, whole flowering tops including the bracts.

Dried linden flowers have a pleasant, distinctive odor different from that of the fresh blossoms. They have pleasant, faintly sweet, mucilaginous taste.

The pleasant taste is based on the interaction of astringent tannins (about 2 %) with mucilage and aromatics. However, the flowers have not been shown to have constituents with a specific diaphoretic action. The diaphoretic effect of linden flower tea (like that of elder flower tea) is based at least partly on the heat of the liquid itself combined with warm bed rest. It should be noted that the response to thermal stimuli follows a marked diurnal pattern. Hildebrandt et al. (1954) found that heat applied in the morning had little or no effect, while heat applied in the afternoon and evening induced profuse sweating.

4.2.1.3 Meadowsweet Flowers

The crude drug consists of the dried flowers of *Filipendula ulmaria* (formerly *Spiraea ulmaria*), an herbaceous perennial of the family Rosaceae native to northern Europe. The dried herb consists mostly of brownish yellow petals accompanied by numerous

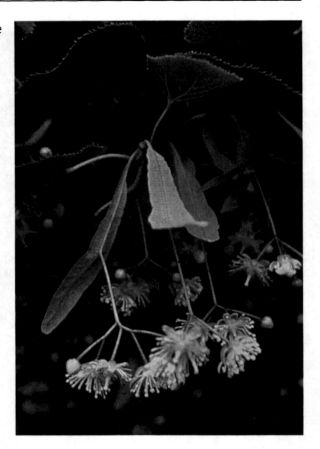

Abb. 4.3. ▶ Drooping cymes of the linden (*Tilia platyphyllos*).

unopened buds. Commercial herb of good quality has a faint odor of methylsalicylate and a bitter, astringent taste. Meadowsweet flowers contain 0.5 % flavonol glycosides, mostly quercetin-4´-glucoside (spiraeoside). The astringent taste is due to the presence of tannins. Hexahydroxydiphenic acid esters of glucose have been identified as components of the tannin fraction. The aromatic fraction consists of salicylaldehyde, phenylethyl alcohol, anisaldehyde, and methylsalicylate (methyl ester of salicylic acid).

Meadowsweet flowers are used in the form of a tea infusion, either alone or mixed with other tea herbs, in the supportive therapy of colds. Infusions contain only trace amounts of salicylates, so meadowsweet tea is considered an aromatic remedy rather than a salicylate medication.

4.2.1.4 Tea Formulas

Indications: **Febrile upper respiratory infections in which diaphoresis is desired.**

Preparation and dosing guidelines: Pour boiling water (about 150 mL) over 1 tablespoon or 1–2 teaspoons of the dried herb, cover and steep for about 10 min, and strain. Drink one fresh cup several times daily.

Directions to patient: Take 1–2 teaspoonsful per cup (about 150 mL) as an infusion several times daily.

Diaphoretic tea according to DRF (German Prescription Formula Index)

Rx	Elder flowers	25,0
	Linden flowers	25.0
	Mix to make tea	
	Directions (see above)	

Diaphoretic tea according to Meyer Camberg

Rx	Linden flowers	30,0
	Elder flowers	aa 30.0
	Chamomile flowers	40.0
	Mix to make tea	
	Directions (see above)	

Diaphoretic tea in Swiss Pharmacopeia 6

Rx	Linden flowers	40.0
	Elder flowers	30.0
	Peppermint leaves	20.0
	Pilocarpus leaves	10.0
	Mix to make tea	
	Directions (see above)	

Cold-relief tea I according to German Standard Registration

Rx	Linden flowers	30.0
	Elder flowers	30.0
	Meadowsweet flowers	20.0
	Rose hips	20.0
	Mix to make tea	
	Directions (see above)	

Cold-relief tea IV according to German Standard Registration

Rx	Willow bark	35.0
	Elder flowers	30.0
	Thyme	20.0
	Rose hips	5.0
	Licorice root	5.0
	Mallow flowers	5.0
	Mix to make tea	
	Directions (see above)	

Diaphoretic tea according to Suppl. Vol.6 (German Pharmacopeia)

Rx	Willow bark	20.0
	Birch leaves	20.0
	Elder flowers	20.0
	Linden flowers	20.0

Meadowsweet flowers	10.0
Chamomile flowers	0.5
Pilocarpus leaves	0.5
Mix to make tea	
Directions (see above)	

Indications: bronchitis symptoms and catarrhal diseases of the upper respiratory tract.

Preparation and directions: Pour boiling water (about 150 mL) over 1 tablespoon of tea, cover and steep for about 10 min, and pass through a tea strainer. Drink one cup of freshly brewed tea slowly several times daily, preferably while the tea is still hot.

Antitussive tea according to German Standard Registration

Rx	Marshmallow root	25.0
	Fennelseed	10.0
	Iceland moss	10.0
	English plantain	15.0
	Licorice root	10.0
	Thyme	30.0
	Directions (see above)	

Chest tea according to German Pharmacopeia

Rx	Marshmallow root	40.0
	Marshmallow leaves	20.0
	Licorice root	15.0
	Mullein flowers	10.0
	Violet root	5.0
	Aniseed, crushed	10.0
	Directions (see above)	

Chest tea according to Swiss Pharmacopeia

Rx	Marshmallow root	10.0
	Licorice root	10.0
	Marshmallow leaves	10.0
	Mullein flowers	15.0
	Cornflower	5.0
	Helichrysum flowers	10.0
	Mallow flowers	10.0
	Aniseed, crushed	15.0
	Senega root	10.0
	Wild thyme flowers	10.0

Cough and bronchial tea I according to German Standard Registration

Rx	Fennelseed	10.0
	English plantain	25.0
	Licorice root	25.0
	Thyme	20.0
	Marshmallow leaves	5.0
	Cornflower	5.0
	Mallow flowers	5.0
	Primrose flowers	5.0

Cough and bronchial tea Ii according to German Standard Registration

Rx	Aniseed	10.0
	Linden flowers	40.0
	Thyme	20.0
	Iceland moss	5.0
	Mallow flowers	5.0
	Primrose flowers	5.0
	Heartsease	5.0

Pectoral tea according to Hager (1893)*)

Rx	Marshmallow leaves	20.0
	Nettle leaves	10.0
	Horsetail	10.0
	English plantain	5.0
	Mallow flowers	5.0
	Linden flowers	5.0
	Fennelseed, crushed	5.0
	Mullein flowers	2.5
	Fenugreek seeds, crushed	2.5

*) Original formula modified by substituting marshmallow leaves for coltsfoot leaves.

4.2.2 Willow Bark and Salicylates

The treatment of inflammatory disorders with salicin-containing plant extracts was known to the physicians of ancient Greece. Dioscorides (ca. 50 CE), in his book *De Materia Medica* recommended willow bark preparations as a remedy for gout and other inflammatory joint diseases, suggesting that it be taken "with some pepper and wine." Extracts from parts of the willow tree (*Salix* species) were also used in medieval folk medicine for their pain-relieving and fever-reducing properties. In 1829, the French pharmacist. Leroux isolated the glycoside salicin as the active principle in these extracts. Six years later the German chemist Löwig was the first to synthesize salicylic acid. Because he had extracted the parent compound, salicylaldehyde, from plants of the genus *Spiraea*, he named the product spiric acid. This name later became the root for aspirin (*a-* acetyl, *-spir-* spiric acid, *-in* suffix), first marketed in 1896. Acetylsalicylic acid (ASA) is better tolerated.

The following calculation illustrates the problems posed by the continued use of willow bark preparations: A single aspirin dose of at least 500 mg is necessary for effective analgesia. Allowing for differences in molecular weights, 500 mg of aspirin is equivalent to 794 mg of salicin – an amount contained in no less than 88 g of willow bark. Moreover, when the powdered herb is used, salicin is not released quantitatively. As far as orthodox scientific medicine is concerned, willow bark is purely of historical interest today. Recent studies on pain-relieving efficacy raise the question of whether the analgesic effects of willow bark preparations are based entirely on the salicylates that they contain (see Sect. 8.4.2).

Willow bark is indicated in phytotherapy for "febrile diseases, rheumatic complaints, and headache" according to the German Commission E monograph of 1992. Accordingly, the herb is a common ingredient in diaphoretic and antirheumatic teas. The source plant, identified simply as willow bark, has not been specifically defined. Various *Salix* species and varieties with a high salicin content are used, most notably *Salix alba* (white willow), *S. fragilis* (brittle willow), and *S. purpurea* (purple willow). In addition to salicin, willow bark contains 8–20 % tannins. Presumably, the bitter taste and known irritant effect of tannins on the gastric mucosa would limit the use of higher doses in the form of powdered herb or infusions.

4.3 Pharmaceutical Preparations with Essential Oils

There is much empirical evidence to show that essential plant oils such as peppermint oil and eucalyptus oil are beneficial for subjective complaints involving the nasopharynx, particularly nasal airway obstruction. Surprisingly, rhinomanometric measurements after menthol inhalation showed no objective change in nasal airflow, which seem to contradict general experience. But when a patient with a stuffy nose has the sensation of being able to breathe more easily after inhaling peppermint oil and is able to sleep better after this therapy, the response must be characterized as something more than a placebo effect (Eccles et al., 1988).

Essential oils can be used in various forms: as a liquid preparation (applied externally or gargled), as nasal ointments or nosedrops, as an ingredient of troches or lozenges, or inhaled in aerosol or vapor form. Also, essential oils or substances derived from them are contained in plant extracts that are present as active ingredients in liquid or solid medicinal products.

4.3.1 Nasal Ointments, Nosedrops, and Rubs

Menthol, camphor, and essential oils are lipophilic substances that, when processed into medicines, can be incorporated only into lipophilic bases. White petroleum jelly or lanolin alcohols are used for nasal ointments, and fatty plant oils are used for nose-drops. As a rule, rhinologic medications should not disrupt the normal protective functions of the nasal mucosa. Hydrophilic preparations are preferable in this regard as they do not disrupt the normal function of the ciliary apparatus. Fatty preparations have two serious disadvantages: they do not mix with the nasal mucous so they do not make adequate contact with the mucosa, and the high viscosity of hydrophobic bases can significantly retard ciliary motion.

The effect of menthol (a pure compound originally derived from peppermint leaf oil, now usually produced synthetically) on the nasal mucosa appears to depend on the concentration. Higher concentrations (>5 %), which generally are not used, cause local irritation. According to Nöller (1967), the application of menthol to the nasal mucosa elicits a two-phase response: an initial phase lasting about 30 min in which the nasal air passage becomes constricted or even obstructed, followed by a period of improved nasal airflow. Despite the initial, objective increase in mucosal swelling, test subjects consistently report a pleasant, cooling sensation and a feeling of being able to breath more easily. This purely subjective improvement in rhinitis-associated complaints by menthol application may relate partly to the action of menthol on temperature and pain receptors (Bromm, 1995; Göbel, 1995). Cold, fresh air has a similar effect on nasal stuffiness, most noticeable on walking outdoors from a heated room (Fox, 1977).

The effects of camphor (a pure compound originally derived from *Cinnamomum camphora* and now produced synthetically) and eucalyptus oil (distilled from the leaves of *Eucalyptus globules*) are similar to those of menthol. Detailed investigations (Burrow et al., 1983; Eccles and Jones, 1987, 1988) showed that all three substances stimulate the cold receptors in the nasal mucosa and lead to subjective improvement of complaints, despite the fact that there is no measurable decongestant effect. The absence of this effect is advantageous, however, when one considers that the inflammatory response is a natural process and that suppressing it could delay or prolong recovery.

Interestingly, Bromm et al. (1995) and Göbel et al. (1995) found significant differences between the effects of peppermint oil (main component: menthol) and eucalyptus oil (main component: cineol) on temperature and pain receptors when applied topically to the scalp.

Most medications classified as chest rubs or cold balsams are ointments; some are oil- or paraffin-base solutions that incorporate essential oils. The designated amount is applied to the skin of the chest and back. As lipophilic compounds, portions of the oils penetrate the skin, enter the circulation, and reach the bronchial mucosa. As unknown percentage evaporates on the warm skin and is inhaled.

Essential oils are available in several forms for adding to bathwater: bath salts, bath oils, and essences (i.e., essential oils without other additives). The very large surface area of exposed skin allows for more extensive absorption and distribution than chest rubs. Portions of the absorbed essential oil components are excreted via the lungs, producing an expectorant action in the bronchial tree. The percutaneously absorbed and exhaled doses are further supplemented by the inhalation of essential oils from the air over the bathwater.

Observations in aromatherapy (Jackson, 1989) are consistent with the dose-response relationship found in experimental animals (Boyd and Sheppard, 1970) and support the value of moderate dosing. Just 7-9 drops of essential oil, equivalent to about 150-200 mg, is recommended for a whole bath consisting of about 30 L water. Favorite essential bath oils for respiratory tract diseases are eucalyptus oil, pine needle oil, spruce needle oil, thyme oil, and cypress oil.

Camphor, menthol, and medications in general that contain strong-smelling compounds or their essential oils should not be used in the facial region of infants or children under 2 years of age due to the risk of glottic spasm or respiratory arrest. In particular, they should not be used intranasally in this subset of patients. Failure to observe this contraindication, especially in self-medication with essential oils, can lead to life-threatening complications (Lübke and Brockstedt, 2001).

4.3.2 Preparations Administered by Inhalation

Essential oils reach the nasal mucosa in much lower concentration when administered by inhalation than when applied topically. It is conceivable, for example, that small amounts of essential oils reaching the mucosa could actually stimulate ciliary motion. In one clinical study, the inhalation of cineol led to significant improvement in ciliary clearance in patients with chronic obstructive bronchitis (Dorow, 1989). Extrapolating observations on the expectorant effects of inhaled alcohol (Boyd and Sheppard, 1970) on the nasal mucosa suggests that essential oils could stimulate the flow of secretions. The fact that secretions inhibit drying of the nasal mucosa is important because mucosal dryness can seriously disable the ciliary apparatus.

Two basic methods are available for administering essential oils by inhalation: steam inhalation and dry inhalation. Steam inhalation is a simple, effective method when applied by any of three techniques:

▶ simmering chamomile, peppermint leaves, or anise in a pot and inhaling the rising vapors while the head is covered with a towel (head steam bath);
▶ adding 1 teaspoon of lemon balm spirit to a steam vaporizer; chamomile extracts and other products containing essential oils can also be used;
▶ taking a hot bath to which a bath salt containing essential oils has been added.

Inhalation devices can be purchased and used for dry inhalation, but a simpler method is to place several drops of peppermint oil on a handkerchief or on the pillow near the head at bedtime and inhale the vapors through the nose. Several breaths should be enough to produce a sensation of easier breathing. As menthol stimulates the cold receptors in the nasal mucosa, it intensifies the patient's sensation and awareness of air streaming through the nose. This is a subjective response that need not be accompanied by an objective change in the nasal air passage (Burrow et al., 1983; Eccles et al., 1987, 1988). Meanwhile, it is a physiological fact that thermoregulation is linked to vasoregulation, i.e., cold stimuli tend to induce vasoconstriction. Therefore, it may be hypothesized that essential oils, by activating cold receptors in the nose, can induce reflex vasoconstriction and thus exert a decongestive effect (Leiber, 1967). Hamann and Bonkowsky (1987) supported this hypothesis by demonstrating objective improvement in the nasal airway.

Spruce needle oil, pine needle oil, and turpentine oil may exacerbate bronchial spasms in asthmatics and in patients with whooping cough.

4.3.3 Lozenges, Troches, and Gargles

Lozenges, troches, and gargles are used to soothe local inflammation in the mouth and throat and inhibit the urge to cough. The cough accompanying a common cold may develop as a result of nasal airway obstruction. As the pharyngeal mucosa dries out, the cough receptors in the throat become more irritable. Even in the absence of objective clinical studies, it is reasonable to assume that lozenges, by promoting the flow of saliva, can keep the mucosa moist and indirectly quiet the cough.

A major ingredient of throat lozenges is sugar, which may be in the form of sucrose, corn syrup, glucose, maltose, fructose, or substitutes like the sugar alcohols sorbitol and xylitol. Troches differ from ordinary tablets in their significantly longer dissolving time, achieved by omitting the disintegration excipients and forming the troches under much higher pressure. Another difference is that the troche masks the taste of the drug substance itself (e.g., plant mucilage). Besides the sugars, essential oils also serve as flavor correctives and thus perform a dual function.

Gum lozenges derive their name from their content of the raw material gum arabic. The base consists of sugar, gum arabic, and possibly other hydrocolloids. The liquid mass is mixed with solid drug substances, plant extracts, and essential oils and formed by pouring into molds. Essential oils may be the only medicinal substances that are incorporated into cough drops and gum lozenges. The most important essential oils for this purpose are anise oil, eucalyptus oil, fennel oil, menthol, peppermint oil, thyme oil, and tolu balsam (Table 4.2).

Cough drops and gum lozenges are held in the mouth for 20–30 min while they dissolve. One function of the essential oils in them is to impart a pleasant flavor that stimulates salivation. The increased salivation promotes more frequent reflex swallowing, although voluntary swallowing is also useful for suppressing an imminent urge to cough.

Gargling involves taking a fluid into the mouth without swallowing it and holding it suspended in the throat by forcing air through it while exhaling. Gargling exerts a massaging action that is mostly confined to the pharyngeal ring and largely spares the tonsils. Thus, gargles are indicated for inflammatory diseases of the oropharynx and have two essential functions: to cleanse the mouth and pharynx while exerting an anti-inflammatory action on inflamed mucous membranes. The most common ingredients in gargles are essential oils and aromatic herbs that contain volatile oils. Herbs with anti-inflammatory properties are also used, most notably chamomile and tannin-containing herbs. Oral antisepsis is no longer considered a therapeutic goal, for it is known that only transient antiseptic effects are obtained even when highly active concentrations are used.

The gargle may be used in the form of a warm tea infusion or a liquid commercial product. The phytotherapeutic components of commercial gargles include essential oils as well as extracts from chamomile (anti-inflammatory), sage (essential oils, bitters, and tannins), or tormentil rhizome (tannins). Partially evaporated aqueous extracts from Iceland moss are also used.

4.4 Essential Oils as Cough Remedies and Expectorants

Throat lozenges and other intraoral cough remedies may contain essential plant oils singly or in combination with other medicinal agents. Anise oil, eucalyptus oil, fennel oil, menthol, peppermint oil, thyme oil, and tolu balsam are commonly used (Table 4.2). The function of the essential oils is to produce a pleasing taste sensation that stimulates

Table 4.2.
Essential oils commonly used in cough remedies.

Essential oil (Latin name)	Source	Main constituents	Sensory qualities
Anise oil (Anisi aetheroleum)	Ripe fruits of *Pimpinella anisum* (aniseed)	90 % *trans*-Anethole	Spicy odor of anise; sweet taste
Eucalyptus oil (Eucalypti aetheroleum)	Fresh leaves of *Eucalyptus* species that contain cineol	70 % Cineole (=eucalyptol)	Camphor-like odor; taste is initially acrid, then cooling
Fennel oil (Foeniculi aetheroleum)	Ripe fruits of sweet fennel, *Foeniculum vulgare var. vulgare*	50–70 % trans-Anethole, 10–23 % fenchone	Odor similar to anise; taste is initially sweet, then becomes bitter and camphor-like
Peppermint oil (Menthae piperitae aetheroleum)	Flowering tops of *Mentha piperita* (peppermint)	40–55 % Menthol, 10 % esters of menthol, 10–35 % menthone	Pale yellowish liquid with the pleasant, refreshing odor of the peppermint plant; taste is initially acrid, then cooling
Thyme oil (Thymi aetheroleum)	Fresh flowering tops of *Thymus vulgaris* (thyme)	30–70 % Thymol, 3–15 % carvacrol	Colorless liquid that gradually turns red; has a phenolic (medicinal) smell and acrid taste
Tolu balsam (Balsamum tolutanum)	Balsamic resin seeps from the damaged bark *Myroxylon balsamum*	Esters of benzoic and cinnamic acid (not well analyzed)	Doughy, reddish-brown mass with an odor reminiscent of vanilla; has a somewhat bitter, acrid taste

the production and secretion of saliva, which in turn activates the swallowing reflex. Voluntary swallowing can also suppress an impending cough. Lozenges and cough drops can aid patients in their efforts at voluntarily controlling the urge to cough (Walther, 1979).

Often in practical use a strict distinction cannot be drawn between antitussives and expectorants. Mucus in the bronchi stimulates coughing, so expectorants produce an indirect antitussive effect. Conversely, vigorous coughing intensifies the secretion of mucus, so antitussives can reduce excess mucus production (Kurz, 1989). According to their pharmacologic definition, expectorants are agents that can influence the consistency, formation, and transport of bronchial secretions.

Herbal expectorants have been used on an empirical basis for centuries. They are believed to act by three mechanisms: a reduction of mucus viscosity (owing partly to the water content of tea preparations), a gastropulmonary reflex mechanism, and the liquefaction of secretions, which is accomplished mainly by direct effects of the essential oils on the bronchial glands. Bronchomucotropic agents (Ziment, 1985) directly stimulate the bronchial glands and increase their activity. These agents may be inhaled externally or administered orally for subsequent excretion (and action) via the bronchial tree. Essential oils and aromatic herbs have bronchomucotropic properties (Ziment, 1985).

The principal essential oils that are used as expectorants are reviewed in Table 4.3. These oils cannot be strictly differentiated from essential oils that are used as antitussives (Table 4.2). The essential oils are well absorbed after oral administration and are

Table 4.3.
Essential oils that are used as expectorants in inhalants, cold ointments, or capsules. See also Table 4.2.

Essential oil (Latin name)	Source plant (family)	Main constituents	Remarks
Spruce-needle oil (Piceae aetheroleum)	*Pinus exelsa, Abies species* (Pinaceae)	20–40 % Bornyl acetate along with α- and β-pinene and β-phellandrene	
Cajuput oil (Cajuputi aetheroleum rectificatum)	Leaves of *Melaleuca species* (Myrtaceae)	65 % Cineole (=eucalyptol)	Reminiscent of eucalyptus oil (see Table 4.1)
Pine-needle oil (Pini aetheroleum)	*Pinus silvestris* (Pinaceae)	80 % Monoterpene hydrocarbons, including α-pinene and 3-carene	
Myrtol	Exact botanical origin unknown	Mainly cineole (=eucalyptol), α-pinene and limonene	
Niaouli oil	*Melaleuca viridiflora* (Myrtaceae)	Like cajuput oil; principal constituent cineole (=eucalyptol)	
Rectified turpentine oil (Terebinthinae aether oleum rectificatum)	*Pinus palustris* and other P. species (Pinaceae)	90 % Monoterpene hydrocarbons: α- and β-pinene	Starting material is the tree trunk gum turpentine
Citronella oil (Citronellae aetheroleum)	*Cymbopogon winterianus* and *C.nardus* (Poaceae)	Monoterpene alcohols such as geraniol, nerol, and corresponding aldehydes such as citral and citronellal	Often sold under the name of lemon grass oil or Indian grass oil

partially excreted via the lungs. As the exhaled molecules pass through the bronchial tree, they can act on the bronchial mucosa to stimulate the serous glandular cells and ciliated epithelium.

4.4.1 Studies with Various Preparations in Patients and Volunteers

Irritation of the mucous membranes is a property shared by all essential oils. Even trace amounts that have little or no detectable odor can exert demonstrable local effects on mucosal surfaces (Boyd and Sheppard, 1970a). The specificity of the effects of essential oils is demonstrated by studies with a turpentine oil that has been purified with oxidants (Ozothine®). Chemically, it represents a mixture of monoterpene alcohols, aldehydes, and ketones, most notably verbenol, verbenone, myrtenol, myrtenal, and pinocarveol. Its actions can be summarized as follows: stimulates serous bronchial gland function and suppresses mucous glandular cell activity following i.v. administration (Bauer, 1973); reduces surface tension (surfactant effect) (Zänker and Blümel, 1983); improves mucociliary activity and tracheobronchial clearance in concentrations of 10^{-7} g/mL or higher (Iravani, 1972). The direct effect on the bronchial glands has also been investigated: while this turpentine oil selectively stimulates the serous glands, it inhibits the function of the mucous glands, resulting in the liquefaction of secretions (Lorenz and Ferlinz, 1985).

Controlled clinical studies have been conducted to test the efficacy of certain medicinal products containing essential oils. A placebo-controlled double-blind study was conducted in patients with chronic obstructive bronchitis who were being managed with theophylline and a beta-adrenergic drug. This regimen was supplemented by treatment with an ointment containing menthol, camphor, eucalyptus oil, and pine oil as its active ingredients. Statistical analysis showed that this regimen was significantly better than a placebo-supplemented regimen in terms of objective parameters (pulmonary function, quantify of sputum) as well as subjective parameters (cough, breathing difficulties, lung sounds) (Linsenmann and Swoboda, 1986). Placebo-controlled double-blind studies in patients with acute tracheobronchitis showed improved mucolysis following the administration of essential oils in capsule form (containing anethole, cineole, and dwarf pine needle oil) compared with a placebo (Stafunsky et al., 1989; Linsemann et al., 1989). Another study in patients with chronic obstructive airway disease showed that an orally administered combination of pine oil, lemon oil, and cineole was effective as ambroxol in increasing mucociliary clearance (Dorow et al., 1987).

Two controlled clinical studies were carried out in a total of 160 patients to test the efficacy and tolerance of a multicomponent essential oil distillate in the treatment of common cold symptoms. Control groups received an ethanol solvent or a placebo, and the tests were blinded by adding orange and vanilla aroma to all the test preparations. Five subjective symptoms were scored by the physician during a 7-day treatment period. A steady decline in mean scores was observed for the symptoms of general malaise, headache and body aches, sore throat, and swallowing difficulties. This decline was significantly greater in the oil-treated group than in the controls. The oil distillate and placebo were equivalent in their effects on the symptoms of cough, hoarseness, and runny nose. These descriptive results were confirmed and differentiated by a statistical factor analysis that included local pharyngeal findings in addition to subjective symptoms (Schneider, 1997).

4.4.2 Cineole (Eucalyptol)

Approximately 70 % of eucalyptus oil is comprised of cineole, hence its synonym, eucalyptol (Table 4.1). Cineole is an ambiguous term, referring either to the pure chemical substance that is isolated from cineole-containing eucalyptus oils by fractional crystallization or distillation, or to the commercial medication known as cineole. The pharmaceutical product has a cineole content of only 80–90 % and is produced simply by treating eucalyptus oils with lye. This yields a clear, colorless liquid with a camphor-like odor and a pungent, cooling taste.

Cineole has antispasmodic, secretagogic, secretolytic, antimicrobial, and fungicidal properties. Experiments with cineole inhalation in rabbits showed that it exerts a surfactant-like action by reducing surface tension (Zänker et al., 1984).

Römmelt et al. (1988) investigated the pharmacokinetics of 1,8-cineole following 10 min exposure to a terpene-containing ointment (9.17 % cineole) administered by steam inhalation. The C_{max} in the venous blood following alveolar absorption was 200 ng/mL; the half-life was 35.8 min. Concentrations as low as 10 ng/mL were associated with an increase in ciliary frequency.

As for adverse effects, rare instances of stomach upset have been reported following the internal use of cineole, and external use occasionally causes hypersensitivity reactions of the skin. The LD_{50} in rats is 3480 mg/kg b.w. Cineole has a wide therapeutic range, and there have been almost no reports of cineole toxicity. Patel and Wiggins (1980) reported one case of medicinal poisoning with eucalyptus oil.

The Commission E monograph on eucalyptus oil for internal use recommends an average daily dose of 0.3–0.5 g in the treatment of upper respiratory infections (Blumenthal et al., 1998).

4.4.3 Anise Oil and Anethole

Anise oil as described in *German Pharmacopeia 9* is the essential oil obtained from the ripe fruits (often called seeds) of *Pimpinella anisum* (family Apiaceae, Fig.4.4) or *Illicium verum* (family Illiciaceae). The principal component (80–90 %) of anise oil is anethole which is obtained from anise oil by freezing.

Anise oil is a clear, colorless liquid with a spicy odor and a sweet, aromatic taste that solidifies to a white crystalline mass when refrigerated. Anethole forms white crystals that melt at 20–22 °C.

The expectorant effects of anise oil and anethole are presumably based on their ability to stimulate the ciliary activity of the bronchial epithelium. Moreover, antispasmodic and antibacterial actions have been demonstrated in vitro.

Figure 4.4. ▶ Anise (*Pimpinella anisum*).

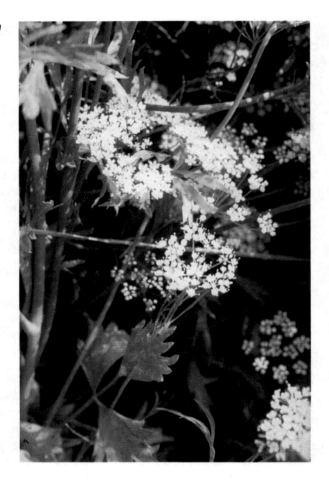

Anethole is rapidly absorbed from the gastrointestinal tract of healthy subjects and is just as rapidly eliminated with the urine (54–69 %) and expired air (13–17 %). Its principal metabolite is 4-methoxyhippuric acid (approximately 56 %); additional metabolites are 4-methoxybenzoic acid and three other metabolites that have yet to be identified (Caldwell and Sutton, 1988; Sangister et al., 1987). Changing the dose does not alter the pattern of metabolite distribution in humans, contrary to findings in the mouse and rat (Sangister et al., 1984). These results do not support the assumption based on animal experiments that higher doses of anethole in humans could block the enzyme system responsible for its degradation.

Adverse effects consist of occasional allergic skin reactions (Opdyke, 1973). The LD_{50} in different animal species (rat, mouse, guinea pig) ranges from 2090 to 3050 mg/kg b.w. for trans-anethole. The *cis* derivative is at least 15 times more toxic. At present there are no regulations specifying a maximum allowable content of *cis*-anethole in anethole or anise oil. Animal studies have refuted speculations about a carcinogenic effect (Drinkwater et al., 1976; Miller et al., 1983; Newberne et al., 1989; Truhaut et al., 1989).

The indications for the internal and external use of anise oil and anethole are catarrhal diseases of the upper respiratory tract. The Commission E monograph on anise recommends an average daily oral dose of 3 g of crude drug or 0.3 g of the essential oil for this indication (Blumenthal et al., 1998).

4.4.4 Myrtol (Gelomyrtol®)

Myrtol (trade name Gelomyrtol®), an essential oil with a pleasant odor reminiscent of turpentine oil and eucalyptus oil. The drug product that has the following manufacturer-listed ingredients: not less than 25 % limonene, 25 % cineole, and 6.7 % (+)-α-pinene. There is no information in the pharmaceutical literature on the botanical origin of the ingredients.

The chemical composition of myrtol is similar to that of eucalyptus oil. The pharmacologic profile of myrtol features mucolytic properties that are supplemented by antioxidative and anti-inflammatory actions (De Mey and Wittig, 2002). Strictly speaking, since myrtol is a artificial mixture derived from specific essential oils, it is not classified as a phytomedicine but belongs to the group of essential oils and essential oil-derived compounds, and, as such, is approved in Germany for use in "acute and chronic bronchitis and sinusitis." Gelomyrtol® is not only among the most commonly prescribed herbal medications in Germany (see Table A3 in the Appendix) but is also the essential oil-based medication whose efficacy has been most convincingly documented by modern clinical studies.

In a multicenter study by physicians in private practice, the efficacy and tolerance of myrtol was tested relative to placebo in 331 patients with acute sinusitis. The severity of the sinusitis was rated with a 0-3 total symptom score based on headache, pain on bending forward with the head down, tenderness to pressure on trigeminal nerve exit points, nasal discharge, quantity of discharge, obstructed nasal breathing, malaise, and fever. The medication consisted of 4 × 300 mg/d myrtol or placebo, and the duration of treatment was approximately 1 week. The symptom score showed a significantly better score reduction in response to myrtol than in the placebo group (10.3 vs. 9 points). Further treatment with antibiotics was necessary in 23 % of the patients who had been treated with myrtol, versus 37 % in the placebo group. Side effects with myrtol consisted of 9 cases of abdominal complaints such as pain or epigastric pressure, bloating, or nausea (Federpil et al., 1997).

In another randomized multicenter double-blind study, myrtol administered in 3 daily doses of 300 mg was tested against a placebo in 246 patients with chronic bronchitis. The duration of treatment was 6 months. Efficacy was evaluated by the exacerbation rate, the need for antibiotics, a symptom score, and a quality-of-life score. The exacerbation rate in the myrtol group was 53 %, compared with 72 % in the placebo group (p<0.01). Quality of life and general well-being tended to be better with myrtol than with the placebo. Adverse events consisted mainly of mild to moderate abdominal discomfort, with no statistical difference between myrtol and placebo (Meister et al., 1999).

Another randomized double-blind study compared the efficacy and tolerance of 2 weeks of treatment with myrtol (4 × 300 mg on days 1–14), cefuroxime (2 × 250 mg/d on days 1–6), ambroxol (3 × 30 mg on days 1–3 and 2 × 30 mg on days 4–14), and a placebo. The patients consisted of 676 male and female outpatients with acute bronchitis of less than 5 days' duration, an $FEV_1 > 75$ %, and no clinical evidence of chronic airway disease. The patients were examined at baseline (visit 1), after 1 and 2 weeks of treatment (visits 2 and 3), and 2 weeks after the treatment was concluded (visit 4). The outcome measures were the responder and nonresponder rates, clinical findings (abnormal auscultation), symptoms (journal entries on coughing at night and during the day, sputum consistency, general well-being), FEV_1, global assessment of efficacy, absence of recurrence, and tolerance. Although the symptoms improved rapidly in all the treatment groups, regression was slower and less complete in the patients treated with placebo. Thirty-six patients in the placebo group (20.9 %) showed an exacerbation of acute bronchitis so severe that the study had to be terminated after 1 week (nonresponders). After another week (visit 3), 19 additional patients in the placebo group (11 %) were classified as nonresponders. In the group of patients treated with standardized essential oil mixture myrtol, the nonresponder rate was only 5.3 % at visit 2 and 1.2 % at visit 3. The responder rates at visit 2 were significantly higher (p<0.001) for myrtol compared with placebo and were similar to those for cefuroxime and ambroxol. The superiority of the active treatments vs. placebo, with little difference among the treatment groups, was confirmed for all of the remaining criteria. The treatments were well tolerated (Matthys et al., 2000; De Mey and Wittig, 2002).

4.5   Mucilaginous Herbs

Coughing as a reflex act is triggered by mechanical irritation of the respiratory mucosa. The pharynx, larynx, and trachea contain receptors that are highly sensitive to mechanical stimuli (Gysling, 1976; Hahn, 1987). The mucilages in plants can inhibit cough by forming a protective coating that shields the mucosal surface from irritants (Kurz, 1989). This effect is limited to the pharynx, however, since plant mucilages probably are not absorbed as macromolecules and thus cannot reach the tracheobronchial mucosa following oral administration. Mucilaginous herbs have not known adverse effects, although coltsfoot leaves may be contraindicated due to their content of pyrrolizidines (hence the omission of this herb from Table 4.4). While it is true that the content of potentially carcinogenic pyrrolizidine alkaloids is very low, implying a very small risk, it is always possible that products may contain varieties of coltsfoot leaves that have a higher alkaloid content or are mixed with butterbur leaves (Petasites hybridus), which also contain pyrrolizidine alkaloids. It should be added that since cultivated varieties of coltsfoot have become available, it is no longer necessary to gather the plant in the wild (Kopp et al., 1997). Other available mucilaginous herbs include mallow leaves and Iceland moss. "Immunomodulating" effects have also been ascribed to polysaccharides isolated from Iceland moss (Ingolfsdottir et al., 1998).

The antitussive efficacy and tolerance of an English plantain preparation were tested in an observational study of 593 patients with acute respiratory infections and bron-

Table 4.4.
Mucilaginous herbs used in teas or lozenges to soothe coughs and sore throat.

Herb (Latin name)	Source plant (family)	Constituents	Preparation
Marshmallow root (Althaeae radix)	Althaea officinalis (Malvaceae)	5–10 % Mucilage	2–5 % Infusion or cold-water maceration (1–2 teaspoons/150 mL)
Iceland moss (Lichen islandicus)	Cetraria ericetorum and C. islandica (Parmeliaceae)	About 50 % mucilage of glucan type, including lichenin as the main component	1–2 % Infusion (1–2 teaspoons/150 mL)
Mullein flowers (Verbasci flos)	Verbascum densiflorum and V. phlomoides (Scrophulariaceae)	3 % Mucilage of unknown structural type	1–2 % Infusion (3–4 teaspoons/150 mL)
Mallow leaf (Malvae folium)	Malva sylvestris and M. neglecta (Malvaceae)	About 8 % mucilage of unknown tertiary structure; arabinose, glucose, galactose, and galacturonic acid also occur as basic components	2–3 % Infusion (3–4 teaspoons/150 mL)
Mallow flowers (Malvae flos)	Malva sylvestris ssp. mauritaniana (Malvaceae)	About 10 % mucilage as in mallow leaves	2 % Infusion (2 teaspoons/150 mL)
Plantain (Plantaginis lanceolatae herba)	Plantago lanceolata (Plantaginaceae)	About 6 % mucilage, including a rhamno-galacturonan, an arabinogalactan, and a glucomannan; iridoid glycosides including 1–2 % aucubin	2 % Infusion (3–4 teaspoons/150 mL)

chitis. The average duration of treatment was 10 days, and the patients ranged from 6 to 70 years of age. Therapeutic efficacy was rated by taking 13 separate scores and adding them to get a total score. The total score decreased by 65 % during the observation period, and the partial scores for cough symptoms and chest discomfort declined by 70–80 %. Only 7 of the 593 patients reported adverse reactions, including 5 cases of diarrhea. None of the patients found the side effects serious enough to discontinue the therapy. Separating the patients into 7 different age groups showed an approximately equal response at all age levels (Kraft, 1997).

4.6 Saponin-Containing Herbs

Saponins are glycosidic plant constituents with a terpenoid agylcone component. They are like detergents in their tendency to form a durable foam when shaken with water.

Saponins have an acrid and/or bitter taste and are irritating to mucous membranes. In finely powdered form, saponins cause sneezing, eye inflammation, and lacrimation. In addition to their surfactant properties, saponins alter the permeability of all biologic membranes. Higher concentrations entering the blood or tissues have a generally toxic effect on cells. Due to their polar nature, saponins are only sparingly absorbed from the gastrointestinal tract so they usually produce no systemic effects when administered orally. Their expectorant action is thought to be mediated by the gastric mucosa, which reflexly stimulates mucous glands in the bronchi via parasympathetic sensory pathways. Higher doses of saponin-containing expectorants cause stomach upset, nausea, and vomiting. All substances that induce vomiting at higher doses can be used at a lower dosage as expectorants (1/10 of the emetic dose). The prototype of this drug is emetine, an alkaloid derived from ipecac root. Even ordinary doses of saponins can cause adverse side effects in patients with a sensitive stomach.

The saponin-containing herbs that are most commonly used as expectorants are listed in Table 4.5. The list does not include licorice root. The glycyrrhizin contained in licorice root is often classified as a saponin, and its chemical composition would support this. But licorice does not have all the biologic and pharmacologic properties that are characteristic of saponins. As a result, licorice root and its preparations are not included in the class of reflex expectorants. This mechanism by which glycyrrhizin exerts its expectorant action requires further study. In any case, licorice and licorice extracts are useful as flavorings in teas and cough syrups.

Table 4.5.
Saponin-containing herbs that are used as expectorants.

Herb (Latin name)	Source plant (family)	Type of saponin	Remarks
Ivy leaf (Hederae folium)	Hedera helix (Araliaceae)	Neutral bis-desmosides, termed hederacosides, with oleanolic and 28-hydroxyoleanolic acid as aglycone; also hederin type of monodesmosides; total saponin content 3–6 %	Not used as an infusion. Extracts used in drug products, with daily dose equal to 0.3 g of crude drug. Fresh leaves can cause skin irritation; the contact allergen is falcarinol, an aliphatic C alcohol with acetylene bonds
Primula root (Primulae radix)	Primula veris and/or P. elatior (Primulaceae)	Monodesmosidic triterpene saponins (5–10 %), including the principal saponin primulic acid A	Used as an infusion or tincture, with daily dose equal to 1 g of crude drug
Soap bark (Quillajae cortex)	Quillaja saponaria (Rosaceae)	Triterpene saponins (10 %)	Single dose of 0.2 g of crude drug corresponds to 10 g of decoction (2 %) or 1.0 g of tincture
Senega snakeroot (Polygalae radix)	Polygala senega (Polygalaceae)	6–10 % Bisdesmosidic triterpene saponins	Single dose of 1 g of crude drug corresponds to 20 g of decoction (5 %) or 2.5 g of tincture (1 : 5)

Some combination products contain preparations from *Gypsophila* species as their saponin component. These plants are perennial herbs or subshrubs that prefer a dry climate (e.g., tall gypsophyll). Gypsophila-derived saponin is a complex chemical mixture. It is the standard saponin used to determine the haemolytic index as described in pharmacy texts.

Small amounts of saponins are also contained in grindelia, a tincture of which is a component of several combination products. The aerial parts of *Grindelia* species, native to the southwestern U.S., are gathered during the flowering season and dried to make the crude drug, which also contains 0.3 % volatile oil. Grindelia is believed to act as an expectorant, although relevant pharmacologic studies have not been performed.

In a controlled multicenter study, 761 private physicians tested a combination product containing 60 mg of cowslip root (*Primula veris*) extract and 160 mg of thyme (*Thymus vulgaris*) extract in a total of 7783 patients with acute bronchitis. More than 2000 of the patients were children under 12 years of age. A total of 4629 patients took the herbal combination product for 10 days, and 3154 patients took reference drugs, mainly *N*-acetylcysteine and ambroxol, for an equal period. Using a standard rating scale, the physicians and the patients rated the signs and symptoms at the beginning and end of the 10-day treatment period. Statistical analysis showed that the herbal combination product was marginally better than *N*-acetylcysteine and ambroxol in its efficacy and was significantly better in its tolerance. This positive outcome occurred equally in the subgroups of children and adults (Ernst et al., 1997b).

4.6.1 Ivy Leaf Extract

The only saponin-containing herb that is widely prescribed as a single-herb preparation (see Table A2) is ivy (*Hedera helix*, Fig. 4.5). The 1988 Commission E monograph states that ivy leaves are for use in the treatment of catarrhal disorders of the upper respiratory tract and in the symptomatic treatment of chronic inflammatory bronchial diseases. The average recommended daily dose is 0.3 g of the dried herb or an equivalent dose of extract (Blumenthal et al., 1998). Four controlled studies in patients with chronic obstructive bronchitis have demonstrated the therapeutic efficacy of a water-ethanol extract (30 % ethanol, herb-to-extract ratio 5–7:1, brand name Prospan) in adults (Meyer-Wegener et al., 1993) as well as children (Gulyas et al., 1997; Mansfeld et al., 1997, 1998). One of these studies was a prospective double-blind study in 99 women and men 25–70 years of age diagnosed with chronic obstructive bronchitis. Four week's treatment with a daily dose of approximately 60 mg of ivy extract (equivalent to about 400 mg of the crude drug) was compared with 90 mg of ambroxol. The key parameters for rating therapeutic efficacy were the spirometrically measured vital capacity and one-second forced expiratory volume, chest auscultation, and a global efficacy rating by the physician. The two pharmacotherapies were rated as equally effective in all test criteria, with no statistically significant differences. Seven patients taking the ivy extract and 6 patients taking ambroxol reported adverse reactions, but only one patient (taking ambroxol) had to drop out because of side effects (Meyer-Wegener et al., 1993).

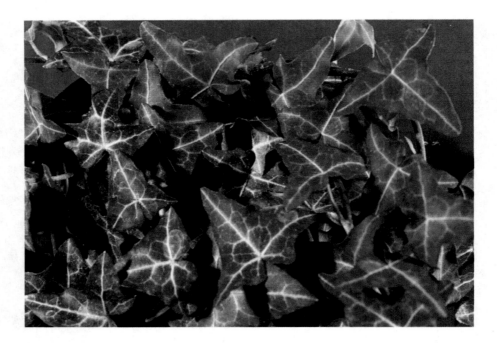

Figure 4.5. ▲ Ivy (*Hedera helix*).

A water-ethanol solution of the same extract was tested in a randomized, double-blind, placebo-controlled, crossover study in 24 children 4–12 years of age with bronchial asthma. The protocol consisted of treatment periods of 3 days alternating with washout periods of 3–5 days. The daily dose of ivy extract was 35 mg, equivalent to 210 mg of the crude drug. All medications were taken and all measurements were performed at the same time of day. The main test parameter was airway resistance. Secondary parameters were intrathoracic gas volume, residual volume, and several other spirometric parameters. Children treated with the ivy extract showed statistically significant and clinically relevant improvements, especially in airway resistance and intrathoracic gas volume, compared with the placebo-treated controls (Mansfeld et al., 1998).

The same group of authors performed another randomized crossover study in 26 hospitalized children 5–11 years of age comparing the efficacy of the alcohol-based solution taken orally and the extract administered in suppository form. The orally and rectally administered extracts were equivalent in their effects when given in a dose ratio of approximately 1:5 (Mansfeld et al., 1997). Another double-blind crossover study investigated the dose equivalence of an alcohol-free juice preparation and the water-ethanol solution in 25 children 10–16 years of age. Surprisingly, it was found that the water-ethanol solution was approximately 2.5 times more effective than the alcohol-free juice preparation (Gulyas et al., 1997). In an observational study of 113 children of both sexes, the juice preparation produced no adverse effects when taken over a period of 3–4 weeks (Lässig et al., 1996).

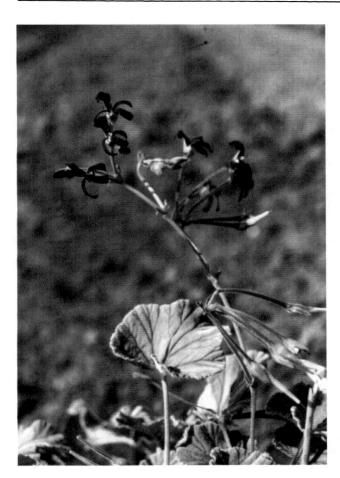

Figure 4.6. ◀ Leaves and flowers of *Pelargonium sidoides.*

When 372 children (average age 5.7 years) with respiratory infections were treated with a standard dose of ivy extract for approximately 7 days in an observational study, only one child experienced an adverse side effect described as "problems in taking the medication" (Jahn and Müller, 2000).

4.7　Pelargonium Root Extract

Extracts obtained from rhizomes of *Pelargonium sidoides* (Fig. 4.6) are used in the treatment of respiratory tract infections. Native to South Africa, this herb was introduced in Europe in 1997 under the brand name "Umckaloabo" (from a Zulu word meaning "severe cough"). An extract manufactured by a special process and designated as EPs 7630 contains cumarins (including umckalin, which is typical of this plant) in addition to tannins. Both groups of compounds have been linked to the antibacterial and immunomodulating properties of the extract. Experimental studies on antimicrobial activity have shown that the minimum inhibitory concentrations of the extract are in the range of 5 to 7.5 mg/mL. The second principle of action is believed to be nonspecific immune stimulation. This is supported by experimental evidence of NO-inducing properties, the formation and release of tumor necrosis factor, and the induction of interferon production. Secretion of the microbicidal effector molecule NO and the observed cytoprotective effects resulting from stimulated cytokine secretion in various in vitro test models document the activation of macrophages. The half-maximum concentrations of active ingredients in the whole extract are in the range of 0.1–0.3 g/mL, which is about one order of magnitude lower than those of the individual fractions or groups of compounds. This suggests that the actions of *P. sidoides* extract, like those of many other phytomedicines, are based on an interaction of the various plant constituents. There is also evidence for a third principle of action: with its high tannin content, the extract appears to interfere with bacterial and viral adhesion to the surfaces of host cells, thereby disrupting the cycle of infection. This "triple action" provides a rationale for the use of *P. sidoides* extract in the treatment of acute respiratory tract infections such as acute bronchitis (Kayser and Kolodziej, 1997; Kolodziej and Kayser, 1998; Kayser et al., 2001).

To date, the results of 5 controlled clinical studies in a total of 854 acutely ill patients, including 263 children 5–12 years of age, have been published. Three of these randomized multicenter studies were double-blind and placebo-controlled (Golovatiouk et al., 2002; Heger et al, 2002, 2003). One study compared pelargonium extract with symptomatic therapy (gargling with fruit vinegar, Priessnitz compresses; Blochin et al., 2000), and one study compared it with acetylcysteine (Blochin et al., 1999). The test medications consisted of water-alcohol solutions. The drug and placebo solutions were identical in appearance. Acetylcysteine was administered in the form of 200-mg bags twice daily. Patients with fever higher than 38.5 °C were also allowed acetaminophen, which was given as 500-mg suppositories in children and as tablets in adults. The use of acetaminophen was taken as a secondary outcome measure. The duration of treatment was 6–7 days in most cases. An initial baseline examination was performed, followed by examinations at 3–5 days and at the end of treatment.

The confirmatory outcome measure in all 5 studies was a decline in the semiquantitative total score for 5 symptoms typical of acute bronchitis and acute tonsillopharyngitis. The change in symptom scores showed a significant advantage for the pelargonium extract EPs 7630 in the 3 placebo-controlled studies. The improvements in symptom scores for all 5 controlled studies are shown in Table 4.6. The total scores with pelargonium declined from about 7–10 points initially to 0–2.4 points after 4–7 days of treatment. The final scores with placebo were approximately 4–6 points. In 2 observational studies, the average total scores in children with acute bronchitis decreased from 6 to 1.4 (Haidvogel et al., 1996) and from 6 to 2.8 (Dorne et al., 1996) following treatment with EPs 7630. Several observational studies have been published on patient tolerance of the commercial product Umckaloabo with therapeutic use. The total incidence of reported adverse events in these studies was only 0.6 % and 2.3 % of the patients treated. Except for 3 cases of skin rash in children, the reported events appear to relate more to the disease than to the medication. Based on experience reported to date, there need be no concern about serious risks or adverse quality-of-life effects with this therapy.

Table 4.6.
Controlled clinical studies with the pelargonium root extract EPs 7630.

First author, year	Indication	Patients (EPs vs. reference)	Duration of therapy (d)	Comparison - of therapies	Symptom score (EPs vs. reference) Before → After	
Blochin, 1999	Bronchitis	60 children (30/30)	4	Acetylcysteine	7/7 →	0/1
Blochin, 2000	Tonsillitis	60 children (30/30)	6	Gargling, Priessnitz wrap	9/9 →	4/6
Heger, 2002	Tonsillitis	143 children (73/70)	6	Placebo	10.3/9.7 →	0.8/6.3
Golovatiouk, 2002	Bronchitis	124 adults (64/60)	7	Placebo	9.0/9.1 →	1.8/4.2
Heger, 2003	Bronchitis	467 adults (233/234)	7	Placebo	8.3/8.1 →	2.4/5.1

The results of other clinical studies are already available or are in preparation (Kolodziej and Schulz, 2003).

4.8 Phytotherapy of Sinusitis

First among the 100 most commonly prescribed herbal medications in Germany (see Appendix) is a combination product, Sinupret, approved by Commission E in 1994 for use in the treatment of "acute and chronic inflammations of the paranasal sinuses." A liquid form of the product has been available since 1934, and the coated tablet was introduced in 1968. The active ingredient in the tablet is a mixture of 5 powdered herbs: 6 mg of gentian root and 18 mg each of primrose flowers, sorrel, elder flowers, and European vervain. The liquid preparation contains a water-and-alcohol extract from the same herbs, also in proportions of 1:3:3:3:3. The Commission E monographs on these 5 herbs state that their actions are chiefly mucolytic, so Sinupret comes under the official heading of herbal expectorants.

A doctoral dissertation (März, 1998) cites more than a dozen pharmacologic and toxicologic studies dealing with the combination product. Of the 12 controlled clinical therapeutic studies, 4 compared Sinupret with a placebo (Table 4.7) and 8 compared it with reference drugs (ambroxol, myrtol, acetylcysteine, and bromhexine).

In the study by Neubauer (1994) in Table 4.7, there was an average difference of only 17 % between the outcomes with Sinupret versus a placebo in patients on a basic regimen of antibiotics and decongestant nosedrops. In the common indications for phytotherapy, it is not unusual to find high success rates with placebos resulting in a relatively small difference between the placebo-treated and herb-treated groups (see Sect. 1.5.6 and Fig. 1.6). But since 3 of the 4 placebo-controlled studies showed a statistically significant superiority of the true drug, and 2 other double-blind studies showed equal or better efficacy and tolerance compared with ambroxol, it is reasonable to conclude that the product is effective for the approved indication, even if the fixed combination

Table 4.7.
Double-blind studies comparing Sinupret (S) with a placebo (P).

First author, year	Number of cases (n)	Indication	Duration of treatment (days)	Study criteria: statistical result
Richstein, 1980	31	Chronic sinusitis	7	Headache: "relieved" + "improved" S vs. P = 12 vs. 6 (p = 0.03); X-ray findings: S vs. P p = 0.035
Lechler, 1986	39	Acute sinusitis (adolescent asthmatics)	?	X-ray findings: "normal" + "improved" S vs. P = 16 vs. 9 (p < 0.05)
Berghorn, 1991	139	Acute sinusitis	14	Total symptom score: outcome tended to be better with S than P, but difference was not statistically significant.
Neubauer, 1994	177	Acute sinusitis (160), chronic sinusitis (17)	14	X-ray findings: "normal" + "improved" S vs. P = 87 % vs. 70 % (p < 0.05). Patient self-rating "relieved" + "improved", S vs. P = 96 % vs. 75 %.

NOTE: The comparison of the statistical results is based on the number of patients in the first two studies and on the percentage of patients in the last study.

of 5 herbal powders is difficult to justify and does not conform to the dosages used in traditional herbal medicine (Sect. 1.5.4). The safety of the product has been well documented by toxicologic studies (März, 1998) and by observational experience. The incidence of mild side effects reported in a recent study was less than 1 % (Ernst et al., 1997a).

4.9 Butterbur Leaf Extract in Allergic Rhinitis

In the past, extracts from the leaves and roots of the butterbur plant (*Petasites hybridus*) have been used mainly to treat spasms of the gastrointestinal and urogenital tract. But data from case reports have led to the incidental discovery that butterbur has an ameliorating effect on hay fever. A leaf extract from a cultivated herb has been specially developed for this indication. The extract Ze 339 is produced by supercritical CO_2 extraction from the leaves of a specially cloned variety. The efficacy of this extract is determined partly by the petasins which it contains. Two pharmacologic actions have been confirmed: the inhibition of leukotriene synthesis in neutrophils and eosinophils from atopics and an inhibition of the stimulated release of the inflammatory mediators histamine and sterotonin. Pharmacokinetic studies have shown good and rapid bioavailability of the petasins, which comprise 14 % of the extract. Absorption kinetics were tested in 24 volunteers (Käufeler et al., 2000).

Clinical efficacy was initially determined in a small group of patients (n=6) by assessing the severity of typical symptoms. Particularly impressive was the rhinomanometric finding that nasal airflow increased from less than 500 mL to more than 800 mL (normal value) within 5 days, indicating a definite anti-inflammatory action of the extract. In a multicenter, double-blind, randomized study, the clinical efficacy of the extract (standardized to 8 mg of petasins per tablet) was compared with that of cetirizine (10 mg) in 125 patients with confirmed allergic rhinitis. Sixty-one of the patients were treated with Ze 339 and 64 with cetirizine for 2 weeks. The results were evaluated primarily with the Medical Outcome Short-Form Health Survey Questionnaire (SF-36), which is validated for allergic rhinitis. Secondary variables were items 1–3 in the Clinical Global Impression (CGI) scale. The response was the same in both treatment groups, with equivalent main outcome measures and secondary variables. The number of adverse events (AEs) was comparable in both groups (16.4 % vs. 17.2 %). It is noteworthy that two-thirds of the AEs in the cetirizine-treated group consisted of sedative effects. The butterbur extract Ze 339 was found to be as effective as the "gold standard" cetirizine in the treatment of seasonal allergic rhinitis (Brattström and Schapowal, 2002; Schapowal, 2002).

Another multicenter, randomized, prospective study investigated the dose-dependent efficacy of the extract Ze 339. The outcome measure was the effect of the extract on the severity of symptoms. A total of 187 patients were enrolled in the three-armed, prospective, randomized, placebo-controlled, multicenter study. Inclusion criteria were preexisting allergic rhinitis with at least 2 of 4 symptoms (runny, itchy, stuffy nose, sneezing) rated as 2 or more on a 0–4 scale and a positive skin test, prick test, or positive RAST. The duration of the study was 2 weeks. Both of the tested medications were significantly superior to placebo, and a dose of 3 tablets was markedly superior to a dose of 2 tablets (Brattström, 2003).

4.10 Ephedra

The crude drug consists of the dried, young stems of *Ephedra sinica* and other *Ephedra* species that contain ephedrine, such as *E. equisetina* and *E. intermedia*. Ephedra species are herbaceous perennials (family Ephedraceae) that grow to a height of 1 m and vaguely resemble horsetail. Ephedra tops contain up to 2 % alkaloids with (–) ephedrine as the principal alkaloid.

Preparations made from ephedra stems exert the peripheral vasoconstricting, bronchodilating, and central stimulatory actions of ephedrine. Whole herb extracts reportedly have a less pronounced hypertensive action than pure (–)-ephedrine (*Brit Herb Pharmacopoeia* 1983, p 83).

Coughing induced by stimulation of the tracheal or bronchial mucosa in anesthetized animals is suppressed by ephedra extracts (Hosoya, 1985) much as it is suppressed by ephedrine itself (0.01 mg/kg b.w.). This suppression of the cough reflex results from the bronchodilating action of ephedrine, although a pronounced antitussive effect is obtained even in nonasthmatic subjects (Aviado, 1972). One disadvantage is that ephedrine lacks an expectorant action and has even been shown to reduce airway secretions in laboratory animals.

The indications for ephedra preparations are mild forms of airway disease, especially those resulting from spastic disorders. A single dose of ephedra extract should deliver 15–30 mg of alkaloids, calculated as ephedrine. According to the Commission E the maximum daily dose for adults for ephedra a quantity equivalent to 300 mg total alkaloids calculated as ephedrine. While this dosage may appear to be relatively high compared to the total dosage of ephedra alkaloids for U.S. FDA-approved OTC drugs – i.e.150 mg/day for pure ephedrine and/or its salts and 240mgday for pseudophedrine and/or its salts, usually in the hydrochloride form (Blumenthal et al., 2003), this dosage is limited to the Commission E approved indication for respiratory tract disorders with mild bronchospasms in adults and children over six (Blumenthal et al., 1998). The maximum daily dose for children is 2 mg/kg body weight. Today ephedrine is usually administered in pure form rather than as one component of a whole plant extract. Potential adverse effects are palpitations, blood pressure elevation, sleeplessness, anorexia, and urinary difficulties.

Conditions that would contraindicate ephedra preparations or limit their use are hypertension, thyrotoxicosis, pheochromocytoma, narrow-angle glaucoma, and prostatic adenoma with urinary retention, anorexia, insomnia, diabetes, cardiac arrhythmias, pregnancy, lactation.

In the United States, the central-nervous-system stimulation effects of ephedra preparations are often potentiated by the addition of caffeine-containing botanicals. Previously, such combination products had frequently been usefd on a chronic basis to promote weight loss or to enhance athletic performance, but ephedra-containing dietary supplements were banned by the U.S. FDA in February 2004 (US FDA, 2004). Relatively high doses of products containing ephedra with other botanicals were also previously employed, especially by teenagers and young adults, as euphoriants or intoxicants, so-called legal highs, although such products are illegal and are seldom seen in the market in the U.S. or Europe The American Herbal Products Association estimates that, based on sales figures provided by 14 companies, 6.8 billion dosage forms of ephedra dietary supplements were sold in the U.S. between 1995 and 1999 (McGuffin, 2000).

As of 1999, the Food and Drug Administration (FDA) had recorded more than 2000 adverse events purportedly attributed to ephedra, but these were not evaluated as to degree of seriousness. All events resulting in illness or injury apparently associated with an ephedra product were listed. Of these, 29 deaths supposedly associated with ephedra or ephedrine were included. The validity of these figures was later questioned by a Congressional committee (Skinner, 1999). More recently, the FDA has claimed that over 16,000 adverse event reports (AERs) were attributable to ephedra, but many of these include so-called "incident reports" made to a large seller of ephedra supplements. An independent, peer-reviewed evaluation of ephedra by the RAND Corporation reviewed all known AERs associated with ephedra, plus the pharmacology and toxicology, and all published clinical trials (Shekelle et al., 2003). The RAND report concluded that the serious AERs were "sentinenl events" but there was not adequate scientific and medical data to establish a causal relationship between the ingestion of ephedra dietary supplements and the serious adverse events.

In 1995 and 1996, the FDA held two meetings of an expert advisory group to make recommendations regarding the continued marketability of ephedra products. As a result of these deliberations, the agency proposed, in 1997, the following rules: prohibit the marketing of dietary supplements (non-drug products) containing 8 mg or more of ephedrine [sic] alkaloids per serving with a maximum daily dosage of 24 mg; require label statements instructing consumers not to use the product for more than 7 days; prohibit the use of ephedrine alkaloids with caffeine or herbs containing caffeine; prohibit labeling claims that require long-term intake to achieve the purported effect; require a statement that "taking more than the recommended serving may result in heart attack, stroke, seizure, or death." Because of industry objections, these rules were never implemented. Whether they ever will be remains in doubt (Huck, 1999). In the meantime, several states have imposed restrictions on ephedra sales.

Because the health problems associated with long-term consumption of ephedra preparations have received widespread publicity, many persons are reluctant to utilize products containing it. Consequently, some manufacturers have substituted *Sida cordifolia* (family Malvaceae), an ancient Ayurvedic remedy, for ephedra. Its seeds contain about 0.3 % of an alkaloid mixture of which ephedrine is the principal constituent. So, the activity is essentially the same as ephedra, but this is not recognized by the uninformed consumer. This herb was specifically listed in the US FDA's ban on ephedra and ephedrine-containing dietary supplements in February 2004 (US FDA, 2004).

There has also been concern expressed in the U.S. that clandestine chemists may use ephedra as a starting material for the synthesis of illegal designer drugs, such as methamphetamine. Although possible, it is not likely because of the difficulty in separating the product from accompanying plant material. A much more likely starting material is pseudoephedrine which is readily available in pure form. Large-scale sales of that alkaloid are now monitored by the Drug Enforcement Agency (Maltz, 1996).

Due to concerns about the reported and potential toxicity of ephedra-containing dietary supplement products sold in the U.S. for purposes other than the traditionally used respiratory indications, i.e., as aids in weight loss and for enhancement of athletic performance, the U.S. Food and Drug Administration (FDA) banned the sale of ephedra supplements in February 2004 (U.S Food and Drug Administration, 2004). FDA exempted ephedra-containing preparations used by licensed acupuncturists and doctors of Oriental medicine for traditional indications (i.e., short-term use for respiratory disorders) so long as these preparations are not labelled as dietary supplements.

4.11 Drug Products

The *Rote Liste 2003* lists well over 100 herbal products under the heading of Antitussives and Expectorants, consisting mostly of fixed combinations of active ingredients along with numerous products containing a single active ingredient (Tables 4.1–4.4). The 100 most commonly prescribed phytomedicines in Germany include 25 herbal antitussive-expectorants, consisting of 10 single-herb products and 15 combination products.

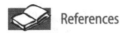 References

AkdÄ - Arzneimittelkommission der deutschen Ärzteschaft: Therapieempfehlungen der Arzneimittelkommission der deutschen Ärzteschaft - Akute Atemwegsinfektionen. Deutscher Ärzte-Verlag, Cologne, 2002, 17-32.

Altiner A, Abholz HH (2001) Akute Bronchitis und Antibiotika: Hintergründe für eine rationale Therapie. Z Allg Med 77: 358-362.

Aviado DM (1972) Antitussives with peripheral actions. In: Pharmacological Principles of Medical Practice. The William & Wilkins Co, Baltimore, pp. 405-407.

Bauer L (1973) Die Feinstruktur der menschlichen Bronchialschleimhaut nach Behandlung mit Ozothin. Klin Wochenschr 51: 450-453.

Bent B, Saint S, Vittinghoff E, Grady D (1999) Antibiotics in acute bronchitis: a meta-analysis. Am J Med 107: 62-67.

Blochin B, Haidvogel M, Heger M (1999) Umckaloabo im Vergleich mit Acetylcystein bei Kindern mit akuter Bronchitis. Der Kassenarzt 49: 46-49.

Blochin B, Heger M (2000) Umckaloabo versus symptomatische Therapie in der Behandlung der Angina catarrhalis. Päd 6: 2-8.

Blumenthal M, Hall T, Goldberg A (2003) The ABC Clinical Guide to Herbs. Austin, TX: American Botanical Council.

Blumenthal M, Busse WR, Goldberg A, Gruenwald J, Hall T, Riggins CW, Rister RS (eds.). Klein S, Rister RS (trans). (1998) The Complete German Commission E Monographs - Therapeutic Guide to Herbal Medicines. American Botanical Council, Austin, Texas. www.herbalgram.org.

Boyd EM, Sheppard E (1970 a) The effect of inhalation of ceitral and geraniol on the output and composition of respiratory tract fluid. Arch Intern Pharmacodyn Ther 188: 5-13.

Boyd EM, Sheppard E (1970 b) Inhaled anisaldehyde and respiratory tract fluid. Pharmacol 3: 345-352.

Brattström A (2003) A newly developed extract (Ze 339) from butterbur (Petasites hybridus L.) is clinically efficient in allergic rhinitis (hay fever).Phytomedicine 10 Suppl IV: 50-52

Brattström A, Schapowal A (2002) RCT Pestwurzextrakt Ze 339 vs. Cetrizin bei allergischer Rhinitis. In: Schulz V, Rietbrock N, Roots I, Loew D (eds) Phytopharmaka VII - Forschung und klinische Anwendung. Steinkopff-Verlag, Darmstadt 2002.

Bromm B, Scharein E, Darsow U, Ring J (1995) Effects of menthol and cold on histamine-induced itch and skin reactions in man. Neuroscience Lett 187: 157-160.

Burrow A, Eccles R, Jones AS (1983) The effects of camphor, eucalyptus and menthol vapur on nasal resistance to airflow and nasal sensation. Acta Otolaryng (Stockholm) 96: 157-161.

Caldwell J, Sutton JD (1988) Influence of dose size on the disposition of trans-[methoxy-14C] anethole in human volunteers. Food Chem Tox 26: 87-91.

De Mey C, Wittig T (2002) Myrtol standardisiert und Antibiotika in der Behandlung der akuten Bronchitis - Eine randomisierte, doppelblinde Vergleichsstudie. In: Schulz V, Rietbrock N, Roots I, Loew D; Phytopharmaka VII - Forschung und klinische Anwendung. Steinkopff-Verlag, Darmstadt, 27-39.

Dome L, Schuster R (1996) Umckaloabo - Eine phytotherapeutische Alternative bei akuter Bronchitis im Kindesalter. Ärztezeitschrift für Naturheilverfahren 37: 216- 222.

Dorow P (1984) Pharmakotherapie der Atmungsorgane. In: Kuemmerle HP, Hitzenberger G, Spitzy KH (eds) Klinische Pharmakologie, Kap IV-4.5, Ecomed, Landsberg München.

Dorow P (1989) Welchen Einfluß hat Cineol auf die mukoziliare Clearance? Therapiewoche 39: 2652-2654.

Dorow P, Weiss Ph, Felix R, Schmutzler H (1987) Einfluß eines Sekretolytikums und einer Kombination von Pinen, Limonen und Cineol auf die mukoziliäre Clearance bei Patienten mit chronisch obstruktiver Atemwegserkrankung. Arzneim Forsch (Drug Res) 37: 1378-1381.

Drinkwater NR, Miller EC, Miller JA, Pitot HC (1976) Hepatocardinogenicity of estragole and 1'-hydroextragole in the mouse and mutagenicity of 1-acetoxystragole in bacteria. J Natl Canc Inst 57: 1323-1331.

Eccles R, Jones AS (1982) The effects of menthol on nasal resistance to airflow. J Laryngology

Otology 97: 705–709.

Eccles R, Lancashire B, Tolley NS (1987) Experimental studies on nasal sensation of airflow. Acta Otolaryngol (Stockholm) 103: 303–306.

Eccles R, Morris S, Tolley NS (1988) The effects of nasal anaesthesia upon nasal sensation of airflow. Acta Otolaryngol (Stockholm) 106: 152–155.

Ernst E, März R, Sieder C (1997a) Akute Bronchitis: Nutzen von Sinupret\R. Forschritte der Medizin 115: 52–53.

Ernst E, März R, Sieder C (1997b) A controlled multi-centre study of herbal versus synthetic secretolytic drugs for acute bronchitis. Phytomedicine 4: 287–293.

Fahey T, Howie J (2001) Reevaluation of a randomized controlled trial of antibiotics for minor respiratory illness in general practice. Fam Pract 18: 246–248.

Federspil P, Wulkow R, Zimmermann T (1997) Wirkung von Myrtol standardisiert bei der Therapie der akuten Sunusitis – Ergebnisse einer doppelblinden, randomisierten Multicenterstudie gegen Placebo. Laryngo-Rhino-Otol 76: 23–27.

Fox N (1977) Effect of camphor, ecalyptol and menthol on the vascular state of the mucous membrane. Arch Otolaryngol 6: 112–122.

Göbel H, Schmidt G, Dworschak M, Stolze H, Heuss D (1995) Essential plant oils and headache mechanisms. Phytomedicine 2: 93–102.

Golovatiouk A, Tschutschalin AG (2002) Wirksamkeit eines Extraktes aus Pelargonium sidoides (EPS 7630) versus Placebo bei akuter Bronchitis. In: Schulz V, Rietbrock N, Roots I, Loew D; Phytopharmaka VII – Forschung und klinische Anwendung. Steinkopff-Verlag, Darmstadt, 3–12.

McGuffin M. Statement before Department of Health & Human Services Office of Public Health & Sciences, Public Meeting on the Safety of Dietary Supplements Containing Ephedrine Alkaloids; 2000 Aug. 8, Washington, D.C.

Gulyas A, Repges R, Dethlefsen U (1997) Konsequente Therapie chronisch-obstruktiver Atemwegserkrankungen bei Kindern. Atemwegs- und Lungenkrankheiten 23: 291–294.

Gysling E (1976) Behandlung häufiger Symptome. Leitfaden zur Pharmakotherapie. Huber, Bern Stuttgart Vienna, p 86.

Hahn HL (1987) Husten: Mechanismen, Pathophysiologie und Therapie. Dtsch Apoth Z 127 (Suppl 5): 3–26.

Haidvogl M, Schuster R, Heger M (1996) Akute Bronchitis im Kindesalter-Multizenter-Studie zur Wirksamkeit und Verträglichkeit des Phytotherapeutikums Umckaloabo. Z Phytotherapie 17: 300–313.

Hamann KF, Bonkowsky V (1987) Minzölwirkung auf die Nasenschleimhaut von Gesunden. Dtsch Apoth Z 125: 429–436.

Heger M et al. (2003) Wirksamkeit und Verträglichkeit eines Extraktes aus Pelargonium sidoides (EPs 7630) bei akuter Bronchitis: Ergebnisse einer multizentrischen, doppelblinden, placebokontrollierten Studie. Phytomedicine 10, 2002, in press.

Heger M, Bereznoy VV (2002) Nicht-streptokokkenbedingte Tonsillopharyngitis bei Kindern: Wirksamkeit eines Extraktes aus Pelargonium sidoides (EPs 7630) im Vergleich zu Placebo. In: Schulz V, Rietbrock N, Roots I, Loew D; Phytopharmaka VII – Forschung und klinische Anwendung. Steinkopff-Verlag, Darmstadt, 13–25.

Hosoya E (1985) Studies of the construction of prescription in ancient Chinese medicine. In: Chang HM, Yeung HW, Tso WW, Koo A (eds) Advances in Chinese Medicinal Material Research. World Scientific Publ, Singapore, pp 73–94.

Huck P (1999) Revisting ephedra. Health Suppl Retailer 5(4): 22–25, 28, 30.

Ing_fsd_tir K, Jurcic K, Wagner H (1998) Immunomodulating polysaccharides from aqueous extracts of Cetraria islandica (Iceland moss). Phytomedicine 5: 333–339.

Iravani J (1972) Wirkung eines Broncholytikums auf die tracheobronchiale Reinigung. Arzneim Forsch (Drug Res) 22: 1744–1746.

Jahn E, Müller B (2000) Efeublättertrockenextrakt – Pädiatrische Therapiestudie zur Wirksamkeit und Verträglichkeit. Deutsche Apotheker Zeitung 140: 1349-52.

Käufeler R, Thomet OAR, Simon HU, Meier B, Brattström A (2000) Der Pestwurzextrakt Ze 339: Wirkprinzipien und klinische Pharmakologie. In: Rietbrock N (ed) Phytopharmaka VI –

Forschung und klinische Anwendung. Steinkopff-Verlag, Darmstadt 2000.

Kayser O, Kolodziej H, Gutmann M (1995) Arzneilich verwendete Pelargonien aus Südafrika. DAZ 135: 853–864.

Kayser O, Kolodziej H, Kiderlen AF (2001) Immunmodulatory principles of Pelargonium sidoides. Phytotherapy Res 15: 122–126.

Kolodziej H Schulz V (2003) Umckaloabo – Von der traditionellen Anwendung zum modernen Phytopharmakon. Deutsche Apotheker Zeitung 143: 1303–12

Kolodziej H, Kayser O (1998) Pelargonium sidoides DC. Neuste Erkenntnisse zum Verständnis des Phytotherapeutikums Umckaloabo. Z Phytotherapie 19: 141–151.

Kopp B, Wawrosch C, Lebada R, Wiedenfeld H (1997) PA-freie Huflattichblätter. Deutsche Apotheker Zeitung 137: 4066–4069.

Kraft K (1997) Therapeutisches Profil eines Spitzwegerichkraut-Fluidextraktes bei akuten respiratorischen Erkrankungen im Kindes- und Erwachsenenalter. In: Loew D, Rietbrock N (Hrsg) Phytopharmaka III: Forschung und klinische Anwendung. Steinkopff Verlag, Darmstadt: 199–209.

Kurz H (1989) Antitussiva und Expektoranzien. Wissenschaftliche Verlagsgesellschaft Stuttgart.

Lässig W, Generlich H, Heydolph F, Paditz E (1996) Wirksamkeit und Verträglichkeit efeuhaltiger Hustenmittel. TW Pädiatrie 9: 489–491.

Leiber B (1967) Dieskussionsbemerkung. In: Dost FH, Leiber B (eds) Menthol and Menthol-Containing External Remedies. Thieme Stuttgart, p 22.

Linsenmann P, Hermat H, Swoboda M (1989) Therapeutischer Wert ätherischer Öle bei chronisch-obstruktiver Bronchitis. Atemw Lungenkrankh 15: 152–156.

Linsenmann P, Swoboda M (1986) Therapeutische Wirksamkeit ätherischer Öle bei chronisch-obstruktiver Bronchitis. Therapiewoche 36: 1162–1166.

Little P, Williamson I, Warner G, Gould C, Gantley M, Kinmonth AI (1997) Open randomised trial of prescribing strategies in managing sore throat. BMJ 314: 722–7.

Lorenz J, Ferlinz R (1985) Expektoranzien: Pathophysiologie und Therapie der Mukostase. Arzneimitteltherapie 3:22–27.

Lübke G, Brockstedt M (2001) Vergiftungen mit ätherischen Ölen. Kinder- und Jugendarzt 32: 1024.

Maltz GA (1996) New rule regulates sales of large amounts of pseudoephedrine. Pharm Today 2(9): 9.

Mansfeld HJ, Höhre H, Repges R, Dethlefsen U (1997) Sekretolyse und Bronchospasmolyse. TW Pädiatrie 10: 155–157.

Mansfeld HJ, Höhre H, Repges R, Dethlefsen U (1998) Therapie des Asthma bronchiale mit Efeublätter-Trockenextrakt. Münchener Medizinische Wochenschrift 140: 26–30.

März RW (1998) Evaluation of a Phytomedicine. Clinical, pharmacological and toxicological data of Sinupret. Dissertation University of Utrecht.

Matthys H, de Mey C, Cars C, Rys A, Geib A, Wittig T (2000) Efficacy and tolerance of myrtol standardized in acute bronchitis – a multicentre, randomized, double-blind, placebo-controlled parallel group clinical trial vs. cefuroxime and ambroxol. Arzneim-Forsch/Drug Res 50: 100–711.

Meister R, Wittig T, Beuscher N, de Mey C (1999) Wirksamkeit und Verträglichkeit von Myrtol standardisiert bei der Langzeitbehandlung der chronischen Bronchitis – Eine placebo-kontrollierte Doppelblindstudie. Arzneim-Forsch/Drug Res 49: 351–8.

Meyer-Wegener J, Liebscher K, Hettich M (1993) Efeu versus Ambroxol bei chronischer Bronchitis. Zeitschrift für Allgemeinmedizin 68: 61–66.

Miller EC, Swanson AB, Phillips DH, Fletcher TL, Liem A, Miller JA (1983) Structure-activity studies of the carcinogenicities in the mouse and rat of some naturally occuring and synthetic alkylbenzene derivates related to safrole and estragole. Cancer Res 34: 1124–1134.

Murray S Del Mar C, O'Rourke (2000) Predictors of an antibiotic prescription by GPs for respiratory tract infections: a pilot study Fam Pract 17: 386–388.

Neubauer N, März RW (1994) Placebo-controlled, randomized double-blind clinical trial with Sinupret sugar-coated tablets on the basis of a therapy with antibiotics and decongestant nasal drops in acute sinusitis. Phytomedicine 1: 177–181.

Newberne PM, Carlton WW, Brown WR (1989) Histopathological evaluation of proliferative lesions in rats fed with trans-anethol in chronic studies. Food Chem Tox 27: 21–26.

Nöller HG (1967) Elektronische Messungen an der Nasenschleimhaut unter Mentholwirkung. In: Menthol and Menthol-Containing External Remedies. Thieme, Stuttgart: 146–153, 179.

Opdyke DLJ (1973) Food cosmet toxicol 11, 865 quoted in Leung AY, Encyclopedia of Common Drugs and Cosmetics. Wiley, Chichester Brisbane Toronto 1980, pp 31–33.

Patel S, Wiggins J (1980) Eucalyptus oil poisoning. Arch Dis Childh 55: 405–406.

Römmelt H, Schnizer W, Swoboda M, Senn E (1988) Pharmakokinetik ätherischer Öle nach Inhalation mit einer terpenhaltigen Salbe. Z Phytother 9: 14–16.

Sangister SA, Caldwell J, Smith RL (1984) Metabolism of anethole. II. Influence of dose size on the route of metabolism of transanethole in the rat and mouse. Food Chem Tox 22: 707–713.

Schapowal A (2002) Randomised controlled trial of butterbur and cetiricine for treating seasonal allergic rhinitis. BMJ 324: 144–146.

Schneider B (1997) Statistische Analyse von Erkältungskrankheiten und ihre Bedeutung. In: Loew D, Rietbrock N (eds) Phytopharmaka III: Forschung und klinische Anwendung. Steinkopff Verlag, Darmstadt: 81–90.

Schwabe U, Paffrath D (Hrsg.) Arzneiverordnungsreport 2001. Springer, Berlin-Heidelberg-New York, p 126.

Shekelle P, Morton S, Maglione M, et al. Ephedra and Ephedrine for Weight Loss and Athletic Performance Enhancement: Clinical Efficacy and Side Effects. Evidence Report/Technology Assessment No. 76 (Prepared by Southern California Evidence-based Practice Center, RAND, under Contract No. 290-97-0001, Task Order No. 9). AHRQ Publication No. 03-E022. Rockville, MD: Agency for Healthcare Research and Quality. February 2003. Available at *http://www.fda.gov/OHRMS/DOCKETS/98fr/95n-0304-bkg0003-ref-07-01-index.htm.*

Skinner W (1999) FDA flunks U.S. House hearings on ephedra. Nat Med Law 3(1): 1, 5–8.

Stafunsky M, Manteuffel GE, Swoboda M (1989) Therapie der akuten Tracheobronchitis mit ätherischen Ölen und mit Soleinhalationen - ein Doppelblindversuch. Z Phytother 10: 130–134.

Truhaut R, LeBourhis B, Attia M, Glomot R, Newman J, Caldwell J (1989) Chronic toxicity/carcinogenicity study of transanethole in rats. Food chem Tox 27:11–20.

U.S. Food and Drug Administration. Sales of Supplements Containing Ephedrine Alkaloids (Ephedra) Prohibited, February 6, 2004. 69 Fed. Reg. 6788 (February 11, 2004). Available at *http://www.fda.gov/oc/initiatives/ephedra/february2004/.*

Walther H (1979) Klinische Pharmakologie. Grundlagen der Arzneimittelanwendung. Volk und Gesundheit, Berlin: 360–364.

Zänker KS, Blümel G, Probst J, Reiterer W (1984) Theoretical and experimental evidence for the action of terpens as modulators in lung function. Prog Resp Res 18: 302–304.

Ziment I (1985) Possible mechanism of action of traditional oriental drugs for bronchitis. In: Chang HM, Yeung HW, Tso WW, Koo A (eds) Advances in Chinese Medicinal Materials Research. World Scientific Publ, Singapore: 193–202.

5 Digestive System

This chapter deals with phytomedicines that are used in the treatment of poor appetite, functional dyspepsia (irritable stomach syndrome), irritable bowel syndrome (irritable colon), gastritis and ulcer disease, acute diarrhea, constipation, and chronic liver disease. These diseases and ailments are based only partly on underlying organic pathology; most are "functional" disturbances of the gastrointestinal tract and bile ducts. The remedies that are used for these indications are not always covered by health insurance in Germany, and certain groups, such as laxatives, have been largely excluded from coverage. The result has been an increase in the self-prescribing of these products by patients with digestive complaints. But functional dyspepsia and irritable bowel syndrome are examples of conditions in which it is imperative that the family doctor continue to provide appropriate counseling and guidance.

5.1 Anorexia

In natural healing, anorexia refers to a syndrome featuring nausea, epigastric pressure, bloating, flatulence, and crampy abdominal pains, presumably due to the deficient secretion of gastric juice, deficient bile production, impaired filling and emptying of the gallbladder (biliary dyskinesia), or the deficient secretion of pancreatic juice (exocrine pancreatic insufficiency) (Fintelmann et al, 1993). Effective herbal remedies may be selected from the categories of bitters, cholagogues, or carminatives, depending on whether the dysfunction involves the stomach, biliary tract, or bowel. In practical terms, however, categorical distinctions of this kind cannot be consistently drawn from either a diagnostic or therapeutic standpoint.

Lack of appetite may be a symptom of organic disease (infectious diseases, gastrointestinal disorders, malignant tumors), or it may be psychosomatic (anorexia nervosa, emotional stress) or drug-induced (cancer chemotherapy, antibiotics). In other cases lack of appetite or early satiety may occur in the setting of a dyspeptic syndrome (see Sect. 5.2), resulting in overlaps in treatment. In psychophysiologic terms, appetite is an instinctive mechanism of which the main locus of control resides in the hypothalamus (limbic system) (Adler, 1979). Mechanisms involved in the anticipatory-metabolic taste reflexes may be even more important in understanding the effects of appetite-stimulating and secretagogic agents, including herbal chalogogues (Nicolaidis, 1969).

5.1.1 Bitter Herbs (Bitters)

Two different interpretations, each supported by experimental data, can be found in the pharmacologic literature regarding the mechanism of action of bitters. Both interpretations agree that stimuli originating in the mouth can reflexively induce gastric secretions. A bitter in the form of an aperitif or stomach bitter, taken in a moderate amount 20–30 min before eating, can stimulate gastric and biliary secretions, increasing the acidity of the gastric juice and aiding digestion (Bellomo, 1939). In one study, 200 mg of gentian root or 25 mg of wormwood herb significantly increased the production of gastric juice even in healthy subjects. The authors concluded that bitters can increase gastric and biliary secretions in healthy subjects compared with the normal volume of secretions induced by food stimuli (Glatzel and Hackenberg, 1967).

These findings are contradicted by other studies showing that bitters taken by healthy subjects with a normal appetite do not increase digestive secretions beyond the reflex secretions that normally occur during the cephalic phase of digestion. The secretory mechanism as a whole is already functioning at an optimum level, and the administration of bitters cannot produce any significant change. In conditions where the reflex secretion of gastric juice is inhibited, however, the administration of bitters can initiate the necessary reflex, leading to gastric secretion of the same intensity and duration (2–3 h) as normal reflex secretion.

There is a definite psychological component to the efficacy of bitters. This was demonstrated by a study in which bitters markedly improved appetite in patients with gastric achylia, despite the fact that increased gastric acid secretion cannot be induced in these patients (Møller, 1947).

Bitters do not invariably act as appetite stimulants. Animals, for example, tend to prefer sweet-tasting foods and avoid bitter-tasting ones (Nachmann and Cole, 1971). Humans are ambivalent toward bitter-tasting foods and beverages, tending to prize the flavor of artichokes, beer, grapefruit, liquors, etc. while disliking the sour taste of pickles and heat-preserved citrus juices. There is also a psychological tendency to associate a bitter taste with the bitterness of an unpleasant experience.

Bitter herbs can be ranked according to the intensity of their bitter taste (Table 5.1) Bitters that are used medicinally to stimulate appetite and digestive secretions are not merely herbs with a bitter taste; they are herbs that can produce a pleasant taste sensation in conjunction with their bitter flavor. Another criterion is that medicinal bitters must cause no systemic side effects when used in the proper concentration. Large amounts of bitters reduce gastric secretions, partly by their direct action on the gastric mucosa, and cause appetite suppression. Very strong wormwood tea, for example, can

Herbs	Relative bitterness
Quassia	40,000–50,000
Gentian	10,000–30,000
Wormwood	10,000–20,000
Condurango bark	10,000–15,000
Devil's claw	ca. 6,000
Lesser centaury	2,000–10,000
Bitter orange peel	600–2,5000
Blessed thistle	800–1,500
Cinchona bark	ca. 1,000

Table 5.1.
Relative bitterness of the principal bitter herbs according to the *Deutsches Arzneibuch* (German Pharmacopeia).

Bitter	Stroke volume: percentage decrease	
	Swallowed at once	Left in Mouth for 30 s
Gentian	8	12
Hops	7	11
Bitter orange	5	13
Rhubarb	4	10
Wormwood	2	21

Table 5.2.
Decrease in cardiac stroke volume after swallowing the bitter immediately and after leaving it in the mouth (for 30 seconds). Decrease is shown as a percentage of the pretreatment value (Glatzel, 1968).

spoil the appetite. Other constituents in bitter herbs are important determinants of taste, and several types of bitter herb are differentiated on that basis:

▶ Simple bitters such as gentian, bogbean, and centaury.
▶ Aromatic bitters that contain volatile oils, such as angelica root, blessed thistle, bitter orange peel, and wormwood.
▶ Astringent bitters that contain tannins, such as cinchona bark and condurango bark.
▶ Acrid bitters such as ginger and galangal.

Besides their action on the digestive glands, bitter principles act reflexively on the cardiovascular system, causing a decrease in heart rate and cardiac stroke volume (Table 5.2). Taking bitters for several weeks can engender an aversion to certain bitter herbs, accompanied by loss of appetite. Bitters, then, differ from other dyspeptics (Sect. 5.2) in that they are generally used for a shorter period of time. The taste of bitter herbs cannot be corrected with raw sugar or other sweeteners. As for adverse effects, bitters occasionally cause headache in susceptible users, and overdoses can induce nausea or vomiting. Because bitters stimulate digestive secretions, they are contraindicated in patients with gastric or duodenal ulcers.

5.1.1.1 Wormwood (Absinthe)

The crude drug consists of the dried aerial parts of *Artemisia absinthium* (of the family Asteraceae, Fig. 5.1), a perennial shrub native to arid regions of Eurasia and naturalized in North and South America and New Zealand. The leaves and flowering tops are harvested from wild and cultivated plants. Wormwood has a penetrating, aromatic odor

Figure 5.1. ▶ Wormwood
(*Artemisia absinthium*).

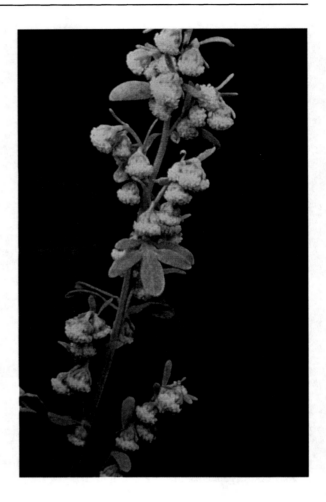

and a spicy, strongly bitter taste. The bitter principles contained in the aerial parts of the plant are classified chemically as sesquiterpene lactones, which occur as monomers such as artabsin or dimers such as absinthin. Wormwood contains about 0.3–0.5 % volatile oil, up to 70 % of which consists of the two stereoisomeric forms of thujone, designated as (–)-thujone and (+)-isothujone; these compounds give the herb its pleasant, fresh, spicy odor. Preparations from the aerial parts of various wormwood species are used in traditional medicine not just as bitters but also for the treatment of widespread infectious diseases such as malaria and hepatitis. The diversified biology and chemistry of the constituents have become a focus of scientific interest and are reviewed in Tan et al. (1998).

When the herb is taken in small doses (e.g., 1.0 g in an infusion or tincture), it acts as an aromatic bitter. As the dosage is increased, the toxic effect of the thujone becomes more pronounced, leading to increased salivation and hyperemia of the mucous membranes and pelvic viscera. The production of pure wormwood liquors is prohibited by law due to the risk of absinthe addiction. Thujone heightens and alters the effects of alcohol, and chronic thujone poisoning leads to cerebral dysfunction with epileptiform seizures, delirium, and hallucinations. Roman wormwood (*A. pontica*) is best for making vermouth wines, as this species has a finer aroma and a much lower thujone content for better tolerance. The leaves of the maritime absinth (*A. maritima*) are also used in making vermouth.

The 1984 German Commission E monograph on wormwood states that the crude drug (dried aerial parts) should have a minimum content of 0.3 % volatile oil and a relative bitterness of at least 15,000. The monograph cites as indications poor appetite, dyspeptic complaints, and biliary dyskinesia, recommending an average daily dose of 2–3 g of the crude drug (Blumenthal et al., 1998).

5.1.1.2 Other Bitter Herbs

Quassia (bitterwood) is a collective term for two herbs: Jamaican quassia obtained from *Picrasma exelsa*, a stately tree native to the Caribbean, and Surinam quassia obtained from *Quassia amara*, a shrub or small tree native to northern South America. Quassia has a lingering, purely bitter taste. Large amounts of quassia tea irritate the gastric mucosa and induce nausea. A mixture of the bitter principles quassin, neoquassin, and 18-hydroxyquassin (0.1–0.2 %) is terpenoid in nature. Quassia is reputed to have value in the treatment of dyspeptic complaints accompanied by constipation. The recommended daily dose is 2–10 mL of a 1:10 tincture.

Gentian root consists of the roots and rhizomes of the yellow gentian (*Gentiana lutea*, family Gentianaceae), an herbaceous perennial growing to 1 m and native to the mountainous regions of central and southern Europe. It grows in the wild and is also cultivated. Gentian root has a distinctive odor, an initial sweet taste, and a persistent, very bitter aftertaste. Gentiopicroside (known also as gentiopicrin) is the most abundant of the bitter principles (2–3 %). Gebhard (1997) showed that an aqueous extract of gentian root causes direct stimulation of acid secretion in cultured rat parietal cells. The Commission E monograph states that gentian root is indicated for poor appetite, flatulence, and bloating; it is contraindicated by gastric and duodenal ulcers. The average single dose is 1 g of the crude drug, and the average daily dose is 3 g (Blumenthal et al., 1998).

Bogbean leaves are obtained from *Menyanthes trifoliata* (family Menyanthaceae, closely related to gentian), a perennial aquatic plant that grows in swampy areas of the northern temperate zone. The leaves are gathered in May or June while the plant is in flower and before the leaves turn dry and brittle later in the summer. Bogbean is odorless and has a strongly bitter taste. The bitter principles of bogbean leaves, like those of gentian root, belong to the class of secoiridoid glycosides.

Hop strobiles, the female flowers of *Humulus lupulus* (family Cannabaceae), are grown commercially and are carefully shielded from pollination by weeding out nearby male plants. This results in larger flowering tops that have strong bitter principles and a powerful aroma. The dried strobile has an aromatic odor and a slightly bitter, acrid taste. The odor changes with prolonged storage, and old hops have the unpleasant smell of isovaleric acid. The bitter taste of hops is due to the presence of so called alpha acids such as humulone, cohumulone, and adhumulone in the hop resin. The bitter principles are susceptible to oxidation and undergo marked chemical changes during storage. While hops has been used as a natural preservative in the brewing industry for centuries, beer no longer contains hops' humulones and lupulones in their original form as the brewing process converts them into water-soluble derivatives. Hops are used in phytotherapy for their calmative properties (Sec. 2.4.3).

Blessed thistle tops are obtained from *Carduus benedictus*, syn. *Cnicus benedictus* (family Asteraceae), an herbaceous plant with spiny leaves native to the Mediterranean region. The dried leaves and flowering tops are almost odorless but have a strongly bitter taste. The bitter principles consist of cnicin and lesser amounts of other sesquiterpene lactones.

Condurango bark consists of dried bark from the stems and branches of *Marsdenia condurango* (family Asclepiadaceae), a climbing vine that grows on the western slopes of the Cordillera range in South America. Condurango bark has a faintly sweet aromatic odor and a slightly bitter, acrid taste. Its main bitter principle is condurangin.

Bitter orange peel is obtained from the fruit of the bitter orange tree *Citrus aurantium* (family Rutaceae). Most of the white, spongy parenchyma is removed during preparation of the crude drug. Bitter orange peel is an aromatic bitter with a spicy, aromatic odor and a spicy, bitter taste. The flavanone glycosides naringin and neohesperidin are responsible for the bitter flavor. The aroma and spicy taste are based on the 1–2 % content of volatile oils, mostly limonene; other constituents such as jasmone, linalyl acetate, geranyl acetate, and citronellal also contribute to the aroma. A dwarf variety of the bitter orange, the chinotte, has an exceptionally bitter peel that is used to aromatize a popular Italian bitter soft drink (Chinotto).

Centaury (Fig. 5.2), a member of the gentian family, is indigenous to Europe (particularly the Mediterranean region) and northern Africa; it has also become naturalized in North America. The crude drug consists of the dried aerial parts of *Centaurium erythraea*. Centaury is nearly odorless and has a strong bitter taste. Some of its bitter principles are identical to those in gentian (gentiopicroside), and some are very closely related chemically (sweroside, centapicrin, swertiamarin).

5.2 Functional Dyspepsia (Irritable Stomach Syndrome)

While the symptom of anorexia simply involves lack of appetite, the term dyspepsia can have various interpretations. In pediatrics, it refers to acute nutritional disturbances in infants occurring as a result of diarrhea. In internal medicine, it refers to a syndrome of functional complaints that emanate from the upper gastrointestinal tract. By contrast, irritable bowel syndrome (IBS, also called irritable colon) is characterized by complaints that arise chiefly from the lower intestinal tract, particularly the colon. A strict

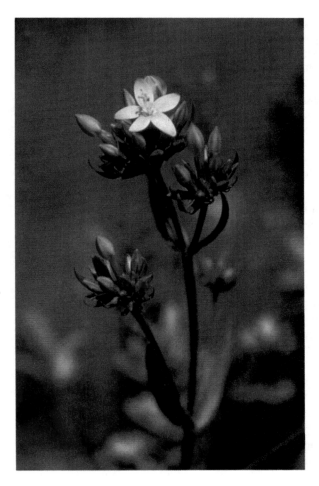

Figure 5.2. ◀ Centaury (*Centaurium erythraea*).

diagnostic distinction cannot always be made, however, and approximately 30 % of these patients have symptoms that are referable to both diagnostic entities (Talley et al., 1999). Overlaps between the two syndromes also occur when herbal remedies are used. For example, peppermint oil (alone or combined with caraway oil) is used successfully both in functional dysplasia and in irritable bowel syndrome.

Functional dyspepsia presents clinically with epigastric pain and pressure, retrosternal burning, nausea, occasional vomiting, early satiety, bloating, and crampy abdominal pain. Based on the Rome II criteria, the complaints should persist or recur over a period of more than 12 weeks (Madisch und Hotz, 2000). Decreased gastric juice secretion, decreased bile formation, biliary tract dyskinesias, and exocrine pancreatic insufficiency have been cited as possible causes (Fintelmann et al., 1993, 1996). The recommended phytomedicines may belong to the categories of "bitters" (see Sect. 5.1.2), "cholagogues," or "carminatives," depending on the dominant functional deficits and complaints. For an optimum response, moreover, the patient must have confidence in the physician and in the selected therapeutic agent. The physician should always take the patient's complaints seriously while guarding against overdiagnosis. The consultation with the physician, along with the selected remedy, should stimulate and promote the patient's self-healing powers. Over a decade ago, a meta-analysis of placebo-controlled clinical trials showed that a successful response to treatment for this indication depends more on the therapeutic context than on the drugs themselves (Dobrilla et al., 1989). In a subsequent meta-analysis of 17 controlled studies, herbal medicines reduced symptoms and complaints in 60–95 % of the patients treated (Coon and Ernst, 2002).

5.2.1 Biliary Remedies (Cholagogues)

Some phytomedicines have proved effective in increasing biliary flow, such as preparations made from artichokes or tumeric. But clinical studies have mainly documented their efficacy in the symptomatic treatment of functional dyspepsia, regardless of their mechanism of action. The classic term "cholagogues" was based on older pathogenetic concepts for this group of herbal remedies, and a more accurate current term is "antidyspeptics." From the standpoint of differential indications, cholagogues are used mainly in the treatment of dyspeptic complaints that are characterized by a feeling of pressure or pain in the right upper quadrant of the abdomen. The term cholagogues in this context is a generic one for choleretics (agents that stimulate bile production in the liver) and cholekinetics (agents that promote emptying of the gallbladder and extrahepatic bile ducts).

Reasoning by analogy with kidney stones and recurrent urinary tract infection, it is plausible that increasing the bile flow would help to cleanse the biliary tract of crystallization nuclei and bacteria that have entered the tract by the retrograde route, but such an assumption is difficult to prove experimentally (Ritter, 1984). Of course, lithiasis might be considered a contraindication to cholagogic therapy since stimulating bile flow or gallbladder contractions could cause a gallstone to become impacted. But bitters can induce a mild, almost physiologic stimulation of bile secretion and biliary tract motility (Sect. 5.1.1) (Glatzel, 1968), and generally a strict distinction cannot be drawn between the classes of bitter and cholagogic remedies in practical therapeutic use. Available information suggests that all these remedies have primarily a subjective mode of action. From a practical standpoint, this means that herbal bitters and cholagogues should not contain any ingredients that might be harmful if used on a long-term basis.

5.2.1.1 Artichoke Leaves

The only herbal preparation in this group of indications (Table 5.3) that has shown choleretic properties in placebo-controlled double-blind studies in humans is an extract from artichoke leaves. The crude drug consists of the fresh or dried foliage leaves of *Cynara scolymus* (Fig. 5.3). Typical constituents are caffeoylquinic acid derivatives, especially cynarin. Besides its choleretic effect, pharmacologic studies with an aqueous artichoke leaf extract have shown inhibitory effects on cholesterol biosynthesis and hepatoprotective effects in isolated liver cells (Gebhardt, 1995 a, b). The inhibitory effect on cholesterol biosynthesis in vitro is consistent with numerous empirical

Table 5.3.
Herbs used as biliary remedies owing to their choleretic, cholekinetic, or antispasmodic properties.

Herb (Latin name)	Key constituents	Daily dose
Artichoke leaf (Cynarae folium)	Cynarin and bitter principales (e.g., cynaropicrin)	6 g of crude drug
Boldo leaf (Boldo folium)	> 0.1 % Alkaloids (main active principle: boldine), 2% volatile oils	3 g of crude drug
Fumitory (Fumariae herba)	> 0.1 % Fumarine and other isoquinoline alkaloids	6 g of crude drug
Turmeric rhizome (Curcumae rhizoma)	> 3 % Curcumin and desmeth-oxycurcumin, > 3 % volatile oils	1.5–3 g of crude drug
Dandelion root and leaf (Taraxici radix cum herba)	Mixture of bitters designated taraxicin, also phytosterols	3–4 g of crude drug
Greater celandine (Chelidonii herba)	> 6 % Total alkaloids, calculated as chelidonine	2–5 g of crude drug or 12–30 mg total alkaloids

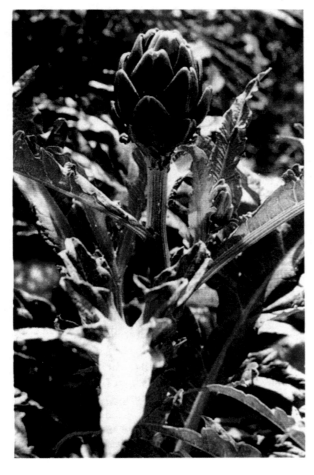

Figure 5.3. ◄ Artichoke (*Cynara scolymus* L.).

reports and with the results of a controlled clinical study (Englisch et al., 2000), indicating that the long-term use of artichoke preparations can help lower serum cholesterol levels in humans (Fintelmann, 1996). Other studies indicate that artichoke leaf extract can also inhibit human LDL oxidation, which has a significant role in the pathogenesis of atherosclerosis (Gebhardt, 1996). Kraft (1997) reviewed the pharmacologic actions of artichoke leaf extract and the most important published results on its clinical efficacy.

The choleretic effects of artichoke leaf extract are documented. Two placebo-controlled studies in humans (Kupke et al., 1991; Kirchhoff et al., 1994) showed increases of 127 % and 152 % respectively, in bile flow 30 min and 60 min after the intraduodenal administration of 1.92 g of a standardized artichoke extract (Fig. 5.4). These findings led the authors to conclude that artichoke extract is beneficial in the treatment of dyspeptic complaints, especially in patients with a suspected dysfunction of bile secretion (Kirchhoff et al., 1994).

The Commission E monograph of July, 1988, cites dyspeptic complaints as the indication for artichoke leaf preparations. The efficacy and tolerance of artichoke leaves for this indication were evaluated in outpatients treated with a mean daily dose of 1500 mg of dry extract from artichoke leaves. A statistically significant and clinically relevant regression of dyspeptic symptoms was documented after 6 weeks of treatment (Fig. 5.5). Significant reductions occurred in 302 of 553 patients whose total serum cholesterol and serum triglycerides were determined at the start and end of the study. The reduction in total cholesterol averaged 11.5 % from an initial baseline of 264 mg/dL, and the average triglyceride reduction was 12.5 % from a baseline of 215 mg/dL. Seven of the 553 patients (1.3 % experienced adverse reactions in the form of bloating (n=5), weakness (n=1), and hunger (n=1) (Fintelmann, 1996). A 6-month treatment study in 203 patients showed that the extract continued to exert antiemetic and carminative effects over this extended period with no decrease in response. No adverse effects were observed in the 6-month study (Fintelmann and Petrowicz, 1998).

A prospective, randomized, placebo-controlled, double-blind, multicenter comparative parallel-group study was carried out to determine whether a regimen of two 320-mg capsules of artichoke leaf extract (ALE) taken 3 times daily was superior to treatment with a pharmacologically inactive placebo. The main inclusion criteria were the diagnosis of chronic digestive complaints that mainly involved the upper abdomen and were at least of moderate severity. Patients with evidence of organic disease or a predominance of reflux symptoms or irritable bowel symptoms were excluded. The patients were questioned about any change in dyspeptic complaints each week during the 6-week treatment period (primary outcome measure). Secondary outcome measures were the severity of symptoms and the rating of efficacy and tolerance by the physician. The main outcome measure was evaluated as a total score summed over the whole treatment period (corresponding to the chronic recurring course of the disease). The study encompassed 247 patients from 30 test centers. The data from 244 patients were available for intent-to-treat analysis. Evaluation of the primary outcome measure indicated a significant superiority of the ALE over placebo during the 6-week period (Fig. 5.5) (Holtmann et al., 2003).

The efficacy of an artichoke leaf extract in hyperlipidemia was tested in another double-blind study, in which 143 patients with a total serum cholesterol > 7.3 mmol/L

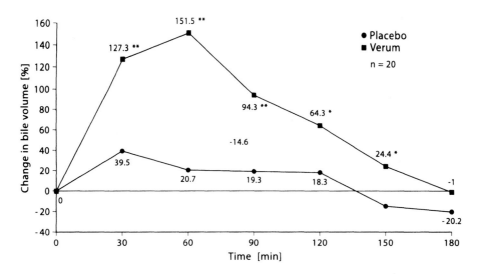

Figure 5.4. ▲ Effect of intraduodenal administration of 1.92 g of a standardized artichoke extract on bile flow. Mean values were measured in 20 healthy subjects. The differences relative to the placebo at 120 and 150 min were statistically significant (* = $p < 0.05$; ** = $p < 0.01$, after Kirchhoff et al., 1994.

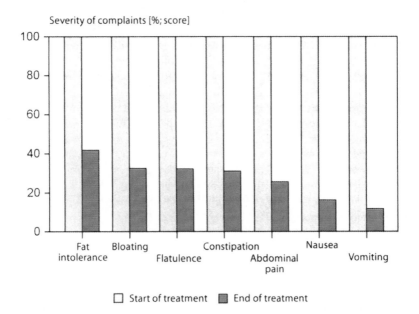

Figure 5.5. ▲ Regression of typical dyspeptic symptoms after six weeks' treatment with an artichoke leaf extract at a daily mean dose of 1500 mg. Mean values observed in 553 patients (Fintelmann, 1996).

(> 280 mg/dL) received 1800 mg/d of artichoke leaf extract or placebo for 6 weeks. The total serum cholesterol level decreased by an average of 18.5 % in the artichoke-treated group compared with 8.6 % in the placebo group (intergroup difference p < 0.0001). No adverse events referable to the artichoke extract were observed (Englisch et al., 2000). This result confirms earlier observations and case reports on the lipid-lowering effects of artichoke, which so far have been tested in only a few pilot studies in human patients (Pittler and Ernst, 1998).

In the Commission E monograph on artichoke leaves, the recommended therapy for "dyspeptic complaints" is an average daily dose of 6 g of the crude drug or an equivalent dose of extract based on the herb-to-extract ratio. The monograph lists biliary tract obstruction and allergy to artichoke or other composite herbs as contraindications. It also states there are no known side effects or drug-drug interactions (Blumenthal et al., 1998).

5.2.1.2 Other Cholagogues

Table 5.3 lists six specific herbs whose preparations are often contained in cholagogic remedies. Most of the commercial products available in Germany are made from extracts. If it is assumed for the sake of simplicity that these products have an extract content on the order of about 20 % (approximately 5:1 herb-to-extract ratio), the dosage of extract would be in the range of about 300–1200 mg daily. In the case of herbs that are consumed in powdered form, the active daily dose would be as high as 1.5–6 g/day. These figures suggest that some 50 % of the most common single-herb biliary remedies sold in Germany, and virtually all the combination products, are underdosed.

Turmeric (curcuma) extract is reported to have choleretic and cholecystokinetic properties (Maiwald and Schwantes, 1991). These are due partly to the presence of curcumins, although whole extracts are thought to be more potent than individual fractions. Curcuma is also described as an anti-inflammatory agent (Ammon and Wahl, 1990). Turmeric has a long tradition as a spice and medicinal herb. *Curcuma longa* is used mainly as a spice (e.g., in curry) while *C. xanthorrhiza* is used more as a medicinal herb. Both plants contain yellow dyes, curcuminoids, and essential oil, with each species showing a typical composition. Both species are equivalent in their long-known cholagogic effects. In addition, curcuma preparations have been described as having carminative, lipid-lowering and antineoplastic properties. Curcuminoids are powerful antioxidants, and this property could form a basis for new therapeutic uses of turmeric. Reviews on the pharmacognosy, pharmacology, and therapeutic use of curcuma can be found in Hänsel (1997) and in Fintelmann and Wegener (2001).

A four-week observational study of a *C, longa* extract (162 mg/d) administered at a dose of 162 mg/d demonstrated curative effects in 440 patients with functional dyspepsia (34 %), irritable bowel (36 %), functional disorders of the lower biliary tract (18 %), or other nonspecific digestive disorders (12 %). The regression of dyspeptic symptoms averaged 68 %. Onset of effect took approximately one week. Adverse events were not observed (Kammerer and Fintelmann, 2001).

Extract of greater celandine, when administered to experimental animals, causes a slow but steady increase in bile flow that is believed to result more from choleretic than cholekinetic effects (Baumann, 1975). The crude drug, consisting of the dried aerial parts of *Chelidonium majus* (family Papayeraceae) harvested while the plant is in bloom, contains 0.1–1 % total alkaloids (approximately 30 in all), including chelidonine, a papaverine-related compound that reportedly acts as an antispasmodic and a weak central analgesic. Overdoses of greater celandine or its preparations can cause stomach pain, intestinal colic, urinary urgency, and hematuria accompanied by dizziness and stupor. Tea preparations are difficult to dose properly, and therefore greater celandine should not be taken in that form. There is recent evidence linking commercial products to hepatotoxic side effects, depending on the alkaloid content, and these effects merit further testing. Schilcher (1997) has reviewed the pharmaceutical and medical aspects of treatment with celandine preparations.

Boldo leaves are obtained from the evergreen shrub *Peumus boldus* (family Monimia-ceae), a relative of the laurel tree that is native to arid regions of Chile. The crude drug has a burning, aromatic taste and odor caused by its content of volatile oil. Its true active principle is boldine, an aporphine alkaloid. Because the herb contains substances that are potentially toxic (Duke, 1985), it is not recommended for long-term use and should not be taken during pregnancy.

Dandelion (*Taraxacum officinalis*, family Asteraceae) extract reportedly leads to an increase in bile flow (Böhm, 1959; Pirtkien et al., 1960). This action may be based on bitter principles contained chiefly in the dandelion root.

Fumitory (*Fumaria officinalis*, family Fumariaceae) is a traditional native European herb whose extracts reportedly relieve spasms of the sphincter of Oddi and exert a general regulatory effect on biliary functions (Fiegel, 1971).

5.2.2 Carminatives

Flatulent states with fullness and nausea are typical complaints of functional dyspepsia and are among the most common presenting complaints that are seen by general practitioners. Their causes are diverse and range from inflammatory gastrointestinal disorders and biliary/pancreatic secretory dysfunction to atherosclerotic lesions of the mesenteric blood vessels. Most cases are thought to be based less an excessive gas formation than on deficient gas absorption. Although bloating and flatulence generally are not painful, they can be very troublesome for the patient. They not only affect mood, appetite, and sleep but can have adverse circulatory effects corresponding to the gastrocardiac symptom complexes described by Roemheld syndrome at the turn of the century.

Herbal preparations play a special role in the treatment of flatulence. Herbs that are useful in expelling gas to relieve flatulence are called carminatives (from the Latin carminare, to cleanse). The pharmacologic literature (Gunn, 1920; Sigmund and

McNally, 1969) defines carminatives as preparations, originally taken with food, that produce a warm sensation when ingested and promote the postprandial elimination of digestive gas by flatus or eructation. These products include essential oils as well as herbal preparations and plant extracts that have a high content of volatile oils, most notably caraway, fennel, and anise as well as peppermint, chamomile. lemon balm, and angelica root.

It has been well established, at least in vitro, that many of the essential oils used as carminatives have antispasmodic actions (Schwenk and Horbach, 1978; Forster, 1983; Reiter and Brandt, 1985). This particularly applies to peppermint oil (Taylor et al., 1983; Hills and Aaronson, 1991). Studies in human subjects have shown that the administration of peppermint oil can relax the lower esophageal sphincter in minutes, equalizing the intraluminal pressures between the stomach and esophagus (Sigmund and McNally, 1969). It has been found that alcoholic extracts of the typical carminative herbs, caraway, fennel, and anise have antispasmodic activity, but their essential oils do not (Forster, 1983); indeed, the latter substances tend to heighten muscle tonus and stimulate bowel motility (Brand, 1988). Thus, while carminatives are unquestionably effective from the standpoint of the user, the mechanisms that underlie their efficacy are not yet fully understood.

5.2.2.1　Typical Carminative Herbs

Caraway (*Carum carvi*, Fig. 5.6): The dried ripe fruits (often called seeds) of this plant of the family Apiaceae are considered the most typical and effective of the carminative

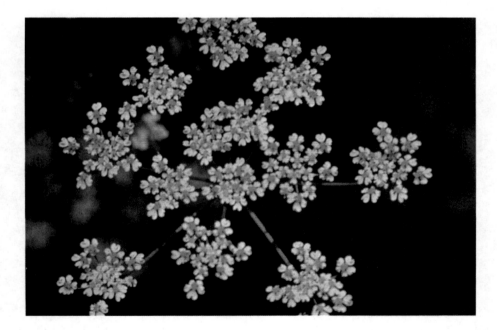

Figure 5.6. ▲ An umbel of caraway (*Carum carvi*).

herbs. Caraway is a biennial plant that grows wild in Europe and Asia, but the herb used for medicinal and seasoning purposes is obtained almost exclusively by cultivation. Caraway fruits contain 2–7 % volatile oil and about 10–20 % fatty oil. The volatile oil consists mainly of carvone (50–60 %) and limonene. Alcoholic caraway extracts have been used for centuries as stomachics.

Fennel (*Foeniculum vulgare*), also a member of the family Apiaceae, grows to 1–2 m and is native to southern Europe. Its fruits (seeds) are used medicinally and contain 2–6 % volatile oil and 9–12 % fatty oil. Fennel volatile oil consists mostly of fenchone and anethole. The fruits are mainly carminative but also act as a mild expectorant, especially in children. Fennel also makes an excellent flavor corrective for carminative tea mixtures. Additionally, fennel tea is a common European remedy for infants with dyspepsia and diarrhea. Allowing only fennel tea during the initial fasting period not only supplies the infants with fluid but also provides a carminative effect that reduces flatulence and eases intestinal spasms.

Anise (*Pimpinella anisum*) is native to the Orient but is also grown in certain regions of Germany. Like caraway and fennel, anise is a member of the family Apiaceae. It has a pungent odor and grows to a height of about ½ m. Anise seed (botanically a fruit) contains 2–3 % volatile oil and about 10 % fatty oil. The main constituent of the volatile oil is anethole. Anise is a less potent carminative than caraway but reportedly has a stronger expectorant action. Weiss (1991) ranks the umbelliferous herbs as follows in order of decreasing carminative effect and increasing expectorant effect: caraway, fennel, anise.

Other herbs considered to have carminative actions are chamomile, peppermint, lemon balm, angelica root, and coriander seeds. Angelica root has an unpleasant odor and a spicy, bitter taste. It contains about 0.4–0.8 % volatile oil. The fruits of coriander, native to the Mediterranean region, have a spicy aromatic odor and a slightly burning taste. Their odor and taste are due to the content of volatile oil, consisting mainly of linalool (60–70 %). The aerial parts of marjoram are also said to have a weak carminative action but are used mainly as a culinary spice.

5.2.2.2 Combination of Peppermint Oil and Caraway Oil

A fixed combination of peppermint oil and caraway oil (90 mg + 50 mg per dose; Enteroplant®) has been approved in Germany in the form of enteric-coated capsules as a remedy for "dyspeptic complaints, especially when associated with bloating, fullness, and mild gastrointestinal spasms." Two controlled studies have been done with this product in healthy subjects, and four therapeutic trials have been conducted in patients with functional dyspepsia (combined with IBS in one study).

The double-blind crossover studies in a total of 30 healthy subjects used a standardized manometric technique to document spasmolytic effects for the two separate components peppermint oil and caraway oil and also for their combination (additive effect) in the human stomach and duodenum (Micklefield, 2000; Micklefield et al., 2000).

A placebo-controlled double-blind study was performed in 45 patients with nonulcerative dyspepsia, combined in some cases with IBS. The treatment regimen consisted of 1 capsule taken 3 times daily for 4 weeks. The primary outcome measures were pain intensity based on a 6-point scale and a global assessment by the physician using the CGI scale. Both criteria after 2 and 4 weeks' therapy demonstrated a statistically significant superiority of the peppermint/caraway oil combination over placebo (May et al., 1996).

In another double-blind study, the combination product Enteroplant (1 capsule b.i.d. + 1 capsule placebo) was compared with the prokinetic agent cisapride (10 mg t.i.d.) in 118 patients with functional dyspepsia. The outcome measures included a pain score (with a visual analog scale), pain frequency, and a total symptom score. The two test medications showed no differences in any of the outcome measures (Madisch et al., 1999).

Another placebo-controlled double-blind study was performed in 96 patients with functional dyspepsia. The primary outcome measure was a decrease in the intensity of epigastric pain during 28 days of treatment with 1 capsule of Enteroplant b.i.d. compared with a placebo. This study, too, demonstrated a significant superiority of the peppermint/caraway oil combination in both the primary outcome measure and in several secondary parameters (May et al., 2000).

The above studies in patients with functional dyspepsia did not include data on quality of life. This aspect was explored in another double-blind multicenter study. A total of 114 patients were admitted to the study and randomized. The severity of dyspeptic symptoms was determined with the validated Nepean Dyspepsia Index (NDI). The primary outcome measures were the difference in total score 1 (NDI subscore based on intensity of epigastric pain, epigastric complaints, epigastric spasms, and epigastric bloated feeling) and total score 2 (NDI subscore based on intensity of epigastric pressure and feeling of fullness after eating or slow digestion) between days 0 and 29. Secondary criteria were the symptom score and total score of the NDI. Intention-to-treat analysis was used for confirmation. As in previous studies, Enteroplant was statistically significantly superior to placebo therapy in all the outcome measures and criteria. Significantly greater reductions were achieved in both total scores (Holtmann, 2003).

5.2.3 Ginger for Nausea and Vomiting

The Commission E monograph on ginger rhizome states that moderate daily doses equivalent to 2–4 g of the crude drug are indicated for the treatment of "dyspeptic complaints" and the "prevention of travel sickness" (Blumenthal et al., 1998). A meta-analysis on efficacy for nausea and vomiting was based on 6 randomized studies – 3 dealing with postoperative nausea and vomiting, one with sea sickness, one with morning sickness, and one with vomiting related to chemotherapy. At a dose of 1 g of pulverized herb, the efficacy in all studies was better than that of placebo or equivalent to metoclopramide. Overall, however, the data from the three postoperative studies showed no statistically significant difference in nausea amelioration by ginger compared with placebo (Ernst and Pittler, 2000).

Another placebo-controlled study was conducted in 70 pregnant Thai women at or before 17 weeks' gestation. Women with nausea or vomiting were randomized to receive either oral ginger 1 g per day or a placebo for 4 days. Graded by a visual analog scale, the symptoms decreased by 2.1 points in the ginger group compared with 0.9 points in the placebo group (p < 0.001). Corresponding differences were also found in the number of vomiting episodes (Vutyavanich et al., 2001).

The results of these controlled treatment studies offer compelling evidence that the antiemetic properties of ginger rhizome, prized by sailors for centuries, still have therapeutic applications today.

5.2.4 *Iberis amara* – Combination

A combination product containing nine 9 ingredients, with the trade name Iberogast®, is among the 10 most commonly prescribed herbal medications in Germany (see Table A3 in the Appendix). The product contains a tincture of two bitter herbs – wild candytuft (*Iberis amara*) and angelica root – along with extracts from chamomile flowers, caraway seeds, milk thistle fruits, lemon balm leaves, peppermint leaves, greater celandine, and licorice root. The dominant therapeutic effect in any given case may be the tonic effect of the candytuft and angelica root extracts or the more spasmolytic effect of the other herbal extracts, depending on the initial pathophysiology (Rösch, 2000). With this action profile, the product has an intermediate classification between bitters and antidyspeptics.

A review of studies on the efficacy of Iberogast (Rösch, 2000) presents data from 8 controlled clinical studies, 4 of which were older studies in a total of 158 patients with "functional or organic gastroenterologic disorders." Three other studies (total of 486 patients) were performed in patients with functional dyspepsia (irritable stomach), each comparing the combination product with a different herbal test combination and with placebo (2 studies) or with the prokinetic agent cisapride (1 study). The duration of treatment was 4 weeks, and outcomes were measured with a complaint score covering 11 symptoms. In these studies Iberogast was significantly superior to placebo or equivalent to cisapride. Another study with a similar design was conducted in 208 patients with IBS. A significant improvement in complaint and pain profiles was achieved after 4 weeks' therapy, with a tolerance comparable to placebo (Rösch, 2000; Madisch et al., 2000; Madisch et al., 2001).

5.2.5 Digestive Enzymes

Replacement therapy with digestive enzymes may be utilized in an attempt to relieve the complaints resulting from excretory pancreatic insufficiency with associated indigestion. This involves the use of combination products containing lipase, amylase, and proteases. Most of these products contain preparations made from animal pancreatic tissue. Some combination products (e.g., Esberizym®) also contain plant proteases – bromelain, which is derived from the fresh juice of the pineapple plant (*Ananas comosus*), and papain, which is obtained from the latex of the fleshy, unripe fruit of ⁺

papaya (*Carica papaya*). Since there is no clinical syndrome that would warrant protease replacement as an isolated therapy, and there seems to be no rationale for combining the proteases bromelain and papain with other preparations in this group, Commission E of the former German Federal Health Agency, now called the German Federal Institute of Drugs and Medical Devices, did not sanction the use of bromelain and papain for the replacement therapy of digestive insufficiency.

5.2.6 Suggested Formulations (for 5.1 and 5.2)

A) For stomach tinctures and teas

Indications: **poor appetite, dyspeptic complaints with bloating and fullness.**
Contraindications: gastric and duodenal ulcers.
Adverse effects: occasional headache in patients sensitive to bitters.

Rx	Bitter tincture according to German Pharmacopeia 6.	
	Directions: Take 10–20 drops in one-half glass of water before meals.	
	Tonic-aromatic stomach remedy for dyspeptic conditions according to Weiss (1982).	
Rx	Gentian tincture	10.0
	Wormwood tincture	10.0
	Peppermint tincture	10.0
	Directions: (same as above).	

Bitter tea according to Austrian Pharmacopeia*)

Rx	Wormwood	20.0
	Centaury	20.0
	Bogbean leaves	15.0
	Gentian root	15.0
	Bitter orange peel	20.0
	Cinnamon bark	10.0
	Mix to make tea	
	Directions: Take 2 teaspoonful in 1 cup as an infusion 30 min before meals several times daily.	

*) Modified to omit calamus root.

Stomach tea I according to German Standard Registration

Rx	Gentian root	20.0
	Bitter orange peel	20.0
	...ry	25.0
	...wood	25.0
	...mon bark	10.0

Stomach tea II according to German Standard Registration

Rx	Angelica root	25.0
	Yarrow	25.0
	Centaury	15.0
	Wormwood	15.0
	Aniseed	5.0
	Cornflower	5.0
	Orange blossoms	5.0
	Rosemary	5.0

Stomach tea III according to German Standard Registration

Rx	Wormwood	25.0
	Yarrow	25.0
	Balm leaves	25.0
	Blackberry leaves	5.0
	Cornflower	5.0
	Orange blossoms	5.0
	Calendula flowers	5.0
	Sage leaves	5.0

Stomach tea IV according to German Standard Registration

Rx	Gentian root	20.0
	Dandelion leaves and root	35.0
	Centaury	30.0
	Basil	5.0'
	Calendula flowers	5.0
	Sage leaves	5.0

Note: Each formula should include (1) mix to make tea and (2) the same directions stated for the Austrian Pharmacopeia tea.

B) Suggested formulation for bile teas

Indications: supportive treatment of noninflammatory gallbladder complaints involving a disturbance of bile flow, also gastrointestinal complaints that involve bloating and digestive problems.

Contraindications: inflammation or obstruction of the bile ducts; bowel obstruction.

Directions to patient: Infuse 1 teaspoonful in 1 cup of water (about 150 mL); drink 1 fresh cup 30 min before meals 3 or 4 times daily.

Bile tea I according to German Standard Registration

Rx		
	Dandelion leaves and root	30.0
	Javanese turmeric rhizome	20.0
	Peppermint leaves	20.0
	Milk thistle fruit	20.0
	Caraway fruit	10.0

Bile tea II according to German Standard Registration

Rx		
	Dandelion leaves and root	15.0
	Javanese turmeric rhizome	20.0
	Peppermint leaves	20.0
	Yarrow	20.0
	Fennelseed	5.0
	Chamomile	5.0
	Calendula	5.0
	Licorice root	5.0
	Wormwood	5.0

C) Complaints such as bloating, flatulence, and mild gastrointestinal cramping; also nervous gastrointestinal complaints

Compound caraway tincture according to German Prescription Formula Index

Rx		
	Caraway volatile oil	2.0
	Valerian tincture	to make 20.0

Directions: Take 30 drops in water 3 times daily.

Carminative rub according to Fintelmann.

Rx		
	Caraway volatile oil	2.0
	Olive oil	to make 20.0

Directions: Use externally for bloating; rub several drops into the periumbilical area.

Tea Mixtures

Preparation and use: Pour boiling water (about 150 mL) over 1–2 teaspoons of the tea mixture, steep for 10 min, and strain. Drink 1 cup warm after every meal.

Carminative tea according to German Prescription Formula Index (DRF, 1950)

Rx		
	Chamomile	
	Peppermint	
	Valerian root	
	Caraway fruit	
	Aniseed	aa, to make 100.00

Directions (see above).

Gastrointestinal tea I according to German Standard Registration

Rx Valerian root
    Caraway fruit
    Peppermint
    Chamomile   aa, to make 100.0
    Directions (see above).

Gastrointestinal tea III according to German Standard Registration

Rx Fennelseed   30.0
    Coriander fruit   30.0
    Calendula flowers   5.0
    Cornflower   5.0
    Directions (see above).

Gastrointestinal tea IX according to German Standard Registration

Rx Aniseseed
    Fennelseed
    Caraway fruit
    Chamomile
    Yarrow   aa, to make 100.0
    Directions (see above).

Gastrointestinal tea XII according to German Standard Registration

Rx Chamomile   30.0
    Licorice root   30.0
    Yarrow   20.0
    Mallow flowers   5.0
    Balm leaves   5.0
    Calendula flowers   5.0
    Cinnamon bark   5.0
    Directions (see above).

5.3 Irritable Bowel Syndrome

5.3.1 Symptoms, Epidemiology, and Approaches to Treatment

Irritable bowel syndrome (IBS, also called irritable colon) is a common, chronic functional disorder defined as a variable combination of chronic and recurring gastrointestinal symptoms with no identifiable structural abnormalities or biochemical pathology. The cardinal symptoms are abdominal pain, constipation, diarrhea, altered defecation, and bloating. Functional disturbances of gastrointestinal motility, generalized hypersensitivity of the visceral smooth muscle, and visceral hyperalgesia have been postulated as pathophysiologic factors. Psychopathologic factors, especially anxiety disorders, also play a role and suggest that IBS is related to the somatoform disorders (F45 in ICD 10 classification). The diagnosis is made by excluding organic disease according to the Manning criteria (Manning et al., 1978) or the Rome diagnostic criteria for functional bowel disorders and functional abdominal pain (Thompson et al., 1992).

IBS is very common. Its prevalence in European countries, the U.S., China, and Japan is estimated at between 10 % and 25 % of the adult population (Camilleri and Choi, 1997). From 30 % to 50 % of patients seen by gastroenterologists have IBS. Symptoms start before age 35 in about 50 % of cases, and another 40 % have their onset between age 35 and 50. Women are affected more frequently than men. The etiology is unknown (Maxwell et al., 1997).

Treatment is symptomatic and depends on individual manifestations. Constipation can be treated with a fiber supplement such as wheat bran, linseed, or psyllium, while diarrhea is managed by reducing dietary fat intake and, if necessary, by taking an antidiarrheal agent that reduces bowel motility. Abdominal pain and spasms can be treated with mebeverine-type antispasmodics, but peppermint oil is equally or more effective (see Sect. 5.4.2.5). Antidepressants are recommended for the treatment of somatoform disorders, especially when significant anxiety is present. In the field of phytotherapy, St. John's wort preparations may be considered for this purpose (see Sect. 2.2). Regardless of the type of pharmacotherapy used, the physician has a responsibility to manage and counsel the patient. It has been estimated that 40–70 % of the success in irritable bowel therapy is based on psychodynamic effects (Friedmann, 1991; Maxwell et al., 1997; Jailwala et al., 2000). Pharmacodynamic effects, which are of secondary importance in overall treatment response, are currently considered to be most favorable for antispasmodic agents and least favorable for bulking agents (Camilleri, 1999; Jailwala et al., 2000).

5.3.2 Peppermint

Medicinal peppermint (*Mentha piperita*; family Lamiaceae) is a hybrid that was first cultivated in late seventeenth-century England; it does not grow in the wild. Cultivation has yielded a number of varieties distinguished by their habit, growth vigor, resistance, and content of volatile oil. Still the most important variety is Mitcham mint, first grown in England more than 200 years ago.

Peppermint is a perennial plant that grows to about 30–80 cm and sends off numerous underground and surface runners (stolons). Related plants that grow in the wild (e.g., water mint, curly-leaved mint) are much inferior to peppermint in their fragrance, taste, and volatile oil content.

5.3.2.1 Crude Drug and Constituents

All the aerial parts of peppermint are machine-harvested shortly before the plant blooms (Fig. 5.7) and are dried a a low temperature. The crude drug should contain at least 1.2 % volatile oil. It also contains 6–12 % tannins along with flavonoids, triterpenes, and bitter principles (Wichtl, 1989). Dried peppermint leaves are used in making teas.

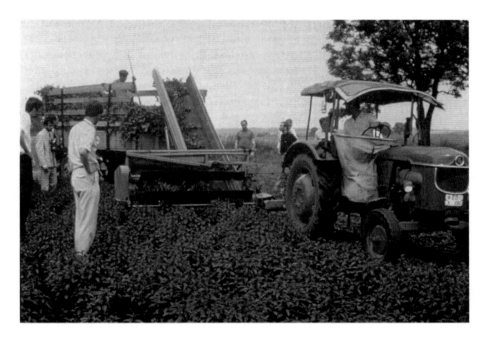

Figure 5.7. ▲ Harvesting peppermint (*Mentha x piperita*).

5.3.2.2 Peppermint Oil

Peppermint oil, obtained by steam distillation of the fresh or dried herb, is a colorless to pale green liquid with a pungent odor of peppermint. It has an initially burning taste and cool aftertaste, especially when air is drawn in through the mouth. To date, 85 chemical compounds have been isolated from peppermint oil. The main constituent (about 50–60 %) is menthol, which partially crystallizes at low temperatures. Peppermint oil also contains menthone (5–30 %), a number of esters (about 5–10 %), and small amounts of cineole and other terpenes.

5.3.2.3 Pharmacokinetics

Studies on the renal excretion of menthol following the oral ingestion of peppermint oil were performed in a total of 25 patients and healthy subjects. One study involved 6 healthy subjects and 6 ileostomy patients, each of whom received 0.4 mL of peppermint oil in 2 different formulations (original form or bound to a macromolecular vehicle). The urinary excretion of menthol (in the form of glucuronide) was then measured over a 24-hour period. Total menthol excretion in the healthy subjects was 35 % of the ingested amount in the original oil formulation and 40 % in the delayed-release capsule formulation. Peak menthol excretion levels were reached at 2 h with the oil formulation and at 4–6 h with the capsule formulation. Urinary menthol excretion in the ileostomy patients was 17 % with the original oil and 35 % with the capsules. This indicates that a significant portion of the ingested peppermint oil reaches the terminal ileum and the colon (Somerville et al., 1984). In a second study, each of 13 healthy subjects received 0.6 mL of peppermint oil in 2 different delayed-release formulations. The urinary excretion of menthol and its glucuronide metabolite was again measured over a 24-hour period. Peak excretion occurred at 5 h with one formulation and at 3 h with the other. The terminal elimination half-life based on urinary excretion was approximately 4 h with both formulations. While 5 subjects who took the faster-absorbing form complained of nausea and mild abdominal discomfort, no patients who took the other form complained of any adverse side effects. This may mean that peppermint oil is tolerated better when taken at a higher dose in a delayed-release formulation (White et al., 1987). It is doubtful whether the therapeutic effect in patients with IBS is favorably influenced by partial absorption in the distal ileum or proximal colon when a delayed-release product is used, because patients who take peppermint oil for acute colicky pain generally experience relief within 30 min after taking the preparation. Peppermint oil is believed to inhibit the activity of cytochrome P 450 (CYP3A4) in the liver and thus can increase the active levels of certain drugs in the body when they are taken concurrently (Dresser et al., 2002).

5.3.2.4 Pharmacology

Peppermint oil has an antispasmodic action on isolated segments of ileum (rabbits and cats) at dilutions no greater than 1:20,000. This effect, which is reversible, is marked by a decline in the number and amplitude of spontaneous contractions, in some cases to the point of complete paralysis. Peppermint oil antagonizes the spasmogenic action of barium chloride, pilocarpine, and physostigmine (Gunn, 1920). It relaxes ileal longitudinal muscle, though it is less potent in this action than papaverine (Brandt, 1988). Peppermint oil acts competitively with nifedipine and blocks Ca^{2+}-exciting stimuli. Thus, the antispasmodic action of peppermint oil is based on properties that are characteristic of Ca^{2+} antagonists (Taylor et al., 1983; Hawthorn et al., 1988; Hills and Aaronson, 1991; Beesley et al., 1996). Menthol-β-glucuronide may act as a prodrug for colonic delivery of the spasmolytic agent menthol (Nolen and Friend, 1994). Alcohol extracts from the aerial parts of peppermint have the most potent effect compared with extracts of other herbs that contain essential oils (lemon balm, rosemary, chamomile, fennel, caraway, and citrus) (Forster et al., 1980).

5.3.2.5 Therapeutic Efficacy

An aqueous suspension of peppermint oil injected along the biopsy tract in 20 patients prevented the colonic spasms that otherwise occur in endoscopic examinations (Leicester and Hunt, 1982). The efficacy of peppermint oil added to a barium sulfate contrast meal was tested in a double-blind study of 141 patients. Following the contrast examination, 60 % of the patients in the group treated with peppermint oil had no residual spasms compared with 35 % of patients in the placebo group (Sparks et al., 1995). Peppermint oil relaxes the esophageal sphincter when administered orally (15 drops of oil suspended in 30 mL of water), eliminating the pressure differential between the stomach and esophagus and allowing reflux to occur (Sigmund and McNally, 1969). The effectiveness of peppermint oil added to barium sulphate suspension in relieving colonic muscle spasm during contrast barium enema examination was assessed in a double-blind study with 141 patients. No residual spasm was evident in a significant proportion of patients in the treated group (60 %) compared with the control group (35 %). There were no adverse effects on the quality of the examination (Sparks et al., 1995). Nine controlled clinical studies were conducted in a total of 366 patients with IBS to test the therapeutic efficacy of peppermint oil (Table 5.4). The total daily dose, taken in 3 divided doses, ranged from 0.6 to 1.2 mL, and the duration of treatment ranged from 14 to 180 days. While 3 of the studies (Nash et al., 1986; Lawson et al., 1988; Shaw et al., 1991) found no therapeutic benefits, the results of the remaining 6 studies in Table 5.4 demonstrated a statistically significant benefit from peppermint oil therapy. A statistical meta-analysis of 8 studies showed that the treatment of IBS with peppermint oil was more effective than treatment with a placebo. It should be noted that some of the older studies had serious methodologic drawbacks including vague inclusion criteria for patients and treatment periods that were too short. Nevertheless, the overall result of the meta-analysis supports the therapeutic efficacy of peppermint oil in IBS (Pittler and Ernst, 1998). A typical result from one treatment study (Liu et al., 1997) is shown graphically in Fig. 5.8. Another placebo-controlled, double-blind study was performed in 39 patients using a combination product containing peppermint oil (90 mg) and caraway oil (50 mg). The main study criterion, a reduction in pain intensity, improved significantly (p=0.025) in comparison with the placebo group (Mey et al., 1996).

The Commission E monograph also ascribes a cholagogic action to peppermint oil (Blumenthal et al., 1998). The analgesic effects of peppermint oil applied externally are discussed in Sect. 8.5.

Table 5.4.
Randomized clinical studies on the treatment of irritable bowel syndrome with peppermint oil.

First author, year	Patients	Daily dose of peppermint oil (mL)	Duration of treatment (days)	Global improvement, drug vs. placebo
Rees, 1979	16	0.6–1.2	21	13/15 vs. 2/16
Dew, 1984	29	0.6–1.2	14	24/29 vs. 5/29
Nash, 1986	33	1.2	14	13/33 vs. 17/33
Lech, 1988	42	0.6	28	13/19 vs. 6/23
Lawson, 1988	25	0.6–1.2	28	n.s. vs. placebo
Carling, 1989	38	0.6–1.2	14	17/30 vs. 5/13
Schneider, 1990	47	?	42	Pain: p<0.01 in favor of test drug
Shaw, 1991	35	0.6	180	3/17 vs. 13/18[1]
Liu, 1997	101	0.6–0.8	28	41/52 vs. 21/49

NOTE: Except for the studies by Lech and Liu et al. (parallel group design) and by Shaw (open study comparing peppermint oil with stress management therapy), the remaining studies were placebo-controlled double-blind studies with a crossover design (after Pittler and Ernst, 1998).
[1] Peppermint oil vs. stress management therapy

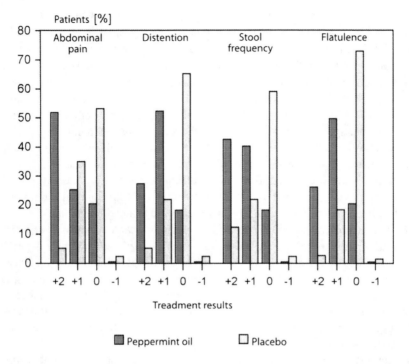

Figure 5.8. ▲ Response of symptoms to 0.6 mL peppermint oil daily for 4 weeks (colored bars) compared with a placebo (gray bars). +2 = significant improvement; +1 = moderate improvement; 0 = no change; -1 = worsening of symptoms. The overall result with peppermint oil was significantly better than with a placebo (p<0.05; Liu et al., 1997).

5.3.2.6 Risks and Side Effects

The long-term use of peppermint tea is not associated with risks or significant side effects.

Peppermint oil should not be applied to the nasal area of small children as it can provoke glottic spasms and respiratory arrest. The ingestion of excessive amounts of peppermint oil has been associated with interstitial nephritis and acute renal failure. The estimated lethal dose of menthol for humans is approximately 2–9 g. No mutagenic or carcinogenic effects of peppermint oil have been reported.

An overview of the risks and side effects of peppermint leaves and oil can be found in Bowen and Cubbin (1993).

5.3.2.7 Indications, Dosages, and Contraindications

The two Commission E monographs of 1986 state that peppermint leaves are indicated for "colicky pains in the gastrointestinal region, gallbladder, or biliary tract", and that peppermint oil can be taken internally for "colicky pains in the upper gastrointestinal tract and biliary tract, irritable colon, and catarrhal diseases of the upper respiratory tract." An average daily dose of 3-6 g is recommended for peppermint leaves taken in tea form. An average dose of 6-12 drops daily is recommended for peppermint oil. An average single dose of 0.2 mL, or average daily dose of 0.6 mL, is recommended for the treatment of IBS. Patients with this condition should take enteric-coated tablets before meals to ensure that the tablet will not dissolve inside the stomach with the chyme (most of the clinical trials with peppermint oil for treating IBS symptoms were conducted with enteric-coated tablets). The Commission states no contraindications to the herb. The oil is contraindicated by biliary tract obstruction, cholecystitis, and severe liver damage, and it should not be applied to the facial region of small children (Blumenthal et al., 1998).

5.4 Gastritis and Ulcer Disease

Inflammations of the gastric mucosa, ranging from relatively mild forms of gastritis to peptic ulcer disease, are treated pharmacologically with acid-neutralizing agents (antacids), agents that inhibit acid secretion (anticholinergics, H_2-antagonists), and with demulcent anti-inflammatory and antibiotic remedies. Phythotherapy has made a significant contribution to anticholinergic therapy, at least from a historical perspective, in that the alkaloids derived from the deadly nightshade (*Atropa belladonna*), atropine and scopolamine, are the prototypes of all anticholinergic drugs. Due to their narrow therapeutic range, however, preparations made from the leaves of deadly nightshade or henbane (*Hyoscyamus niger*) (0.2-0.3 % hyoscyamine and scopolamine) cannot be recommended today, i.e., for these indications (they are still approved and appropriate for other, non g.i., uses).

Some mucilaginous herbs have demulcent properties that can reduce local irritation in acute gastritis, particularly linseed, marshmallow leaves and roots, and common mallow leaves. A proven home remedy in this regard is linseed, which should be presoaked in water for about 30 min, similar to its mode of use as a laxative (Sect.5.8.2.1). Linseed can also be combined with chamomile preparations.

The main phytomedicines in use today for gastritis relief are chamomile and its preparations and licorice root preparations. Their effects are assumed to be based on anti-inflammatory and demulcent actions.

5.4.1 Chamomile

German chamomile (*Matricaria recutita*) is one of the best known and most versatile medicinal plants. Its many dermatologic uses are reviewed in Chap. 8.

Today it is believed that chamomile owes its therapeutic properties to three groups of active principles. First, there are the terpenoid volatile oils (content 0.25-1 %), especially bisabolol and chamazulene, both of which show a mild anti-inflammatory action in experimental animals (Isaak, 1980). Next come the flavonoids (content about 2.4 %), with apigenin showing particular activity as an antispasmodic agent. Finally, chamomile flowers have a 5–10 % content of pectin-like mucilages. It is believed that these substances are preferentially released during the infusion process and act swiftly to soothe irritation of the gastric mucosa.

Chamomile flowers prepared as an infusion or contained in an ethanolic extract-based product have mild anti-inflammatory and antispasmodic activity. This lends credence to physicians' observations that the therapeutic use of chamomile in acute flare-ups of chronic ulcer disease promotes ulcer healing. Chamomile no longer has a role in the treatment of chronic gastritis, Crohn's disease, or ulcerative colitis. It should be noted that the pharmacologic actions of various commercial products are affected by the solvent that was used in making the product. For example, while an aqueous infusion will extract no more than 15 % of the volatile oil contained in the dried herb, this process will extract almost all of certain flavonol glycosides and mucilaginous principles. Alcoholic extracts, in turn, are associated with a different spectrum of constituents. Thus, the results of several clinical studies in the late 1950s documenting the efficacy of a certain chamomile extract in acute gastritis and parapyloric ulcer disease (surveyed in Schilcher, 1987) cannot be readily applied to other types of preparations.

5.4.2 Licorice Root

Licorice root consists of the dried rhizome and roots of *Glycyrrhiza glabra* (Fig. 5.9). The genus name is derived from the Greek *glykos* (sweet) and *rhiza* (root). The crude drug contains two types of active principles: glycyrrhizin (5–15 %) and the flavonoids liquiritin and isoliquiritin. Orally administered glycyrrhizin is believed to relieve gastric inflammation by its inhibition of prostaglandin synthesis and lipoxygenase (Inoue et al., 1986; Tamura et al., 1979). A controlled clinical study with nearly 900 peptic ulcer patients resulted in similar efficacy of deglycyrrhizinated liquorice compared to antacids and cimetidine (Kassir, 1955). Because of the mineralocorticoid-like action of glycyrrhizin, the average daily dose should not exceed 5–15 g of the dried herb (equivalent to 200–600 mg glycyrrhizin), and the course of treatment should not exceed 4–6 weeks. A higher dosage or longer use could lead to adverse effects consisting of sodium and water retention, blood pressure elavation, potassium loss, and edema. These side effects should be absent or minimal with licorice root extracts that have a low glycyrrhizin content. Bielenberg (1998) has reviewed all reports on licorice toxicity and on additional pharmacologic actions of licorice root preparations and glycyrrhizin.

Licorice root preparations are contraindicated by cholestatic liver disorders, cirrhosis of the liver, hypertension, hypokalemia, severe renal failure, and pregnancy.

Drug Products (for 5.1 to 5.4)

Liquid preparations are the recommended dosage form for administering bitters. Teas can be prepared at home as an alternative to ready-made products, provided this can be

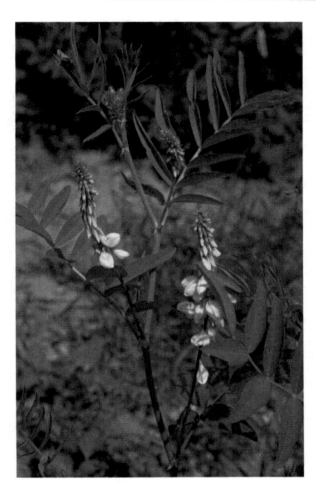

Figure 5.9. ◄ Flowering tops of the licorice plant (*Glycyrrhiza glabra*).

done with an acceptable therapeutic risk (see wormwood). Digestive aids, cholagogues, and carminatives are no longer covered by health insurance in Germany in accordance with 1999 Drug Guidelines. This is a circumstance that emphasizes rather than reduces the need for physician guidance in these important indications for self-medication.

The *Rote Liste 2003* lists a total of three single-herb products under the category of medications that affect gastrointestinal motility.

 References (for 5.1 to 5.4)

Adler M (1979) Physiologische Psychologie, Teil II: Spezielle Funktionssysteme, Enke Stuttgart, 177–185.
Ammon HPT, Wahl MA (1990) Pharmacology of Curcuma longa. Planta Med 57: 1–7.
Anonymus (1999) Schöllkraut – rezeptfrei und lebertoxisch. Arzneitelegramm 6/99: 65.
Baumann J (1975) Über die Wirkung von Chelidonium, Curcuma, Absinth und Carduus marianus

auf die Galle- und Pankreassekr tion bei Hepatopathien. Med Mschr 29: 173.

Bellomo A (1939) Ricerche cliniche. Giorn cad Med Torino 52: 181.

Bielenberg J (1998) Die Süßholzwurzel. Wirkungen und Anwendungen unter dem Aspekt neuer pharmakologischer Erkenntnisse. Zeitschrift für Phytotherapie 19: 197–208.

Blumenthal M, Busse WR, Goldberg A, Gruenwald J, Hall T, Riggins CW, Rister RS (eds.). Klein S, Rister RS (trans). (1998) The Complete German Commission E Monographs – Therapeutic Guide to Herbal Medicines. American Botanical Council, Austin, Texas. *www.herbalgram.org.*

Böhm K (1959) Untersuchungen über choleretische Wirkungen einiger Arzneipflanzen. Arzneim Forsch/Drug Res 9: 376.

Bowen IH, Cubbin IJ (1993) Mentha piperita and Mentha spicata. In: De Smet PAGM, Keller K, Hänsel R, Chandler RF (eds) Adverse Effects of Herbal Drugs 1. Springer Verlag, Berlin Heidelberg New York: 171–178.

Brandt W (1988) Spasmolytische Wirkung ätherischer Ole. In: Phytotherapie, Hippokrates Stuttgart, 77–89.

Brandt W (1988) Spasmolytische Wirkung ätherischer Öle. In: Phytotherapie, Hippokrates Stuttgart, 77–89.

Braun JE, Rice-Evans CA (1998) Luteolin-rich artichoke extract protects low-density lipoprotein from oxidation in vitro. Free Radical Research 29: 247–255.

Camilleri M (1999) Therapeutic approach to the patient with irritable bowel syndrome. Am J Med 107: 27S-32S.

Camilleri M, Choi MG (1997) Review article: irritable bowel syndrome. Aliment Pharmacol Ther 11: 3–15.

Carling I, Svedberg LE, Hulten S (1989) Short term treatment of the irritable bowel syndrome: a placebo-controlled trial of peppermint oil against hyoscyamine. OPMEAR 34: 55–57.

Coon JT, Ernst E (2002) Systematic review: herbal medicinal products for non-ulcer dyspepsia. Alment Pharmacol Ther 16: 1689–99.

Dew MJ, Evans BK, Rhodes J (1984) Peppermint oil for the irritable bowel syndrome: a multicentre trial. Br J Clin Pract 38: 394–395.

Dobrilla G, Comberlato M, Steele A, Vallaperta P (1989) Drug treatment of functional dyspepsia. A meta-analysis of randomized controlled clinical trials. J Clin Gastroenterol 11: 169–77.

Dresser GK, Wacher V, Ramtoola Z, Cumming K, Bailey D (2002) Peppermint oil increases the oral bioavailability of felodipine and simvastatin. Clin Pharmacol Ther 71: P67.

Duke JA (1985) CRC Handbook of medicinal Herbs. CRC Press, Boca Raton (USA): 358–359.

Englisch W, Beckers C, Unkauf M, Ruepp M, Zinserling V (2000) Efficacy of artichoke dry extract in patients hyperlipoproteinemia. Arzneim-Forsch/Drug Res 50: 260–5.

Ernst E, Pittler MH (2000) Efficacy of ginger for nausea and vomiting: a systematic review of randomized clinical trials. Br J Anaesth 84: 367–71.

Fiegel G (1971) Die amphocholeretische Wirkung der Fumaria officinalis. Z Allg Med 34: 1819.

Fintelmann V (1996) Klinische Bedeutung der lipidsenkenden und antioxidativen Wirkung von Cynara scolymus (Artischocke). In: Loew D, Rietbrock N (eds) Phytopharmaka II: Forschung und klinische Anwendung. Steinkopff Verlag, Darmstadt: 145–159.

Fintelmann V, Menßen HG, Siegers CP (1993) Phytotherapie Manual. Pharmazeutischer, pharmakologischer und therapeutischer Standard. 2nd Ed. Hippokrates Verlag Stuttgart.

Fintelmann V, Petrowicz O (1998) Langzeitanwendung von Hepar-SL forte bei dyspeptischem Symptomenkomplex: Ergebnisse einer Beobachtungsstudie. Natura med 13: 17–26.

Fintelmann V, Wegener T (2001) Curcuma longa – eine unterschätzte Heilpflanze. Deutsche Apotheker Zeitung 141: 3735-43.

Forster H (1983) Spasmolytische Wirkung pflanzlicher Carminativa. Allgemeinmedizin 59: 1327–1333.

Forster HB, Niklas H, Lutz S (1980) Antispasmodic effects of some medicinal plants. Planta med 40: 309–319.

Friedman G (1991) Treatment of the irritable bowel syndrome. Gastroenterology Clinics of North America 20: 325–333.

Gebhardt R (1997 a) Stimulation of acid secretion by extracts of Gentiana lutea L. in cultured cells from rat gastric mucosa. Pharm Pharmacol Lett 7: 106–108.

Gebhardt R (1997 b) Antioxidative and protective properties of extracts from leaves of the artichoke (Cynara scolymus L.) against hydroperoxide-induced oxidative stress in cultured rat hepatocytes. Toxicol Appl Pharmacol 144: 270–286.

Gebhardt R (1998) Inhibition of cholesterol biosynthesis in primary cultured rat hepatocytes by artichoke (Cynara scolymus L.) extracts. J Pharmacol Exp Ther 286: 1122–1128.

Gebhardt R, Fausel M (1997) Antioxidant and hepatoprotective effects of artichoke extracts and constituents in cultured rat hepatocytes. Toxicology in Vitro 11: 669–672.

Glatzel H (1968) Die Gewürze. Ihre Wirkungen auf den Menschen. Nicolaische Verlagsbuchhandlung, Herford: 170.

Glatzel H, Hackenberg K (1967) Röntgenuntersuchungen der Wirkungen von Bittermitteln auf die Verdauungsorgane. Planta Med 15: 223–232.

Gunn JWC (1920) The carminative action of volatile oils. J Pharmacol Exp Ther 6: 93–143.

Gunn JWC (1920) The carminative action of volatile oils. J Pharmacol Exp Ther 16: 93–143.

Guttenberg A (1926) Das Cholagogum Curcumen. Klin Wschr 5: 1998–1999.

Hänsel W (1997) Die Gelbwurzel – Curcuma domestica Val., Curcuma xanthorrhiza Roxb. Portrait zweier Arzneipflanzen. Zeitschrift für Phytotherapie 18: 297–306.6.

Hawthorn M, Ferrante J, Luchowski E, Rutledge A, Wei XY, Triggle DJ (1988) The actions of peppermint oil and menthol on calcium channel-dependent processes in intestinal, neuronal and cardiac preparations. Aliment Pharmacol Therap 2: 101–118.

Hills JM, Aaronson PI (1991) The mechanism of action of peppermint oil on gastrointestinal smooth muscle. Gastroenterology 101: 55–65.

Hills JM, Aaronson PI (1991) The mechanisms of action of peppermint oil on gastrointestinal smooth muscle. Gastroenterol 101: 55–65.

Holtmann G, Gschossmann JM, Buenge L, Wieland V, Heydenreich CJ (2003) Effects of a fixed combination of peppermint oil and caraway oil on symptoms and quality of life in patients suffering from functional dyspepsia. Phytomedicine 10 Suppl IV: 56–57

Inoue H, Saito K, Koshihara Y, Murota S (1986) Inhibitory effect of glyzyrrhetinic acid derivatives of lipoxygenase and prostaglandin synthetase. Chem Pharm Bull 34: 897.

Isaac D (1980) Die Kamillentherapie – Erfolg und Bestätigung. Dtsch Apoth Ztg 120: 567–570.

Jailwala J, Imperiale TF, Kroenke K (2000) Pharmacologic treatment of the irritable bowel syndrome: a systematic review of randomized, controlled trials. Ann Intern Med 133: 136–47.

Jenss H (1985) Zur Problematik funktioneller Magen-Darm-Krankheiten am Beispiel des Colon irritabile. In: Oepen I (Hrsg) An den Grenzen der Schulmedizin, eine Analyse umstrittener Methoden. Deutscher Ärzte-Verlag Cologne: 197–212.

Kammerer E, Fintelmann V (2001) Curcuma-Wurzelstock bei dyspeptischen Beschwerden – Ergebnisse einer Anwendungsbeobachtung an 440 Patienten. NaturaMed 16: 18–24.

Kassir ZA. Endoscopic controlled trial of four drug regimens in the treatment of chronic duodenal ulceration. Irish Med J. 1985; 78: 153–156.

Kirchhoff R, Beckers CH, Kirchhoff GM, Trinczek-Gärtner H, Petrowicz O, Reimann HJ (1994) Increase in choleresis by means of artichoke extract. Phytomedicine 1: 107–115.

Kohlstaedt E (1947) Choleretika, Cholekinetika und Cholagoga. Pharmazie 2: 529–536.

Kraft K (1997) Artichoke leaf extract – recent findings reflecting effects on lipid metabolism, liver and gastrointestinal tracts. Phytomedicine 4: 369–378.

Kupke D, Sanden H, Trinczek-Gärtner H, Lewin J, Blümel G, Reimann HJ (1991) Prüfung der choleretischen Aktivität eines pflanzlichen Cholagogums. Z Allg Med 67:1046–1058.

Lawson MJ, Knight RE, Tran K, Walker G, Roberts-Thomson IC (1988) Failure of enteric-coated peppermint oil in the irritable bowel syndrome: a randomized, double-blind crossover study. J Gastroenterol Hepatol 3: 235–238.

Lech AY, Olesen KM, Hey H et al. (1988) Behandling af colon irritable med pebermynteolie. Ugeskr Laeger 150: 2388–2389.

Leicester RJ, Hunt RH (1982) Peppermint oil to reduce colonic spasm during endoscopy. Lancet: 989.

Liu JH, Chen GH, Yeh HZ, Huang CK, Poon SK (1997) Enteric-coated peppermint-oil capsules in the treatment of irritable bowel syndrome: A prospective, randomized trial. J Gastroenterol 32: 765–768.

Madisch A, Heydenreich CJ, Wieland V, Hufnagel R, Hutz J (1999) Treatment of functional dyspepsia with a fixed peppermint oil and caraway oil combination preparation as compared to cisapride. Arzneim-Forsch/Drug Res 49: 925-32.

Madisch A, Hotz J (2000) Therapie von Reizmagen- und Reizdarmsyndrom aus klinischer Sicht. In: Rietbrock N (ed) Phytopharmaka VI - Foerschung und Praxis. Steinkopff, Darmstadt, pp. 193-200.

Madisch A, Melderis H, Mayr G, Sassin I, Hotz J (2001) Ein Phytotherapeuticum und seine modifizierte Rezeptur bei funktioneller Dyspepsie. Ergebnisse einer doppelblinden placebokontrollierten Vergleichsstudie. Z Gastroenterol 39: 511-7.

Madisch A, Plein K, Mayr G, Burchert D, Hotz J (2000) Benefit of a herbal preparation in patients with irritable bowel syndrome: results of a blind, randomized, placebo-controlled multicenter trial. Gastroenterology 118: A4440.

Maiwald L, Schwantes PA (1991) Curcuma xanthorrhiza Roxb., eine Heilpflanze tritt aus dem Schattendasein. Z Phytother 12: 35-445.

Manning AP, Thompson WG, Heaton KW, Morris AF (1978) Towards positive diagnosis of the irritable bowel. BMJ 2: 653-654.

Maxwell PR, Mendall MA, Kumar D (1997) Irritable bowel syndrome. The Lancet 350: 1691-1695.

May B, Köhler S, Schneider B (2000) Efficacy and tolerability of a fixed combination of peppermint oil and caraway oil in patients suffering from functional dyspepsia. Aliment Pharmacol Ther 14: 1671-7.

May B, Kuntz HD, Kieser M, Köhler S (1996) Efficacy of a fixed peppermint oil/caraway oil combination in non-ulcer dyspepsia. Arzneim-Forsch/Drug Res 46: 1449-53.

May B, Kuntz HD, Kieser M, Köhler S (1996) Efficacy of a fixed peppermint oil/caraway oil combination in non-ulcer dyspepsia. Arzneim-Forsch/Drug Res 46: 1149-1153.

Micklefield GH (2000) Fixe Kombination aus Pfefferminzöl und Kümmelöl: Übersicht zur Pharmakologie und Klinik. In: In: Rietbrock N (Hrsg.) Phytopharmaka VI - Foerschung und Praxis. Steinkopff, Darmstadt, S. 209-217

Micklefield GH, Greving I, May B (2000) Effects of peppermint oil and caraway oil on gastroduodemal motility. Phytother Res 14: 20-23.

Möller K (1947) Pharmakologie, Benno Schwabe + Co Verlag Basel, 133-136.

Nachmann M, Cole LP (1971) Role of taste in specific hungers. In: Beidler LM (ed) Handbook of Sensory Physiology, Vol IV, Chemical Senses 2, Taste, Springer. Berlin Heidelberg New York: 337-362.

Nash P, Gould SR, Barnardo DE (1986) Peppermint oil does not relieve the pain of irritable bowel syndrome. Br J Clin Pract 40: 292-293.

Nicolaidis S (1969) Early systemic responses in the regulation of food and water balance: functional and electrophysiological data. In: Neurol regulation of food and water intake. Ann NY Acad Sci 157: 1176-1203.

Nolen HW, Friend DR (1994) Menthol-β-Glucuronide: A potential prodrug for treatment of the irritable bowel syndrome. Pharmaceutical Research 11: 1707-1711.

Pirtkien R, Surhe E, Seybold G (1960) Vergleichende Untersuchungen über die choleretischen Wirkungen verschiedener Arzneimittel bei der Ratte. Med Welt 1: 1417.

Pittler MH, Ernst E (1998) Artichoke leaf extract for serum cholesterol reduction. Perfusion 11: 338-40.

Pittler MH, Ernst E (1998) Peppermint oil for irritable bowel syndrome: a critical review and meta-analysis. The American Journal of Gastroenterology 93: 1131-1135.

Rees WDW, Evans BK, Rhodes J (1979) Treating irritable bowel syndrome with peppermint oil. Brit med J II: 835-838.

Reiter M, Brandt W (1985) Erschlaffende Wirkungen auf die glatte Muskulatur von Trachea und Ileum des Meerschweinchens. Arzneim-Forsch/Drug Res 35: 408-415.

Ritter U (1984) Therapie mit Choleretika und Cholekinetika. Med Mo Pharm 7: 99-104.

Rösch W (2000) Stellenwert von Iberogast® beim Reizmagen- und Reizdarmsyndrom. In: Rietbrock N (Hrsg.) Phytopharmaka VI - Foerschung und Praxis. Steinkopff, Darmstadt, pp. 201-207.

Schilcher H (1987) Die Kamille. Handbuch für Ärzte, Apotheker und andere Naturwissenschaftler.

Wissenschaftliche Verlagsgesellschaft, Stuttgart.

Schilcher H (1997) Schöllkraut – Chelidonium majus L. Portrait einer Arzneipflanze. Zeitschrift für Phytotherapie 18: 356–366.

Schneider MME, Otten MH (1990) Efficacy of Colpermin in the treatment of patients with irritable bowel syndrome. Gastroenterology 98: A389.

Schwenk HU, Horbach L (1978) Vergleichende klinische Untersuchung über die Wirksamkeit von Carminativum-Hetterich bei Kindern mittels wiederholter Sonographie des Abdomens. Therapiewoche 28: 2610–2615.

Shaw G, Scrivastava ED, Sadlier M et al. (1991) Stress management for irritable bowel syndrome: a controlled trial. Digestion 50: 36–42.

Sigmund ChJ, McNally EF (1969) The action of a carminative on the lower esophageal sphincter. Gastroenterol 56: 13–188

Sommerville KW, Richmond CR, Bell GD (1984) Delayed-release peppermint oil capsules (Colpermin) for the spastic colon syndrome: a pharmacokinetic study. Br J Clin Pharmac 18: 638–640.

Talley NJ, Stanghellini V, Heading RC et al. (1999) Functional gastroduodenal disorders. Gut 45 (Suppl II) II37–II42.

Tamura Y, Nishikawa T, Yamada K, Yamamoto M, Kumagai A (1979) Effects of glyzyrrhetinic acid and its derivatives on $\Delta 4$-5α- and 5β-reductase in rat liver. Arzneimittel Forsch/Drug Res 29: 647.

Tan RX, Zheng WF, Tan HQ (1998) Biologically active substances from the genus Artemisia. Planta Med 64: 295–302.

Taylor BA, Luscombe DK, Duthie HL (1983) Inhibitory effect of peppermint on gastrointestinal smooth muscle. Gut 24: A992 (Abstract).

Thompson WG, Creed F, Drossman DA, Heaton KW, Mazzacca G (1992) Functional bowel disease and functional abdominal pain. Gastroenterology International 5: 75–91.

Vutyavanich T, Kraisarin T, Ruangsri RA (2001) Ginger for nausea and vomiting in pregnancy: randomized, double-masked placebo-controlled trial. Obstet Gynecol 97: 577–82.

Weiß RF (1991) Lehrbuch der Phytotherapie. 7th Ed. Hippokrates Verlag Stuttgart.

White DA, Thompson SP, Wilson CG, Bell GD (1987) A pharmacokinetic comparison of two delayed-release peppermint oil preparations, Colpermin and Mintec, for treatment of the irritable bowel syndrome. Int J Pharmaceutics 40: 151–155.

Wichtl M (ed) (1989) Teedrogen. Wissenschaftliche Verlagsgesellschaft mbH Stuttgart: 372–374.

5.5   Acute Diarrhea

Diarrhea refers to the frequent (more than 3 times daily) passage of a liquid or semi-liquid stool. Acute diarrhea has an abrupt onset, usually lasts only 3–4 days, often has an infectious cause, and tends to be self-limiting. Chronic diarrhea persists longer than 4 weeks and may be symptomatic of a chronic underlying illness such as ulcerative colitis, Crohn's disease, or hyperthyroidism. Causal treatment of the underlying disease is essential in all chronic forms of diarrhea. Brief episodes of acute diarrhea in particular warrant the use of symptomatic measures that may be both dietary and pharmacologic. Phytomedicines have a significant role, both as traditional home remedies and as galenic preparations, in the symptomatic treatment of diarrhea. Three groups of preparations are particularly important: tannin-containing herbs, pectins, and a special strain of live dried yeast.

5.5.1 Tannin-Containing Herbs

Tannins have a protein-precipitating action. When applied to mucous membranes, tannins cause proteins to be deposited on the epithelial surface, the precipitate forming a stable, coherent membrane. Particularly in the intestinal tract, this process could line the bowel lumen with a protective film that would hamper the absorption of toxins, blunt the action of local irritants, and normalize hyperperistalsis (Sollmann, 1948). This classic hypothesis on the mechanism of action of tannins is plausible but still needs to be confirmed by controlled clinical studies.

Table 5.5 reviews the tannin-containing herbs and preparations that are most commonly used in the treatment of acute diarrhea. Most tannins in this series are chemical derivatives of the pentahydroxyflavanol catechin. They are water-soluble oligomeric or polymeric products that are resistant to acid hydrolysis. Some herbs contain both catechins and gallotannins. Tannic acid, a mixture of the tannins found in oak bark, is a pure gallotannin. Pure gallotannins are extensively hydrolyzed in the upper small bowel, so they can produce little if any astringent action in the colon. Reportedly, tannins can be bound to albumin (tannalbin) to make them bioavailable in the colon as well.

5.5.1.1 Green and Black Tea

By far the most pleasant way to take tannins is to ingest them in the form of green or black tea. The tea should be steeped for 15–20 min, however, to release as much of the tannins as possible; this will necessarily impart a bitter taste to the beverage.

Black and green tea are both derived from the tea shrub (*Camellia sinensis*, formerly known also as *Thea sinensis*), an evergreen woody plant that is native predominantly to southeastern Asia and can grow to 5 m (Fig. 5.10). The cultivated plant is pruned to a bushy shrub to facilitate harvesting. The leaves are harvested and dried to yield the crude drug. The quality and action of a tea depend on the provenance and age of the

Table 5.5.

Tannin-containing herbs and preparations for the treatment of acute diarrhea.

Herb or preparation	Active constituents	Average daily dose
Green or black tea	5.20 % Tannins 2–5 % Caffeine 1 % Volatile oil	3–10 g of crude drug[1]
Bilberry	5–10 % Tannins 1 % Fruits acids	20–60 g of berries[2]
Witch hazel leaf and bark	5–15 % Tannins	0.1–1 g of crude drug[3]
Tormentil root	15–20 % Tannins	2–6 g of crude drug[1]
Oak bark	10–20 % Tannins	2–6 g of crude drug[1]
Albumin tannate	ca. 50 % Tannins	2–4 g

[1] prepare as infusion (tea); [2] dried berries; use about 5 times more fresh berries; [3] for external use only.

tea leaves (young shoots > younger leaves > older leaves) and on their initial processing:

▶ Green tea consists of leaves that are heated immediately after harvesting, mechanically rolled and crushed, and then dried to prevent enzymatic changes. In this way
the natural constituents and color of the tea leaf are essentially preserved. As a result,
green tea (haysan, gunpowder, imperial, etc.) has a particularly high tannin content
and is strongly astringent.
▶ Black tea is produced by fermentation. The leaves are wilted before they are rolled
and then left in a humid environment for several hours to promote enzymatic changes in the herb, which gradually turn reddish brown. The herb is then dried to yield
the black leaf that has a distinctive varietal flavor (e.g., pekoe, souchong, congo).

In 12 healthy test subjects who consumed 2 L of tea daily (containing 8 g of herb), intestinal transit time after 4 days was significantly prolonged relative to a group taking a
placebo (Hojgaard, 1981). The excretion of bile acids in the stool was decreased, and
increased amounts of oxalic acid were excreted in the urine. In interpreting the results,
the authors attributed the constipating action less to the tannin content of the tea than
to its theophylline content, reasoning that the increased glomerular filtration led to extracellular dehydration resulting in greater fluid absorption from the bowel. However,
the very small amount of theophylline (5–10 mg/L) casts doubt on this interpretation,
and it appears more likely that tannins are the key active principle (Table 5.5.1).

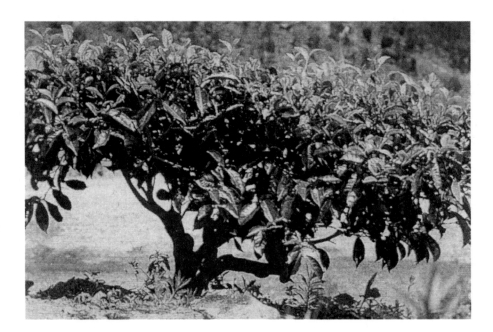

Figure 5.10. ▲ The tea shrub (*Camellia sinensis*).

When proper attention is given to the caffeine content of tea (Sect. 2.2.1.1), the usage risks are minimal. The tannins could become hepatotoxic if tea were consumed to excess by an individual with preexisting liver damage. For example, one woman who consumed an amount of tea equivalent to 65 g of tea leaves daily for 5 years developed liver dysfunction. But splenomegaly and ascites resolved after the tea was withdrawn (Martindale, 1989).

Ludewig (1995) and Scholz and Bertram (1995) have published up-to-date reviews of the actions and side effects of black and green tea for culinary and medicinal use. Blumenthal et al. (2003) have reviewed 29 clinical trials on the actions of green and black tea and related tea-based phytomedicinal preparations (Blumenthal et al., 2003).

5.5.1.2 Other Tannin-Containing Herbs

Bilberries (European blueberries) are the dried ripe fruit of *Vaccinium myrtillus*, a dwarf shrub of the family Ericaceae. Dried bilberries contain 5–10 % catechins, about 30 % invertose, and small amounts of flavonone glycosides and anthocyanosides, particularly glycosides of malvidin, cyanidin, and delphinidin.

Bilberries are used either by soaking 20–60 g of dried berries (daily dose) in water or red wine, then chewing well and swallowing, or by consuming fresh or freshly preserved berries in an amount 5–10 times the quantity of the dried herb. Bilberries are a home remedy for the treatment of acute, nonspecific diarrhea and are particularly recommended in school-age children.

Tormentil rhizome, known also as cinquefoil or potentilla, is the dried rhizome of *Potentilla erecta*, an herbaceous plant of the family Rosaceae that is widely distributed in Europe and North America. Tormentil is odorless and has a strongly astringent taste. The herb contains catechins (15–20 %) and tannins (1–2 %), including agrimoniin as the main component (Lund and Rimpler, 1985). It is used chiefly as a tea (2–3 g herb in 1 cup water 150 mL). The recommended dose for acute nonspecific diarrhea is 1 cup 2–3 times daily between meals. Nausea or vomiting may occur in sensitive individuals.

Oak bark consists of the dried bark of young twigs of *Quercus robur* harvested in the spring. It contains 1–20 % tannins, including a high content of gallotannins. The Commission E monograph states that oak bark is used externally for inflammatory skin diseases and internally for nonspecific acute diarrhea; it is also applied locally for mild inflammatory conditions involving the mouth, throat, genitalia, or anal region (Blumenthal et al., 1998). Patients with diarrhea should take oak bark for no longer than 3–4 days. Oak bark is reported to have antiviral activity in addition to its astringent properties.

5.5.1.3 Tannic Acid and Albumin Tannate

Tannic acid, obtained from nutgalls, is a heterogeneous mixture of various esters of gallic acid with glucose. The brownish yellow powder, which has a faint but characteristic odor and a puckery taste, disperses readily in water to form a colloid. Tannic acid has an astringent action when applied locally in concentrations of 1:20,000 to 1:50,000.

Higher concentrations can be cytotoxic, and oral administration may irritate the gastric mucosa and cause vomiting.

Gallotannins are hydrolyzed in the small intestine, forming free gallic acid that does not have an astringent action. Therefore, they are administered therapeutically in the form of albumin tannate, a protein-tannic acid compound with a tannin content of about 50 %. Heating the reaction product to 110–120 °C makes it resistant to gastric juices and delays tannin release until the product reaches the alkaline medium of the intestine; there the tannin is released gradually, producing an astringent action in the small intestine and colon. Whereas orally administered tannin does not enter the stool, free tannin is detected in the stool following the administration of albumin tannate. The average single dose is 0.5–1 g; the daily dose for adults is 2–4 g.

5.5.2 Pectins

Pectins are biopolymers with molecular weights of 60,000 to 90,000. Their basic structural framework is formed by galacturonic acid molecules. Numerous acid groups give pectins their ability to hold water and form gels. These gels are not attacked by digestive enzymes and pass unchanged into the colon, where they are broken down by colonic bacteria. In the small intestine, pectin gels can form a protective film on the mucosa. But bacterial degradation precludes this type of action in the colon, so a different antidiarrhetic mechanism is required. One hypothesis is that the short-chain fatty acids released from the microbial breakdown of pectins in the colon have an inhibitory action on colonic motility (Yajima, 1985).

Pectins consistently accompany cellulose, so they contribute much to the structural integrity of the cell and of the plant in general. Pectins are present to some degree in all plant products but are particularly abundant in fleshy fruits and storage roots. Rich commercial sources are sugar beet fragments, apple residue, orange and lemon waste product, and carrots. The following "home remedies" are dietary constituents have proven useful in the treatment of diarrhea:

▶ 1–1,5 kg of raw greated apples, eaten throughout the day;
▶ bananas, cut into small pieces and eaten as often as desired (particularly recommended for children);
▶ carrot preparations are suitable for infants and small children, e.g.: boil 500 g of peeled carrots in 1 L of water for 1–2h, pour through a strainer, and puree in a blender. Add water to make 1 L, and add 3 g of table salt (Schulte and Spranger, 1988)

5.5.3 Live Dried Yeast

While traveling through Indochina in 1923, the French mycologist Henri Boulard noticed that the native population used the skins of tropical fruits as a remedy for diarrhea. Boulard found that a yeast isolated from the surface of these fruits had antidiarrheal properties. The Centraalbureu voor Schimmelcultures in the Netherlands classifies this tropical wild yeast as *Saccharomyces cerevisiae* Hansen CBS 5926, but it is known internationally as *S. boulardii*.

Yeasts occur ubiquitously in nature wherever there are fermentable juices with a high sugar content. The best known variety is brewer's yeast (*Saccharomyces cerevisiae*) Unlike bacteria, yeasts have a true cell nucleus and are classified as fungi. This makes *S. boulardii* a member of the plant kingdom, so its medicinal use is a form of phytotherapy.

For commercial production the yeast strain is grown in large fluid cultures and freeze-dried; the lyophilization preserves the viability of the cells. The optimum development temperature is 30–40 °C, corresponding to the normal temperature range in the bowel. Lactose is added to the lyophilisate for technical reasons (to allow the precise filling of capsules). Microbiologic and microscopic quality control measures are conducted to check the purity of the cultures and the viability of the cells.

5.5.3.1 Pharmacology and Toxicology

The antidiarrheal action of *S. boulardii* is based on its antagonistic effects on pathogenic microorganisms and its stimulatory effect on the enteric immune system. Its therapeutic efficacy depends on the viability of the yeast cells (Massot et al., 1982), which must be sustained as the cells pass through the intestinal tract. On entering the colon, however, the cells undergo a bacterial breakdown that leaves only 0.05 % of the ingested dose of yeast cells to be excreted in the stool. *S. boulardii* is antagonistic to a number of pathogenic microorganisms, which are damaged or destroyed by the presence of the cells (Böckeler and Thomas, 1989). One study showed that mannose structures on the surface of the yeast cells enable them to bind and entrap fimbriated pathogenic *E. coli* (Gedek, 1989). *S. boulardii* can also reduce the activity of bacterial toxins (Czerucka et al., 1994). Other experimental studies showed that the yeast has a stimulatory effect on the natural immune system of the bowel (Jahn and Zeits, 1991).

According to the Commission E monograph of 1994, no toxic reactions were observed in mice and rats given a single oral dose of 3 g/kg (Blumenthal et al., 1998). Similarly, doses of approximately 330 mg/kg given to dogs for 6 weeks and doses of 100 g/kg given to rats and rabbits for 6 months caused no adverse changes. The Ames test showed no evidence of mutagenicity.

5.5.3.2 Therapeutic Efficacy

Five double-blind studies were performed between 1983 and 1993 to test the therapeutic efficacy of Perenterol 5, a standardized preparation of *S. boulardii*, in various forms of acute diarrhea.

Tempé et al. (1983) tested the efficacy of *S. boulardii* in preventing nutritionally related diarrhea in 40 patients fed by gavage. When the yeast preparation was added prophylactically to the nutrient solutions, the incidence of diarrhea averaged 8.7 % compared with 16.9 % in patients given a placebo. The difference between the two treatment groups was statistically significant.

Kollaritsch et al. (1988) tested the efficacy of *S. boulardii* in preventing travel-related diarrhea. In a group of 1231 travelers, 406 were given a placebo, 426 received the yeast preparation in a dose of 250 mg/day, and 399 received a dose of 500 mg/day. The treatment was started 5 days before the subjects began their travels and was continued throughout their stay in tropical or subtropical regions. The incidence of diarrhea was 42.6 % in the placebo group, 33.6 % in the low-dose treatment group, and 31.8 % in the higher-dose treatment group. The reduction in both treatment groups was statistically significant relative to the placebo.

Surawicz et al. (1989) tested the efficacy of *S. boulardii* in preventing antibiotic-associated diarrhea. The 180 patients in the study were divided into two groups, one receiving a placebo and the other receiving 500 mg/day of the yeast preparation during at least a 3-day course of antibiotic therapy. The incidence of diarrhea was 22 % in the placebo-treated group versus only 9.5 % in the yeast-treated group. Again, the difference between the groups was statistically significant ($p<0.04$).

Höchter et al. (1990) performed a study in 92 ambulatory patients with acute diarrhea. One group was given a daily dose of 300–600 mg of *S. boulardii*, the other a placebo. The patients treated with *S. boulardii* showed a significantly greater reduction in their stool-frequency and -quality score (the main study criterion) than the placebo group after 4 days' treatment (respective score changes of –17.2 and –13.6; $p<0.04$).

Plein and Hotz (1993) conducted a pilot study in 20 patients with Crohn's disease. First, all the patients were given 750 mg of *S. boulardii* daily for 14 days. The average frequency of bowel movements declined during this period from 5 to 4.4 per day. At 14 days, half the patients continued to receive *S. boulardii* while the other half were switched to a placebo. The frequency of bowel movements continued to decline in the yeast-treated group (to 3.3/day) but returned to the initial value (5/day) in the control group.

5.5.3.3 Indications, Dosages, Risks, and Contraindications

The Commission E monograph of 1994 states that the dried yeast *Saccharomyces boulardii* is used for the symptomatic treatment of acute diarrhea and the prevention and symptomatic treatment of diarrhea associated with travel or feeding by gavage (Blumenthal et al., 1998). The monograph also notes its adjunctive use in the treatment of chronic forms of acne.

The recommended dose is 250–500 mg/day, with a daily dose of 500 mg recommended for diarrhea related to feeding by gavage. For the prevention of travel-related diarrhea, treatment should be initiated 5 days before the start of the trip. In cases of acute diarrhea, treatment should be continued for several days after symptoms have abated.

There have been reports of bloating and sporadic intolerance reactions in the form of itching, urticaria, and generalized skin eruptions. Yeast sensitivity is a contraindication. A fall in blood pressure may occur as a drug interaction in patients who are also taking a monoamine oxidase inhibitor.

5.5.4 Other herbal Antidiarrheals

Opium the air-dried milky sap obtained from the unripe capsules of the opium poppy (*Papaver somniferum*), has a powerful constipating effect. Opium contains 20–25 %

alkaloids, including 7–20 % morphine, which is chiefly responsible for this action. Opium does not actually immobilize the bowel; it intensifies its contractions (segmental constrictions), producing a state of spastic constipation (Ewe, 1983). Opium and its derivative morphine are not herbal medications in the true sense (they are plant-derived conventional drugs; see Sect.1.2) and are outside the scope of this volume.

Calumbo root is obtained from *Jateorrhiza palmata*, a woody vine (liana) native to tropical eastern Africa. Pieces of the bulbous, fleshy roots are dug up, washed, sliced, and dried, yielding a crude drug that contains 1–2 % berberine-type alkaloids along with bitter principles. As for therapeutic applications, it is interesting to note older pharmacologic results indicating that the herb is similar to morphine in its ability to increase resting tonus. Because the side effects of calumbo root are comparable to those of morphine, the herb is no longer important as an antidiarrheal.

Uzara root is obtained from *Xysmalobium undulatum*, a native South African herb that apparently has been used for centuries as a remedy for diarrhea. The underground parts are harvested from 2- to 3-year-old plants. Alcohol-water extracts from uzara roots were introduced to Germany in 1911 as an herbal remedy for acute diarrhea. The crude drug contains at least 6 % glycosides, the most important of which are uzarin and uzarigenin, the latter resembling digitoxigenin in its chemical structure. Uzara root extracts act mainly by inhibiting the motility of the visceral smooth muscle, probably via the local stimulation of sympathetic nerves. This action is qualitatively similar to that of papaverine. At higher doses, the uzara glycosides exert digitalis-like effects on the heart. The lethal dose of dry extract in dogs is approximately 100–200 mg/kg body weight (Schmitz et al., 1992). The Commission E monograph of 1990 states that uzara root preparations are used for treating nonspecific acute diarrhea and cites concomitant treatment with cardioactive glycosides as a contraindication (Blumenthal et al., 1998). The monograph further states that the single adult dose should be equivalent to 500–100 mg of total glycosides. An observational study in 552 patients published by the manufacturer of an uzara product showed surprisingly good tolerance after 2–6 days' treatment with an average total dose of 200 mg of extract, which is equivalent to approximately 60 mg of total glycosides. Only one patient (0.18 %) experienced an adverse reaction (pruritus) that prompted the discontinuation of treatment. Measured by a total score for diarrhea symptoms, the treatment was effective in approximately 80 % of all patients (Anonymous, 1994).

Carob bean or St. John's bread is obtained from the evergreen tree *Ceratonia siliqua*, native to the Mediterranean region. A meal made from carob seeds makes a safe, natural antidiarrheal that is particularly useful in infants, toddlers, and children. A special extraction process is used to produce this meal from portions of the carob seed. Carob seed meal consists of galactomannoglycans (about 88 %) and other polysaccharides (5 %) in addition to proteins and minerals. Its molecular weight is 310,000 daltons, signifying a high degree of polymerization (d.p. 19,000). A branched linear heteropolysaccharide, it has a high water-holding capacity even in low concentrations (50 to 100 times its dry weight). Besides its use as an antidiarrheal, carob seed meal is also used as a component of low-calorie diets.

5.5.5 Suggested Formulations

Antidiarrheal tea

Rx	Black tea leaves	40.0
	Balm leaves	20.0
	Fennelseed, crushed	20.0
	Centaury	20.0
	Mix to make tea	

Directions: Prepare 2 teaspoons in 1 cup as an infusion; steep 10–20 min.

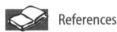 References

Anonymus (1994) Anwendung von Uzarabei unspezifischen Durchfallerkrankungen. Wissenschaftlicher Abschlußbericht, STADA Arzneimittel AG.

Blumenthal M, Hall T, Goldberg A. (eds.) (2003) The ABC Clinical Guide to Herbs. Austin, Tex: American Botanical Council.

Blumenthal M, Busse WR, Goldberg A, Gruenwald J, Hall T, Riggins CW, Rister RS (eds.). Klein S, Rister RS (trans). (1998) The Complete German Commission E Monographs – Therapeutic Guide to Herbal Medicines. American Botanical Council, Austin, Texas. *www.herbalgram.org.*

Böckeler, W. Thomas G (1989) In-vitro-Studien zur destabilisierenden Wirkung Lyophilisierter Saccharomyces cereviseae Hansen CBS 5926-Zellen auf Enterobakterien. Läßt sich diese Eigenschaft biochemisch erklären? In: Müller J, Ottenhann R, Seifert J (eds) Ökosystem Darm. Springer Verlag, pp 142–253.

Czerucka D, Roux I, Rampal P (1994) Sacccharomyces boulardii inhibits secretagogue-mediated adenosine 3',5'-cyclic monophosphate induction in intestinal cells. Gastroenterology 106: 65–72.

Ewe K (1983) Obstipation – Pathophysiologie, Klinik, Therapie. Int Welt 6: 286–292.

Gedek B, Hagenhoff G (1989) Orale Verabreichung von lebensfähigen Zellen des Hefestammes Saccharomyces cerevisiae Hansen CBS 5926 und deren Schicksal während der Magen-Darm-Passage. Therapiewoche 38 (special issue): 33–40.

Höchter W, Chase D, Hagenhoff G (1990) Saccharomyces boulardii bei akuter Erwachsenendiarrhoe. Münch Med Wschr 132: 188–192.

Hojgaard I, Arffmann S, Jorgenson M, Krag E (1981) Tea consumption: a cause of constipation. Br Med J 282: 864.

Jahn HU, Zeitz M (1991) Immunmodulatorische Wirkung von Saccharomyces boulardii beim Menschen. In: Seifert J, Ottenhann R, Zeitz M, Brockenmühl J (eds). Ökosystem Darm III. Springer Verlag, pp 159–164.

Kollaritsch HH, Tobüren D, Scheiner O, Wiedermann G (1988) Prophylaxe der Reisediarrhoe. Münch Med Wschr 130: 671–673.

Ludewig R (1995) Schwarzer und Grüner Tee als Genuß- und Heilmittel. Dtsch Apoth Z 135: 2203–2218.

Lund K, Rimpler H (1985) Tormentillwurzel. Dtsch Apoth Z 125: 1105–107.

Reynolds JEF (ed) (1989) Martindale. The Extra Pharmacopoeia. 29th Ed. The Pharmaceutical Press, London, p 1535.

Massot J, Desconclois M, Astoin J (1982) Protection par Saccharomyces boulardii de la diarrhée à Escherichia coli du souriceau. Ann Pharm Fr 40: 445–449.

Plein K, Hotz J (1993) Therapeutic effect of Saccharomyces boulardii on mild residual symptoms in a stable phase of Crohn's disease with special reference to chronic diarrhea – a pilot study. Z. Gastroenterol 31: 129–134.

Schmitz B, El Agamy R, Lindner K (1992) Uzarawurzel – seit 80 Jahren bewährt bei akuten Druchfallerkrankungen. Pharmazeutische Zeitung 137: 1697–1713.

Scholz E, Bertram B (1995) Camelia sinensis (L.) O. Kuntze – Der Teestrauch. Z Phytother 17: 235–250.

Schulte FJ, Spranger J (1988) Lehrbuch der Kinderheilkunde. Fischer, Stuttgart, p 320.

Sollmann T (1948) A Manual of Pharmacology. 7th Ed. Saunders Company, Philadelphia London, p 110.

Surawicz C, Elmer GW, Speelman P, McFarland LV, Chinn J, van Belle G (1989) Die Prophylaxe Antibiotika-assoziierter Diarrhöen mit Saccharomyces boulardii. Eine prospektive Studie. Gastroenterol 96: 981–988.

Tempé JD, Steidel AL, Blehaut H, Hasselmann M, Lutun P, Maurier F (1983) Prévention par Saccharomyces boulardii des diarrhées de l'alimentation entérale à débit continu. La Semaine des Hôpitaux de Paris 59: 1409–1412.

Yajima T (1985) Contractile effect of short-chain fatty acids on the isolated colon of the rat. J Physiol 368: 667–678.

5.6 Constipation

5.6.1 Symptoms, Causes, General Measures

Constipation is characterized by findings and complaints that are based largely on the frequency and difficulty of bowel movements. Constipation is considered to be present when the frequency of bowel movements is less than once in 2–3 days. But constipation assumes pathologic significance by its subjective features, i.e., straining heavily at stool, painful defecation, and a feeling of incomplete evacuation (Table 5.6). Constipation is often accompanied by other types of discomfort such as abdominal cramping, a feeling of fullness, or autonomic dysfunction. Constipation alternating with bouts of diarrhea is a feature of irritable colon (IBS) (Sect.5.4).

Constipation of acute onset may have a trivial cause such as a change in diet, travel, or a febrile illness with confinement to bed. Numerous drugs, including antacids and anticholinergics, can also lead to constipation. A new irregularity in bowel habits with no obvious cause should always be investigated due to the risk of malignant disease, e.g., colon cancer. But in the great majority of cases, the cause of chronic constipation is functional in nature. The following factors are important in the pathogenesis of constipation:

▶ a faulty lifestyle (lack of exercise) and poor eating habits (low-fiber diet, hasty or irregular meals);
▶ psychological factors such as ignoring the urge to defecate due to emotional stress or an exaggerated personal cleanliness;
▶ fear of disease or self-poisoning leading to pseudoconstipation (Ewe, 1983).

Thus, the treatment of chronic constipation should always start with dietary counseling and, where appropriate, psychotherapeutic counseling. Dietary counseling should include specific recommendations for increasing the intake of dietary fiber, increasing fluid intake (4–6 glasses of water during the morning hours) and, when increased use

Table 5.6.
Syndrome of constipation (Ewe, 1988).

Findings and complaints	Explanations
Infrequent passage of stool	Less than three bowel movements a week
Difficult passage of stool	Straining at stool
Passing stools of hard consistency	Small, hard stools
Passing scant stool	Small stool volume (<50g)
Subjective sensations	Sense of delayed, difficult, and incomplete evacuation

Table 5.7.
Herbs used as bulk laxatives for the treatment of constipation.

Herbs	Daily dose[1]	Remarks
Linseed	30–50 g	Take in the form of crushed whole seeds
Wheat bran	20–40 g	Not for use in small children or patients with glutin-induced enteropathy
Psyllium	5–10 g	Husks have 3 times the fiber content of the seeds (reduce daily dose to 3 g)
Agar	5–10 g	Bulk laxative stimulates peristalsis by increasing the stool volume

[1] Should be taken with liquid volume equal to about 10 times the dose volume

of bulking agents and fiber are not successful, resorting to stimulant laxatives (e.g., the anthronoid-containing herbs like rhubarb root, cascara sagrada, senna leaf or fruit) is recommended. Physical measures should include an exercise program to strengthen the abdominal muscles, perhaps abdominal-wall massage, and a general recommendation for more exercise. Phytotherapy starts with a recommendation and prescription for bulk-forming agents. Stimulant laxatives, especially anthranoid-containing herbs, are agents of second choice.

5.6.2 Bulk-Forming Agents

These products (Table 5.7), consisting of bulking and swelling agents, are gentle, low-risk laxatives that stimulate the physiologic effects of a high-fiber diet. Their water-binding capacity also makes them useful for the symptomatic treatment of diarrhea in some patients. Bulk-forming agents are also widely recognized for their value in the long-term management of IBS and chronic diverticulitis.

5.6.2.1 Mechanism of Action

The term bulking agent is used synonymously in this chapter with bulk materials and dietary fiber. Bulking agents are normally ingested as components of food. They are composed of indigestible carbohydrates, which may undergo complete (pectins) or partial breakdown (bran) by colonic bacteria. These substances stimulate bowel activity through their mechanical, bulk-producing action and hasten the transit of fecal material through the intestinal tract. All bulking agents can swell to a degree through the uptake of water, and the distinction from swelling agents in purely quantitative. Swelling agents in the strict sense are distinguished by their capacity to form mucilages or gels. They are virtually synonymous with the thickening agents used in food processing and with the mucilaginous agents used in pharmacy and medicine (Hutz and Rösch, 1988). Mucilaginous swelling agents usually are not contained in foods but are taken in medicinal form (e.g., psyllium husks) or in the form of a crude herbal product (e.g., karaya gum). Like bulking agents, they are composed of indigestible carbohydrates, but they differ from bulking agents in that they undergo little or no degradation by intestinal flora.

To understand the mechanism of action of bulk-forming agents, it is helpful to know the relationships between stool weight, intestinal transit time, and the quantitative composition of the feces. Intestinal transit time is the period that elapses between the ingestion of food and the excretion of its indigestible components as feces. Transit time is greatly influenced by the content of indigestible food constituents.

Bulk materials have little effect on transit time through the small intestine, but they do affect colonic transit. The heavier the stool weight, the shorter the transit time. Besides their absolute quantity, the composition of indigestible materials is also important. Surprisingly, the increase in fecal bulk caused by water absorption appears to be less crucial to the action of bulk-forming agents than their content of pentosans. For example, 20 g of wheat bran increases stool weight by 127 % whereas 5 g of guar, despite its high water-binding capacity, increases stool weight by only 20 % (Cummings, 1978).

Therefore, it appears that the stimulation of bowel motility caused by an increase in fecal bulk is not the only determinant of efficacy. Another key factor is the modification of the intestinal flora. The colon is inhabited by more than 400 bacterial species, whose precise makeup is determined by the nature of the available substrate. Bacteria constitute more than 50 % of the total dry mass of the feces (Stephen and Cummings, 1980). Bulk materials provide the bacterial flora with a substrate for their proliferation, causing an increase in bacterial mass and stool weight. Because the bacteria are specific to particular substrates, a latent period of 4–6 weeks is needed to establish a more suitable intestinal flora. This concept is supported by studies in healthy subjects in which a 3-week period of increased dietary fiber intake was necessary before significant changes occurred in transit time and stool weight (Cummings et al., 1978).

The celluloses, hemicelluloses, lignins, and pectins contained in bulk-forming agents are resistant to human digestive enzymes so they pass unchanged through the small intestine into the colon. The colonic bacteria can then break down all or part of the bulk materials, mainly releasing short-chain fatty acids (particularly acetic, propionic, and butyric acids) along with methane, carbon dioxide, and molecular hydrogen. It has been suggested that the metabolism of short-chain fatty acids in the colonic mucosa may have a protective role in maintaining normal mucosal function (bibliography in Kasper, 1985). But the main significance of the short-chain fatty acids is their ability to promote the absorption of salts and water (Ruppin et al, 1980) and to provide osmotic stimuli that promote colonic motility (Yajima, 1985). Swelling agents make the stool softer and enable it to pass through the bowel more easily. It has also been postulated that swelling agents stimulate intrinsic intestinal activity by causing distention of the bowel wall.

Gases generated by bacterial breakdown in the lower bowel may cause bloating and flatulence, and constipation may worsen during the first two weeks following initial consumption of bulking agents. Generally these symptoms resolve once a new intestinal flora has been established. It may be useful to start treatment with one-half the normal dosage. A change of product may become necessary in some cases (Fingl, 1980).

It is imperative that bulk-forming agents be taken with sufficient liquid. The amount of liquid depends on the swelling capacity of the agent and generally is 5 to 10 times the dry weight of the agent. Stenotic lesions of the gastrointestinal tract contraindicate the use of bulk-forming agents. Even in the absence of such lesions, treatment with bulking agents may rarely lead to bowel obstruction, underscoring the urgency of an adequate fluid intake. Bulk-forming agents should not be taken at bedtime or while the patient is lying down. They should not be used in conjunction with an antiperistaltic (e.g., loperamide).

5.6.2.2 Linseed

Linseed consists of the dried, ripe seeds of flax (*Linum usitatissimum*, Fig. 5.11), one of the world's oldest cultivated plants. Linseed is grown for its oil-bearing seeds and for its fiber. The seeds of the annual herb are odorless and, when placed in the mouth, slowly acquire a mucilaginous taste. The main constituents are mucilages (7-12 %), fatty oil (about 40 %), protein (about 23 %), as well as crude fiber, minerals, and cyanogenic glycosides (about 1 %).

The key swelling constituents of linseed are the mucilages, which are located in the epidermis of the seed husk. The seed must be ground, or preferably cracked, so that it can absorb fluid and swell. Cracking or crushing allows rapid swelling without releasing large amounts of fatty oil (about 500 kcal in 100 g linseed) for intestinal absorption. The whole seeds have a significantly longer shelf life, for the highly unsaturated fatty acids in linseed meal quickly become rancid when exposed to atmospheric oxygen.

The seeds swell to several times their dry volume. Linseed mucilage retains its colloidal structure even in the acid milieu of the stomach, and its swelling and lubricating properties are undiminished by the weakly alkaline medium of the small intestine. The bulk materials are also thought to contribute to the stimulation of peristalsis. Onset of action is preceded by a latent period of several days (Sewing, 1986).

Risk from Hydrogen Cyanide
Due to its content of linamarin, a cyanogenic glycoside, linseed (along with bitter almonds) was long considered a potential source of dietary hydrogen cyanide (HCN) poisoning. One hundred grams of linseed contains approximately 30 mg of HCN (by comparison, 100 g of bitter almonds contains about 250 mg). The lethal dose of HCN for humans is approximately 50–100 mg. But while HCN is absorbed in minutes through the gastric mucosa when administered in, say, cyanogenic salts such as potassium cyanide, only very low blood levels of HCN were found after the ingestion of 100 g linseed. Similarly low levels were detected after the consumption of 10 bitter almonds, but eating 50 bitter almonds produced blood levels that were life-threatening in one test subject (Schulz et al., 1983) (Fig. 5.12).

Figure 5.11. ▶ Flowering tops of linseed (*Linum usitatissimum*).

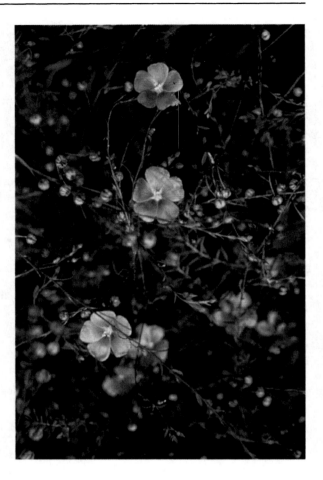

One reason for the nonlinear absorption and elimination kinetics of HCN in the body lies in the enzyme-dependency of the release of HCN from its glycosidic bond. In the case of linseed, this cleavage is catalyzed by the plant enzyme linamarase; the acidic gastric juice partially inactivates this enzyme, slowing the release of HCN. Once it is absorbed, HCN is subject to transformation by the enzyme rhodanase, which is present in the mitochondria of all somatic cells and rapidly converts small amounts of HCN into the harmless compound thiocyanate. The rhodanase detoxification system has a limited capacity, however. The sudden ingestion of large amounts of HCN can easily overwhelm this system, leading to swift and fatal poisoning (Schulz, 1984).

In a controlled study, 20 healthy subjects ingested 30 or 100 g of cracked linseed acutely followed by 45 g daily over a period of 4 weeks. None of the subjects showed a significant rise in HCN blood levels. The HCN metabolite thiocyanate did show rising serum levels during the course of the treatment period, accompanied by an average 75 % increase in the urinary excretion of thiocyanate, comparable to the elevations typically measured in heavy smokers. This moderate accumulation of thiocyanate did not imply any special risks or contraindications (Schulz et al., 1983).

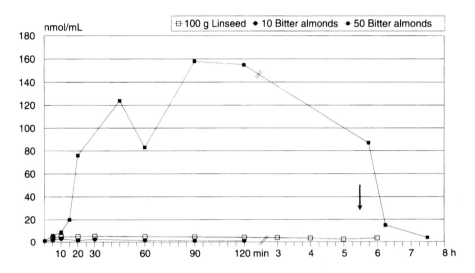

Figure 5.12. ▲ Cyanide level in a volunteer who ingested linseed and bitter almonds. At 5.5 hours (↓), 1 g of sodium thiosulfate was administered by intravenous infusion as an antidote (Schulz et al., 1983).

5.6.2.3 Wheat Bran

Wheat bran is a byproduct formed in the manufacture of wheat flour from the grain of *Triticum aestivum*. It consists mainly of the outer layers of the wheat kernel, including the aleurone layer, i.e., the husk, seed coat, and germ. Because there is no natural demarcation between the starch-containing endosperm and the bran layers, the composition of the bran can vary somewhat, depending on the milling process. A dietary bran for long-term use must meet certain criteria. First, dietary bran must conform to the provisions of food regulations, especially in terms of its pesticide content. It must not be contaminated by actinomyces or other bacteria. Moreover, the size of the bran particles must be defined and standardized, and their water content must be substantially lower than in unprocessed bran. Finally, bran products are deemed acceptable only if the trypsin inhibitors present in unprocessed bran have been inactivated.

The composition of wheat bran is shown in Table 5.8. The protein fraction contains gluten, which is why wheat bran should not be used in patients with gluten-induced enteropathies. The gluten content also contraindicates the use of bran in children younger than 2 years of age. Some bran constituents are digestible, but the calorific value, at 150–175 kcal, is low. The remaining components enter the colon unchanged, where especially the pentosans and other hemicelluloses are broken down by bacteria. The increase in stool bulk is based on three factors: the swelling capacity of the pentosans, the bulk characteristics of indigestible materials (fibers and lignin), and the proliferation of intestinal bacteria. Additionally, short-chain acids are released that cause chemical irritation of the intestinal mucosa.

Bran is also useful for preventing inflammation in patients with diverticulosis. In one study, 70 patients received 12–14 g bran daily as a supplement to their low-fiber diet. Following a latent period of 2–4 weeks, 62 of the patients were free of complaints

Table 5.8.
Chemical composition of wheat bran (Huth et al., 1980).

Components	%
Water	10
Protein	15
Fat	5
Carbohydrates	55
– Starch	12
– Cellulose	21
– Hemicelluloses	22
Lignin	8
Vitamins and minerals	7

(Weinreich, 1980). The desired therapeutic effects, especially in terms of shortening intestinal transit time, appear to depend strongly on the particle size of the bran. Coarse particles larger than 1 mm in diameter are the most effective (Smith et al., 1981).

The administration of bran (2 × 15 g/day) to healthy test subjects for 6 weeks led to significant changes in the relative proportions of bile acids, marked by a decrease in deoxycholic acid and an increase in chenodeoxycholic acid (Kasper, 1980). However, the clinical relevance of this observation is unclear. The use of wheat bran carries a risk of bowel obstruction only if fluid intake is inadequate.

5.6.2.4 Psyllium Seed and Husk

Psyllium seed consists of the ripe seed obtained from several *Plantago* species. The seeds are elliptical and about 2–3 mm long; they are odorless, bland-tasting, and become mucilaginous when chewed. The mucilaginous husk of the Indian variety separates fairly easily from the rest of the seed, so these husks constitute a separate commercial product (psyllium husk). The important swelling agents (mucilages, hemicelluloses) are located in the epidermis of the husk, making the husks about five times more active than the seeds themselves.

The whole seeds or husks are soaked in water for several hours and are then taken with a copious amount of liquid. The mucilage retains the moisture during gastrointestinal transit, promoting the passage of a soft stool after a transit time of 6–12 h. It has also been suggested that the laxative action involves a purely mechanical irritation of the bowel wall causing a reflex stimulation of peristalsis (USD, 1967).

Rare cases of allergic reactions have been reported. In animal studies, feeding powdered psyllium seeds to rats for 18 weeks and to dogs for 4 weeks led to the deposition of a brownish black pigment in the proximal renal tubules with no associated impairment of renal function. Similar phenomena were not observed following the long-term use of whole psyllium seeds (Leng-Peschlow and Mengs, 1990).

5.6.2.5 Agar and Karaya Gum

Agar (or agar agar) is a dried, hydrophilic, colloidal substance obtained by extracting various red algae, usually *Gelidium* or *Gracilaria* species. The main constituents of the product are two polysaccharides:

▶ agarose, a long-chain compound in which about 10 % of the chains are esterified with sulfuric acid;

▶ agaropectin, which differs from agarose in its significantly higher degree of esterification with sulfuric acid. The molecule also contains pyruvic acid in a ketal bond.

Agar is sold commercially in the form of pale yellow strips or pieces or as a yellowish powder. The products are odorless and tasteless. Agar is indigestible and passes through the gastrointestinal tract almost unchanged. It undergoes little if any breakdown by intestinal microorganisms, which may account for its relatively low activity in regulating the bowel. It acts solely by its ability to absorb water and swell within the intestine.

Karaya gum, known also as karaya, sterculia gum, or Indian tragacanth, is a substance that exudes from the incised tree trunks of *Sterculia urens*, *Cochlospermum gossypium*, and related species of these genera. The crude drug consists of yellow-brown, yellowish, or reddish pieces that have a marked acetic acid smell when pulverized. Karaya gum is also composed of polysaccharides, and its macromolecular structure is similar to that of pectins. The product has a great swelling capacity, and a 10 % solution will expand to form a homogeneous, sticky gelatinous mass.

5.6.3 Osmotic Agents

The prototypes of osmotic laxatives are certain salts that are highly water-soluble but poorly absorbable, such as sodium sulfate and magnesium sulfate. These salts retain water in the bowel purely by their osmotic action, thereby increasing the water content of the stool. If they are administered in hypotonic solution, water is quickly absorbed from the intestines until the administered solution becomes isotonic. If a hypertonic solution is administered, water is drawn from the body and retained in the bowel.

The same mechanism underlies the action of nonabsorbable sugars (manose) and sugar alcohols (mannitol and sorbitol) of plant origin. With these compounds, however, a second mechanism is operative as well: the unabsorbed sugars enter the colon unchanged, where they are broken down into short-chain fatty acids. This process releases acetic, lactic, and butyric acids that stimulate peristalsis and promote osmotic water retention. The proliferation of normal intestinal flora probably also contributes to bowel regulation by increasing the fecal mass.

The prototype of this laxative group is lactulose, a partially synthetic transformation product of lactose that is not an herbal substance.

Mannitol is of plant origin, however, and occurs widely throughout the plant kingdom. Seaweed contains significant amounts of mannitol (up to 20 %), and manna, the dried sap of the manna ash (*Fraxinus ornus*), contains up to 13 %. Medicinal mannitol is a partially synthetic agent produced by the hydration of invertose.

Sorbitol is a sugar alcohol that also occurs in the plant kingdom. Relatively high concentrations are present in apples, pears, plums, apricots, cherries, and especially mountain ash berries (*Sorbus aucuparia*). Again, the commercial product is a partially synthetic agent produced by the reduction of glucose. Sorbitol acts as a mild laxative when taken in an oral dose of 20–30 g.

5.6.4 Anthranoid-Containing Herbs

While bulk-forming agents act mainly through physical effects within the bowel lumen, stimulant laxatives, particularly those containing, anthranoids, act directly on the intestinal mucosa. The stimulant laxatives usually induce an unphysiologic bowel movement with loose stools and frequent griping (Gysling, 1976).

Several mechanisms are involved in this effect:

▸ Reflexes elicited by the stimulation of receptors in the mucosa and submucosa, leading to increased propulsive colonic motility, a shortened transit time, and a net decrease in the absorption of water and electrolytes.
▸ An increase of cyclic AMP (cAMP) in the enterocytes. As the intracellular calcium concentration changes, chloride enters the intestinal lumen; sodium and water follow for osmotic reasons and to maintain electroneutrality (= secretagogic action).
▸ Leakage of the junctional complexes (terminal bars) between the endothelial cells of the large intestine. Sodium and water that have already been absorbed can re-enter the lumen through the incompetent junctional complexes.
▸ Blockage of the sodium pump (sodium-potassium-ATPase) on the bowel epithelium facing away from the lumen. This inhibits the absorption of sodium and water (= antiabsorptive action).

The laxative effect of anthranoid-containing herbs is caused by the presence of chemically defined anthranoid compounds. Accordingly, commercial products are standardized on the basis of their anthranoid content. This group of phytomedicines should not be dosed according to their quantity of dried herb or raw extract, but only by the quantity of the key active constituents, i.e., anthranoids. The corresponding pharmaceutical dose equivalents are given in Table 5.9.

Knowledge of the pharmacokinetics of anthranoid-containing herbs is fragmentary, sennosides being the only compounds for which studies are available. Anthranoids bound to sugars are pharmacoligically inert and enter the colon unchanged. There they are metabolically altered by intestinal bacteria, yielding products that include free

Table 5.9.
The dosage of an anthranoid-containing herb is based on its total anthranoid content, the daily dose of which should not exceed 20–30 mg of anthranoids.

Herb	Total anthranoids (%)	Daily dose (g)
Rhubarb	2–3	1
Senna leaf	2–3	1
Buckthorn berries	3–4	1
Senna pods	3–6	0.5–1
Buckthorn bark	6–9	0.5
Cascara	> 8	0.5
Aloe	20–40	0.1

anthrones, which are considered the true active principles. Most of the metabolites are excreted in the stool; a quantitatively undetermined fraction is absorbed and appears as glucuronide or sulfate conjugates in the urine, turning the urine a dark yellow or even red if there is a positive alkaline reaction. In nursing mothers, anthranoid metabolites can enter the milk and give it a brownish tinge. There is debate as to whether the active ingredients become sufficiently concentrated in breast milk to cause diarrhea in nursing infants (Curry, 1982). A study was performed to test the absorption of aloe-emodin and rhein in 12 subjects following a single dose of senna extract and after taking the extract for several days. The single dose corresponded to 20 mg of hydroxyanthracene derivatives, calculated as sennoside B. While the maximum plasma levels of rhein after 4 days' ingestion ranged from 60 to 90 ng/mL, no trace of the potentially mutagenic aloe-emodin (Mengs, 1996) could be detected in the plasma of any of the 12 subjects at any time during the study (Schulz et al., 1998).

The principal adverse effect that can occur with occasional use is colicky abdominal pain, or griping. The susceptibility to this complaint varies greatly among different individuals. Anthranoids, particularly aloe, can cause a reflex engorgement of abdominal blood vessels throughout the pelvis, with a substantial augmentation of blood flow to the uterus and its appendages. This can increase the intensity of menstrual bleeding, and in pregnancy it can heighten the risk of fetal loss. Melanosis coli develops in about 5 % of long-term anthranoid users over a period of 4–13 months, but this condition has no clinical importance and resolves in 6–12 months after the laxative is discontinued (Weber, 1988).

True adverse side effects result almost entirely from long-term abuse leading to severe electrolyte and water losses and eventual hyperaldosteronism (Ewe, 1988). The chronic hypokalemia worsens constipation and may cause damage to the renal tubules. These toxic side effects should not occur when anthranoid laxatives are taken intermittently and at low doses. Recent studies cast doubt on the notion that chronic laxative abuse causes irreversible damage to intramural ganglia and nerves of the intrinsic mucosal plexus (Dufour and Gendre, 1988).

Anthranoid preparations are contraindicated in partial or complete bowel obstruction, pregnancy, and lactation. Interactions with cardiac glycosides and other drugs may occur indirectly as a result of electrolyte imbalance (hypokalemia).

Chronic laxative use is undesirable by its very nature, but prolonged laxative use under the supervision and guidance of a physician (e.g., potassium replacement) is justified in severe forms of constipation (Ewe, 1988). The same applies to colonic inertia in the elderly. There is no apparent reason to discount the importance of laxatives more than any other symptom-relieving medication (Müller-Lissner, 1987). Recent clinical and epidemiologic studies have allayed fears that the melanosis coli caused by anthranoid laxatives is a premalignant condition or that the chronic use of anthranoid laxatives predisposes to colorectal tumors (Nusko et al., 1996; Loew et al., 1996; Brunswick et al., 1997). A review of studies on the mutagenic risk of senna extracts, sennosides A, B, C and D, rhein, and aloe-emodin revealed no evidence of mutagenic or carcinogenic effects on mammalian cells aside from some positive findings in the Ames test. The authors concluded that the use of senna laxatives in particular did not pose an increased risk of mutagenicity or carcinogenicity in human patients (Brusick and Mengs, 1997).

5.6.4.1 Rhubarb Root

Rhubarb root consists of the dried underground parts of medicinal rhubarb (*Rheum* spp.) (Fig. 5.13), native to the mountainous regions of western China and cultivated in Europe. The dried herb has a faint aromatic odor and a bitter, slightly astringent taste. Chewing the root produces a gritty sensation between the teeth caused by large calcium oxalate crystals, and it turns the saliva yellow. The crude drug contains about 2.5 % anthranoids (calculated as rhein), consisting mostly of anthraquinone glycosides (60–80 %) with lesser amounts of anthrone glycosides (10–25 %) and free anthraquinones (about 1 %). Rhubarb also contains about 5 % tannins of the gallotannin and catechin type along with flavonoids, pectins, and minerals.

Besides the anthranoids, which have a cathartic action, rhubarb also contains tannins and pectins, which produce an antidiarrheal effect. Both actions are superimposed during use. The overall effect is dose-dependent because emodins and tannins appear to have different dose-response characteristics. Rhubarb taken in smaller doses (0.1–0.3 g) has an astringent action in gastritis and dyspepsia and an antidiarrheal action in

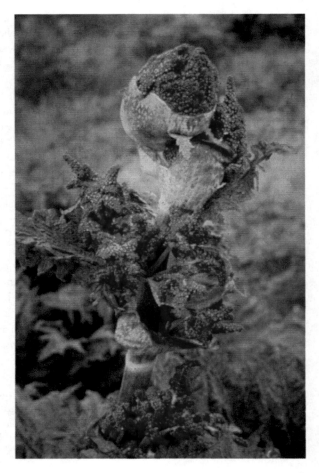

Figure 5.13. ▶ Flower head of medicinal rhubarb (*Rheum* sp.).

mild forms of diarrhea. Higher doses (1.0–4.0 g) produce a mild laxative effect. Since the relative contents of emodins and tannins are variable, the laxative action is somewhat uncertain. The *German Pharmacopeia* describes a rhubarb root extract that is made with 70 % alcohol. This extract is adjusted with lactose as needed to obtain a 4–6 % anthranoid content. Rhubarb extract is a brown, hygroscopic, powdered material with a distinctive odor and the bitter taste of rhubarb root.

5.6.4.2   Buckthorn Bark

This herb consists of the dried bark from the trunk and branches of the buckthorn (*Rhamnus frangula*). This deciduous shrub or small tree (family Rhamnaceae) is widely distributed in Europe and western Asia. The common German name for buckthorn, *Faulbaum*, means the "rotten tree", and refers to the offensive odor of the friable wood (frangere = "break").

Buckthorn bark contains 6–9 % anthraquinone glycosides, the most important of which are glucofrangulin A and B. The bark differs from other anthranoid, containing herbs in that its active constituents occur mainly as anthraquinones, which have less powerful antiabsorptive and hydragogic properties. This accounts for the relatively mild action of buckthorn bark.

The cut and dried herb is a frequent ingredient in commercially produced specialty teas. Additionally, powdered extracts are used for instant teas, and solid or powdered extracts are used as ingredients in combination products that are usually sold in capsule or tablet form.

The anthrones in the freshly dried herb are extremely potent, and the bark should be stored for at least 1 year before use or aged artificially by heating it while exposing it to the air. Use of the untreated fresh bark can cause severe vomiting and spasms.

Cascara bark, which is related to alder buckthorn bark, is obtained from *Rhamnus purshianus*, a tree resembling the buckthorn and native to the Pacific Northwest in North America. Cascara bark contains at least 8 % total anthranoids, approximately two-thirds of which are cascarosides. Preparations in the form of extracts and fluidextracts are used as ingredients in pharmaceutical products. Because of its disagreeable odor, the bark is not suitable for use in teas. Cascara bark was formerly widely used in over-the-counter (OTC) stimulant laxative drug products in the United States, but was recently removed from the market by the U.S. Food and Drug Administration (FDA) due to the lack of submissions by manufacturers of modern clinical and safety data to confirm the herb's safety (USFDA, 2002). To clarify, the FDA did not find cascara bark to be unsafe; rather, due to the peculiarities of the regulatory system, a lack of affirmative data confirming the drug's safety results in its removal from the market (Bayne, 2002). The same process occurred for aloe, used as a laxative (see 5.6.4.4).

5.6.4.3   Senna Pods and Leaves

Senna pods and leaves are obtained from two different senna species: *Cassia senna* and *Cassia angustifolia*. The former species is a small shrub of the family Fabaceae that reaches a height of 60 cm. It grows along the Nile in Egypt and Sudan. The seed pods of

Cassia senna (Alexandrian senna pods) have a bittersweet, mucilaginous taste. They contain 3.5–5.5 % anthranoids, principally sennosides A and B.

Cassia angustifolia is a shrub growing to 2 m that is native to the region about the Red Sea. Its seed pods (Tinnevelly senna pods) are cultivated in India and Indonesia. The anthranoid spectrum of *C. angustifolia* is mostly identical to that of *C. senna*, but its total anthranoid content, at 2–3 %, is considerably lower, so it must be given in a higher dose. Senna leaves can be harvested from both *Cassia* species. In fact, some modern taxonomists now place both species in a single taxon *Senna alexandrina*. However, in this volume, the classic nomenclature has been retained. The crude drug consists of the stripped leaflets rather than whole leaves and should contain at least 3 % total anthranoids including the key active constituents, sennosides A and B. Senna leaves are most commonly used in the form of teas, but extracts are frequently used in a wide variety of laxative products.

5.6.4.4 Aloe

The genus *Aloe* includes more than 300 species, all of which are native to tropical countries, especially eastern and southern Africa. *Aloe barbadensis* Mill. (synonym: *Aloe vera* L.) is the species that is most widely used for medicinal purposes. Some commercial products are made from the dried juice of the aloe leaf. This is not an herb in the usual sense but an herbal preparation, which is also known as cape aloe in Europe because it originates in southern Africa.

Cape aloe is obtained by cutting off the leaves and holding the cut surface down to drain the juice from the base of the leaf. The collected juice is thickened by heating over an open fire or by allowing the semisolid latex to harden in a canister. This yields a homogeneous, vitreous mass that is sold commercially under the brand name Lucida. Alternatively, the juice can be slowly evaporated (e.g., by letting it stand in the sun), causing the aloin (a mixture of anthraquinones) to crystallize out. This product has a flat, lusterless appearance and is sold under the brand name Hepatica. Powdered aloe is greenish-brown, has a pungent odor and a bitter, unpleasant taste. Key active constituents are the anthraquinoid compounds aloin A and B, barbaloin, and emodin, which together make up 20–40 % of the preparation. The product is used medicinally for relief of constipation. Dosage and risks of therapy are discussed in Sect. 5.6.4.

The latex preparation described above is distinguished from aloe gel. The gel is obtained by other means, such as by grinding the leaves. The main constituents of the gel are polysaccharides such as glucomannan and acemannan, but the gel contains almost no anthranoids. It is considered to have anti-inflammatory properties and is used chiefly as a topical treatment for wound healing problems or psoriasis (see Sect. 8.2.4).

Aloe is the most powerful herbal anthranoid laxative and also the most widely used in Europe. Because of its drastic cathartic action it is not commonly employed in the United States, and its status as an approved OTC stimulant laxative drug was recently withdrawn by the FDA for the same reasons as cascara (see Sect. 5.6.4.2). Research on the long-term toxicity and pharmacokinetics of aloe is still incomplete. In particular, it is not known what portions of the relatively lipophilic aloins undergo unwanted absorption. An accurate risk assessment cannot be made on the basis of available information.

5.6.5 Castor Oil

Castor oil is the oil that is mechanically pressed from the seeds of *Ricinus communis* (Fig. 5.14), family Euphorbiaceae, without heating. Cold pressing is carried out to keep the highly toxic protein ricin from entering the expressed oil. Castor oil has a very faint but characteristic odor; it has a mild initial taste and an acrid aftertaste.

In contrast to most fatty oils, which are composed of mixed-acid triglycerides, up to 80 % of castor oil consists of triricinolein, which is broken down by saponification into glycerol and ricinoleic acid. Ricinoleic acid, or the sodium salt that forms from it, is the actual laxative agent. Because castor oil, like other triglycerides, is readily attacked by lipases and bile acids, its laxative action affects both the small and large intestine. The high polarity of the acid distinguishes it from other fatty acids and allows large portions of the acid to enter the colon.

A powerful cathartic, castor oil has a recommended dose of 5–10 g (1–2 teaspoons) for adults. It takes about 8 h to act. If more rapid catharsis is desired, the dose can be

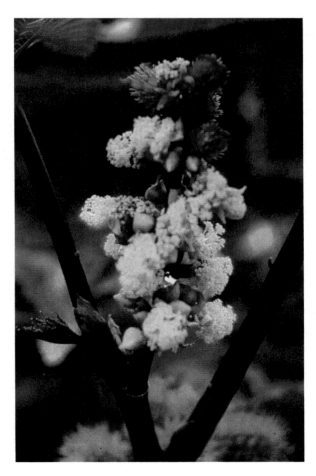

Figure 5.14. ◄ Raceme of castor (*Ricinus communis*).

increased to a maximum of 30 g (6 teaspoons). Castor oil is most effective when taken on an empty stomach. Use in the form of gelatin capsules avoids the unpleasant taste, but a large number of capsules must be taken.

The contraindications and risks are similar to those of other laxatives. Because castor oil is a powerful stimulant of bile flow, it is also contraindicated by biliary tract obstructions and other biliary disorders. The laxative use of castor oil is contraindicated in poisonings with lipid-soluble agents because the oil can promote their absorption.

5.6.6 Suggested Formulation

Laxative tea I according to German Standard Registration

Rx	Senna leaves	60.0
	Fennelseed	10.0
	Chamomile	10.0
	Peppermint leaves	20.0
	Mix to make tea	

Directions: Prepare 1–2 teaspoons as an infusion, steep for 10 min. Drink 1 cup every evening.

Laxative tea according to R.F. Weiss (1982)

Rx	Senna leaves	25,0
	Buckthorn bark	25.0
	Chamomile	25.0
	Fennelseed, crushed	25.0
	Mix to make tea	

Directions: Prepare 1–2 teaspoons as an infusion, drink 1 cup every evening.

5.6.7 Drug Products

The *Rote Liste 2003* contains a number of single-herb laxatives, which consist mostly of bulk-forming agents. With anthranoid-containing herbs, the dosage of a given product is measured by the amount of hydroxyanthracene derivatives that it contains. A 1993 Commission E recommendation states that the daily dose of hydroxyanthracene derivatives should not exceed 20–30 mg

References

Bayne HJ. FDA Issues Final Rule Banning Use of Aloe and Cascara Sagrada in OTC Drug Products. *HerbalGram.* 2002; 56: 56

Brunswick D, Mengs K (1997) Assessment of the genotoxic risk from laxative senna products. Environmental and Molecular Mutagenesis 29: 1–9

Cummings JH, Southgate DAT, Branch W, Houston H, Jenkins DJA, James WPT (1978) Colonic response to dietary fiber from carrot, cabbage, apple, bran, and guar gum. Lancet I: 5.

Curry CE (1982) laxative products. In: Handbook of Nonprescription Drugs. Am Pharmac Assoc, Washington, pp 69–92.

Dufour P, Gendre P (1988) Long-term mucosal alterations by sennosides and related compounds. Pharmacology 36 (Suppl 1): 194–202.

Ewe K (1988) Schwer therapiebare Formen der Pbstipation. Verhandl dtsch Ges Inn Med 94: 473–480.

Ewe K (1983) Obstipation – Pathophysiologie, Klinik, Therapie. Int Welt 6: 286–292.

Fingl E (1980) Laxatives and cathartics. In: Goodman AF, Goodman L, Gilman A (eds) The Pharmacological Basis of Therapeutics. 6th Ed. Macmillan, New York Toronto London, p 1004.

Gysling E (1976) Behandlung häufiger Symptome. Leitfaden zur Pharmakotherapie. Huber, Basel Bern Stuttgart Vienna.

Huth K, Pötter C, Cremer CD (1980) Füll- und Quellstoffe als Zusatz industriell hergestellter Lebensmittel. In: Rottka H (ed) Pflanzenfasern-Ballaststoffe in der menschlichen Ernährung. Thieme, Stuttgart New York, pp 39–53.

Hutz J, Rösch W (eds) (1987) Funktionelle Störungen des Verdauungstrakts. Springer-Verlag, Berlin Heidelberg New York, pp 200, 222.

Kasper H (1980) Der Einfluß von Gallstoffen auf die Ausnutzung von Nährstoffen und Pharmaka. In: Rottka H (ed) Pflanzenfasern-Ballastoffe in der menschlichen Ernährung. Thieme, Stuttgart New York, pp 93–112.

Kasper H (1985) Ernährungsmedizin und Diätetik 5th Ed. Urban & Schwarzenberg. Munich Vienna.

Leng-Peschlow E, Mengs U (1990) No renal pigmentation by Plantago ovata seeds or husks. Med Sci Res 18: 37–38.

Loew D, Bergmann U, Dirschedl P, Schmidt M, Melching K, Hues B, Überla K (1996) Retro- und prospektive Fall-Kontroll-Studien zur Anthranoidlaxanzien. In: Loew D, Rietbrock N (Hrsg) Phytopharmaka II, Forschung und klinische Anwendung. Steinkopff, Stuttgart: 175–184.

Mengs U (1996) Zur Sicherheit von Sennalaxanzien. In: Loew D, Rietbrock N (Hrsg) Phytopharmaka II, Forschung und klinische Anwendung. Steinkopff, Stuttgart: 161–166.

Müller-Lissner S (1987) Chronische Obstipation. Dtsch Med Wschr 112: 1223–1229.

Nusko G, Schneider B, I, Wittekind CH, Hahn EG (1996) Prospektive klinische Studie zur Sicherheit von Anthranoidlaxanzien. In: Loew D, Rietbrock N (Hrsg) Phytopharmaka II, Forschung und klinische Anwendung. Steinkopff, Stuttgart: 167–174.

Ruppin, H, Bar-Meir S, Soergel KH, Wood CM, Schmitt MG (1980) Absorption of short-chain fatty acids by the colon. Gastroenterol 78: 1500–1507.

Schulz HU, Schürer M, Silber W (1998) Pharmakokinetische Untersuchungen eines Sennesfrüchte-Extraktes. Zeitschrift für Phytotherapie 19: 190–194.

Schulz V, Löffler A, Gheeorghiu T (1983) Resorption von Blausäure aus Leinsamen. Leber Magen Darm 13: 10–14.

Schulz V (1984) Clinical pharmacokinetics of nitroprusside, cyanide, thiosulphate, and thiocyanate. Clinical Pharmacokinetics 9: 239–251.

Sewing KFR (1986) Obstipation. In: Fülgraff G, Palm D (eds) Pharmakotherapie, Klinische Pharmakologie. 6th Ed. Fischer, Stuttgart, pp 162–168.

Smith AN, Drummond E, Eastwood MA (1981) The effect of coarse and fine wheat bran on colonic motility in patients with diverticular disease. Am J Clin Nutr 34: 2460–2464.

Stephen AM, Cummings JH (1980) The microbial contribution to human fecal mass. J Med Microbiol 13: 45–66.

USD (1967) The United States Dispensatory and Physicians' Pharmacology. In: Osol R, Pratt R, Altschule MD (eds) Lippincott, Philadelphia Toronto, p 917.

US Food and Drug Administration. 67 *Federal Register* 31125 (May 9, 2002).

Weber E (1988) Taschenbuch der unerwünschten Arzneiwirkungen. Fischer, Stuttgart New York.

Weinrich J (1980) Therapy of colon disease with a fiber-rich diet. In: Rottka H (ed) Pflanzenfasern-Ballaststoffe in der menschlichen Ernährung. Thieme, Stuttgart New York, pp 154–157.

Yajima T (1985) Contractile effect of short-chain fatty acids on the isolated colon of the rat. J Physiol 368: 667–678.

5.7 Liver Diseases

Most liver remedies were introduced into therapeutic use because they were found to have protective properties in certain animal species. The experimental agent (drug substance) was administered to the laboratory animal for a specified period of time, then a hepatotoxic agent was administered. In some models, the protective and toxic agents were administered concurrently. There have been studies in which liver damage was induced first and the experimental agent was administered afterward to test its curative properties, but in most cases the agent did not favorably affect the course of the hepatotoxicity. Even when curative effects were seen, experimental designs based on the administration of a hepatotoxic substance (carbon tetrachloride, galactosamine, thioacetamide, phalloidin) are not a valid model for studying liver diseases in humans. The main problem is that the alcohol-related liver damage so common in humans cannot be adequately reproduced in experimental animals except for certain species of higher apes (Bode, 1981). Thus, the antihepatotoxic and hepatoprotective effects seen in animal studies do not allow for the prediction of therapeutic efficacy in human patients with liver disease (alcoholic liver disease, hepatitis, fatty degeneration). A far more useful indicator is the finding that certain agents promote hepatic regeneration, as in the case of silymarin, which is described below (Sect.5.7.1.4).

The following therapeutic goals have been defined as criteria for the clinical testing of hepatic remedies (Bode, 1986):

▶ improving the patient's subjective symptoms,
▶ shortening the duration of the disease, and
▶ reducing the number of fatal outcomes.

A very important criterion for the patient is the relief or improvement of complaints: anorexia, nausea, vomiting, epigastric pain and pressure, flatulence, and itching. This is a critical point in the objective assessment of drug actions, for an improvement in complaints is not necessarily linked to an objective amelioration of the disease process. The problem of assessment is made even more difficult by the extreme fluctuations that can occur in the spontaneous course of liver diseases.

The best criteria to use in the objective assessment of therapeutic response are (Bode, 1986): the regression of clinical symptoms of functional decompensation and laboratory findings.

It is commonly argued that the course of liver diseases cannot be significantly influenced by therapy (Dölle and Schwabe, 1988; Martini, 1988). However, molecular biochemical studies on the regeneration-promoting action of silybinin (Sonnenbichler et al., 1984, 1987, 1988) and supporting clinical reports (survey in Reuter, 1992) suggest that adequate doses of silymarin preparations can inhibit the progression of liver diseases when combined with appropriate general measures.

5.7.1 Milk Thistle Fruits, Silymarin

The majority of all biochemical, pharmacologic, and clinical tests of herbal liver remedies have employed a fraction extracted from the fruits ("seeds") of the milk thistle. Seventy percent of this fraction consists of silymarin, a mixture of four isomers including the main active constituent silybinin.

5.7.1.1 Medicinal Plant and Crude Drug

Milk thistle (*Silybum marianum*, Fig. 5.15) is an annual to biennial plant of the family Asteraceae growing to 2 m. It is native principally to southern Europe and northern Africa and grows in warm, dry locales. The milk thistle is a protected plant in Germany and is cultivated for medicinal purposes mainly in northern Africa and South America. It blooms in July and August at Central European latitudes.

The crude drug consists of the ripe fruits from which the pappus has been removed. Each fruit is about 6–7 mm long and 3 mm wide with a glossy, brownish black to grayish brown husk. The freshly milled fruits have a cocoa-like odor and an oily taste.

5.7.1.2 Components and Active Constituents

Milk thistle fruits contain 15–30 % fatty oil and about 20–30 % proteins. The true active constituents constitute only about 2–3 % of the dried herb. The mixture of active principles, called silymarin, consists of four isomers: silybinin (about 50 %) and lesser amounts of isosilybinin, silydianin, and silychristin (Pelter et Hänsel 1968; Arnone et al., 1979; Wagner, 1976). Silymarin is most concentrated in the protein layer of the seed husk.

5.7.1.3 Pharmacokinetics

About 20–50 % of silymarin is absorbed following oral administration in humans. About 80 % of the dose, whether administered orally or by intravenous injection, is excreted in the bile (Mennicke, 1975); about 10 % enters the enterohepatic circulation. With repetitive use, the circulating levels of silybinin reach an equilibrium state after just one day (Lorenz et al., 1982). The absorption rate depends on the galenic form of the preparation and can vary by a factor of at least two among different commercial products (Schulz et al., 1995).

5.7.1.4 Pharmacology and Toxicology

Pharmacologic studies have been performed on silymarin and its main component silybinin. It was found that silymarin mainly exerts antitoxic effects and promotes the

Figure 5.15. ▶ Milk thistle
(*Silybum marianum*).

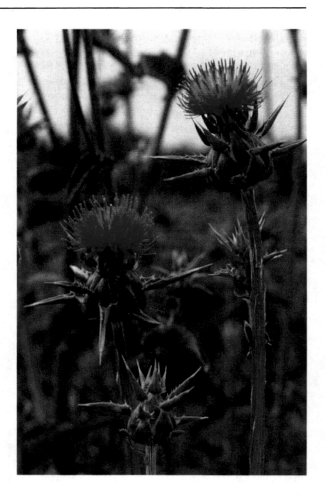

regeneration of liver tissue. The antitoxic effects are based in part on membrane-stabi-
lizing and radical-antagonizing actions. The regeneration-promoting effects are attributed to the stimulation of protein biosynthesis (survey in Reuter, 1992).

Antitoxic effects: Silymarin premedication in rats was found to prevent the injurious
effects of various liver toxins such as carbon tetrachloride, galactosamine, thioacetamide, and praseodymium (Hahn et al., 1968; Rauen and Schriewer, 1971). Silymarin
also protects the liver from drug toxicity (Martines et al., 1980; Leng-Perschlow et al.,
1991). Particularly impressive are experimental reports of protective effects against the
toxins of the mushroom *Amanita phalloides*, phalloidin and α-amanitin which attack
the liver at various sites. Silymarin forms the basis for the only antidote to amanita poisoning (Sect.5.7.1.6).

It is believed that the antidotal efficacy of silymarin against phalloidin, hepatotoxic
chemicals, and alcohol is based on its tendency to bind to proteins and receptors on cell
membranes, displacing toxic substances and preventing their entry into the cells.

Regeneration-promoting action: Silymarin may derive its curative properties from
the capacity, especially of its silybinin component, to stimulate the regeneration of liver

cells (Sonnenbichler and Zetl, 1988). In biochemical terms, the regenerative capacity of a tissue is based on stimulation of the cell metabolism and of macromolecular synthesis. Silybinin induces a global increase in cellular protein synthesis (Sonnenbichler and Zetl, 1986, 1987). The mechanism for stimulating protein synthesis is based on the ability of silybinin to bind to a subunit of the RNA polymerase of the cell nucleus, taking the place of an intrinsic cell regulator. The presence of the silybinin stimulates the polymerase to synthesize more ribosomal RNA, whose rate of transcription is increased. This leads to an increase in ribosome formation and, as a secondary effect, to an augmentation of cellular protein synthesis (Sonnenbichler and Zetl, 1988).

In evaluating silybinin-containing drugs, it is important to consider that silybinin not only protects the liver when administered prophylactically but also acts curatively to promote the regeneration of cells that are already damaged. It is also noteworthy that silybinin exerts its regeneration-promoting action at a 10 times lower concentration than is needed for antihepatotoxic membrane effects, and that the regenerative action is less structure specific. The regeneration-promoting action of silybinin may well account for the clinically observed acceleration of liver cell regeneration in response to silymarin preparations (Fintelmann and Albert, 1980).

Antifibrotic effect: Fibrotic transformation plays a key role in the pathogenesis of hepatic cirrhosis. Two study groups performed tests in rats to investigate the antifibrotic effect of silymarin, a standardized plant extract containing 60 % silybinin. Experimental cirrhosis was induced in both studies by injecting sodium amidotrizoate (Ethibloc) to produce complete bile duct occlusion. The resulting periductal inflammation causes a progressive, fibrotic expansion of the portal vessels culminating in secondary biliary cirrhosis. Schuppan et al. (1994) used this model to investigate silymarin and compare it with D-penicillamine and colchicine for antifibrotic efficacy. Only the animals treated with silymarin had a 50 % decrease in hepatic collagen content after 6 weeks, regardless of whether silymarin was administered from weeks 1 to 6 (prophylactic) or from weeks 4 to 6 (therapeutic). Boigk et al. (1997) confirmed these results in another series of tests comparing treated animals with a sham-operated control group of Wistar rats. The dose dependence of the antifibrotic effect was also tested. A highly significant reduction in hepatic collagen accumulation was obtained with a dose of 50 mg silybinin/kg/day but not with 25 mg/kg/day.

5.7.1.5   Therapeutic Efficacy in Chronic Liver Diseases

By far the most frequent cause of chronic liver disease is alcohol abuse. The regular consumption of more than 50 g of ethanol per day is sufficient to pose an excess risk. The most effective therapeutic measure is abstinence from alcohol. Alcohol-related fatty liver changes, for example, will regress in most patients within a few months after alcohol is withdrawn.

Seven controlled clinical studies have been performed in patients with alcohol-related toxic liver damage using a standardized product with the brand name Legalon® (Varis et al., 1978; Fintelmann and Albert, 1980; Benda et al., 1980; Salmi and Sarna, 1982; Feher et al., 1988, 1989; Ferenci et al., 1989). Most of the studies involved about 50–100 patients, and one study included 170 patients (Ferenci et al., 1989). Two studies (Benda et al., 1980; Ferency et al., 1989) involved treatment periods of up to 4 years and used survival rate as their confirmatory parameter. Both of these studies showed a significant (p<0.05) improvement in survival rate in the silymarin-treated group versus a placebo (Fig. 5.16). Most of the other studies also showed statistically significant gains in patients treated with the milk thistle preparation. A systematic review of the literature identified a total of 14 placebo-controlled double-blind studies and 15 studies without placebo control. Five of 7 studies in patients with chronic alcoholic liver disease showed improvement in at least one parameter in response to silymarin therapy. Three of 4 studies in patients with hepatic cirrhosis indicated positive trends, and two studies documented significant superiority. Four studies in patients with viral hepatitis yielded only contradictory results (Ernst et al., 2001).

The tolerance toward silymarin preparations was very good. One observational study in 2160 patients revealed 21 cases (1 %) of reported side effects, consisting mainly of transient gastrointestinal complaints (Reuter, 1992). Another observational study was done with the product Legalon 140 in 998 patients with chronic liver disease (fatty liver, fatty liver with hepatitis, cirrhosis due to various causes). Over a treatment period of 3 months, 20 patients (2 %) reported a total of 32 adverse side effects: 8 diarrhea, 6 flatulence, 4 bloating, 4 abdominal pain, and 1 each of dizziness, nausea, vomiting, sweating, hot flashes or allergic reaction. The attending physicians concluded that 12 of these reports may have related to the test medication, 9 were probably related, and 6 were probably unrelated. The physicians rated the tolerance as good to excellent in 98 % of the patients treated (Schuppan, 1998).

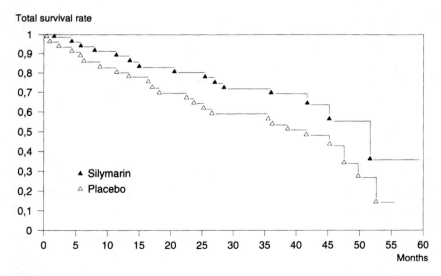

Figure 5.16. ▲ Survival rates of 170 patients with hepatic cirrhosis treated with silymarin or a placebo. The Kaplan-Meier method was used for statistical analysis. Significantly better survival rates (p<0.05) were observed in the group treated with silymarin (Ferenci et al., 1989).

5.7.1.6 Use in Mushroom Poisoning

More than 90 % of all fatal mushroom poisonings are caused by ingestion of the death cup mushroom *Amanita phalloides*. A death cup of moderate size contains about 10 mg of amanitin – a potentially lethal quantity for an adult. The toxins in amanita mushrooms block the RNA polymerase in liver cells, culminating in cell death after a typical latent period of about 12–24h. It is believed that silybinin competitively displaces the amanitin from the enzyme, thereby reactivating the process of protein biosynthesis (Sonnenbichler, 1988).

Placebo-controlled double-blind studies in humans are prohibited for this indication. To date, some 150 case reports have been published on the therapeutic use of silybinin in patients with amanita poisoning. While older publications cited mortality rates of 30–50 % from this type of poisoning, studies using silybinin infusion therapy reported dramatically lower death rates: 1 death in 18 patients (Hruby et al., 1983) and 1 death in 13 patients (Marugg and Reutter, 1985).

5.7.1.7 Indications, Dosages, Risks, and Contraindications

The Commission E monograph of March, 1986, states that milk thistle is used for "dyspeptic complaints". If cites the following indications for silymarin preparations: "toxic liver damage; also the supportive treatment of chronic inflammatory liver diseases and hepatic cirrhosis" (Blumenthal et al., 1998).

There are no known contraindications, side effects, or interactions with other drugs. The recommended average daily dose is 12–15 of the dried herb or 200–400 mg silymarin, calculated as silybinin.

The recommended regimen for amanita poisoning is infusion therapy with a silybinin derivative (brand name Legalon SIL). The manufacturer recommends a total dose of 20 mg silybinin per kg body weight over a 24-h period, divided into 4 infusions, each administered over a 2-h period.

5.7.2 Soybean Phospholipids

The term essential phospholipids (EPLs) denotes a soybean lecithin fraction that the manufacturer describes as a "choline phosphoric acid glyceride ester of natural origin containing predominantly unsaturated fatty acids, specifically linolenic acid (about 70 %), linoleic acid, and oleic acid." Phospholipids are an integral component of biomembranes and are involved in numerous membrane-dependent metabolic processes. It is postulated that phospholipids with polyunsaturated fatty acids prevent the hydrocarbon chains of the membrane phospholipids from assuming a parallel alignment owing to the *cis* double bonds of their polyunsaturated fatty acids. This would reduce the packing density of the micellar phospholipid structure, thereby increasing the rate of transmembrane exchange processes. This hypothesis underlies the presumed ability of soybean phospholipids to enhance the biochemical functioning of the liver parenchyma (Vogel and Görler, 1981; Peeters, 1976).

EPLs reportedly are absorbed unchanged after oral administration (Koch, 1980). Pharmacologic studies in rats showed a 100 % absorption of orally administered EPLs within 24 h, which reached the liver almost entirely by the lymphatic pathway. The liver absorbs 10–25 % of administered EPLs, which are gradually excreted via the urine and bile.

A total of 10 controlled therapeutic studies have been performed in patients with chronic liver disease. A review of these studies by Commission E in May of 1994 stated that 4 of the 10 studies demonstrated statistically significant benefits from EPL therapy (Blumenthal et al., 1998). The Commission concluded that EPL preparations are indicated "for the improvement of subjective complaints such as anorexia and pressure in the right upper abdomen due to toxic-nutritional liver damage or chronic hepatitis." The recommended dose is 1.5–2.7 g of soybean phospholipids containing 73–79 % phosphatidylcholine. There have been rare reports of gastrointestinal complaints; there are not known contraindications or drug-drug interactions.

5.7.3 Drug Products

The *Rote Liste 1998* lists 33 single-herb products under the heading of liver remedies, consisting of 30 standardized silymarin preparations and one soybean phospholipid preparation, in addition to numerous combinations. None of the combination products is included among the 100 most commonly prescribed herbal medications (see Appendix).

 References

Arnone A, Merlini L, Zanarotti A (1979) Constituents of Silybum marianum. Structure of isosilybin and stereochemistry of isosilybin. J Chem Soc (Chem Commun): 696–697.

Benda L, Dittrich H. Ferenzi P, Frank H, Wewalka F (1980) The influence of therapy with silymarin on the survival rate of patients with liver cirrhosis. Wien Klin Wschr 92 (19): 678–683.

Blumenthal M, Busse WR, Goldberg A, Gruenwald J, Hall T, Riggins CW, Rister RS (eds.). Klein S, Rister RS (trans). (1998) The Complete German Commission E Monographs – Therapeutic Guide to Herbal Medicines. American Botanical Council, Austin, Texas. *www.herbalgram.org.*

Bode JC (1986) Arzneimittel für die Indikation "Lebererkrankungen". In: Dölle W, Müller-Oerlingshausen, B, Schwabe U (eds) Grundlagen der Arzneimitteltherapie. Entwicklung, Beurteilung und Anwendung von Arzneimitteln, B.I.-Wissenschaftsverlag, Mannheim Vienna Zurich, pp 202–211.

Bode JC (1981) Die alkoholische Hepatitis, ein Krankheitsspektrum. Internist 220: 536–545.

Boigk G, Stroedter L, Herbst H, Waldschmidt J, Riecken EO, Schuppan D (1997) Silymarin retards collagen accumulation in early and advanced biliary fibrosis secondary to complete bile duct obliteration in rats. Hepatology 26: 643–649.

Dölle W, Schwabe U (1988) Leber- und Gallenwegstherapeutika. In: Schwabe U, Paffrath D (eds) Arzneiverordnungsreport 88. Gustav Fischer, Stuttgart New York, pp 242–253.

Ernst E, Pittler MH, Stevinson C, White A (2001) The Desktop Guide to Complementary and Alternative Medicine – an evidence-based approach. Mosby, Edingurgh London New York, pp 134–5.

Feher J, Deak G, Muezes G, Lang I, Niederland V, Nekam K, Karteszi M (1989) Hepatoprotective activity of silymarin Legalon therapy in patients with chronic alcoholic liver disease. Orv Hetil 130 (51): 2723-2727.

Ferenci P, Dragosics B, Dittrich H, Frank H, Benda L, Lochs H, Meryn S, Base W, Schneider B (1989) Randomized controlled trial of silymarin treatment in patient with cirrhosis of the liver. J Hepatol 9 (1): 105-113.

Fintelmann V, Albert A (1980) Nachweis der therapeutischen Wirksamkeit von Legalon bei toxischen Lebererkrankungen im Doppelblindversuch. Therapiewoche 30 (35): 5589-5594.

Hahn G, Lehmann HD, Kürten M et al. (1968) Zur Pharmakologie und Toxikologie von Silymarin, des antihepatotoxischen Wirkprinzips aus Silybum marianum (L.) Gaertn. Arzneim Forsch/Drug Res 18: 696-704.

Hruby K, Fuhrmann M, Csomos G, Thaler H (1983) Pharmakotherapie der Knollenblätterpilzvergiftung mit Silibinin. Wien Klin Wschr 95 (7): 225-231.

Koch H (1980) Leberschutz-Therapeutika. Pharmazie in unserer Zeit 9: 33-44, 65-74.

Leng-Peschlow E, Strenge-Hesse A (1991) Die Mariendistel (Silybum marianum) und Silymarin als Lebertherapeutikum. Z Phytother 12: 162-174.

Lorenz D, Mennicke WH, Behrendt W (1982) Untersuchungen zur Elimination von Silymarin bei cholecystektomierten Patienten. Planta Med 45: 216-233.

Martines G, Copponi V, Cagnetta G (1980) Aspetti del danno epatico dopo somministrazione sperimentale diarrhea alcuni farmaci. Arch Sci Med 137: 367-386.

Martini GA (1988) Hepatocelluläre Erkrankungen, Leberkrankheiten. In: Riecker G (ed) Therapie innerer Krankheiten. Springer, Berlin Heidelberg New York, pp 638-652.

Marugg D, Reutter FW (1985) Die Amanita-phalloides-Intoxikation. Moderne therapeutische Maßnahmen und klinischer Verlauf. Schweiz Rundschau Med (Praxis) 14 (37): 972-982.

Mennicke WH (1975) Zur biologischen Verfügbarkeit und Verstoffwechselung von Silybin. Dtsch Apoth Z 115 (33): 1205-1206.

Peeters H (ed) (1976) Phosphatidylcholine. Biochemical and Clinical Aspects of Essential Phospholipids. Springer-Verlag, Berlin Heidelberg New York.

Pelter A, Hänsel R (1969) The structure of silybin (Silybum substace E_6), the first flavonolignan. Tetrahedron Letters 25: 2911-2916

Rauen HM, Schriewer H (1971) Die antihepatotoxische Wirkung von Silymarin bei experimentellen Leberschäden der Ratte durch Tetrachlorkohlenstoff, D-Galaktosamin und Allylalkohol. Arzneim Forsch/Drug Res 21: 1194-1201.

Reuter HD (1992) Spektrum Mariendistel und andere leber- und gallewirksame Phytopharmaka. In: Bundesverband Deutscher Ärzte für Naturheilverfahren (ed). Arzneimitteltherapie heute. Aesopus Verlag, Basel.

Salmi HA, Sarna S (1982) Effect of silymarin on chemical, functional und morphological alterations of the liver. A double-blind controlled study. Scand J Gastroenterol 17 (4): 517-521.

Schulz HU, Schürer M, Krumbiegel G, Wächter W, Weyhenmeyer R, Seidel G (1995). Untersuchungen zum Freisetzungsverhalten und zur Bioäquivalenz von Silymarin-Präparaten. Arzneim Forsch/Drug Res 45: 61-64.

Schuppan d, Lang T, Gerling G, Leng-Peschlow E, Krumbiegel G, Riecken EO, Waldschmidt J (1994) Antifibrotic effect of silymarin in rat secondary biliary fibrosis induced by bile duct obliteration with ethibloc. Z jGastroenterol 32: 45-46.

Schuppan D, Strösser W, Burkard G, Walosek G (1998) Verminderung der Fibrosierungsaktivität durch Legalon bei chronischen Leberererkrankungen. Z Allg Med 74: 577-584.

Sonnenbichler J, Zetl I (1984) Untersuchungen zum Wirkungsmechanismus von Silibinin, Einfluß von Silibinin auf die Synthese ribosomaler RNA, mRNA und tRNA in Rattenlebern in vivo. Hoppe-Syler's Physiol Chem 365: 555-566.

Sonnenbichler J, Zetl I (1986) Biochemical effects of the flavonolignane silibinin in RNA, protein and DNA synthesis in rat livers. Prog Clin Biol Res 213: 319-331.

Sonnenbichler J, Zetl I (1987) Stimulating influence of a flavonolignane on proliferation, RNA synthesis and protein synthesis in liver cells. In: Okoliczányi L, Csomós G, Crepaldi G (eds) Assessment and Management of Hepatobiliary Disease. Springer, Berlin Heidelberg New York, pp 265-272.

Sonnenbichler J, Zetl I (1988) Specific binding of a flavonolignane to an estradiol receptor. In:

Plant Flavonoids in Biology and Medicine II: Biochemical, Cellular, and Medicinal Properties. Alan R Liss, New York, pp 369-374.

Varis K, Salmi HA, Siurala M (1978) Die Therapie der Lebererkrankung mit Legalon; eine kontrollierte Doppelblindstudie. In: Aktuelle Hepatologie, Third International Symposoium, Cologne, Nov. 15-17, 1978. Hanseatisches Verlagskontor. Lübeck, pp 42-43.

Vogel G, Görler K (1981) Lebertherapeutika. In: Ullmanns Enzyklopädie der technischen Chemie. Vol.18, 4th Ed. Verlag Chemie, Weinheim New York, pp 132-136.

Vogel G (1980) The anti-amanita effect of silymarin. In: Faulstich et al. (eds) Amanita toxins and poisoning. Witzstrock, Baden-Baden Cologne New York, pp 132-136.

Vogel G (1980) The anti-amanita effect of silymarin. In: Faulstich et al. (eds) Amanita toxins and poisoning. Witzstrock, Baden-Baden Cologne New York, pp 180-187.

Wagner H, Seligmann O, Seilz M, Abraham D, Sonnenbichler J (1976) Silydianin und Silychristin, zwei isomere Silymarine aus Silybum marianum L. Gaertn. (Mariendistel). Z Naturforsch 31b: 876-884.

6 Urinary Tract

The two main urologic indications for plant drugs are inflammatory urinary tract diseases and benign prostatic hyperplasia (BPH). The first of these indications includes renal gravel and more severe types of lithiasis. Herbal remedies for these conditions consists mainly of kidney and bladder teas, most of which are relatively heterogeneous mixtures of various herbs. Four herbs are commonly used in the treatment of BPH: saw palmetto berries, nettle root, pumpkin seeds, and pygeum bark. The compound β-sitosterol, a plant sterol derived from *Hypoxis rooperi*, is also used. In Germany, the nonsurgical treatment of BPH relies predominantly on herbal medications (Schmitz, 1998).

6.1 Inflammatory Diseases of the Urinary Tract

In Germany, inflammatory urinary tract disorders are treated mainly with medicinal teas. The designation kidney and bladder teas is somewhat misleading, for while the herbal ingredients of these teas are often purported to have a diuretic action, this has never been proven conclusively. Juniper berries are the only herb deemed likely to have a direct action the renal parenchyma. As for the other herbs used in urologic teas (Table 6.1), it is probable that they derive most or all of their aquaretic effect (Schilcher, 1987, 1992) from the fluid that is ingested with the tea. Although various plant constituents were described as diuretic in the older literature (flavonoids, phenols, volatile oils, silicic acid), their low concentrations alone make it unlikely that they could produce a significant diuretic action (Nahrstedt, 1993; Veit, 1994).

The Ger,man Commission E, after reviewing mostly reports of traditional use, has declared the herbs listed in Table 6.1 to be effective in the treatment of inflammatory urinary tract diseases. Most of these herbs have also been declared useful in the treatment of mild renal stone disease (gravel). It appears that positive experience with the use of these herbal teas, especially in relieving dysuric complaints associated with inflammatory urinary tract diseases and infections, is reflected in current medical prac-

Table 6.1.
Twelve tea herbs recognized by Commission E as having value in the treatment of inflammatory urinary tract disorders and mild renal stone disease.

Herb	Pharmacopeial name	Daily dose (g)
Birch leaf	Betulae folium	12
Dandelion herb and root	Taraxaci herba cum radice	3
Field Horsetail	Equiseti herba	6
Goldenrod and Early Goldenrod	Virgaurea herba and Virgaurea giganteae herba	6-12
Lovage root	Levistici radix	4-8
Nettle leaf	Urticae herba	8-12
Orthosiphon leaf	Orthosiphonis folium	6-12
Parsley herb and root	Petroselini herba cum radice	6
Petasite rhizome	Petasitidis rhizoma	5-7
Red Sandalwood	Santali lignum rubri	10
Restharrow root	Ononidis radix	12
Triticum rhizome	Graminis rhizoma	6-9
Uva Ursi leaf	Uvae ursi folium	3

tice as significant numbers of these preparations are still being recommended and prescribed by German doctors (see Appendix).

In patients with urinary tract infections or with stone-related and other inflammatory irritations of the urinary tract, increasing the output of a hypo-osmolar urine appears to be an effective way to clear ascending bacteria, crystallization nuclei, and other inflammatory agents from the urinary tract, thus protecting the damaged epithelium. While this parmacodynamic principle has been challenged with respect to the prevention of urolithiasis (Ljunghall, 1988), the plausibility of flushing out the urinary tract as a general treatment strategy in inflammatory urinary tract diseases should not be dismissed. A related question is whether urologic teas owe their therapeutic effect to the fluid intake or to specific aquaretic actions of the administered herbs, provided the latter have a reasonable cost and can be used with an acceptable level of potential risk. In 1992, Commission E reversed its position on madder root (*Rubia tinctoria*), which was formerly recommended for the prevention of stone disease, and and removed the herb from approved status due to suspicion of excessive therapeutic risk. Madder root contains lucidin. A number of experimental studies, including the Ames mutagenicity test, strongly suggest that lucidin has mutagenic and carcinogenic properties.

Two herbs from this group (Table 6.1) have more specific actions: uva ursi (bearberry) leaves, whose hydroquinone constituents give it demonstrable antibacterial properties, and petasite rhizome, whose antispasmodic actions are beneficial in relieving spasmodic flank pain, especially when caused by urinary stones. Both herbs are discussed below in greater detail.

6.1.1 Uva Ursi Leaves

This herb consists of the dried leaves of the uva ursi or bearberry shrub (*Arctostaphylos uva-ursi*, family Ericaceae, Fig. 6.1). The trailing, perennial ground cover is similar to the cranberry in appearance and is widely distributed in the cool, temperate, forested zones of the northern hemisphere. Uva ursi leaves are odorless and have a bitter, astringent taste.

The key constituents of the herb are phenolic heterosides such as arbutin (5–12 %), small amounts of the free aglycone hydroquinone (0.2–0.5 %), tannins (10–20 %), and flavonoids. The relatively high tannin content of the herb limits the duration of its use to about 2–3 weeks. The antibacterial principle is arbutin or its hydrolysis product hydroquinone. Relatively little is known about the pharmacokinetics of arbutin; all data are based essentially on studies by Frohne (1986). Arbutin itself is poorly absorbed from the gastrointestinal tract. The aglycone hydroquinone is well absorbed following hydrolytic cleavage of the glycosidic bond by intestinal flora. Hydroquinone is probably conjugated in the intestinal mucosa or liver and excreted as a conjugate via the renal pathway. If the urine is alkaline, it is believed that hydroquinone reforms from the conjugates and, when present in sufficient quantities, acts as a urinary antiseptic. According to this line of reasoning, the urine should be adjusted to a slightly alkaline pH (about 8) through dietary measures. These concepts, though plausible, are supported only by scant experimental data. Meanwhile, phenols normally are antimicrobial in an undissociated state, which requires an acidic urinary pH. Thus, one authoritative

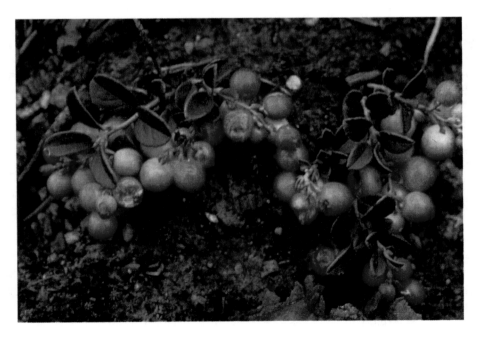

Figure 6.1. ▲ Fruits of bearberry (*Arctostaphylos uva-ursi*).

researcher has stated that an urgent need exists for new studies on the antibacterial properties of uva ursi (Nahrstedt, 1993). However, recent discoveries indicate that hydroquinones are ingested -by bacteria in conjugated form and are deconjugated while inside the bacteria. This means that alkalization of the urine is not necessary in order for arbutin to become active (Siegers et al., 2003).

So far, there have been no statistically and medically valid studies on the clinical use of uva ursi leaves administered as a single-herb preparation. There is a pressing need for up-to-date, controlled clinical studies using a high-dose, single-herb product. Nevertheless, documented experience, several clinical reports, and a number of experimental studies attest to the efficacy of the herb in bacterial inflammatory diseases.

No studies have yet been conducted on the acute and chronic toxicity, mutagenicity, or carcinogenicity of uva ursi leaves or their preparations. There is reason to suspect, however, that hydroquinone, which is partially derived from arbutin, does have mutagenic and carcinogenic effects. This prompted Commission E in 1993 to re-evaluate uva ursi leaves as part of a general review of hydroquinone-containing drugs. While the Commission affirmed the value of uva ursi leaves for "inflammatory diseases of the urinary tract," it cautioned against use of the herb in pregnancy, lactation, or in children under 12 years of age. This caution was based primarily on theoretical concerns, ie, speculative, based on the known pharmacology of hydroquinone, even though there was no direct evidence on uva ursi. The recommended dosage is 3 g of the dried herb, or 400–800 mg of hydroquinone derivatives, taken up to 4 times daily. Due to the risk potential, uva ursi leaves and their preparations should not be taken for more than one week without the advice of a physician, and they should be used no more than five times in one year.

Several therapeutic trials have been carried out on the use of cranberry juice for the same indication and in the prevention of infections of the lower urinary tract. In one randomized trial, 150 women with recurrent urinary tract infections drank 50 mL of cranberry juice or 100 mL of a lactobacillus drink daily for 12 months or received no intervention. The results: 36 % and 39 % of the women in the control and lactobacillus groups, respectively, had at least one recurrence during the treatment period, compared with only 16 % in the cranberry group. The difference was significant (Kontiokari et al., 2001). On the other hand, a Cochrane analysis of four other studies on cranberry juice for this indication did not result in a positive overall assessment (Jepson und Mihaljewic, 2000).

6.1.2 Petasite Rhizome, Ammi Fruit

Petasite rhizome consists of the dried underground parts of *Petasites hybridus*, a native European perennial that flourishes along the banks of streams and other moist areas. The active principles are a group of sesquiterpene compounds, the petasins, which are reputed to have antispasmodic and analgesic actions based on earlier studies (Bucher, 1951). The herb also contains pyrrolizidine alkaloids.

Based on medical experience with petasite rhizome and the results of several experimental studies, Commission E in 1990 recognized the herb as being useful for the "supportive treatment of acute colicky urinary tract pain, especially when due to stone disease", recommending a daily dose of about 5-7 g of the dried herb. Given the possible therapeutic risk, however, the daily dose should not exceed 1 µg pyrrolizidine alkaloids, and the duration of use should not exceed 4-6 weeks per year. The efficacy of butterbur leaf extract in allergic rhinitis is discussed in Sect. 4.9.

Another herb traditionally used to relieve the pain of renal colic and spastic urinary tract disorders, ammi fruit (*Ammi visnaga*), was not approved by Commission E in 1994 because of its excessive therapeutic risk and unproven efficacy. Consequently, preparations made from ammi fruits may no longer be prescribed in Germany for this or any other indication (Blumenthal et al., 1998).

6.2　Benign Prostatic Hyperplasia

Benign prostatic hyperplasia (BPH) is the most important urologic disorder affecting males. It generally affects men over 40 years of age and is present in more than 90 % of men over age 65. Only about 50 % of patients develop symptoms and complaints, however. The main obstructive signs of BPH are hesitancy in initiating the urinary stream, a weak and/or intermittent stream, and the terminal dribbling of urine. Up to 80 % of patients also have irritative symptoms such as pollakiuria, urgency, nocturia, pressure over the bladder, and a feeling of incomplete bladder emptying (Dreikorn et al., 1990). The anatomic cause is an enlargement of the prostate due to hyperplastic changes in the periurethral glands, causing narrowing of the urethra and voiding difficulties. The Vahlensieck classification (Table 6.2) is one of several staging systems that have been developed for diagnostic and therapeutic purposes.

The etiology and pathogenesis of BPH are not fully understood, so a causal medical treatment is not yet available. BPH is generally regarded as an endocrine disorder of older males caused by changes in the hormone balance associated with aging (Ekman, 1989). Three specific hypotheses on the pathogenesis of BPH will be reviewed below to help clarify the mechanisms of actions of herbal remedies.

Table 6.2.
Stages of benign prostatic hyperplasia (Vahlensiek, 1985).

Stage I	Stage II
▸ No voiding difficulties	▸ Transient voiding difficulties
▸ Urine flow > 15 mL/s	▸ Urine flow > 10-15 mL/s
▸ No residual urine	▸ Little or no trabeculation of the bladder
Stage III	**Stage IV**
▸ Permanent voiding dysfunction	▸ Permanent voiding dysfunction
▸ Urine flow < 10 mL/s	▸ Urine flow < 10 mL/s
▸ Residual urine > 50 mL	▸ Residual urine > 100 mL
▸ Trabeculated bladder	▸ Bladder dilatation
	▸ Urinary retention

The most widely favored hypothesis is based on an increase in the prostatic synthesis of dihydrotestosterone (DHT) accompanied by an increase in the estrogen: androgen ratio. The best known therapeutic approach based on this hypothesis is to inhibit the two prostatic enzymes 5α-reductase (which converts testosterone to DHT) and aromatase (which converts testosterone to estrogens). It has also been suggested that an increased production of prolactin may contribute to prostatic hyperplasia (Costello und Franklin, 1994; Nevalainen et al., 1997). A further hypothesis holds that elevated levels of inflammatory mediators (prostaglandins and leukotrienes) are partly responsible for the development of BPH. This multifactorial pathogenesis suggests that plant constituents with anti-inflammatory and antiedematous properties would be of therapeutic benefit in BPH patients (Koch, 1995).

BPH does not require treatment unless it is associated with irritative urinary symptoms (urgency, frequency, nocturia) or obstructive symptoms (weak urinary stream, hesitancy, incomplete voiding). BPH becomes symptomatic in approximately 40 % of males over age 70. While prostatectomy has traditionally been the treatment of choice in the U.S. (Flanigan et al., 1998), stage II and stage III BPH (Table 6.2) are most often treated conservatively with herbal medications in Germany, Austria, Switzerland, and Italy. The use of saw palmetto extracts as self-selected dietary supplements in the U.S. has increased dramatically in recent years, however (Wilt et al., 1998). Two classes of conventional synthetic drugs, the 5-α-reductase inhibitors and alpha$_1$-receptor blockers, are also available as alternatives to herbal prostate remedies. The synthetic drugs are comparable to the herbal products in efficacy, but the herbals are associated with fewer and milder adverse side effects, particularly with regard to sexual function (Bach et al., 1996; Carraro et al., 1996).

Besides the pharmacodynamic effects of the active constituents, the therapeutic context has a significant impact on treatment response in BPH as it is in other conditions. Placebo-controlled studies show that this effect accounts for approximately 30–60 % of the attainable therapeutic response, depending on the outcome measures that are used. This means that, beyond the medications themselves, counseling of the patient by the physician with regard to living habits is a key factor in improving the patient's complaints. To reduce congestion and bladder irritation, the patient should urinate promptly when the urge is felt, avoid overdistending the bladder by rapidly drinking large amounts of fluid, and avoid prolonged sitting or excessive cold. Emphasis is also placed on regular bowel habits and ample physical exercise; excessive alcohol intake, cold carbonated beverages, and pungent spices should be avoided (Sökeland, 1987). It should be noted that adrenomimetic drugs such as ephedrine in cough syrups and phenylephrine in nosedrops (no longer widely available in OTC drugs) can exacerbate voiding difficulties, as can anticholinergics and antihistamines.

Synthetic conventional preparations are also available for the pharmacotherapy of BPH; their role is discussed in Sect. 6.3.

6.2.1 Saw Palmetto Berries

The use of preparations made from the ripe fruits (berries) of a small fan palm known as saw palmetto or sabal (*Serenoa repens*, Fig. 6.2) for the treatment of BPH can be traced back to the early 1900's (Harnischfeger and Stolze, 1989). Saw palmetto berries are about 1–2 cm long and are usually gathered in the wild. The sole supplier of the raw berries is the United States, to which the berries re native to the Southeastern region; standardized extracts are available from European and American suppliers. Commercial preparations contain only lipophilic (fat-soluble) extracts, which are obtained from the powdered herb by extraction with hexane or liquid carbon dioxide. The principal ingredients in these extracts are saturated and unsaturated fatty acids, which occur mostly in free form. Free and conjugated plant sterols are also key constituents.

6.2.1.1 Pharmacology

The results of animal studies and in vitro experiments with saw palmetto extracts have been published in numerous original papers (surveys in Hänsel et al., 1994, and Koch, 1995; Plosker and Progden, 1996; Coppenolle et al., 2000). Studies in mice and rats demonstrated antiandrogenic actions in various models. Several in vitro studies confirmed inhibitory effects of saw palmetto extracts on 5 α-reductase. A comparison of relative efficacies showed that saw palmetto extract was some 6000 times less potent than an equal weight of the synthetic inhibitory agent finasteride (Proscar®) (Rhodes et al., 1993), but allowance for the therapeutic dosage of both agents narrowed the potency difference by a factor of 100 (Koch, 1995). In experiments on live rats, however, saw palmetto extract caused an equivalent inhibition of hormone-induced enlargement of the lateral prostate compared with finasteride in a dose proportional to that used in

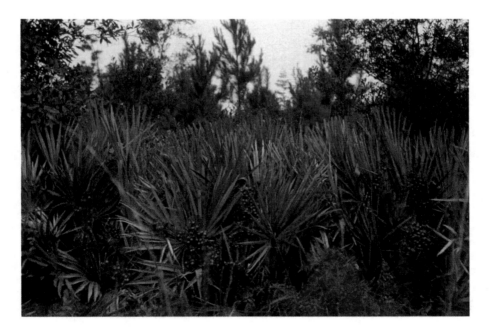

Figure 6.2. ▲ Saw palmetto (*Serenoa repens*).

humans (Coppenolle et al., 2000). The inhibition of 5 α-reductase by saw palmetto extract is partly due to its content of free fatty acids. One study compared the effect of saw palmetto extract with that of free fatty acids of various chain lengths. It was found that several common dietary fatty acids (e.g., linoleic acid) exerted stronger inhibitory effects on 5 α-reductase than equivalent concentrations of saw palmetto extract (Niederprüm et al., 1994), raising some unanswered questions regarding this mechanism of action. Saw palmetto extracts have other effects as well. For example, saw palmetto extract in rats was found to inhibit sulpiride-induced hyperprolactinemia and the associated prostatic hyperplasia – an effect that could not be achieved with finasteride (Coppenolle et al., 2000). In addition, fractions from saw palmetto berries as well as commercial saw palmetto extracts demonstrated anti-inflammatory and antioxidant actions in typical experimental models of inflammation (carrageenan-induced rat's paw edema) (Koch, 1995).

6.2.1.2 Therapeutic Efficacy

Two meta-analyses on 18 randomized controlled clinical studies in a total of 2939 patients were published between 1983 and 1998 (Table 6.3). Sixteen of the studies had a double-blind design, and 11 of those used an identical extract (Wilt et al., 1998, 2001; Boyle et al., 2000) Three studies published since 1996 (Carraro et al., 1996; Metzker et al., 1996; Sökeland and Albrecht, 1997) are based on a validated, WHO-recommended symptom index for evaluating benign prostatic hyperplasia. The evaluation is based on several total scores. The first score is the International Prostate Symptom Score (IPSS); it contains questions on the seven most common subjective complaints (incomplete emptying, frequency, intermittency, urgency, weak stream, straining to initiate the stream, and nocturia), each of which is rated on a 0–5 scale. An IPSS score of 10–20 indicates moderate symptoms, and a score of 20–30 indicates severe symptoms. The other total scores include a quality-of-life scale, which has ratings from 0 (no impairment) to 6 (severe impairment), and a 0–5 scale for rating sexual function (Barry et al., 1992). The corresponding results of a 6-month double-blind randomized equivalence study that compared the efficacy of a saw palmetto extract (320 mg/d) with that of a 5-α-reductase inhibitor (5 mg/d finasteride) in 1098 men with BPH are summarized in Table 6.4 and Figs. 6.3 and 6.4. As Table 6. shows, the plant extract and synthetic drug were equivalent in their effects on IPPS, quality of life, and average urinary flow. Finasteride was borderline superior (p<0.05) in its effect on peak urinary flow, and the saw palmetto extract was markedly superior (p<0.01) in its effect on sexual function (Fig. 6.4) (Carraro et al., 1996).

Another randomized double-blind study was performed to test the therapeutic equivalence of finasteride with a product containing saw palmetto extract (test dose 320 mg/d) in addition to a small amount of nettle root extract (test dose 240 mg/d). This study was done in a total of 543 patients over a 48-week period. The IPSS in the saw palmetto group decreased from 11.3 to 8.2 (week 24) and then to 6.5 (week 48), while in the finasteride group it decreased from 11.8 to 8.0 and finally to 6.2 in the same intervals. The quality of life score (lower = better) decreased from 7.5 to 4.3 in the saw palmetto group and from 7.7 to 4.1 in the finasteride group. Peak urinary flow increased by 1.9 mL/s in the saw palmetto group and by 2.4 mL/s in the finasteride group. A statisti-

Table 6.3.
Review of 19 randomized controlled studies of saw palmetto extract preparations in a total of 3129 men.

First author	Year	Cases (n)	Duration (d)	Extract dose (mg/d)	Reference therapy	Outcome measures
Emili	1983	30	28	320	Placebo	UF, PV, RU, N
Boccafoschi	1983	22	60	320	Placebo	UF, symptoms
Madressi	1983	60	28	320	Placebo, Pygeum	RU, N, symptoms
Champault	1984	110	28	160	Placebo	UF, RU, N
Tasca	1985	30	56	320	Placebo	UF, N, symptoms
Reece	1986	80	84	320	Placebo	UF, RU, symptoms
Cukier	1985	168	69	320	Placebo	RU, N, symptoms
Pannuzio	1986	60	56	320	Depostat®	UF, PV, N, symptoms
Carbin	1990	55	84	80 + 80	Placebo	UF, RV, N, symptoms
Mattei	1990	40	91	320	Placebo	PV, RU, N, symptoms
Löbelenz	1992	60	35	300	Placebo	UF
Roveda	1994	30	28	640	Rektal	PV, RU, symptoms
Descotes	1995	215	28	320	Placebo	UF, N, symptoms
Carraro	1996	1098	180	320	Placebo, Finasteride	IPSS, QLS, SES, UF, RU, RV
Metzker	1996	40	336	320 + 240	Placebo	IPSS, UF, RU
Sökeland	1997	543	336	320 + 240	Placebo, Finasteride	IPSS, QLS, UF, PV, RU
Braeckman	1997	238	84	320	Placebo	UF, PV, RU
Bauer	1999	101	168	320	Placebo	IPSS, QLS, UF, PV
Bondarenko	2003	140	420	320 + 240	Tamsulosin	IPSS, QLS

NOTE: Metzger (1996), Sökeland (1997), and Bondarenko (2003) used a combination product containing saw palmetto seed extract and nettle root extract. Carbin (1990) tested a combination product containing saw palmetto seed extract and pumpkin seed extract. The reference-therapy doses were as follows: pygeum 100 mg extract/day; Depostat® 200 mg/day gestonorone i.m.; Rektal 640 mg/day saw palmetto extract rectally; finasteride 5 mg/day.
Abbreviations: IPSS = International Prostate Symptom Scale; QLS = Quality of Life Score; SFS = Sexual Function Score; N = nycturia; UF = urine flow; PV = prostate volume; RU = residual urine.

cal comparison of the efficacy parameters confirmed therapeutic equivalence of the two test preparations. Marked differences were found, however, in the incidence of certain adverse side effects (saw palmetto vs. finasteride): decreased ejaculatory volume 0 vs. 5, erectile dysfunction 1 vs. 7, joint pain 1 vs. 5, headache 2 vs. 6, and gastrointestinal complaints 10 vs. 13 (Sökeland and Albrecht, 1997). These results were independent of the initial prostatic volume (Sökeland, 2000).

In another prospective, randomized, reference-controlled, multicenter double-blind study, a combination product of saw-palmetto and urtica extract (PRO) was compared with tamsulosin in 140 patients with symptomatic BPH. A 2-week placebo run-in was followed by 60 weeks of treatment with 1 capsule of PRO 160/120 mg twice daily (n=71) or 1 capsule of tamsulosin (TAM, n=69) in a double-dummy format. Outcomes were measured with the IPSS. Patients were classified as responders if they displayed only mild symptoms (IPSS 7 points) at the conclusion of treatment. Another target parame-

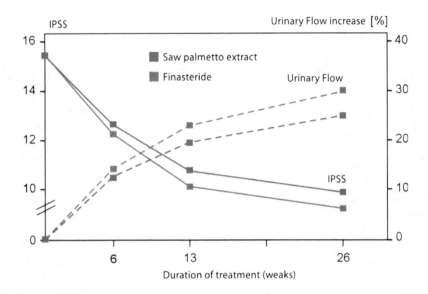

Figure 6.3. ▲ Study from Table 6.3, showing the mean values in 553 patients (saw palmetto extract) and 545 patients (finasteride) for the International Prostate Symptom Score (IPSS) and the percentage increase in urinary flow rate during 26 weeks of treatment (after Carraro et al., 1996).

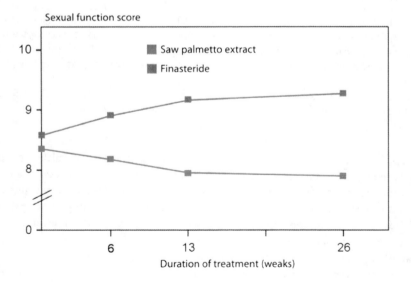

Figure 6.4. ▲ Same study in Fig. 6.3, showing the progression of mean scores for impairment of sexual function (after Carraro et al., 1996).

Table 6.4.

Results of a randomized double-blind study comparing the efficacy of 320 mg/day saw palmetto extract with 5 mg/day finasteride in 1098 patients with BPH (Carraro et al., 1996).

Parameters	Initial	At 26 weeks	% Change	Group comparison
IPSS				
Saw palmetto extract	15,7	9,9*	– 37	n. s.
Finasteride	15,7	9,5*	– 39	
Quality of life				
Saw palmetto extract	3,63	2,25*	– 38	n. s.
Finasteride	3,66	2,15*	– 41	
Sexual function				
Saw palmetto extract	8,4	7,9 n. s.	– 6	$p < 0.001$
Finasteride	8,6	9,3**	+9	
Peak urinary flow				
Saw palmetto extract	10,6	13,3*	+25	$p < 0.05$
Finasteride	10,8	14,0*	+30	
Average urinary flow				
Saw palmetto extract	5,4	6,2*	+15	n. s.
Finasteride	5,5	6,6*	+20	

NOTE: The results for IPSS, quality of life, and sexual function are given as scores (lower = better); urinary flow is stated in mL/sec.
Abbreviations: IPSS = International Prostate Symptom Score, * = $p<0.05$, ** = $p<0.01$, n.s. = not significant.

ter was quality of life (QoL). All 140 patients were candidates for intention-to-treat analysis. During the 60-week treatment period, the IPSS in both groups improved by a median value of 9 points from a baseline of 20 points. At the end of the study (n=136), 22 of the PRO patients (32.4 %) and 19 of the TAM patients (27.9 %) displayed only mild symptoms (p=0.03; noninferiority test, 10 % limit). With regard to QoL, the PRO group improved by 2 points from a baseline of 3 while the TAM group improved by 1 point from a baseline of 4 (median values). Adverse events were slightly more frequent in the TAM group than the PRO group (Bondarenko et al., 2003).

In a meta-analysis of 18 controlled clinical studies of saw palmetto extracts with treatment periods of 4 to 48 weeks, the extracts were significantly better than placebo and comparable to finasteride in their therapeutic efficacy. (Wilt et al., 1998, 2001). Another meta-analysis of 11 of these studies, all using an identical extract (Permixon®, Pierre Fabre, Toulousse, France), yielded a similar result. The best response was achieved in maximum urinary flow, while the frequency of nocturia showed a less pronounced change relative to placebo (Boyle et al, 2000). The distribution of the daily dose (2 × 160 mg in the morning and evening or 320 mg of extract taken as a single morning dose) does not appear to affect treatment response (Stepanov et al., 1999).

6.2.1.3 Tolerance

Two meta-analyses on saw palmetto demonstrate the general safety of this herb. Adverse side effects from the saw palmetto extracts were generally mild and were comparable in incidence to the adverse effects associated with a placebo. Of the 2939 total men studied in all of the 18 trials reviewed the dropout rate due to adverse effects was 7 % with placebo, 9.1 % with saw palmetto extract, and 11.2 % with finasteride. The incidence of erectile dysfunction was 0.7 % with placebo, 1.1 % with saw palmetto extract, and 4.9 % with finasteride. Gastrointestinal complaints occurred in 0.9 % of the placebo patients, 1.3 % of the saw palmetto patients, and 1.5 % of the finasteride patients (Wilt et al., 1998, 2001). In a 3-year prospective study, 34 of the 435 patients (7 %) reported a total of 46 mild adverse reactions, approximately one-third of which were gastrointestinal. Adverse urologic events were observed in a total of 9 patients: 4 cases of prostatic carcinoma, 3 urinary tract infections, 1 case of impotence, and 1 case of ejaculatory problems (Bach, 1996). There has been one case report of severe intraoperative hemorrhage occurring in a 53-year-old man during a meningioma resection. Preoperative tests had shown normal coagulation parameters, but the postoperative bleeding time was prolonged to 21 min. Because the patient had been taking saw palmetto extract for some time, it was reasonable to assume that the extract had adversely affected platelet aggregation due to inhibitory effects on cyclooxygenase (Cheema et al., 2001).

To date, almost all of the research on saw palmetto has conducted in western Europe, mainly France, Germany, and Italy. However, in the past few years there have been two papers based on research conducted in the U.S. In one trial (Marks et al., 1999) 44 men (ages 45-85) who were diagnosed with BPH underwent prostate biopsies to establish a baseline of prostate tissue parameters. They were given a combination product containing saw palmetto (106 mg), nettle root extract (80 mg), pumpkin seed oil extract (160 mg), bioflavonoids (33 mg) and vitamin A (as beta-carotene, 190 mg) (Nutrilite, Buena Park , California, USA) three times daily, or placebo. The saw palmetto blend group had non-statistically significant improvement versus the placebo in clinical parameters (e.g., IPSS, uroflowmetry, residual urine volume, prostate volume). After 6 months, the saw palmetto blend was associated with prostate epithelial contraction, notably in the transition zone where the epithelial contraction changed from 17.8 % at baseline to 10.7 % after 6 months of saw palmetto herbal blend (p<0.01), suggesting a possible mechanism for clinical significance found by other studies. No serious adverse effects were associated with SP blend. This is the first time a study has determined that a saw palmetto preparation actually may shrink prostate tissue.

Another trial by some of the same investigators (Marks et al., 2001), attempted to determine the effects the same saw palmetto combination compared to finasteride on testosterone and dihydrotestosterone (DHT) levels in prostate tissue. A total of 244 biopsied prostate tissue samples from 3 separate trials were analyzed for the androgen levels. The study concluded that for control versus finasteride-treated men, the tissue androgen values obtained with needle biopsy specimens were similar – both for absolute values and the percentage of change – to those previously reported using surgically excised volumes of prostatic tissue. They concluded that quantification of prostatic androgens by assay of needle biopsies is thus feasible and offers the possibility of serial studies in individual patients. The saw palmetto blend induced suppression of prostatic DHT levels, at modest but significant levels in a randomized trial. This conclusion supports the hypothesis that inhibition of the enzyme 5-alpha reductase is a mechanism of action of the saw palmetto blend. Unfortunately, since the product contained 3 phytomedicines used for BPH, it is not possible to determine from this research if the observed effect is a result of the activity of one of the phytomedicines, or of an additive or synergistic combination of all three.

The Commission E monograph on saw palmetto in its January, 1991, revision states that certain preparations made from saw palmetto berries are indicated for "urination problems in benign prostatic hyperplasia stages I and II," recommending a daily dose of 1–2 g of the crude drug or 320 mg of an extract made with lipophilic solvents (Blumenthal et al., 1998). As for side effects, there have been rare reports of gastric upset. There are no known contraindications to saw palmetto preparations.

6.2.2 Nettle Root

Familiar to everyone, nettle (*Urtica dioica*) is a traditional medicinal plant cited in medieval herbals for its usefulness as a diuretic and a remedy for joint ailments. It is only since around 1980 that nettle root and its preparations have been applied to the treatment of benign prostatic hyperplasia (Nöske, 1994). All experimental pharmacologic studies and several clinical studies of nettle root have used hydroalcoholic extracts prepared with relatively hydrophilic solvents, i.e., methanol or ethanol in concentrations of 20–60 %. The main components of these extracts include phytosterols, triterpene acids, lignans, polysaccharides, and simple phenol compounds.

Numerous experimental pharmacologic studies (survey in Koch, 1995) have shown that nettle root extracts inhibit prostatic aromatase and 5-α-reductase, interact with sex-hormone-binding globulin, and exert multiple inhibitory effects on inflammatory mediators (Hryb et al., 1995; Hartmann et al., 1996). An aqueous extract of nettle root showed weak anti-inflammatory activity when tested in the model of carrageenan-induced rat's paw edema. The authors attributed the anti-inflammatory action to an acid polysaccharide fraction in the extract (Wagner et al., 1994).

The positive effects of nettle root extract in patients with BPH have been attributed in part to the competitive displacement of sex-hormone-binding globulin (SHBG) (Schmidt, 1983). However, such an effect requires extract concentrations on the order of 1–10 mg/mL (Hryb, 1995), which probably are too high to be attained with therapeutic doses.

In addition to 8 open and observational studies, a total of 4 placebo-controlled, double-blind studies have been published on the therapeutic efficacy of nettle root extract (Vontobel et al., 1985; Dathe and Schmid, 1987; Fischer and Wilbert, 1992; Engelmann et al., 1996). All 4 studies employed a methanol-water extract of nettle root (20 % v/v, herb-to-extract ratio approximately 10:1).

Vontobel et al. (1985) performed their study in 50 patients with BPH (25 nettle root extract, 25 placebo). The daily dose was 600 mg of extract, and the treatment period was 9 weeks. The authors found a statistically significant reduction of SHBG and a significant increase in urinary output (44 %) and peak urinary flow (9 %) compared with a placebo.

Dathe and Schmid (1987) conducted a double-blind study in a total of 79 patients over a period of 4–6 weeks. The patients received the same preparation at the same dosage (600 mg/day extract) as in the study of Vontobel et al. The patients had BPH, but the stage was not specified. Response was assessed by the measurement of urinary flow rate, which increased significantly by 2 mL/s (14 %) relative to the placebo-treated group.

Fischer and Wilbert (1992) performed a study in 40 patients with BPH. After 4 weeks' treatment with a placebo, the patients were randomly divided into 2 groups, one of which received a daily dose of 1200 mg of nettle root extract for 24 weeks. A symptom score devised by Boyarski was used to evaluate efficacy. Laboratory measurements were also performed, including an SHBG assay. Comparison of the Boyarski scores in the nettle root and placebo groups showed significant improvements starting in week 4 of treatment. A significant reduction in SHBG was also found in the patients treated with nettle root extract.

Engelmann et al. (1996) tested a liquid nettle root extract in 41 patients with BPH. The daily dose was equivalent to approximately 5–6 g of nettle root, and the duration of treatment was 12 weeks. The IPSS, quality-of-life score, peak urinary flow rate, and post-void residual urinary volume were used to evaluate response. The IPPS of the patients treated with nettle root extract decreased by 9.5 units from 18.2 to 8.7, compared with an average decrease of only 4.7 in the placebo group. The difference between the groups was statistically significant ($p < 0.002$). Quality of life, peak urinary flow, and residual urinary volume were better in the group treated with nettle root extract, but the differences were not statistically significant.

The tolerance to nettle root extract is demonstrated by an observational study in 4087 patients with BPH who took 600–1200 mg of the extract daily for 6 months. Only 35 of the patients reported side effects, with 33 citing gastrointestinal complaints (0.65 %), 9 noting skin allergies (0.19 %), and 2 reporting hyperhidrosis (Sonnenschein, 1987).

The Commission E monograph on nettle root in its January, 1991, revision states that the herb is indicated for "difficulty in urination in benign prostatic hyperplasia stages 1 and 2" recommending a daily dose equivalent to 4–6 g of the crude drug (Blumenthal et al., 1998). No contraindications are stated. Occasional, mild gastrointestinal complaints are mentioned as possible side effects.

6.2.3 Pumpkin Seeds

Seeds of the pumpkin, *Cucurbita pepo* (family Cucurbitaceae), have long been used in folk medicine, especially in southeastern Europe, as a remedy for irritable bladder and BPH. The soft-shell varieties are particularly recommended and are the only ones for which scientific data have been acquired.

The seeds, which have a sweet, oily taste, contain fatty oil consisting mainly of linoleic acid (64 %) in addition to plant sterols, tocopherols, carotenoids, and minerals. The identity of the constituents responsible for the therapeutic efficacy of pumpkin seeds remains to be established (Schilcher, 1987, 1992).

Pumpkin seeds are used medicinally in various forms. The most common practice is to use the whole or ground seeds. Expressed oils and dry extracts are also used. An isolated protein known as pumpkin globulin is employed mainly in combination products.

How the different preparations may differ in their pharmacologic actions is unknown (Koch, 1995).

The use of pumpkin seeds and their preparations in the treatment of BPH is based almost entirely on empirical knowledge. One experimental study showed that the Δ-7 sterols contained in pumpkin seeds have the ability to displace DHT from androgen receptors on human fibroplasts. In an open clinical study, 6 patients with BPH each received 90 mg of an isolated pumpkin sterol mixture 3 and 4 days before undergoing a radical prostatectomy. Examination of the excised tissue showed a highly significant decline in the DHT levels of the prostatic tissue compared with an untreated control group (Schilcher, 1987, 1992).

In a randomized double-blind study, the efficacy and tolerance of an ethanol pumpkin seed extract were tested in 476 patients with BPH (233 received the extract and 243 a placebo). The patients took one 500-mg capsule of the extract b.i.d. (equivalent to approximately 20 g/d of pumpkin seed) or the placebo for 12 weeks. Efficacy was evaluated by the IPSS (see Sect. 6.1.2.2), with a reduction of at least 5 points defined as the response criterion. After 3 months of treatment, this criterion was met by 65 % of the patients in the pumpkin seed group and 54 % of the patients in the placebo group. The difference was statistically significant (p<0.02). Five patients each experienced an adverse event that may have been related to the pumpkin seed therapy: hot flashes, headache, stomach ache, gastrointestinal complaints, and gout (Bach, 2000).

The 1985 Commission E monograph states that pumpkin seeds are indicated for "irritated bladder condition, micturition problems of benign prostatic hyperplasia stages 1 and 2," recommending a daily dose of 10 g of ground seeds or corresponding preparations (Blumenthal et al., 1998). There are no known side effects or herb-drug interactions.

6.2.4 Grass Pollens

In 1994, Commission E recommended a preparation for the treatment of BPH whose active ingredient is a complex extract of 92 % rye pollen (*Secale cereale*), 5 % timothy pollen (*Phleum pratense*) and 3 % corn pollen (*Zea mays*). The herbs are extracted with a water and acetone mixture, yielding a product with an herb-to-extract ration of 2.5:1. This extract has been the subject of numerous pharmacologic studies. One in vitro study showed a dose-dependent inhibition of inflammatory mediators (Loschen and Ebeling, 1991); another demonstrated growth-inhibiting effects in cultured prostatic epithelial cells and fibroplasts (Habib et al., 1992). Toxicologic studies showed no evidence of increased therapeutic risks or mutagenic effects.

The therapeutic efficacy of the pollen extract in BPH was tested in two placebo-controlled, double-blind studies in patients with Vahlensieck stage II or stage III disease. The first was a multicenter study involving a total of 103 patients from 6 urologic practices. The extract was administered in a dose of 138 mg/day for 12 weeks. Response was assessed on the basis of FDA-recommended criteria for voiding difficulties (residual urine volume, urine flow, palpable findings, and overall rating by the physician and patient). Comparison of the extract-treated and placebo-treated groups showed a statistically significant improvement in nocturia (in 69 % vs. 37 % of cases, respectively, p<0.005) and in residual urine volumes (reduced by 24 mL vs. 4 mL in the placebo group). There was no significant difference in urine flow (Becker and Ebeling, 1988, 1991).

In the second placebo-controlled, double-blind study, 60 patients with BPH received a daily dose equivalent to 92 mg of the pollen extract for 6 months. The parameters of interest were urine flow, urinary output, ultrasound-determined residual urine volume, transrectal palpation of prostate size, and clinical symptoms. Fifty-three of the patient protocols were deemed satisfactory for analysis. The extract showed statistically significant advantages over the placebo in the total complaint score (69 % vs. 29 % with a placebo, p<0.01), residual urine, and prostate volume. Neither group showed significant changes in urine flow (Buck et al., 1990).

A meta-analysis of 4 studies (2 placebo-controlled) in a total of 444 patients showed significant improvements in subjective symptoms but not in urine flow. Tolerance was good in all the studies (MacDonald et al, 2000).

Based largely on the results of the two placebo-controlled, double-blind studies, which meet current minimum standards for such research, Commission E declared the pollen extract to be useful in the treatment of "micturition difficulties associated with Alken stage I–II benign prostatic enlargement (BPH)." The recommended daily dose is 80–120 mg of the extract taken in 2 or 3 divided doses. As for side effects, rare instances of gastrointestinal complaints or allergic skin reactions have been reported. There are no contraindications. At least a 3-month course of treatment is advised.

6.2.5 Phytosterols from Hypoxis rooperi

The tuber of the South African plant *Hypoxis rooperi* (family Hypoxidaceae) was used by the natives and later by European immigrants as a natural remedy for ailments of the bladder and prostate. Extraction of the herb with lipophilic solvents yields a β-sitosterol fraction that contains 10 % β-sitosterolin (a glycoside of sitosterol).

β-Sitosterol resembles cholesterol in its chemical structure and interferes with the intestinal absorption of cholesterol, so it is also useful in the treatment of hypercholesterolemia. Pharmacologic studies have shown that prostatic tissue tends to bind sitosterol, which then acts on prostaglandin metabolism (Pegel and Walker, 1984). Besides β-sitosterol, β-sitosterolin is also considered a key active ingredient of *H. rooperi* preparations.

One placebo-controlled, double-blind study showed a beneficial effect of β-sitosterol on residual urine volume and urine flow (Ebbinghaus and Baur, 1977). Another double-blind study using ultrasonography showed a significant improvement in the internal echo pattern of prostatic adenoma, which was interpreted as a reduction of interstitial edema by β-sitosterol (Szutrely, 1982).

Another placebo-controlled, double-blind study applied the test criteria of the International Consensus Conference on Benign Prostatic Hyperplasia (Aso et al., 1993) to 200 patients with BPH. When the treatment period was concluded at 6 months, 96 of the patients receiving sitosterol (60 mg/day β-sitosterol) and 91 of those given the placebo were deemed satisfactory for evaluation. Efficacy was judged using a modification of the Boyarsky symptom score (Boyarsky, 1977) in addition to urine flow and prostate volume. On average, the symptom score improved by 6.7 points in the sitosterol-treated group vs. 2.1 points in the placebo group. The difference between the groups was statistically significant (p<0.01). Significant intergroup differences were also seen in maximum urine flow and residual urine volume, but not in prostate volume. No significant side effects were noted during the 6-month course of treatment (Berges et al., 1995). In another placebo-controlled, double-blind study, 177 patients received a daily dose of 130 mg sitosterol for a period of 24 weeks. All three target parameters (IPSS, quality-of-life score, residual urinary volume) improved significantly in the sitosterol group compared with a placebo (Klippel et al., 1997).

A meta-analysis of 4 double-blind studies in a total of 519 patients showed an average improvement of 4.9 points in the IPSS relative to placebo (35 %), a 34 % increase in urine flow, and a 24 % decrease in residual urine volume (Wilt et al., 1999).

The medicinal preparations used in the studies cited above, like the products currently marketed in Germany, contain isolated β-sitosterol rather than actual extracts from *H. rooperi*. But pure compounds, even when of botanical origin, are no longer considered phytomedicines as the term is defined in this book and generally elsewhere in phytotherapy. As for the therapeutic effects shown in clinical studies, critics point out that 150–300 mg of sitosterol is ingested daily in foods, which is equivalent to 2–10 times the amount recommended for commercial herbal products (Schmitz, 1998).

6.2.6 Pygeum

The bark of pygeum (*Prunus africana*, syn., *Pygeum africanum*) has long been used as a bladder and urinary remedy in southern and central Africa, where originally the bark was ground to a fine powder and stirred into milk. Pygeum is an evergreen tree that is related botanically to fruit trees occurring at western latitudes (apricot, cherry, almond, plum, pear, sloe). Lipophilic extracts from pygeum bark contain at least three different classes of active compounds that may be responsible for its therapeutic effect: phytosterols (present in both free and conjugated form), pentacyclic terpenes, and ferulic acid esters (Hass et al., 1999). Relatively low doses of a lipophilic pygeum bark extract have been shown to inhibit 5-α-reductase from rat prostatic homogenate and also aromatase from the human placenta (Hartmann et al., 1996). One study compared a pygeum extract with 320 mg/d of a lipophilic saw palmetto extract and with a placebo. Sixty patients with BPH were enrolled and treated for 4 weeks. Efficacy was evaluated by improvements noted in specific clinical symptoms. Improvement in the frequency of nocturia was particularly evident relative to placebo, but no differences were seen between pygeum extract and saw palmetto extract (Mandressi et al., 1983). A controlled double-blind study was performed in 134 patients with BPH using a combined preparation containing a lipophilic pygeum extract and a hydrophilic extract of stinging nettle root (urtica). Significant improvements were found in a number of symptoms as well as residual urinary volume (Krzeski et al., 1993).

One meta-analysis covered 18 randomized studies (17 double-blind) in a total of 1562 patients. The average doses of pygeum extract in these studies ranged from 75 to 200 mg/d (in some cases combined with other phytomedicines). The average duration of the studies was 64 days. Six studies that used an identical extract compared with placebo achieved an average reduction of 19 % in the frequency of nocturia, a 24 % decrease in residual urine, and a 23 % increase in urine flow (Ishani et al., 2000).

Pygeum preparations were not evaluated by Commission E as pygeum-based phytomedicines were not sold in Germany during the time the Commission was evaluating the safety and efficacy of botanical drugs, i.e., between 1978 and 1994. Currently there are no pygeum products being marketed in Germany. Pygeum extracts are widely used for the treatment of BPH in Italy, Switzerland, and France, especially in products that combine pygeum with nettle root and/or saw palmetto berries. These products are also widely marketed in the U.S. as dietary supplements.

6.3 Therapeutic Significance

Herbal medications are frequently prescribed urinary remedies in Germany, and plant drugs are used mostly in patients treated for benign prostatic disorders.

The preparations, whether by virtue of their fluid content or specific pharmacodynamic actions, are considered beneficial adjuncts in the symptomatic treatment of mild forms of inflammatory urinary tract disease. Of course, there are far more potent synthetic drugs available for the treatment of pain, spasms, and bacterial infections, and the prescribing physician must decide on an individual basis whether such products are preferred. Moreover, there is no rigorous scientific proof that any of the tea herbs listed in Sect. 6.5 are effective in treating urologic disorders. Thus, the supportive use of these teas in inflammatory urinary tract diseases can be justified only if their use does not pose any additional risk. This policy would contraindicate the use of tea therapy in patients with advanced cardiac or renal failure. It also justifies the actions of Commission E in withdrawing its approval of two herbs (madder root and ammi fruit) for urologic indications because of their unacceptable risks.

In Germany, phytomedicines have come to be preferred over synthetic drugs in the treatment of BPH. In assessing the efficacy of the medical or surgical treatment of BPH, and in selecting patients for a specific type of therapy, the physician's task is made difficult by the fact that purely obstructive symptoms, which today can be verified by urodynamic studies, are generally associated with marked subjective complaints that are very difficult to evaluate and confirm objectively. To resolve this dilemma, many studies make provide scoring systems and rating scales (Boyarsky, 1977; Aso et al., 1993). The International Prostate Symptom Score (IPSS) recommended by the WHO has proven most useful in studies of herbal prostate remedies (Wilt et al., 1998). But even when studies are properly designed and conducted, it is likely that 30–60 % of the results will be related to placebo effects. To produce a significant., demonstrable therapeutic change, the tested therapeutic agent must achieve an improvement rate on the order of at least 70–80 % (Dreikorn et al., 1990). Moreover, evaluations of subjective symptoms are subject to considerable spontaneous variation during the initial months of therapy, and a valid assessment requires treatment periods of at least 6 months' and preferably 12 months' duration (Aso et al., 1993).

An obvious alternative to phytotherapy in stage I–III BPH is synthetic drugs, specifically α-reductase inhibitors (e.g., finasteride) or α-adrenergic antagonists (e.g., prazosin). When recent study results with standard synthetic drugs are compared with a typical herbal prostate remedy, no fundamental differences in therapeutic efficacy are found (Wilt et al., 1998, 2001). Tolerance to phytomedicinal preparations for BPH is better than with synthetic drugs, especially in the case of saw palmetto extracts and most notably with regard to sexual dysfunction. For the present, both groups of medications can only provide a symptomatic therapy for BPH. The treatment costs with the two groups of synthetic agents are three times higher than those associated with herbal remedies (Mühlbauer and Osswald, 2002). These boundary conditions are sufficient to justify the preference that many physicians have developed for herbal prostate remedies. This pragmatism of office practitioners has become a constant target of criticism by orthodox medicine, however (Dreikorn et al., 1990, 1995, 2002; Mühlbauer and Osswald, 2002). This attitude is less a matter of the need to prove safety and efficacy than a deep-seated discomfort with the definition and composition of phytotherapeutic agents, their active constituents, and their mechanisms of action, all of which, in the view of many critics, make it impossible for these products to have uniform effectiveness. At the same time, herbal remedies are recommended by physicians on the condition that patients pay for the products themselves (Dreikorn, 2002), as most phytomedicines are usually not covered by conventional medical insurance plans. With all due respect, these arguments against the use of phytomedicines in BPH lack the critical attitude toward the value of synthetic drugs in the treatment of BPH-related complaints that has been shown toward phytomedicines In dealing with this controversy, the question arises regarding what portion of the treatment response achieved under the guidance of a family physician can be strictly credited to the pharmacology of modern conventional drugs, and to what extent this minor therapeutic component can continue to justify the adverse side effects and higher costs both to patients and their insurers (who cover the costs of the conventional medicines but not the phytomedicines).

6.4 Drug Products Other than Teas

The *Rote Liste 2003* includes herbal medications for inflammatory urinary tract diseases under the headings "Therapeutic agents for urinary tract infection" and "Urolithiasis remedies." A total of 23 single-herb products are listed for these indications, 14 of them containing goldenrod extract, 5 containing uva-ursi leaf extract, 2 containing Java tea (orthosiphon) leaf extract, and 1 each containing birch leaf and horsetail extract. Given the major importance of fluid intake for this type of disorder (see Sect. 6.1), tea preparations (see Sect. 6.5) are recommended in preference to extract-based products.

For the treatment of benign prostatic hyperplasia, the *Rote Liste 2003* lists a total of 46 single-herb products under the headings "Micturition remedies" and "Prostate remedies." Fifteen of these products are based on saw palmetto berries, 17 on nettle root, 11 on pumpkin seeds, 2 on grass pollens, and 1 on *Hypoxis rooperi*/sitosterol. Also, the list of the 100 most commonly prescribed herbal medicines in Germany (see Appendix) includes 2 combination products for inflammatory urinary tract diseases and 2 for benign prostatic hyperplasia.

6.5 Bladder and Kidney Teas

More than 100 medicinal herbs, including those listed in Table 6.1, are said to promote the flow of urine when administered in the form of an infusion or decoction. The patient should be taken off the medicinal tea at periodic intervals to ensure that the tea remains palatable. Alternatively, the daily dose can be reduced and supplemented by other forms of fluid intake. Infusions can be prepared from black or green tea, maté, or hibiscus flowers, or mineral water can be taken to provide fluid supplementation.

Patients with a sensitive stomach may find it difficult to tolerate teas with a high tannin content, including tea made from uva ursi leaves.

Suggested tea formulations. These teas are based on herbs that are reputed to have antibacterial and/or diuretic actions. To make the appearance of the tea mixtures more appealing or to improve the taste of the infusion, bladder and urine teas also contain one or more of the following herbs as correctives: calendula flowers, rose hips, fennel seed, peppermint leaves, and licorice root.

Suggested Formulations
Note: The provisions of the German Standard Registration specify the quantitative proportions of key active ingredients and correctives in urologic teas. The total content of flavor correctives may not exceed 30 %, and the content of any one corrective may not exceed 5 %.

General Information
Preparation and use: Pour boiling water (about 150 mL) over 2–3 teaspoons of the tea mixture, cover and steep for about 10 min, and pour through a strainer. Prepare the tea fresh for each use.
Directions to patient: Drink 1 cup 3 or 4 times daily between meals.

Urologic tea according to German Prescription Formula Index		
Rx	Maté leaves	10.0
	Orthosiphon leaves	10.0
	Uva ursi leaves	20.0
	Kidney bean pods	20.0
	Horsetail tops	20.0
	Birch leaves	20.0
	Directions (see above).	

Bladder tea according to Swiss Pharmacopeia 6

Rx	Uva ursi leaves	40.0
	Birch leaves	20.0
	Licorice root	25.0
	Couch grass rhizome	15.0
	Directions (see above).	

Urologic tea according to Austrian Pharmacopeia

Rx	Uva ursi leaves	35.0
	Birch leaves	30.0
	Rupturewort	35.0

Bladder and kidney tea I according to German Standard Registration

Rx	Birch leaves	
	Couch grass rhizome	
	Early goldenrod	
	Restharrow root	
	Licorice root	aa to make 100.0

Bladder and kidney tea II according to German Standard Registration

Rx	Uva ursi leaves	35.0
	Birch leaves	20.0
	Kidney bean pods	20.0
	Horsetail	15.0
	Nettle herb	5.0
	Licorice root	5.0
	Directions (see above).	

Bladder and kidney tea III according to German Standard Registration

Rx	Birch leaves	20.0
	Early goldenrod	20.0
	Restharrow root	20.0
	Horsetail	20.0
	Fennelseed	5.0
	Licorice root	5.0
	Rose hips	5.0
	Calendula flowers	5.0
	Directions (see above).	

Bladder and kidney tea III according to German Standard Registration

Rx	Birch leaves	20.0
	Early goldenrod	20.0
	Restharrow root	20.0
	Orthosiphon leaves	30.0
	Peppermint leaves	5.0
	Red sandalwood	5.0
	Directions (see above).	

Bladder and kidney tea IV according to German Standard Registration

Rx	Uva ursi leaves	35.0
	Kidney bean pods	20.0
	Early goldenrod	25.0
	Orthosiphon leaves	20.0
	Directions (see above).	

Bladder and kidney tea according to Pahlow

Rx	Dandelion root and herb	30.0
	Horsetail	20.0
	Restharrow root	20.0
	Birch leaves	20.0
	Goldenrod	20.0
	Directions (see above).	

Bladder tea according to W. Zimmermann

Rx	Marshmallow leaves	10.0
	Uva ursi leaves	20.0
	Speedwell	20.0
	Sage leaves	20.0
	Horsetail	30.0
	Directions (see above).	

Diuretic tea according to W. Zimmermann

Rx	Heather	20.0
	Kidney bean pods	10.0
	Lovage root	10.0
	Parsley fruit	20.0
	Horsetail	20.0
	Early goldenrod	10.0
	Hops	10.0
	Directions (see above).	

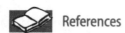 References

Aso Y, Boccon-Gibob L, Brendler CB, et al. (1993) Clinical research criteria. In: Cockett AT, Aso Y, Chatelain C, Denis L, Griffith K, Murphy G (eds) Proceedings of the Second International Consultation on Benign Prostatic Hyperplasia (BPH). Paris, SCI: 345–355.

Bach D (2000) Placebokontrollierte Langzeittherapiestudie mit Kürbissamenextrakt bei BPH-bedingten Miktionsbeschwerden. Urologe 40: 437–43.

Bach D, Ebeling L (1996) Long-term drug treatment of benign prostatic hyperplasia – results of a prospective 3-year multicenter study using Sabal extract IDS 89. Phytomedicine 3: 105–111.1.

Bach D, Schmitt M, Ebeling L (1996) Phytopharmaceutical and synthetic agents in the treatment of benign prostatic hyperplasia (BPH). Phytomedicine 3: 309–313.

Barry MJ, Fowler FJ Jr, O'Leary MP, Bruskewitz RC, Holtgrewe HL, Mebust WK, Cockett ATK (1992) Measurement Committee of the American Urological Association: The American Urological Association symptom index for benign prostatic hyperplasia. J Urol 148: 1549-1557.

Becker H, Ebeling L (1988) Konservative Therapie der benignen Prostata-Hyperplasie (BPH) mit Cernilton - Ergebnisse einer placebokontrollierten Doppelblindstudie. Urologe [B] 28: 301.

Becker H., Ebeling L. (1991): Phytotherapie der BPH mit Cernilton - Ergebnisse einer kontrollierten Verlaufsstudie. Urologe [B] 31: 113.

Berges RR, Windeler J, Trampisch HJ, Senge Th (1995) Randomised, placebo-controlled, double-blind clinical trial of β-sitosterol in patients with benign prostatic hyperplasia. Lancet 345: 1529-1532.

Blumenthal M, Busse WR, Goldberg A, Gruenwald J, Hall T, Riggins CW, Rister RS (eds.). Klein S, Rister RS (trans). (1998) The Complete German Commission E Monographs - Therapeutic Guide to Herbal Medicines. American Botanical Council, Austin, Texas. *www.herbalgram.org.*

Boyle P, Robertson C, Lowe F, Roehrborn C (2000) Meta-analysis of clinical trials of permixon in the treatment of symptomatic benign prostatic hyperplasia. Urology 55: 533-9.

Bondarenko B, Walther C, Schläfke S, Engelmann U (2003) Langzeitstudie zur Wirksamkeit und Verträglichkeit von PRO 160/120 (Kombination aus Sabalfrüchten und Brennesselwurzel und Tamsulosin bei Patienten mit LUTS - Eine placebokontrollierte randomisierte Doppelblindstudie. Phytomedicine, in press

Boyarsky S (1977) Guidelines for investigation of benign prostatic hypertrophy. Trans Am Assoc Gen Urin Surg 68: 29-32.

Bucher K (1951) Über ein antispastisches Prinzip in Petasites officinalis Moendi. Arch Exp Path Pharmacol 213: 69.

Buck AC, Cox R, Rees RWM, Ebeling L, John A (1990) Treatment of Outflow Tract Obstruction due to Benign Prostatic Hyperplasia with the Pollen-Extract "Cernilton". A Double-blind, Placebo-controlled Study. Br J Urol 66: 398.

Carraro JC, Raynaud JP, Koch G, Chisholm GD, Di Silverio F, Teillac P, Da Silva FC, Cauquil J, Chopin DK, Hamdy FC, Hanus M, Hauri D, Kalinteris A, Marencak J, Perier A, Perrin P (1996) Comparison of phytotherapy (Permixon) with finasteride in the treatment of benign prostate hyperplasia: a randomized international study of 1,098 patients. The Prostate 29: 231-240.

Casarosa C, Cosci M, o di Coscio, Fratta M (1988) Lack of effects of a lyposterolic extract of Serenoa repens on plasma levels of testosterone, follicle-stimulating hormone and luteinizing hormone. Clin Ther 10: 5.

Cheema P, El-Mefty O, Jazieh AR (2001) Intraoperative haemorrhage associated with the use of extract of saw palmetto herb: a case report and review of literature. J Intern Med 250: 167-9.

Coppenolle FV, Bourhis XL, Carpentier F et al. (2000) Pharmacological effects of the lipidosterolic extract of Serenoa repens (Permixon®) on rat prostate hyperplasia induced by hyperprolactinemia: comparison with finasteride. Prostate 43: 49-58.

Costello LC, Franklin RB (1994) Effect of prolactin on the prostate. Prostate 24: 162-6.

Dathe G, Schmid H (1987) Phytotherapie der benignen Prostatahyperplasie (BPH). Doppelblindstudie mit Extraktum Radicis Uricae (ERU). Urologe [B] 27: 223-226.

Dreikorn K (2002) The role of phytotherapy in treating lower urinary tract symptoms and benign prostatic hyperplasia. World J Urol 19: 426-35.

Dreikorn K, Richter R, Schönhöfer PS (1990) Konservative, nicht-hormonelle Behandlung der benignen Prostatahyperplasie. Urologe [A] 29: 8-16.

Dreikorn K, Schönhöfer PS (1995) Stellenwert der Phytopharmaka bei der Behandlung der benignen Prostatahyperplasie (BPH). Urologe 34: 119-29.

Ebbinghaus KD, Baur MP (1977) Ergebnisse einer Doppelblindstudie über die Wirksamkeit eines Medikaments zur konservativen Behandlung des Prostata-Adenoms. Z Allg Med 53: 1054-1058.

Ekman P (1989) BPH epidemiology and risk factors. Prostate (Suppl 2): 3-31.

Engelmann U, Boos G, Kreis H (1996) Therapie der benignen Prostatahyperplasie mit Bazoton Liquidum. Urologe [B] 36: 287-291.

Fischer M, Wilbert D (1992) Wirkprüfung eines Phytopharmakons zur Behandlung der benignen Prostatahyperplasie (BPH). In: Rutishauser G (ed) Benigne Prostatahyperplasie III / 3. Klinisch-Experimentelle Konferenz zu Fragen der Benignen Prostatahyperplase. W. Zuckschwerdt Verlag: 79–84.

Flanigan RD, Reda DJ, Wasson JH, Anderson RJ, Abdellatif M, Bruskewitz RD (1998) Five-year outcome of surgical resection and watchful waiting for men with moderately symptomatic benign prostatic hyperplasia: a Department of Veterans Affairs cooperative study. J Urol 160: 12–16.

Frohne D (1986) Arctostaphylos uva-ursi: Die Bärentraube. Z Phytother 7: 45.

Habib FK (1992) Die Regulierung des Prostatawachstums in Kultur mit dem Pollenextrakt Cernitin T60 und die Wirkung der Substanz auf die Verteilung von EGF im Gewebe. In: Vahlensieck W, Rutishauser G (Hrsg) Benigne Prostatopathien. Thieme, Stuttgart: 120.

Hänsel R, Keller K, Rimpler H, Schneider G (eds) (1994) Hagers Handbuch der Pharmazeutischen Praxis. 5th Ed., Vol. 6, Drogen P-Z. Springer Verlag, Berlin Heidelberg New York: 680–687.

Harnischfeger G, Stolze H (1989) Serenoa repens – Die Sägezahnpalme. Z Phytother 10: 71–76.

Hartmann RW, Mark M, Soldati F (1996) Inhibition of 5 α-reductase and aromatase by PHL-00 801 (Prostatonin), a combination of PY 102 (Pygeum africanum) and UR 102 (Urtica dioica) extracts. Phytomedicine 3: 121–128.

Hass MA, Nowak DM, Leonova E, Levin RM, Longhurst PA (1999) Identification of components of Prunus africana extract that inhibit lipid peroxidation. Phytomedicine 6: 379–388.

Hryb DJ, Khan MS, Romas NA, Rosner W (1995) The effect of extracts of the roots of the stinging nettle (Urtica dioica) on the interaction of SHBG with its receptor on human prostatic membranes. Planta Med 61: 31–32.

Ishani A, MacDonald R, Nelson D, Rutks I, Wilt TJ (2000) Pygeum africanum for the treatment of patients with benign prostatic hyperplasia: a systematic review and quantitative meta-analysis. Am J Med 109: 654–64.

Jepson RG, Mihaljewic L (2000) Cranberries for preventing urinary tract infections. The Conchrane Library 2000; 1; 1–13.

Klippel KJ, Hiltl DM, Schipp B (1997) A multicentric, placebo-controlled, double-blind clinical trial of rb-sitosterol (phytosterol) for the treatment of benign prostatic hyperplasia. Brit J Urol 80: 427–432.

Koch E (1995) Pharmakologie und Wirkmechanismen von Extrakten aus Sabalfrücten (Sabal fructus), Brennesselwurzeln (Urticae radix) und Kürbissamen (Cucurbitae peponis semen) bei der Behandlung der benignen Prostatahyperplasie. In: Loew D, Rietbrock N (Hrsg) Phytopharmaka in Forschung und klinischer Anwendung. Steinkopff Verlag, Darmstadt: 57–79.

Kontiokari T, Sundquist K, Nuutinen M et al. (2001) Randomized trial of cranberry-lignonberry juice and Lactobacillus GG drink for the prevention of urinary tract infections in woman. BMJ 322: 1571–3.

Krzeski T, Kaz_ M, Borkowski A, Witeska A, Kuczera J (1993) Comparison of efficacy and tolerance of two dosages of a combined preparation of extracts of stinging nettle root (UR 102) and Pygeum africanum (PY 102): a double-blind study in 134 patients with benign prostatic hyperplasia. Clinical Therapeutics 15: 1011–1020.

Ljunghall S, Fellström B, Johansson G (1988) Prevention of renal stones by a high fluid intake? Eur Urol 14: 381–385.

Loschen G, Ebeling L (1991) Hemmung der Arachidonsäure-Kaskade durch einen Extrakt aus Roggenpollen. Arzneim Forsch/Drug Res. 41 (I) 2: 162.

MacDonald R, Ishani A, Rutks I et al. (2000) A systematic review of cernilton for the treatment of benign prostatic hyperplasia. BJU Int 85: 836–41.

Mandressi S, Tarallo U, Maggioni A (1983) Terapia medica dell'adenoma prostatico: confronto della efficacia dell'estratto di Serenoa repens (Permixon) versus l'estratto di Pigeum Africanum e placebo: Valutazione in doppio cieco. Urologia 50: 752–8.

Marks LS, Partin AW, Epstein JI, et al. Effects of a saw palmetto herbal blend in men with symptomatic benign prostatic hyperplasia. J Urol. 2000 May; 163(5): 1451–6.

Marks LS, Hess, DL, Dorey FJ, Macairan ML, Santos PBC, Tyler VE. Tissue effects of saw palmetto and finasteride: Use of biopsy cores for in situ quantification of prostatic androgens. Urology 2001; 57: 999–1005.

Metzker H, Kieser M, Hölscher U (1996) Wirksamkeit eines Sabal-Urtica-Kombinationspräparates bei der Behandlung der benignen Prostatahyperplasie (BPH). Urologe (B) 36: 292–300.

Mühlbauer B, Osswald H (2002) Urologica. In: Schwabe U, Paffrath D (eds) Arzneiverordnungs-report 2002. Springer Berlin Heidelberg New York, S. 734–41.

Nahrstedt A (1993) Pflanzliche Urologica – eine kritische Übersicht. Pharm Z 138: 1439–1450.

Nevalainen MT, Valve EM, Ingleton PM et al. (1997) Prolactin and prolactin receptors are expressed and functioning in human prostate. J Clin Invest 99: 618–27.

Nickel JC (1998) Placebo therapy of benign prostatic hyperplasia: a 25 month study. Brit J Urol 81: 383–7.

Niederprüm HJ, Schweikert HU, Zänker KS (1994) Testosterone 5α-reductase inhibition by free fatty acids from Sabal serrulata fruits. Phytomedicine 1: 127–133.

Nöske HD (1994) Die Effektivität pflanzlicher Prostatamittel am Beispiel von Brennesselwurzel-extrakt. ÄrzteZ Naturheilverfahren 35 (1): 18–27.

Pegel KH, Walker H (1984) Neue Aspekte zur benignen Prostatahyperplasie (BHP). Die Rolle der Leukotriene und Prostaglandine bei der Entstehung sowie bei der konservativen Therapie der durch sie verursachten Symptome. Extr Urologica 7 (Suppl 1): 91–104.

Plosker GL, Brogden RN (1996) *Serenoa repens* (Permixon®). Drugs & Aging 9: 379–91.

Rhodes L, Primka RL, Berman Ch, Vergult F, Gabriel M, Pierre-Malice M, Gibelin B (1993) Comparison of finasteride (Proscar), a 5α reductase inhibitor, and various commercial plant extracts in in vitro and in vivo 5α reductase inhibition. Prostate 22: 43–51.

Schilcher H (1987 a) Pflanzliche Diuretika. Urologe [B] 27: 215–222; (19877 b) Möglichkeiten und Grenzen der Phytotherapie am Beispiel pflanzlicher Urologika. Urologe [B] 27: 316–319.

Schilcher H (Hrsg) (1992) Phytotherapie in der Urologie. Hippokrates Verlag Stuttgart.

Schmidt K (1983) Die Wirkung eines Radix Urticae-Extrakts und einzelner Nebenextrakte auf das SHGB des Blutplasmas bei der benignen Prostatahyperplasie. Fortschr Med 101: 713–716.

Schmitz W (1998) Urologika. In: Schwabe U, Paffrath D (eds) Arzneiverordnungs-Report '98. Springer Verlag: 534–537.

Siegers JP, Bodinet C, Syed AS, Siegers CP (2003) Bacterial deconjugation of arbutin by *Escherichia coli*. Phytomedicine 10: 58–60.

Sökeland J (1987) Urologie. Thieme, Stuttgart: 258, 260.

Sökeland J (2000) Combined sabal and urtica extract compared with finasteride in men with benign prostatic hyperplasia: analysis of prostate volume and therapeutic outcome. BJU International 86: 439–442.

Sökeland J, Albrecht J (1997) Kombination aus Sabal- und Urticaextrakt vs. Finasterid bei BPH (Stad. I bis II nach Alken). Vergleich der therapeutischen Wirksamkeit in einer einjährigen Doppelblindstudie. Urologe (A) 36: 327–333.

Sonnenschein R (1987) Untersuchung der Wirksamkeit eines prostatotropen Phytotherapeutikums (Urtica plus) bei benigner Prostatahyperplasie und Prostatitis – eine prospektive multizentrische Studie. Urologe [B] 27: 232–237.

Stepanov VN, Siniakova LA, Sarrazin B, Raynaud JP (1999) Efficacy and tolerability of the lipidosterolic extract of *Serenoa repens* (Permixon®) in benign prostatic hyperplasia: a double-blind comparison of two dosage regimens. Advances in Therapy 16: 231–41.

Szutrely HP (1982) Änderung der Echostruktur des Prostataadenoms unter medikamentöser Therapie. Med Klin 77: 42–46.

Vahlensiek W (1985) Konservative Behandlung der benignen Prostatahyperplasie (BPH). Therapiewoche 35: 4031–4040.

Veit M (1994) Probleme bei der Bewertung pflanzlicher Diuretika. Z Phytother 16: 331–341.

Vontobel HP, Herzog R, Rutishauser G, Kres H (1985) Ergebnisse einer Doppelblindstudie über die Wirksamkeit von ERU-Kapseln in der konservativen Behandlung der benignen Prostatahyperplasie. Urologe [A] 24: 49.51.

Wagner H, Willer F, Samtleben R, Boos G (1994) Search for the antiprostatic principle of stinging nettle (Urtica dioica) roots. Phytomedicine 1: 213–224.

Wilt TJ, Isahni A, Stark G, MacDonald R, Lau J, Mulrow C (1998) Saw palmetto extracts for treatment of benign prostatic hyperplasia. A systematic review. JAMA 280: 1604–1609.

Wilt TJ, Ishani I, Stark G et al. (2001) Serenoa repens for benign prostatic hyperplasia (Conchrane Review). In: The Conchrane Library, Issue 1, 2001, Oxford: update software.

Wilt TJ, MacDonald R, Ishani A (1999) β-Sitosterol for the treatment of benign prostatic hyperplasia: a systematic review. BJU Int 83: 976–83.

7 Gynecologic Indications for Herbal Remedies

Herbal remedies are used in the treatment of menstrual irregularities, premenstrual syndrome (PMS), dysmenorrhea, and menopausal complaints in cases where stronger-acting drugs are not indicated or are declined by the patient. Two medicinal plants stand out in the frequency with which they are prescribed for gynecologic complaints: chasteberries (used chiefly for PMS) and black cohosh rhizome (used principally for menopausal complaints) (Schwabe and Rabe, 1998). Table 7.1 also lists four other herbs recommended by the German Commission E as having gynecologic indications. It can be seen that the range of recommended dosages (column 3 in Table 7.1) is greater for gynecologic herbal remedies than for any other class of phytomedicenes. Some of the dosages are many times lower than the traditional single dose of about 1–4 g of crude drug (i.e., dried herbal material) taken in a cup of medicinal tea. There is an urgent need for pharmacologic and clinical studies to investigate the dose-dependency of the actions and efficacy of these herbal drugs.

Historically, most herbal remedies for gynecologic problems were classified as emmenagogues. Hippocrates mentioned a number of herbs that were reputed to induce menstruation or increase menstrual flow. It was recognized in ancient times that regular menstruation was important in the preservation of health, and conversely a variety of ailments were attributed to the absence or irregularity of menstrual bleeding. Classic emmenagogic herbs included locally irritating essential oils and a number of cathartics. With the estrogens and progestins available today, there is no longer a need to use plant drugs for this indication, and indeed the risks of many herbal drugs (abortion in undetected pregnancy) would contraindicate their use.

Herbal remedies continue to be of benefit in PMS, a symptom complex that commonly appears several days before the onset of menstrual bleeding. Many women experience an array of physical and behavioral symptoms that usually subside with the start of menstruation. The physical symptoms are mostly congestive in nature and consist of painful breast swelling and tension (mastodynia); abdominal discomfort with fullness, bloating, and constipation; and edema that typically involves the ankles, the area around the eyes, and the hands. Behavioral symptoms are also a common feature of PMS.

Table 7.1.

Herbal drugs used for gynecologic indications.

Herbs	Indications*	Daily dose*
Black cohosh (Cimicifugae racemosae rhizoma)	Premenstrual, dysmenorrheic, and menopause-related neuroautonomic complaints	40 mg
Bugle weed (Lycopi herba)	Breast pain and tension; mild hyperthyroidism with neuroautonomic disturbances	0.02–2 g
Chasteberry (Agni casti fructus)	Abnormal frequency of menstrual bleeding, premenstrual complaints, mastodynia	30–40 mg
Sheperd's purse	Symptomatic treatment of mild menorrhagia and metrorrhagia	5–15 g
Silverweed (Potentillae anserinae herba)	Mild dysmenorrheic complaints	4 g
Yarrow (Achilleae millefolii herba)	In sitz baths: painful spastic conditions of psychoautonomic origin involving the lesser pelvis	100 g per 20 L water

* according to the monograph of Commission E

The breast discomfort in PMS is believed to relate causally to a latent hyperprolactinemia (Halbreich et al., 1976; Schneider and Bohnet, 1981). Falling estradiol and progesterone levels combined with stress can lead to an increased pituitary secretion, thus providing an experimental approach to confirming the efficacy of chasteberry and other herbal preparations (Wuttke et al., 1995).

The waning of ovarian function that occurs at about age 50 is marked by a number of physical and psychologic complaints collectively referred to as menopausal syndrome. The most frequent and characteristic symptom is hot flashes, which occur in about three-fourths of affected women. Some 50 % of women also experience psychologic complaints such as nervousness, irritability, sleeplessness, or depression (Bates, 1981). Since menopausal discomforts are the result of declining hormone production, hormone replacement can be an effective therapy but is associated with various risks and side effects that many women find objectionable. The need for an alternative therapy with gentle-acting agents forms the basis for the second major indication for gynecologic herbal remedies: menopausal complaints.

7.1   Chasteberry

This herb consists of the dried, ripe fruits of the Chaste tree, *Vitex agnus-castus* (Fig. 7.1), a shrub of the family Verbenaceae that is native to the Mediterranean region. The hard, grey, round berries are about 0.5 cm in size and contain 4 seeds. They have an aromatic odor and an acrid, slightly peppery taste. Chasteberry contains about 0.5 % volatile oil along with the iridoid glycosides agnuside and aucubin. Some of the con-

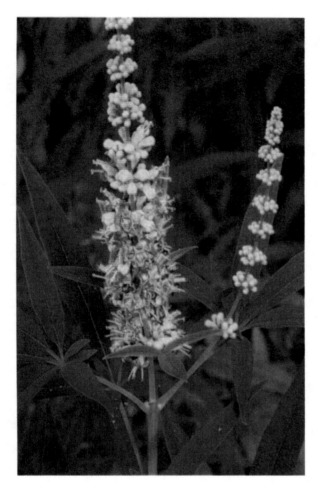

Figure 7.1. ◀ Chasteberry plant (*Vitex agnus-castus*).

stituents responsible for the actions and efficacy of the herb have been identified as bicyclic diterpene derivatives.

The Greek physician Dioscorides mentioned chasteberry as a medicinal plant some 2000 years ago, noting that its Latin name *agnus castus*, meaning chaste lamb, referred to the property of its seeds, when taken as a drink, to reduce sexual desire. Reportedly, the herb aided medieval monks in keeping their vow of chastity; hence, the common name Monk's pepper.

Experimental studies in vitro and in live animals have shown that chasteberries have a prolactin-inhibiting action. This effect is described more specifically as a dopaminergic action based on the selective stimulation of D_2-type dopamine receptors (Jarry et al., 1991, 1994; Winterhoff, 1993). Regarding the dosage used in human beings (see Table 7.1), it is noteworthy that experimental studies had to use extract concentrations of 3.3 mg/mL in vitro (Fig. 7.2) and single doses of 60 mg injected intravenously in experimental rats (Fig. 7.3) in order to achieve significant effects (Wuttke et al., 1995).

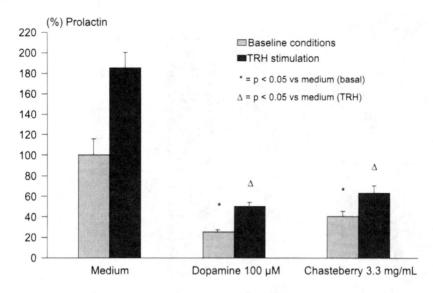

Figure 7.2. ▲ Release of prolactin from cultured pituitary cells under baseline conditions, after stimulation with thyrotropin-releasing hormone (TRH), and after incubation with dopamine and chasteberry extract (Wuttke et al., 1995).

A placebo-controlled, double-blind study was performed in 20 healthy male subjects to test the effect of chasteberry on prolactin levels in humans. A cross-over design was used in which the subjects took an extract in doses equivalent to 120 mg, 240 mg, or 480 mg of the crude drug. The study did not show any definite dose-dependent changes in the 24-h serum prolactin profile. The changes that occurred during the treatment period depended strongly on the baseline values of the individual subjects (Merz et al., 1995; Vogel, 2001). On the other hand, a pilot study in 56 women with mastodynia showed that a chasteberry combination product taken for three menstrual cycles significantly reduced serum prolactin levels in comparison with a placebo (Wuttke et al., 1995). A double-blind study in 52 women with abnormal menstrual patterns due to latent hyperprolactinemia treated for 3 months with 20 mg of extract or placebo showed significant reductions in serum prolactin levels and significant increases in luteal progesterone levels in the serum (Milewicz et al., 1993). Therapeutic efficacy in patients with PMS could not be documented in an initial randomized study (Turner and Mills, 1993), but further studies dealing with the same indication yielded positive results.

In a multicenter double-blind study, a 3-month regimen of 4 mg/day of a chasteberry extract equivalent to 40 mg of the crude drug was compared with 200 mg of pyridoxine in a total of 175 women. The women in the study ranged from 18 to 45 years of age, and all had been diagnosed with premenstrual syndrome. The main confirmatory parameter was the change in a total symptom score (PMTS scale). In patients treated with the chasteberry preparation, the total score decreased from 15 to 5 points while the score in patients treated with the vitamin preparation decreased from 12 to 5 (Reuter et

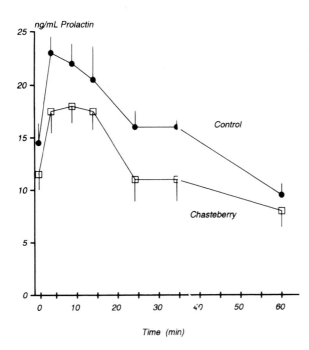

ng/mL Prolactin

Control

Chasteberry

Time (min)

Figure 7.3. ◀ Prolactin blood levels in male rats that were stressed with and without prior treatment with 60 mg chasteberry extract per animal (Wuttke et al., 1995).

al., 1995). In another study, the Clinical Global Impression Scale (CGI) improved in 77 % of patients treated with chasteberry and in 61 % of patients treated with pyridoxine. This led the authors to conclude that chasteberry is at least as effective as pyridoxine in the treatment of premenstrual syndrome, but they also noted that the high placebo responder rate in premenstrual syndrome could account for up to 70 % of therapeutic efficacy even in women treated with pyridoxine (Lauritzen et al., 1997).

In another study, 170 women with PMS were treated with 20 mg/d of an ethanol agnus castus extract (n=86) or placebo (n=84). The primary outcome measure was a total score based on the self-assessment of 6 different symptoms (irritability, mood changes, tension/anger, headache, breast fullness, and other premenstrual symptoms such as bloating and breast tension) from baseline to end point of the 3-month treatment period. Each symptom was scored from 0 (not present) to 10 (unbearable) using a visual analog scale (VAS). Secondary outcome measures were changes in CGI severity of complaints and global improvement) and the responder rate, defined as more than a 50 % reduction in symptoms during treatment. Statistical analysis showed a significant ($p<0.001$) superiority in the total symptom score, the individual symptom scores except for "other" symptoms, and the CGI. The responder rates were 52 % for active agent and 24 % for placebo (Schellenberg, 2001).

Two other studies were conducted in 104 patients and 97 patients who had complaints mainly relating to premenstrual mastodynia. Treatment with 20 mg/d of an ethanol agnus castus extract was continued for three menstrual cycles. Again, a VAS was used to rate the severity of mastodynia. Figure 7.4 shows the results. The differences between the agnus castus extract and placebo were statistically significant ($p<0.05$) at all three visits in the first study by Wuttke et al. (1997) and at the end of cycles 2 and 3 in the study by Halaska et al. (1999).

In a pilot study in 96 women with fertility problems (38 with secondary amenorrhea, 31 with luteal insufficiency, 27 with idiopathic infertility) treated for 3 months with 20 drops of an agnus castus preparation or a placebo t.i.d., significant improvements were noted in 58 % of the agnus castus patients versus 36 % of the placebo group. Of the patients with amenorrhea and luteal insufficiency, 8 became pregnant during treatment with agnus castus compared with only 3 of the placebo-treated women (Gerhard et al., 1998).

No studies have yet been published on the pharmacokinetics and toxicology of agnus castus preparations. To date there have been no reports of serious side effects in any of the available studies or from therapeutic use. A clinical pharmacologic study using significantly higher doses of agnus castus extract did find a number of non-dose-dependent side effects, but the authors did not believe they were serious enough to cause tolerance problems at therapeutic doses (Merz et al., 1995; Vogel, 2001). Besides the results of controlled clinical studies, there have been a number of individual case reports and results of observational studies with agnus castus extract that attest to its therapeutic efficacy. A review of these studies can be found in Gorkow (1999). A comprehensive review of chaste tree pharmacological and clinical studies has been published in an unofficial monograph from the American Herbal Pharmacopoeia (Upton, 2002a).

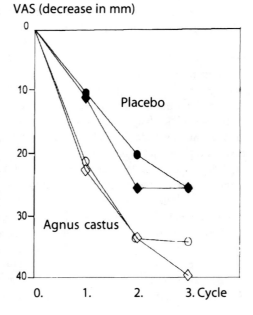

Figure 7.4. ▶ Results of two placebo-controlled studies in 104 and 97 patients complaining of premenstrual mastodynia. The women were treated with 20 mg/day of an chasteberry extract for three cycles. A visual analog scale (VAS) was used to rate the severity of breast complaints. The differences between the extract and placebo groups were statistically significant (p < 0.05) at all three assessment points in one of the studies (Wuttke et al., 1997: ◆) and at the end of cycles 2 and 3 in the other study (Halaska et al., 1999: ●) (after Wuttke et al., 2003a).

7.2 Black Cohosh

Black cohosh (Fig. 7.5), known also as black snakeroot or cimicifuga, is a native North American herbaceous plant (*Actaea racemosa* syn. *Cimicifuga racemosa*) of the family Ranunculaceae. The crude drug, consisting of the dried rhizome and roots, is nearly odorless and has a bitter, acrid taste. The drug contains triterpene glycosides, including actein and cimicifugoside, which are considered the key constituents. Researchers have also isolated from the botanical very small amounts of the isoflavonoid compound for-mononetin, an active principle that possesses hormonal activity (Jarry et al, 1995). Reviews of the medicinal herb, its pharmacology, and its therapeutic uses can be found in Beuscher (1995), Foster (1999), Upton (2002b), Blumenthal et al. (2003), and Lowdog et al., (2003).

The endocrine effects of *Cimicifuga racemosa* extracts, which presumably are exerted on the pituitary, have been investigated in vitro, in ovariectomized rats, and in patients with menopausal complaints. Unlike synthetic estrogens, which affect follicle

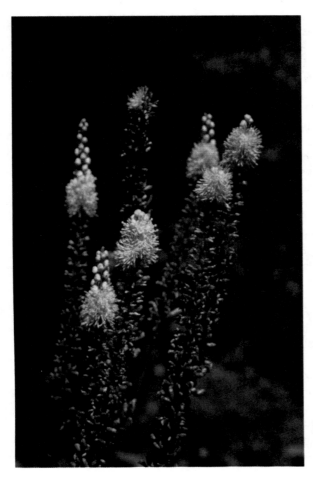

Abb. 7.5. ◀ Black cohosh (*Actacea racemosam* syn. *Cimicifuga racemosa*).

stimulating hormone (FSH), luteinizing hormone (LH), and prolactin release, the investigated black cohosh extract only reduced the serum levels of LH. Estrogen-binding studies in vitro and evidence of antiproliferative effects on the growth of breast carcinoma cells suggest that black cohosh acts on hormonal regulation. Studies of various extracts indicate that the lipophilic fraction contains the hormonally active principle (Jarry et al., 1985; Düker et al., 1991; Winterhoff, 1993; Jarry et al., 1995). While there has been no evidence of estrogen-like effects on the uterus of experimental animals, alcoholic extracts of Cimicifuga racemosa have in some cases produced marked central effects such as a fall in body temperature and an increase in ketamine-induced sleeping time. Both effects could be abolished with the receptor antagonist sulpiride (Löhning et al., 1998). In another model, a lipophilic fraction of the extract had no effect on uterine weight but significantly reduced the LH level. It also significantly increased the expression of estrogen receptors in the central nervous system and bone. It was concluded from these results that constituents of black cohosh act as selective estrogen-receptor modulators in the central nervous system and bone tissue (Jarry et al., 1999).

In connection with the effects of black cohosh on hormonal regulation, a study was done to investigate the effects of cimicifuga rhizome extracts on bone mineral density in ovariectomized and sham-operated rats. Some of the ovariectomized animals received the extracts in doses of 50–200 mg/kg daily for 6 weeks. The ovariectomy caused a significant decline in bone mineral density during this period compared with the sham-operated animals. This density loss could be partially offset by the administration of cimicifuga extracts. The difference was statistically significant compared with untreated ovariectomized animals but was less pronounced in comparison with the sham-operated animals. The authors recommended testing the therapeutic efficacy of cimicifuga extracts in the prevention and treatment of postmenopausal osteoporosis (Li et al., 1996). It should be added that the extracts used in this study were obtained from C. heracleifolia and C. foetida, rather than from C. racemosa, and were effective only at very high pharmacologic doses.

The clinical efficacy of black cohosh extracts is based not just on older studies and anecdotal reports but on five controlled studies comparing the extract with a placebo or with estrogen therapy in women with physical, psychologic, and neuroautonomic complaints relating to menopause (Vorberg, 1984; Warnecke, 1985; Lehmann-Willenbrock, 1988; Daiber 1983; Düker, 1991). Unfortunately, none of these studies employed a double-blind design. But significant changes in the Kupperman index and a series of standard psychometric scales (CGI, POMS, HAMA, STS) do support the therapeutic efficacy of black cohosh extract in menopausal women. All the studies used doses equivalent to 40 mg/day of the crude drug.

In a study of 140 patients with menopausal complaints, the Kuppermann Menopause Index (the severity of 10 symptoms assessed by physician interview) was used to determine whether there was any difference in efficacy between 40 mg/d and 127 mg/d of a cimicifuga root extract after 24 weeks of treatment. This was not the case: in both treatment groups the index fell from approximately 30 points initially to less than 10 points after 4–8 weeks' treatment. A placebo group was not used (Liske et al., 2000).

A three-armed double-blind study was conducted to test for improvement of postmenopausal complaints in 62 women treated for 12 weeks with a cimicifuga root extract compared with conjugated estrogens and a placebo. A Menopause Rating Scale (MRS) was used to assess the frequency and severity of symptoms. The thickness of the endometrium and effects on bone metabolism were also measured. No difference was found between the cimicifuga root extract and conjugated estrogens with regard to the MRS scale, but both agents were significantly better than placebo (p<0.05). Endometrial thickness increased significantly only in the patients treated with conjugated estrogens. Bone metabolism was favorably influenced by the cimicifuga root extract (Wuttke et al, 2003).

Mild side effects were noted in two of the above studies, consisting of gastrointestinal complaints, headache, dizziness, and weight gain. The toxicology of the cimicifuga extract has been partially investigated, and no evidence of toxicity was found in rats treated for 6 months with approximately 100 times the therapeutic dosage used in humans. There has been no reported evidence of mutagenicity or carcinogenicity, and there is no likelihood of specific toxicity for any of the constituents that have been identified thus far (Liske and Wüstenberg, 1998). Recently, however, a case report was published in which a woman required a liver transplant for necrotizing hepatitis after she had taken an unspecified black cohosh preparation for one week. No evidence of infectious or toxic causes was found (Whiting et al., 2002). The German Commission E monograph on cimicifuga rhizome states that a daily dose equivalent to 40 mg of the crude drug leads to occasional gastric complaints and recommends that the duration of treatment not exceed 6 months (Blumenthal et al., 1998). This 6 month duration has been misinterpreted to.suggest that there may be some safety basis in the Commission's 6-month duration recommendation, and that use of black cohosh for treatment of menopause symptoms for longer periods may entail some risk. This is not the case. The Commission E established the 6-month duration to ensure that women return to their gynecologists for a periodic examination; a similar duration is routine with the use of conventional hormone replacement therapies (Blumenthal et al., 2003).

7.3 Phytoestrogens

A number of plants contain isoflavones with estrogen-like properties (Kitaoka et al., 1998). Certain leguminous herbs, including soybeans and red clover, are very rich in these compounds (Zava et al., 1998). The dietary intake of plant estrogens varies greatly in different geographic regions. It is estimated, for example, that dietary phytoestrogen intake is up to 30 times higher in Eastern Asia than in Europe and North America. Because these substances have a relatively weak receptor affinity, it is assumed that they cannot exert their hormone-like effects as long as endogenous estrogens and progestins are predominant. But as the production of these hormones wanes with the onset of menopause, phytoestrogens can help compensate for the hormone deficits and thereby moderate the withdrawal symptoms. This could explain why, for example, only 25 % of menopausal women in Japan suffer hormone withdrawal symptoms as compared with 85 % of women in the U.S. (Notelovitz, 1989).

To test this hypothesis, a placebo-controlled, double-blind study was performed in 104 women in early postmenopause. Fifty-one patients took 60 g of a soy extract daily and 53 patients took 60 g of placebo (casein) daily for 12 weeks. The authors analyzed changes from baseline in the mean number of hot flashes experienced during the treatment period. They found that soy was significantly superior to the casein placebo in reducing the frequency of hot flashes. The overall rates of adverse effects were similar for soy and placebo, and the dropout rates were similar in each group (Albertazzi et al., 1998).

Evidence is also beginning to accumulate that the phytoestrogenic isoflavones of soy in combination with soy protein produce reductions in total and LDL cholesterol levels in moderately hypercholesterolemic persons. A total of 156 such individuals were randomized into 5 groups. Four of the groups consumed daily for 9 weeks a beverage containing 25 g of soy protein and various levels (trace, 25 mg, 42 mg, and 58 mg) of soy isoflavones. The fifth group consumed a placebo consisting of casein.

The soy protein containing 58 mg of isoflavones reduced both total (8 %) and LDL (10 %) cholesterol levels in persons with initially high baseline LDL (>160 mg/dl). Effects were decremental with decreasing isoflavones (Crouse et al., 1998). Additional research is required to determine the beneficial effects, if any, of pure soy isoflavones without accompanying protein on hypercholesterolemic persons (Liebman, 1998). All other potentially beneficial effects of soy isoflavones are less well documented. At this time, it is still impossible to state definitively whether the compounds can reduce the risk of breast or prostate cancer, osteoporosis, or hot flashes. However, this is a very fast-moving research field, and many present conclusions will almost certainly be subject to change as additional data become available.

The hypothesis that phytoestrogens may be beneficial in reducing the incidence of prostate cancer is based largely upon observations that populations having increased concentrations of lignans and isoflavones in their plasma and prostatic fluid have a lower incidence of prostate disease. In a sampling of 50 men from Portugal, 58 from Hong Kong, and 36 from the United Kingdom, much higher concentrations of isoflavones were found in the plasma and prostatic fluid of the participants from Hong Kong than from the other two countries. Because Chinese man have a relatively low incidence of prostate disease, these findings tend to support the conclusion that high concentrations of soy isoflavones in the prostatic fluid may have a protective role (Morton et al., 1997).

A recent randomized placebo-controlled open clinical trial tested the influence of daily doses of mixtures of isoflavones from red clover (*Trifolium pratense*) on arterial compliance, an index of the elasticity of large arteries, in 17 (14 active, 3 placebo) menopausal women. After a 5-week run-in period, the active group took 2 placebo tablets daily for 5 weeks, then one 40 mg isoflavone tablet and 1 placebo daily for the next 5 weeks, and then 2 80 mg isoflavone tablets daily for the final 5 weeks. Systemic arterial compliance was estimated at the end of each period by measuring volumetric blood flow and associated driving pressure. Arterial compliance rose by 28 % relative to the placebo with the 80 mg isoflavone dose and slightly less with the 40 mg dose (Nestel et al., 1999). An important cardiovascular risk factor was significantly diminished by administration of red clover isoflavones.

Soybean preparations of the type tested are sold as dietary products in Europe. In Australia and North America, red clover extracts are available in the form of 500-mg tablets that have a relatively high content (40 mg/tablet) of isoflavones with estrogen-like activity (Kelly et al., 1997). At present it is difficult to reliably evaluate the efficacy of these products. The same applies to the presumed decline in breast cancer risk that has been attributed to the use of phytoestrogens (Dallacker, 1995; Davis, 2001).

In view of the fact that the rapidly developing knowledge of the risk:benefit ratio of phytoestrogens is still evolving, it has been suggested that a much closer study in experimental animals and populations exposed to them is required to determine their true safety and utility (Sheehan, 1998). However, a recent comprehensive review from the British government has confirmed the general safety of dietary isoflavones and other phytoestrogens sold as foods and dietary supplements (Committee on Toxicity, 2003). Another critical review focusing on the efficacy of 29 complementary and alternative treatments used in the U.S. for moderating symptoms of menopause, including phytoestrogenic dietary supplements, has found varying levels of evidence to support some modalities; the phytoestrogens appeared to be safe but do not have as much evidence to support their efficacy as the most well-researched botanical, i.e., black cohosh (Kronenberg and Fugh-Berman, 2003).

7.4 Other Herbs

Several other herbs used for gynecologic indications are listed in Table 7.1. Only some are available as proprietary products (Sect.7.5).

The aerial parts of the bugle weed (*Lycopus* spp., family Lamiaceae) are harvested just before the plant blooms. Tinctures and infusions of it were used in nineteenth-century America as a remedy for bleeding, especially nosebleeds and menorrhagia. Experimental pharmacologic studies have demonstrated antigonadotropic actions (Gumbinger et al., 1981; Winterhoff et al., 1983), antithyrotropic actions (Frömling-Borges, 1987), and a lowering of serum prolactin levels (Sourgens et al., 1982). The clinical relevance of these studies is unclear. Therapeutic trials have not been conducted in patients. Based largely on pharmacologic studies, Commission E recognized these indications for bugle weed in 1990: "mild thyroid hyperfunction with disturbances of the vegetative nervous system. Tension and pain in the breast (mastodynia)" (Blumenthal et al., 1998). In rare cases, thyroid enlargement can occur with long-term use. Sudden withdrawal should be avoided, because it may lead to increased prolactin secretion. Dose recommendations cover an extremely broad range from 0.2 to 2 g/day of the crude drug or equivalent.

The dried aerial parts of silverweed (*Potentilla anserina*, family Rosaceae) contain at least 2 % tannins and have been approved for use in the supportive treatment of nonspecific diarrhea and for the local treatment of oropharyngeal inflammations. In 1985, Commission E additionally recognized the use of silverweed for "mild . dysmenorrheal disorders" (Blumenthal et al., 1998). The recommended daily dose is 4–6 g of the crude drug. Stomach irritation has been reported as a possible side effect. The gynecologic indication for silverweed is based on pharmacologic studies showing that the herb increases the tonus of the isolated uterus in various animal species.

The aerial parts of shepherd's purse (*Capsella bursa-pastoris*, family Brassicaceae) are used in folk medicine for preventing or arresting hemorrhage. Commission E, in its 1986 monograph, recommends daily oral doses equivalent to 10–15 g of the crude drug for mild gynecologic bleeding. The active hemostatic principle in shepherd's purse is believed to be a peptide whose structure is still unknown.

The aerial parts of yarrow (*Achillea millefolium*, family Asteraceae) are used in folk medicine for the topical treatment of wounds and for gynecologic disorders. The Commission E monograph of February, 1990, approves its use in sitz baths for the treatment of "painful, cramp-like conditions of psychosomatic origin (in the lower part of the female pelvis)" and in oral dosage forms for dyspeptic complaints (Blumenthal et al., 1998). The herb is reputed to have antispasmodic activity.

Rhapontic rhubarb root (*Rheum rhaponticum*, family Polygonaceae), besides containing small quantities of laxative principles (anthraquinone glycosides), also contains 4–1 % stilbene derivatives, including the characteristic compound rhapontin, which reportedly has weak estrogenic effects. Given the risks posed by stilbene derivatives, the therapeutic use of this herb can no longer be recommended. Only one product containing the herb is still marketed in Germany.

Hops, the strobiles of *Humulus lupulus*, family Cannabinaceae) was found to have some estrogenic activity in earlier studies on small rodents (Koch and Heim, 1953). The authors believed that this accounted for the old observation that menstrual periods tended to arrive early in female hop pickers. Other investigators could not reproduce the results of Koch and Heim, however, and today it is generally agreed that hop does not have estrogenic effects (Fenselau et al., 1973). The psychotropic actions of hops are discussed in Sect.2.4.2.

Wild Yam, the root of various species of *Dioscorea* (family Dioscoreaceae) is involved in a deceptive practice that has been widely perpetrated upon consumers in the United States during recent years. This fraudulent scheme has become known in scientific circles as the "wild yam scam." Various oral and topical dosage forms, but particularly creams containing extracts of wild yam, have been promoted to the public as natural sources of progesterone and recommended as treatments for conditions ranging from menopausal and menstrual symptoms to osteoporosis.

This assertion is based on the mistaken belief that diosgenin, a steroidal saponin present in wild yam, can be converted in the body to progesterone, just as it is in the chemical laboratory. No evidence supporting this conversion in humans has ever been obtained (Barron, Vanscoy, 1993).

Some women claim to have obtained beneficial results from the use of such products. In all probability, these are due to creams containing additions of pure progesterone produced by conventional techniques. Such a practice is referred to as "spiking", unless the presence of progesterone is actually honestly declared on the label, which appears to be the case with most of the products in this category. The entire situation speaks to the need for addressing ways to appropriately regulate non-oral phytomedicinal preparations in the United States, which, since they are not orally ingested, are not "dietary supplements" but must be viewed legally as cosmetics or drug products.

St. John's wort. In a pilot study, 19 women with PMS were treated with 300 mg/d St. John's wort extract for three menstrual cycles. Two-thirds of the women had more than 50 % improvement in symptom scores by the end of the trial. The authors recommended conducting a randomized study to test the efficacy of hypericum extract as a treatment for PMS (Stevinson and Ernst, 2000).

7.5   Therapeutic Significance

Gynecologic herbs cannot replace sex hormones, anti-infectious agents, or antispasmodic drugs that are medically indicated. So far, therapeutic efficacy has not been established for any herbal gynecologic remedies in a way that would satisfy current standards. In the treatment of premenstrual and menopausal syndromes, however, preparations made from chasteberries and black cohosh offer an alternative to higher-risk hormone therapies for a number of patients, especially when one considers that the subjective complaints of the syndromes in particular show a placebo response rate of approximately 50 %. Given the considerable practical importance of these preparations, further reliable evidence is needed to document their safety and efficacy.

7.6   Drug Products

The *Rote Liste 2003* includes a total of 20 single-herb products for gynecologic indications. Nine are preparations made from chasteberry, seven from black cohosh rhizome, two from silverweed extract, and one each from bugle weed and rhapontic rhubarb. The chasteberry preparations are offered mainly for premenstrual complaints, the black cohosh preparations for menopausal discomforts, and the remaining three for dysmenorrheic complaints (silverweed), mastodynia and mild hyperthyroidism (bugle weed), and follicular hormone therapy (rhapontic rhubarb). Three of these products are among the 100 most commonly prescribed herbal medications in Germany (see Appendix).

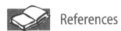 References

Albertazzi P, Pansini F, Bonaccorsi G, Zanotti L, Forini E, De Aloysio D (1998) The effect of dietary soy supplementation on hot flushes. Obstetrics + Gynecology 91: 6–11.
Bates GW (1981) On the nature of the hot flash. Clinical Obstetrics and Gynecology 24: 231–241.
Beuscher N (1995) *Cimicifuga racemosa* L. – Die Traubensilberkerze. Z Phytother 16: 301–310.
Blumenthal M, Hall T, Goldberg A et al. (eds). (2003) The ABC Clinical Guide to Herbs. Austin, TX: American Botanical Council.

Blumenthal M, Busse WR, Goldberg A, Gruenwald J, Hall T, Riggins CW, Rister RS (eds.). Klein S, Rister RS (trans). (1998) The Complete German Commission E Monographs – Therapeutic Guide to Herbal Medicines. American Botanical Council, Austin, Texas. *www.herbalgram.org.*

Committee on Toxicity of Chemicals in Food, Consumer Products and the Environment. (2003) Phytoestrogens and Health. London: The Foods Standards Agency. *http://www.food.gov.uk/multimedia/pdfs/phytoreport0503.*

Crouse JR III, Terry JG, Morgan TM, McGill BL, Davis DH, King T, Ellis JE, Burke GL (1998) Soy protein containing isoflavones reduces plasma concentrations of lipids and lipoproteins. Circulation 97: 816.

Dallacker F (1995) Brustkrebs, Förderung und Hemmung durch Lebensgewohnheiten und Umweltfaktoren. Wissenschaft und Umwelt 2: 99–117.

Davis SR (2001) Phytoestrogen therapy for menopausal symptoms? There's no good evidence that it's better than placebo. BMJ 323: 354-5.

Düker EM, Kopanski L, Jarry H, Wuttke W (1991) Effects of extracts from cimicifuga racemosa on gonadotropin release in menopausal women and ovariectomized rats. Planta Med 57: 420–424.

Fenselau C, Talalay P (1973) Is estrogenic activity in hops? Fd Cosmet Toxicol 11: 597–603.

Foster S (1999) Black cohosh: a literature review. HerbalGram 45: 35–49.

Frömbling-Borges A (1987) Intrathyreoidale Wirkung von Lycopus europaeus, Pflanzensäuren, Tyrosinen, Thyroninen und Lithiumchlorid. Darstellung einer Schilddrüsensekretionsblockade. Inauguraldissertation, Westfälische Wilhelms-Universität Münster.

Gerhard I, Patek A, Monga B, Blank A, Gorkow C (1998) Mastodynon® bei weiblicher Sterilität. Randomisierte, placebokontrollierte, klinische Doppelblindstudie. Forsch Komplementärmed 20: 272–8.

Gorkow C (1999) Klinischer Kenntnisstand von Agni-casti fructus. Klinisch-pharmakologische Untersuchungen und Wirksamkeitsbelege. Zeitschrift für Phytotherapie 20: 159–168.

Gumbinger HG, Winterhoff H, Sourgens H, Kemper FH, Wylde R (1981) Formation of compounds with antigonadotropic activity from inactive phenolic precursors. Contraception 23: 661–666.

Halaska M (1999) Treatment of cyclical mastalgia with a solution containing a Vitex agnus castus extract: results of a placebo-controlled double-blind study. Breast 8: 175–181.

Halbreich U, Assad M, Ben-David M, Bornstein R (1976) Serum prolactin in women with premenstrual syndrome. Lancet: 654–656.

Jarry H, Gorkow Ch, Wuttke W (1995) Treatment of menopausal symptoms with extracts of cimicifuga racemosa: In vivo and in vitro evidence for estrogenic activity. In: Loew D, Rietbrock N (eds) Phytopharmaka in Forschung und klinischer Anwendung. Steinkopff Verlag, Darmstadt: 99–112.

Jarry H, Harnischfeger G (1985) Studies on the endocrine effects of the contents of Cimicifuga racemosa: 1. Influence on the serum concentration of pituitary hormones in ovariectomized rats. Planta Med 51: 46–49.

Jarry H, Harnischfeger G, Düker, E (1985) Studies on the endocrine effects of the contents of Cimicifuga racemosa: 2. In vitro binding of compounds to estrogen receptors. Planta Med 51: 316–319.

Jarry H, Leonhardt S, Düls C, Popp M, Christoffel V, Spengler B, Theiling K, Wuttke W (1999) Organ-specific effects of Cimicifuga racemosa (CR) in brain and uterus. Poster-Abstract. 23rd International LOF-Symposium "Phyto-Estrogens", Gent 1999.

Jarry H, Leonhardt S, Gorkow C, Wuttke W (1994) In vitro prolactin but not LH and FSH release is inhibited by compounds in extracts of Agnus castus: direct evidence for a dopaminergic principle by the dopamine receptor assay. Exp Clin Endocrinol 102: 448–454.

Jarry H, Leonhardt S, Wuttke W, Behr B, Gorkow C (1991) Agnus castus als dopaminerges Wirkprinzip in Mastodynon N. Z Phytother 12: 77–82.

Kelly G, Husband A, Waring M (1997) Promensil™: Hormone supplement designed by nature. Company Monograph of Novogen Limited, Australia.

Kitaoka M, Kadokawa H, Sugano M, Ichikawa K, Taki M, Takaishi S, Iijima Y, Tsutsumi S, Boriboon M, Akiyama T (1998) Prenylflavonoids: A new class of nonsteroidal phytoestrogens (part 1). Isolation of 8-isopentenylnaringenin and an initial study on its structure-activity relationship.

Planta Med 64: 511–515.

Kronenberg F, Fugh-Berman A. Complementary and Alternative medicine for menopausal symptoms: A review of randomized, controlled trials. *Annals of Internal Medicine*. 2002; 137(10): 805–814.

Lauritzen CH, Reuter HD, Repges R, Böhnert KJ, Schmidt U (1997) Treatment of premenstrual tension syndrome with Vitex agnus castus. Controlled, double-blind study versus pyridoxine. Phytomedicine 4: 183–189.

Lehmann-Willenbrock E, Riedel HH (1988) Klinische und endokrinologische Untersuchungen zur Therapie ovarieller Ausfallserscheinungen nach Hysterektomie unter Belassung der Adnexe. Zent Gynäkol 110: 611–618.

Li JX, Kadota S, Li HY, Miyahara T, Wu YW, Seto H, Namba T (1996/97) Effects of Cimicifugae rhizoma on serum calcium and phosphate levels in low calcium dietary rats and on bone mineral density in ovariectomized rats. Phytomedicine 3: 379–385.

Liebmann B (1998) The soy story. Nutr Action Health1 25(7): 3–7.

Liske E Wüstenberg P (1998) Therapy of climacteric complaints with *Cimicifuga racemosa:* herbal medicine with clinically proven evidence. Menopause 5: 250.

Liske E, Boblitz N, von Zeppelin HHH (2000) Therapie klimakterischer Beschwerden mit *Cimicifuga racemosa* – Daten zur Wirkung und Wirksamkeit aus einer randomisierten kontrollierten Doppelblindstudie. In: Rietbrock N (ed) Phytopharmaka VI – Forschung und Praxis. Steinkopff-Verlag, Darmstadt, pp. 247–257.

Löhning A, Verspohl EJ, Winterhoff H (1998) Pharmacological studies on the central activity of Cimicifuga racemosa in mice. Abstract J10. 46th Annual Congress of the Society of Medicinal Plant Research, Vienna 1998.

Lowdog T, Powell KL, Weisman SM. Critical evaluation of the safety of Cimicifuga racemosa in menopause symptom relief. Menopause. 2003; 10: 299–313.

Merz PG, Schrödter A, Rietbrock S, Gorkow Ch, Loew D (1995) Prolaktinsekretion und Verträglichkeit unter der Behandlung mit einem Agnus-castus-Spezialextrakt (B1095E1). Erste Ergebnisse zum Einfluß auf die Prolaktinsekretion. In: Loew D, Rietbrock N (eds) Phytopharmaka in Forschung und klinischer Anwendung. Steinkopff Verlag, Darmstadt: 93–97.

Milewicz A, Gejdel E, Sworen H et al. (1993) Vitex agnus cactus extract in the treatment of luteal phase defects due to latent hyperprolactinemia: results of a randomised, placebo-controlled, double-blind study. Arzneim-Forsch/Drug Res 43: 752–6.

Morton MS, Chan PSF, Cheng C, Blacklock N, Matos-Ferreira A, Abranches-Monteiro L, Correia R, Lloyd S, Griffiths K (1997) Lignans and isoflavonoids in plasma and prostatic fluid in men: samples from Portugal, Hong Kong, and the United Kingdom. Prostate 32: 122–128.

Nestel PJ, Pomeroy S, Kay S, Komesaroff P, Behrsing J, Camron JD, West L (1999) Isoflavones from red clover improve systemic arterial compliance but not plasma lipids in menopausal women. J Clin End Met 84: 895–899.

Notelovitz M (1989) Estrogen replacement therapy indications, contraindications, and agent selection. Am J Ostet Gynecol 161: 8–17.

Schellenberg R for the study group (2001) Treatment for the premenstrual syndrome with agnus castus fruit extract: prospective, randomised, placebo controlled study. BMJ 322: 134–7.

Schneider HPG, Bohnet HG (1981) Die hyperprolaktinämische Ovarialinsuffizienz. Gynäkologe 14: 104–118.

Schwabe U, Rabe T (1998) Gynäkologika. In: Schwabe U, Paffrath D (eds) Arzneiverordnungs-Report '98. Springer Verlag: 299–302.

Sheehan SM (1998) Herbal medicines, phytoestrogens and toxicity: risk: benefit considerations. Proc Soc Exp Biol Med 217: 379–385.

Sourgens H, Winterhoff H, Gumbinger HG, Kemper FH (1982) Antihormonal effects of plant extracts. THS- and prolactin-supressing properties of Lithospermum officinale and other plants. Planta Med 45: 78–86.

Stevinson C, Ernst E (2000) A pilot study of *Hypericum perforatum* for the treatment of premenstrual syndrome. Br J Obstet Gynecol 107: 870–6.

Stoll W (1987) Phytotherapeutikum beeinflußt atrophisches Vaginalepithel: Doppelblindversuch Cimicifuga vs. Östrogenpräparat. Therapeutikum 1: 23–32.

Turner S, Mills S (1993) A double-blind clinical trial on a herbal remedy for premenstrual syndrome: a case study. Complement Ther Med 1: 73–77.

Vogel G (2001) Vergleichende Untersuchungen eines Agnus castus-Spezialextraktes und Bromocriptin auf Prolaktin, Gonadotropine und Sexualhormone bei männlichen Versuchspersonen. Inaugural-Dissertation, Universität Frenkfurt am Main.

Upton R. (ed.) (2002a) Chaste Tree Fruit (*Vitex agnus-castus*). Santa Cruz, CA: American Herbal Pharmacopoeia.

Upton R. (ed.) (2002b) Black Cohosh Rhizome (*Actaea racemosa*). Santa Cruz, CA: American Herbal Pharmacopoeia.

Warnecke G (1985) Beeinflussung klimakterischer Beschwerden durch ein Phytotherapeutikum. Erfolgreiche Therapie mit Cimicifuga-Monoextrakt. Med Welt 36: 871–874.

Whiting PW, Clouston A, Kerlin P (2002) Black cohosh and other herbal remedies associated with acute hepatitis. MJA 177: 432–4.

Winterhoff H (1993) Arzneipflanzen mit endokriner Wirksamkeit. Z Phytother 14: 83–94.

Winterhoff H, Sourgens H, Kemper FH (1983) Pharmacodynamic effects of Lithospermum officinale on the thyroid gland of rats; comparison with the effects of iodide. Horm metabol Res 15: 503–507.

Wuttke W, Gorkow C, Christoffel V, Jarry H, März RH (2003) The Cimicifuga preparation BNO 1055 vs. conjugated estrogens and placebo in a double-blind placebo controlled study – clinical results and additional pharmacological data. Maturitas 33: 1–11

Wuttke W, Gorkow Ch, Jarry J (1995) Dopaminergic compounds in vitex agnus castus. In: Loew D, Rietbrock N (eds) Phytopharmaka in Forschung und klinischer Anwendung. Steinkopff Verlag, Darmstadt: 81–91.

Wuttke W, Splitt G, Gorkow C, Sieder C (1997) Behandlung zyklusabhängiger Brustschmerzen mit einem Agnus castus-haltigen Arzneimittel. Ergebnisse einer randomisierten, placebokontrollierten Doppelblindstudie. Geb Fra 57: 569–74.

Zava DT, Dollbaum CM, Blen M (1998) Estrogen and progestin bioactivity of foods, herbs, and spices. Proc Soc Exp Biol Med 217: 369–378.

8 Skin, Trauma, Rheumatism, and Pain

This chapter deals first with plant drugs that are commonly used for dermatologic indications (local inflammations, eczema, neurodermatitis, acne, wound healing problems). A separate section deals with herbal remedies that are used externally or in some cases internally for the treatment of trauma and its sequelae (bruises, contusions, hematomas, fracture edema) and of osteoarthritis and rheumatic complaints. The chapter concludes with a look at the potential uses of externally applied preparations of essential oils in the treatment of pain. One phytomedicine taken orally for the prophylaxis of migraine headache is also included. Given the medical and economic importance of analgesic remedies, it is important to give due attention to possible phytotherapeutic alternatives.

8.1 Dosage Forms and Preparations

Every medication consists of the active drug and one or more excipients or diluting agents to give the drug a suitable form (see Sect.1.4). With remedies for external use, the action of the medication depends much more on the vehicle than in the case of orally administered drugs. First, the vehicle may produce a marked effect of its own (cooling, drying, moisturizing, occluding) that contributes more to the overall effect of the medication than the drug substance itself. Second, the percutaneous absorption of the drug substance depends critically on the nature of the vehicle (Fig. 8.1).

For example, petroleum jelly produces a strong occlusive effect that promotes absorption by increasing the degree of hydration of the epidermis. Other vehicles such as powders or detergents that draw moisture from the stratum corneum tend to retard penetration. Ethanol is a penetration enhancer, explaining why, for example, tincture of arnica has a much greater allergenicity than arnica cream.

As noted above, the vehicle can greatly affect the moisture content of the stratum corneum. Because of these intrinsic physicochemical actions, dermatologic agents

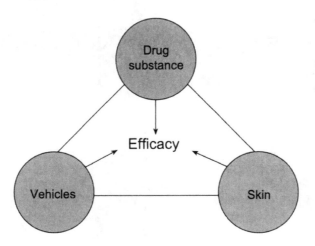

Figure 8.1. ▲ The efficacy of medications for topical use does not depend on the drug substance alone.

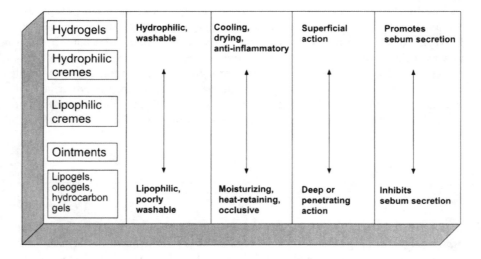

Figure 8.2. ▲ Types of vehicles and excipients used in topical medications (after Beck, 1991).

should be administered in a base that is appropriate for the patient's skin type and for the particular stage of a skin disease. The basic rule is that formulations with a high water content, which have a cooling and drying action, are indicated for oily skin and acute inflammatory conditions, whereas fatty occlusive bases should be used for treating chronic or subcutaneous skin disorders (Fig. 8.2).

An important aspect in the treatment of inflammatory skin diseases is to protect the skin from external injury or irritation. This applies particularly to the various eczematous diseases, all of which, regardless of etiology, cause progressive damage to the stratum corneum. As the protective function of the epidermis is lost, the skin becomes increasingly susceptible to irritation. Demulcents and protectants serve to protect the skin, especially of the hands, from chemical agents and soap solutions. Plant oils, usually mixed with petroleum jelly or lanolin to form a fatty cream, are suitable for this purpose. Protection from organic solvents is afforded by botanically derived film-forming agents such as tragacanth and alginates. The galenic formulations for externally applied herbal remedies basically correspond to those of topically applied synthetic products. Plant extracts are generally more sensitive to environmental influences than synthetic drugs, however, and a highly skilled compounding pharmacist is needed to prepare topical herbal remedies that are stable. Years of experience and development are often necessary, and it is wise to use "time-tested" preparations as long as their pharmacologically active components and dosages conform to the principles of rational phytotherapy.

8.2   Inflammations and Injuries of the Skin

Several dermatologic products contain active ingredients of plant origin that today can be isolated as pure compounds or produced synthetically in a modified form. These include compounds such as β-carotene, chrysarobin, anthralin, methoxsalen, and salicylates, which by definition are outside the bounds of phytotherapy (Chap. 1).

Of the approximately 300 medicinal herbs and herbal products that have been officially evaluated by the German Commission E, 47 herbs have been approved for dermatologic indications. The Commission has given a positive rating to 25 of these herbs, but only about half of the 25 play a significant role in therapeutic practice. Ten important herbs and herbal preparations that are used topically for dermatologic indications are reviewed in Table 8.1. A Commission E monograph was not issued for evening primrose oil, which was approved on a product-specific basis for the treatment of atopic eczema.

Seven herbs with traditional applications in dermatology were given a negative rating because of serious risks and side effects. These are hound's tongue (contains hepatotoxic pyrrolizidine alkaloids), walnut hulls (contain the potentially carcinogenic juglone), pulsatilla (can cause very severe skin irritation), bilberry leaves (not the fruit, which is well known for its safety) and oleander leaves (toxic), and common periwinkle leaves (hermatologic changes). These herbs and their preparations should no longer be used. Commission E has published neutral monographs on 15 other traditional herbs, stating that their efficacy is unproven due to a lack of sufficient scientific evidence but there are no problems regarding their relative safety. Additionally, there are herbs that have received a positive rating from the Commission but have gained little practical therapeutic importance. Recent survey works may be consulted for further information on dermatologic plant drugs, particularly herbs that are not covered in this chapter (Hormann and Korting, 1994; Mennet-von Eiff and Meier, 1995; Willuhn, 1995).

Table 8.1.
Ten important herbs and herbal preparations for external use, shown with year of publication of the Commission E monograph and the indications stated therein.

Monograph, source plant	Year*	Dermatologic indications
Chamomile (Matricariae flos)	1984	Skin and mucosal inflammations and bacterial skin diseases; diseases involving the anal and genital region (baths and douches)
Witch hazel leaves and bark (Hamamelidis folium et cortex)	1985	Mild skin injuries, local inflammations of the skin and mucous membranes; hemorrhoids, varicose veins
Evening primrose oil (Oenotherae seminis oleum)	-	Atopic eczema (neurodermatitis)
Bittersweet stem (Dulcamarae stipides)	1990	Supportive treatment of chronic eczema
Calendula flowers (Calendulae flos)	1986	Wounds, including poorly healing wounds; crural ulcers
Purple coneflower (Echinacea purpureae herba)	1989	Poorly healing superficial wounds
St. John's wort oil (Oleum hyperici)	1984	Primary and secondary treatment of sharp and blunt injuries, myalgias, and first degree burns
Arnica flowers (Arnicae flos)	1984	Used externally for trauma-related conditions and for rheumatic conditions of the muscles and joints
Comfrey leaves and root (Symphyti herba/folium/radix)	1990	Bruises, strains, sprains
Bromelain (from Ananas comosus, pineapple)	1994	Acute postoperative and post-traumatic swelling

NOTE: There is no monograph for evening primrose oil.

8.2.1 Chamomile Flowers

Used medicinally since ancient times, chamomile flowers were mentioned in the works of the classic Greco-Roman physicians Hippocrates, Dioscorides, Galen, and Asclepius. Their use continued into the Middle Ages, and they are still considered to have therapeutic value today (Schilcher, 1987). A number of studies on the pharmacology of chamomile flowers, particularly their anti-inflammatory and antispasmodic properties, have been published in recent decades (Ammon and Kaul, 1992). By contrast, very few controlled therapeutic studies have been published on their clinical efficacy. The virtually unquestioned effectiveness of chamomile for a number of dermatologic indications is still based largely on empirical evidence, i.e., the experience of patients and physicians.

8.2.1.1 Crude Drug, Constituents, and Preparations

The genus *Matricaria* (family Asteraceae) includes several species of annual herbaceous plants, most of which have numerous scientific synonyms. German chamomile

(*Matricaria recutita* L., Fig.8.3) is preferred in central Europe and the United States, while Roman or English chamomile derived from *Chamaemelum nobile* (syn. *Anthemis nobilis*), which has larger flower heads, and usually costs more than German, is increasingly used in other countries. Originally native to the Near East and Eastern Europe, German chamomile now occurs throughout Europe, Australia, and North America. German chamomile is distinguished from the other chamomiles, and especially from the unpalatable and allergenic dog fennel (*Anthemis cotula*), by the conical receptacle on which the florets are arranged – it is hollow, not solid like that of the other chamomiles.

The active constituents of chamomile can be divided into two groups of compounds, one lipophilic and the other hydrophilic. The lipophilic group mainly includes the components of the volatile oil, whose content in the crude drug (dried flower heads) is 0.3–1.5 %. The volatile oil, in turn, consists mainly (about 15 %) of the dark blue chamazulene; the plant itself contains very little of this oil, most of which forms from its colorless precursor matricin during steam distillation. Another important component of chamomile oil is α-bisabolol, which is accompanied by its more oxygen-rich derivatives bisabololoxides A, B, and C. Different cultivated varieties of chamomile are characterized by different concentrations of the bisabolol derivatives (Mennet-von Eiff and Meier, 1995).

The most important hydrophilic constituents are flavonoids, and mucilages. The total flavonoid content of the crude drug ranges from 1 % to 3 %. Experimental pharmacologic studies in isolated intestine indicate that the flavonoids, particularly apigenin, are chiefly responsible for the antispasmodic effects of chamomile preparations.

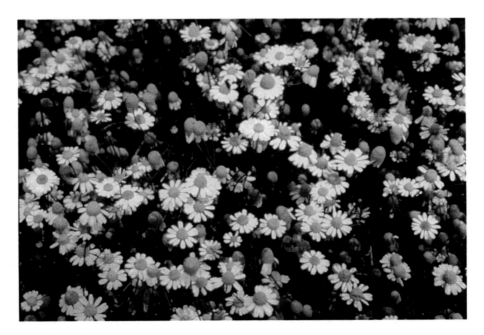

Figure 8.3 ▲ German chamomile (*Matricaria recutita*).

Today, chamomile flowers are obtained almost exclusively by cultivation of selected varieties. About 5000 tons are produced annually throughout the world, with an estimated 3000 tons being exported to Germany. The principal supplier is Argentina; Spain is one of several European countries that also grows chamomile. The *German Pharmacopeia* specifies that the crude drug must contain a least 0.4 % volatile oil. It is used either in the form of aqueous preparations (chamomile tea: 1–2 teaspoons dried chamomile flowers in 200 mL boiling water, steeped for 10 min) or in the form of alcoholic extracts. The latter have a significantly higher content of the lipophilic constituents, that have proven particularly active in pharmacologic models (Schilcher, 1987; Hänsel et al., 1992a).

8.2.1.2 Pharmacology and Toxicology

Chamomile preparations are used mainly for their anti-inflammatory, antispasmodic, and carminative properties. Also, in vitro studies have demonstrated bacteriostatic and fungistatic actions that presumably contribute to the dermatologic uses of chamomile.

Anti-inflammatory effects have been demonstrated both for whole alcoholic extracts and for constituents isolated from them. The compounds have been tested in a number of standard pharmacologic models of inflammation (UV erythema, carrageenan-induced rat's paw edema, cotton-pellet granuloma, adjuvant arthritis in rats) using both topical and oral administration. Chamazulene, α-bisabolol, and flavones such as apigenin were the single components that were found to have the strongest anti-inflammatory properties, but most studies found that the whole extracts were more active than their individual components . The chamomile preparations and their isolated constituents acted mainly on the inflammatory mediators of the arachidonic acid cascade. They had an inhibitory effect on 5-lipoxygenase and cyclooxygenase (Schilcher, 1987).

Besides anti-inflammatory effects, alcoholic extracts of chamomile and isolated flavonoids have also exhibited antispasmodic properties in models such as the guinea pig intestine. When tested on spasms of isolated guinea pig ileum induced by barium chloride, 10 mg apigenin showed an antispasmodic potency roughly equivalent to that of 1 mg papaverine.

Chamomile preparations have also shown antibacterial and fungicidal activity, mainly against gram-positive organisms and *Candida albicans*, in microbial plate tests. Chamomile oil was active at concentrations of 25 mg/mL or higher, and bisabolol at concentrations of 1 mg/mL or higher. This could account for the positive therapeutic effects obtained with chamomile preparations applied topically to infected wounds, for example.

More information on the pharmacologic actions of chamomile and its preparations can be found in Schilcher (1987), Ammon and Kaul (1992), and Hänsel et al. (1992a).

Experiments with chamomile oil in rabbits showed that the acute oral LD_{50} and acute dermal LD_{50} were greater than 5 g/kg, and the constituent α-bisabolol showed equally good tolerance (Jakovlev et al., 1983). There was no evidence of phototoxic effects, skin irritation, or allergenicity. Favorable findings such as these have prompted FDA approval of chamomile as a food ingredient in the United States. It therefore appears on the Generally Recognized as Safe (GRAS) list.

8.2.1.3 Therapeutic Efficacy

Chamomile preparations are used internally for inflammatory disorders and colicky gastrointestinal complaints (see Sect.5.3), and they are administered by inhalation for inflammatory diseases and irritations of the respiratory tract (see Sect.4.2). Chamomile preparations are also used to treat bacterial and nonbacterial inflammations of the skin, poorly healing wounds, abscesses, fistulae, and inflammations of the oral cavity and gums. Other indications are radiation-induced dermatitis and dermatologic conditions in children.

To date, specific evaluations of efficacy in the form of documented case reports, observational studies, and several controlled clinical trials have been based largely on one chamomile product, which has been marketed in Germany under the brand name Kamillosan® since 1921. The case reports and studies have consistently shown positive results in the treatment of acute weeping skin disorders, decubitus ulcers, and dermatitis due to various causes (Schilcher, 1987).

Kamillosan has also been the subject of several controlled therapeutic studies (Albring et al., 1983; Aertgeerts et al., 1985; Nissen et al., 1988; Maiche et al., 1991). Though all these studies did not have a double-blind design with statistical analysis, most documented the therapeutic efficacy of a cream preparation of the standardized product in healthy subjects (cellophane tape stripping test) and in patients with contact dermatitis, various forms of eczema, and postirradiation dermatitis (survey in Hörmann and Korting, 1994).

8.2.1.4 Indications, Dosages, Side Effects, and Risks

The Commission E monograph of 1984 states that chamomile is indicated for "inflammations of the skin and mucous membranes and bacterial diseases involving the skin, oral cavity, or gums; also inflammatory diseases and irritations of the respiratory tract (administered by inhalation) and diseases of the anogenital region (administered by bathing or douching)."

In a supplement to its 1990 monograph, the Commission gives these dosage recommendations: use a 3–10 % infusion for douches; as a bath additive, use 50 g of crude drug per 10 L of water; semisolid preparations should have a 3–10 % content of the crude drug (Blumenthal et al., 1998).

No contraindications, side effects, or drug-drug interactions have been associated with chamomile. As for the risk of allergic reactions, Hausen et al. (1984) reviewed 50 scientific publications and concluded that contamination by dog fennel (which contains the allergenic compound anthecotulide) could account for many cases of so-called chamomile allergy reported in the literature, particularly considering the poor documentation of the identity of the putative chamomile material consumed in many of the case reports. Several true cases of sensitization by German chamomile have been documented, but the overall risk of allergy appears to be very low, especially with preparations made from specific varieties (e.g., Degumille) (Schilcher, 1987; Hörmann and Korting, 1994), and considering the high volume of chamomile teas consumed worldwide.

8.2.2 Witch Hazel and Other Tannin-Containing Herbs

Witch hazel (*Hamamelis virginiana*, family Hamamelidaceae, Fig. 8.4) is a deciduous shrub or small tree that usually grows to 2–3 m and rarely may reach 7 m. Originally native to eastern North America, witch hazel was introduced to England in 1736 and since then has become a popular winter-flowering shrub in parks and gardens of central Europe. The leaves, bark, and twigs are processed to make the crude drug. The bark is particularly rich in tannins (hamamelitannin, gallotannins), containing up to 12 %.

Tannins have strong astringent properties. Applied topically to broken skin or mucous membranes, they induce a protein precipitation that tightens up superficial cell layers and shrinks colloidal structures, causing capillary vasoconstriction (hemostyptic action). The decrease in vascular permeability is tantamount to a local anti-inflammatory effect. The tightening (astringent) action on the tissues deprives bacteria of a favorable growth medium, producing an indirect antibacterial effect. Tannins also have a mild topical anesthetic action that soothes pain and itching. A number of other tannin-containing herbs besides witch hazel are used in the treatment of diarrhea and other ailments that respond to astringent medications (see Sec. 5.5.1 and Table 5.4). The usual preparations for external use (Table 8.1) have a yellow or brown color due to the presence of the tannins. The higher the tannin content, the darker the coloration. This may be why most witch hazel products are based on a distilled extract (hamamelis water) made by soaking the crude drug in water for about 24 h, then distilling the maceration and adding ethanol to the distillate. Unfortunately, these distillates contain

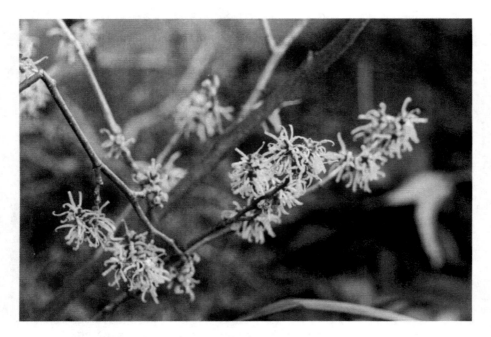

Figure 8.4 ▲ Inflorescence of witch hazel (*Hamamelis virginiana*).

almost no active tannins. It is surprising, however, that preparations of these distillates have shortened bleeding time and shown vasoconstrictive effects in experimental rabbits (Hänsel et al., 1993 a), but this activity may be due to the presence of the ethanol.

When tested in 22 healthy subjects and in 5 patients with atopic neurodermatitis, the same preparation showed anti-inflammatory effects and reduced cutaneous hyperemia (Sorkin, 1980). In two randomized double-blind studies, a hamamelis distillate cream significantly inhibited the development of erythema induced on the skin of the back by UV irradiation and cellophane tape stripping in two groups of 24 healthy subjects (Korting et al., 1993). The same authors performed a double-blind, randomized paired trial in 72 patients with moderately severe atopic eczema. All the patients received a hamamelis distillate cream (5.35 g of hamamelis distillate/100 g) on one side of the body for 14 days. The patients were divided into two groups of 36 patients each, and the corresponding drug-free vehicle or 0.5 % hydrocortisone cream was applied on the other side of the body. The effects were evaluated at 7 and 14 days using a semiquantitative clinical scoring system. Hydrocortisone proved significantly more effective than the hamamelis distillate, which in this study did not differ significantly from the plain base cream (Korting et al., 1995).

The same preparation was found to reduce inflammation and cutaneous hyperemia in 22 healthy subjects and 5 patients with atopic neurodermatitis (Sorkin, 1980). Another randomized double-blind study compared hamamelis ointment with a glucocorticoid ointment in 22 patients with neurodermatitis. After 3 week's treatment, both ointments produced a significant (at least 50 %) improvement in cutaneous symptoms.

A common indication for hamamelis extracts and other preparations made from tannin-containing herbs is stage I or stage II hemorrhoidal disease. The efficacy of a combination product with a high content (10 %) of hamamelis bark extract (an ointment with the brand name Eulatin) was tested in two controlled clinical trials in 75 patients and 90 patients with stage I hemorrhoidal disease. A three-week course of therapy led to dramatic improvement in typical symptoms (bleeding, soreness, itching, burning) in 70–90 % of the patients. The potency of the hamamelis ointment was comparable to that of a corticoid ointment also tested in the double-blind studies (Knoch, 1991; Knoch et al., 1992).

The 1985 Commission E monograph with its 1990 supplement states the following indications for preparations made from hamamelis leaves, bark, and twigs: "mild skin injuries, local inflammations of the skin and mucous membranes, hemorrhoids, and complaints due to varicose veins." The recommended dosage is equivalent to 0.1–1.0 g of the crude drug applied topically to the skin and mucous membranes several times daily. No contraindications, side effects, or herb-drug interactions are known (Blumenthal et al., 1998)

8.2.3　Evening Primrose Oil

Evening primrose (*Oenothera biennis*, family Onagraceae) is a biennial herb that grows to about 1 m. The plant is infertile for the first year, producing only a rosette of leaves close to the ground. During its second year, the plant bears seeds containing up to 25 %

of a fatty oil that is extracted with hexane for medicinal purposes. This extract contains 60–80 % γ-linoleic acid plus 8–14 % γ-linolenic acid (GLA), an omega-6 fatty acid that is formed in the human body by the desaturation of linoleic acid. Reportedly, patients with neurodermatitis are deficient in the enzyme responsible for this conversion (Δ-6-desaturase), accounting for the therapeutic efficacy of evening primrose oil for that indication (Manku et al., 1984; Morse et al., 1989).

Ten placebo-controlled studies, 5 parallel and 5 crossover, were reviewed and evaluated in a meta-analysis (Morse et al., 1989. These studies included a total of about 200 patients with atopic eczema. The duration of treatment in most of the studies was 8 or 12 weeks, and the daily dose ranged from 2 to 6 g of evening primrose oil (EPO, brand name Epogam®), equivalent to 160–480 mg of GLA. Efficacy was rated using a total clinical score based on degree of inflammation, dryness, scaliness, itching, and overall skin involvement. In 4 of the 5 parallel studies, both patient and physician scores showed a highly significant improvement in symptom scores compared with the placebo group. The effects on itching were particularly striking. A breakdown of the results by daily dose showed that the treatment response was dose-dependent (Fig. 8.5). Also, a positive correlation was noted between the improvement in clinical symptoms and a rise in plasma levels of dihomo-γ-linolenic acid (DGLA) and arachidonic acid (AA) (Fig. 8.6), which is consistent with the presumed biochemical mechanism of action. The crossover studies showed a significant hangover effect in patients treated first with evening primrose oil, and this was interpreted as further evidence of therapeutic efficacy. The global improvement rate based on total therapeutic score was a significant 25 % in four of the parallel studies vs. 2 % in the placebo controls. This compared with a placebo improvement rate of 31 % in the only nonsignificant parallel study (Bamford, 1985). The latter study also differed from the other studies in finding marked elevations of plasma DGLA and AA in the placebo-treated patients, and therefore its results must be considered separately. Two later placebo-controlled therapeutic trials in patients with chronic dermatitis could not confirm the positive results of earlier years, and so efficacy for this indication continues to be in question (Berth-Jones and Brown, 1993; Whitaker et al., 1996).

In a long-term uncontrolled multicenter study, 179 patients with atopic eczema were treated with a daily dose of 4 g EPO , equivalent to 320 mg of GLA, for periods ranging from 3 months to 4 years. Symptoms improved in 111 of the 179 patients during treatment. A total of only two adverse effects were reported in this study: one patient complained of abdominal discomfort during treatment, and a second patient experienced mild fluid retention (Stewart et al., 1991).

The effect on barrier function of topical EPO in atopic dermatitis was studied in a vehicle-controlled trial with two populations of 20 atopic patients Evening primrose oil proved to have a stabilizing effect on the stratum corneum barrier, but this was apparent only with the water-in-oil emulsion, not in the amphiphilic emulsion. The choice of vehicle is therefore an important factor in the efficacy of topically applied EPO (Gehring et al., 1999).

Apart from dermatologic indications and a number of other uses, the prophylactic use of GLA in premenstrual syndrome is being discussed on the basis of pathogenetic considerations (König et al., 1999). The result of a 1996 meta-analysis of controlled clinical studies on this indication was less convincing, however (Budeiri et al., 1996).

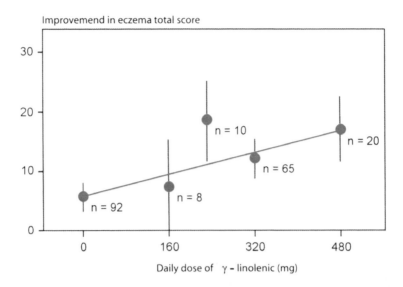

Figure 8.5. ▲ Clinical improvement in eczema patients as a function of the dose of γ-linolenic acid ingested with evening primrose oil. Result of a meta-analysis of 4 clinical studies (after Morse et al., 1989).

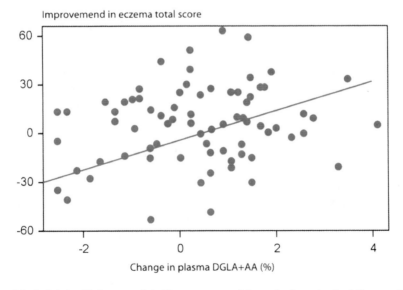

Figure 8.6. ▲ Relationship between clinical improvement and change in plasma levels of dihomo-γ-linolenic acid (DGLA) and arachidonic acid (AA). Same patients as in Fig. 8.5 (after Morse et al., 1989).

In Germany, capsules containing 0.5 g of EPO (corresponding to 40 mg GLA) have been approved for the treatment and symptomatic relief of atopic eczema. The adult dosage is 2–3 g of EPO daily. Occasional side effects are nausea, digestive upset, and headache (Hänsel et al., 1993 b).

8.2.4 Other Dermatologic Herbs (listed alphabetically)

Aloe. Various herbal preparations from the genus *Aloe* are used as laxatives (aloe latex) or for the topical treatment of inflammatory skin conditions (aloe gel). The origin of the plant and the manufacturing processes used for both preparations are discussed in Sect. 5.6.4.4. Aloe gel is an anthranoid-free preparation that mainly contains polysaccharides. Experiments have documented its antimicrobial and anti-inflammatory properties. It is used in ointments, rubs, or gels for the treatment of conditions such as poor wound healing, psoriasis, and herpes. A systematic review of 10 controlled clinical studies (7 with topical use) showed evidence of therapeutic efficacy in patients with psoriasis and genital herpes (Vogler and Ernst, 1999). Use for the prevention of radiation-induced skin lesions did not show convincing proof of efficacy. Allergic skin reactions were reported as adverse events.

Bittersweet (dulcamara) is derived from the stems of the common nightshade (*Solanum dulcamara*, family Solanaceae) gathered in the spring and late fall after the plant has shed its leaves. Extracts of the herb contain steroidal saponins, which showed cortisone-like actions in experimental animals (Frohne, 1992). A multicenter clinical trial showed marked symptom relief in patients with chronic eczema and pruritic skin conditions (Hölzer, 1992). The 1990 Commission E monograph states that dulcamara is indicated for the "supportive therapy for chronic eczema" (Blumenthal et al., 1998). The recommended oral dose is 1–3 g of the dried herb daily. The monograph does not give specific dosage recommendations for the topical use of dulcamara in ointment form, and it mentions no known side effects or herb-drug interactions.

Calendula flowers (*Calendula officinalis*, family Asteraceae) are used in the form of an infusion, tincture, fluidextract, cold infused oil (calendula oil), or ointment to promote the granulation and facilitate healing of skin inflammations, wounds, burns, or eczema. Experiments in various wound models have demonstrated significant wound-healing properties, especially for a hydroalcoholic extract of the herb. The stimulation of new blood vessel formation by calendula accounts for some of these properties (Patrick et al., 1996). The active principle that promotes wound healing has not been identified. One hypothesis is that this action is based on synergistic effects of the volatile oil and the relatively high concentrations of xanthophylls that are present in the herb.

The Commission E monograph of 1986 states that calendula flower preparations are used internally for inflammatory conditions of the oral and pharyngeal mucosa and externally for crural ulcers and for wounds with a poor healing tendency (Blumenthal et al., 1998). The recommended dosage for internal use is 1–2 g of the dried herb. An ointment utilizing 2–5 g of the dried herb in 100 g of a suitable base is applied externally. No contraindications, side effects, or herb-drug interactions are known.

Isaac (1992) may be consulted for a comprehensive review of the pharmacy, pharmacology, and therapeutic use of calendula flower preparations.

Echinacea (Coneflower) is an herbaceous plant of the family Asteraceae originally native to North America, where American Indians used the herb for a wide variety of conditions ranging from snakebite to infected wounds. A German settler, Dr. H.C.F. Meyer, used this Indian herb in 1871 to produce the first commercial echinacea product. By the early 1900's, the herb was known in Europe as well. The original species (*Echinacea angustifolia* and *E. pallida*) were not grown in Europe, but the common purple coneflower (*E. purpurea*) was cultivated instead and used in various pharmaceutical products. According to the Commission E monograph of 1996, semisolid preparations containing at least 15 % of the juice expressed from the aerial parts of the common purple coneflower are applied locally for the treatment of superficial, poorly healing wounds. Both the external use of echinacea and its internal use as an immune stimulant (Sect. 9.2) are contraindicated by progressive systemic diseases such as tuberculosis, leukoses, collagen disorders, and multiple sclerosis. (Blumenthal et al., 1998) However, these contraindications are based on speculative and theoretical considerations, and not on any documented clinical data (Blumenthal et al., 2003). Also, Commission E recommends the duration of use be limited to a maximum of 8 weeks. The reason for this has been misinterpreted by some authors as evidence that use of Echinacea preparations for longer periods produces some higher likelihood of risk. This is not the case. The Commission E established the 8-week duration limit because it considered that all of the approved indications for Echinacea should be treatable within an 8-week period, and if symptoms persist for a longer time, then more aggressive therapy is presumably warranted (Blumenthal et al., 2003).

Hypericum oil is prepared by crushing the flowers of St. John's wort (*Hypericum perforatum*, family Clusiaceae), placing them in olive oil (25:100 ratio), and steeping the herb in a warm place or letting it stand in sunlight for about 6 weeks until the oil acquires a reddish color. The exact composition of this "red oil" is unknown, but its ruddy color is caused not only by the original hypericins but by various naphthodianthrone derivatives in the final product.

Hypericum oil is a traditional remedy for burns, and in former times, every village blacksmith kept a supply on hand for emergencies. The 1984 Commission E monograph on St.John's wort (SJW) states that hypericum oil is used externally for the secondary "treatment and post-therapy of acute and contused injuries, myalgia and first-degree burns" (Blumenthal et al., 1998). Today, however, the treatment of burns with a fatty oil is considered obsolete.

Hypericum ointment. An ointment preparation based on a 1:9 alcoholic extract of St. John's wort (SJW) was tested in 8 subjects for its immune-modulating properties when applied topically to the skin. Both the extract and the constituent hyperforin had an inhibitory effect on the lymphocytic reaction in the epidermis and the proliferation of local T cells. The authors interpreted this as a rationale for the use of SJWpreparations in inflammatory skin diseases (Schempp et al., 2000). As a follow-up to this study, a prospective, randomized, placebo-controlled, double-blind study was conducted to test the efficacy of a SJW cream standardized to hyperforin versus placebo in the treatment of subacute atopic dermatitis in a half-side comparison. In 21 patients with mild to moderate atopic dermatitis (mean SCORAD 44.5), either SJW cream (hypericum extract cream standardized to 1.5 % hyperforin) or a placebo (color-matched base) was applied to the right or left side of the body based on a random selection process. Eighteen of the 21 patients completed the study. Skin condition was evaluated separately for each side of the body using a modified SCORAD index (main outcome measure). Skin condition improved on both sides of the body, but the hyperforin cream was significantly superior to the base at all clinical visits (7, 14, and 28 days) (p<0.05). Both agents reduced skin colonization by *Staphylococcus aureus*, but the hyperforin cream tended to show better antibacterial activity than the placebo (p=0.064). Skin tolerance and cosmetic acceptability were rated as good or excellent for both the hyperforin cream and the placebo (Schempp et al., 2003).

The antidepressant effects of alcoholic extracts of SJW are discussed in Sect.2.2.

Lemon balm leaves (*Melissa officinalis*, family Lamiaceae) exhibited powerful virostatic properties in a study of tissue cultures treated with aqueous extracts from 178 medicinal plants (May and Willuhn, 1978). The active principle was thought to consist of tannins unique to the Lamiaceae. Based on these investigations, a cream was prepared from a balm leaf extract and tested in patients with herpes simplex (Vogt et al., 1991). The 1984 Commission E monograph on balm leaves and its 1990 supplement do not name herpes simplex as an indication, however.

Mahonia root and bark *Mahonia* spp. are closely related to the barberry (*Berberis* spp.). Various parts of the plant, especially the root, have been used in folk medicine for the treatment of psoriasis and other skin conditions. Extracts and individual constituents (i.e., the isoquinoline alkaloids like berberine) have anti-inflammatory properties, which would explain their use for this indication. However, two placebo-controlled studies using an ointment preparation of mahonia bark in psoriasis patients (Wiesenauer and Lüdtke, 1996) were unable to show definite therapeutic efficacy. Isolated berberine has been shown to be mutagenic in in vitro assays, but this has not been demonstrated in mahonia extracts. Given the potential problems with safety and lack of demonstrated efficacy, allopathic (as distinguished from homeopathic) mahonia products are no longer approved for use in Germany (Hänsel et al., 1993 d).

Medicinal yeast consists of the fresh or dried cells of *Saccharomyces cerevisae*, family Saccharomycetaceae. The Commission E monograph of 1988 states that medicinal yeast is approved as an adjunct in the treatment of chronic forms of acne and furunculosis when taken in an average daily dose of 6 g. Side effects consisting of migraine-like headache or flatulence may occur in susceptible individuals.

The use of live dried yeast as an antidiarrheal is discussed in Sect. 5.5.3.

Podophyllin, or podophyllum resin, is obtainend from the rhizome and roots of the mayapple, also called American mandrake (*Podophyllum peltatum*, family Berberidaceae), a perennial plant native to the woodlands of eastern North America. The jointed and branched rhizome with attached roots is up to 1 m long and contains at least 4 % resin with podophyllotoxin as the main constituent. Podophyllotoxin has a purgative action and is highly embryotoxic but nonteratogenic in experimental animals. The Commission E monograph of 1986 states that podophyllum resin is used externally for the removal of condylomata acuminata (venereal warts). It is applied locally once or twice a week in the form of a 5–25 % alcoholic solution or equivalent ointment. The treated skin area should not exceed 25 cm², and adjacent skin areas should be carefully covered. There is evidence that preparations with a substantially lower concentration may be equally effective (Edwards et al., 1988).

Tea tree oil is a volatile oil distilled with steam from the leaves of several species of Australian trees belonging to the genus *Melaleuca* (family Myrtaceae), principally *M. alternifolia*. These trees are native to the coastal regions of northeast New South Wales and are now cultivated there for commercial purposes. The early Australian settlers are said to have learned of the antiseptic properties of the oil from the aboriginals. The Australian Aborigines prized the tea tree as a remedy for cuts, burns, and insect bites. In vitro experiments later showed that tea tree oil inhibits the growth of numerous bacterial and fungal species (Saller et al., 1998). This discovery has led to the worldwide use of tea tree oil in cosmetics and topical medications.

The constituents of tea tree oil are numerous and complex. Current Australian standards specify that it should contain a maximum of 15 % 1,8-cineole and a minimum of 30 % (+)-terpinen-4-ol, the principal germicidal ingredient (Olsen, 1997). Other constituents, including α-terpineol and linalool, also contribute to the antimicrobial activity (Carsen and Riley, 1995). An Australian standard adopted in 1995 requires that tea tree oil contain at least 30 % terpinen-4-ol and 15 % cineole.

A few clinical studies testify to the antibacterial and antifungal activity of tea tree oil. Its efficacy was compared to that of 1 % clotrimazole in a multicenter, randomized, double-blind trial of 117 patients with toenail onchomycosis. After two applications daily for a 6-month period, the two treatments were found to be comparable in efficacy of cure (Buck et al., 1994). Another study compared the efficacy of a 5 % tea tree oil gel to 5 % benzoyl peroxide lotion in 124 patients with mild to moderate acne. The single-blind, randomized clinical trial compared daily application to similar subject groups for a period of 3 months. Both treatments produced a significant improvement in number of both non-inflamed and inflamed lesions, but the benzoyl peroxide was more effective with non-inflamed lesions. However, fewer patients reported unwanted effects, such as dryness, stinging, redness, etc., with the tea tree oil (44 % vs 79 %) (Bassett et al., 1990). A meta-analysis of the relatively few clinical studies that had been published on tea tree oil (cutaneous fungal infections in three studies, acne in one) rated the results as very promising but not yet conclusive (Ernst and Hantley, 2000). There is a risk of allergic skin reactions to tea tree oil, and 3 of 28 volunteers tested strongly positive to patch testing (Rubel et al., 1998). Tea tree oil is toxic when taken orally and should never be administered by that route (Del Beccaro, 1994).

8.3 Post-traumatic and Postoperative Conditions

Mild injuries sustained as a result of blunt trauma (bruises, contusions, strains, sprains) are associated with neurovascular injuries, hematomas, and edema leading in turn to painful limitations of motion. Physical therapy consists of immobilizing and elevating the injured part and may include the use of cold packs. Analgesics and anti-inflammatory agents may also be administered for swelling and inflammation. Two medicinal herbs – arnica and comfrey – have a long tradition in European folk medicine for external use in the treatment of injuries. Crude bromelain (from pineapple fruitstalk) and other herbal enzyme preparations are taken internally and are used mainly for the treatment of postoperative swelling.

8.3.1 Bromelain

Crude bromelain is a mixture of proteolytic enzymes derived from the pineapple plant (*Ananas comosus*, family Bromeliaceae) and especially from the fruiting stems. Although it is widely believed that high-molecular-weight proteins must be broken down before they can be absorbed from the gastrointestinal tract, there is evidence that a certain percentage of orally administered bromelain enters the lymph and bloodstream unchanged in rats, dogs, and human beings (Seifert, 1983; Steffen and Menzel, 1983). The absorption rate in rats is approximately 50 %. No data are yet available on the absolute bioavailability of bromelain in humans.

Orally administered bromelain has displayed anti-inflammatory and antiexudative actions in experimental models (rat's paw edema). Studies in rabbits and humans have shown a prolongation of prothrombin time and bleeding time (Hänsel et al., 1992c). In 1993, Commission E reviewed a total of 9 controlled clinical studies performed in patients with post-traumatic and postoperative edema. Of the 5 studies that could be statisically evaluated, 3 yielded a positive result and 2 a negative result. The Commission concluded that therapeutic efficacy had been satisfactorily established for "acute postoperative and post-traumatic swelling, especially of the nose and paranasal sinuses." The recommended daily dose is 80–320 mg bromelain taken in 2 or 3 divided doses. The duration of use generally should not exceed 8–10 days Blumenthal et al., 1998).

Hypersensitivity to bromelain is noted as a contraindication; side effects consist of gastric upset, diarrhea, and occasional allergic reactions. Bromelain may potentiate the effects of anticoagulants and platelet aggregation inhibitors. The biochemistry, bioavailability, and clinical use of bromelain and other enzyme preparations are reviewed in VanEimeren et al. (1994).

8.3.2 Comfrey

Comfrey (*Symphytum officinale*, family Boraginaceae) is an indigenous European herbaceous plant growing to 50–100 cm with rough, hairy leaves and large purple-red flowers. The leaves and roots have a high mucilage content and also contain allantoin (up to 1.5 % in the root). The mucilages have local demulcent properties, while allantoin promotes wound healing and accelerates the regeneration of cells. The 1990 Commission E monograph states that the aerial parts and roots are indicated for the treatment of bruises, strains, and sprains (Blumenthal et al., 1998). Ointments or other preparation for external use only should contain up to 20 % of the dried herb or equivalent amounts of extract. Comfrey contains unsaturated pyrrolizidine alkaloids (Pas), which have shown hepatotoxic, carcinogenic, and mutagenic properties in rats. Internal consumption of the herb has also been shown to induce hepatic veno-occlusive disease in humans. Thus, the monograph cautions against the external use of more than 1 mg of PAs daily or similar use of the herb for more than 4–6 weeks per year. If the PA content of a product is not standardized or stated, it is best not to use comfrey or any other PA-containing herbs. Because the content of PAs is highly variable and can vary naturally in the crude drug by a factor of approximately 10, only comfrey products that have a declared content of PAs should be used therapeutically (Michler and Arnold, 1996).

8.3.3 Arnica

Arnica flowers are obtained from *Arnica montana* of the family Asteraceae (Fig. 8.7), an herbaceous perennial growing to 30–60 cm that is native to mountainous regions of Europe. Its large, orange flowers bloom from June to August. According to the 1996 *German Pharmacopeia*, the flowers of *A. chamissonis* (subsp. *foliosa*) can be used in place of *A. montana* which is protected and cannot be cultivated. The crude drug contains 0.2–0.3 % volatile oil. The constituents of arnica include helenalin and other sesquiterpene lactones that may be the active principles. The herb also contains about 0.4–0.6 % flavones. Arnica has traditionally been used in the form of tinctures, particularly for external application. Several arnica-based ointments are currently marketed in Germany.

Experimental studies on the effects of arnica preparations have demonstrated antimicrobial, anti-inflammatory, respiratory-stimulant, positive inotropic, and tonus-increasing (uterus) actions. The therapeutically important anti-inflammatory effects of arnica preparations are attributed to helenalin, whose actions include a marked anti-edemic effect that has been confirmed in experimental models (carrageenan-induced paw edema and adjuvant arthritis in rats). The external use of arnica preparations can cause contact dermatitis in individuals sensitized by sesquiterpenes of the helenalin type. The allergenic potential of arnica products depends both on the helenalin concentration and on the vehicle. The pharmacology and toxicology of arnica preparations have been reviewed by Hänsel et al. (1992b) and by Hörmann and Korting (1995). Today, arnica preparations are regarded somewhat critically in terms of their risk-to-benefit ratio (Hörmann and Korting, 1994).

The 1984 Commission E monograph states that arnica flower preparations are indicated for external use in the treatment of post-traumatic and postoperative conditions such as hematomas, sprains, bruises, contusions, fracture-related edema, and rheumatic ailments of the muscles and joints (Blumenthal et al., 1998). Other indications are

Figure 8.7 ► Arnica (*Arnica montana*).

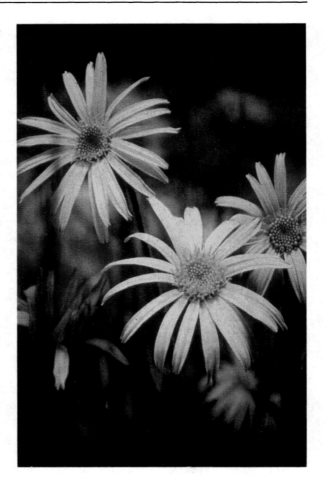

oropharyngeal inflammations, furunculosis, insect bites and stings, and superficial phlebitis. Allergy to arnica contraindicates its use. Edematous dermatoses and eczema may occur as side effects with long-term usage. Tinctures for compresses should be used in a 3:1 to 10:1 dilution, and ointments should contain a maximum of 20–25 % tincture or 15 % arnica oil.

Note: Internal use of arnica (except in highly diluted homeopathic preparations) is not advised. The effects of arnica on the respiratory center, heart, and uterus have not been sufficiently tested to justify the risks associated with oral use.

8.4 Rheumatic Conditions and Degenerative Joint Diseases

Compared to steroidal and nonsteroidal anti-inflammatory agents, phytomedicines play only a minor role in the treatment of rheumatic conditions and osteoarthritis.

Some herbal preparations have displayed marked in vitro and in vivo effects in pharmacologic models of inflammation. Among European herbs, this applies particularly to preparations made from willow, aspen and ash bark and from nettle tops. Among the non-European herbs, pharmacologic and some clinical data have been published on the actions and efficacy of African devil's claw and boswellin (Indian frankincense). Chrubasik and Wink (1997) have reviewed available pharmaceutical, pharmacologic, and clinical data on the treatment of rheumatism with phytomedicines. The sequence in which the herbs are presented corresponds roughly to their importance as phytomedicines in Germany.

8.4.1 Devil's Claw

Devil's claw (*Harpagoghytum procumbens*, Fig. 8.8) is a native South African plant of the family Pedaliaceae. The peripheral tubers of the plant grow up to 3 cm thick and 20 cm long and form the raw material for the crude drug. The tubers are chopped and dried in the sun for about three days. Native Africans used the herb as a bitter tonic (bitterness value 6000, see Sect. 5.1.2), antipyretic, and analgesic. Several iridoid glycosides occur in devil's claw, most notably the key active principle harpagoside, whose content in the crude drug is 0.5–1.6 %. The *German Pharmacopeia 10* requires a minimum content of 1 % harpagoside based on the dried herb.

Crude drug preparations and harpagoside itself have low toxicity. The acute and subacute toxicity of hydrophilic and lipophilic whole extracts was tested in rats and mice (LD_{50} < 5–10 g/kg body weight). The LD50 in mice following the intraperitoneal

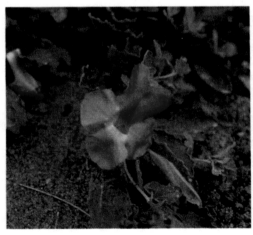

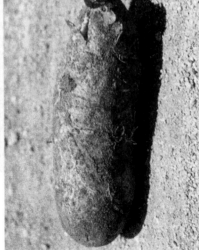

Figure 8.8.
▲ Devil's claw in bloom (*Harpagophytum procumbens*).
▶ Storage roots of devil's claw (crude drug).

administration of isolated harpagoside was 1–3 g/kg body weight (Erdös et al., 1978). To date, about 10 original studies have been published on the pharmacologic actions of harpagophytum preparations. These works are summarized in Wenzel and Wegener (1995), Fleurentin and Mortier (1997), and Wegener (1998, 2000). Analgesic and anti-inflammatory effects were tested in known animal models such as the radiant heat test, rat's paw edema, adjuvant arthritis, UV erythema, and cotton-pellet granuloma test. Most of the studies showed positive analgesic and anti-inflammatory effects, but the anti-inflammatory effect per unit dose was at least 10 times weaker than that of indomethacin (Fleurentin and Mortier, 1997).

The pharmacokinetics of the key constituent harpagoside was tested in 10 volunteers. Seven of the subjects took a single dose of 400 mg or 600 mg of a special extract containing 25 % harpagoside, and 3others took 600 mg, 1200 mg, or 1800 mg of an extract containing 9 % harpagoside. The maximum serum levels (approximately 10–50 ng/mL, depending on the dose) were reached at 1.3 to 3.5 h after administration. The elimination half-life ranged from 3.7 to 6.4 h. Plasma tests revealed a biphasic, dose-independent inhibition of specific inflammatory mediators (Loew et al., 2001).

About 20 publications consisting of controlled studies, uncontrolled studies, observational studies and reports of clinical experience deal with the therapeutic efficacy of devil's claw in patients with active osteoarthritis, low back pain, and rheumatic complaints (surveys by: Wegener, 1998 and 2000, Chrubasik and Wink, 1998; Ernst and Chrubasik, 2000; Chrubasik et al., 2003). 5 placebo-controlled double-blind studies have been published. One study involved 89 patients with rheumatic complaints who received 2 g of the powdered crude drug daily for 2 months. The main test criteria were sensitivity to pain (scored on a 0–10 scale) and fingertip-to-floor distance (in cm). Both parameters showed significant improvement at 30 days and 60 days compared with a placebo (Lecomte and Costa, 1992). In another placebo-controlled, double-blind study, 118 patients with chronic back pain were treated with 2.4 g of harpagophytum extract (equivalent to 50 mg harpagoside) daily for 4 weeks. The protocols of 109 patients could be statistically evaluated. The confirmatory parameter was the Arhuser back pain index. The index improved in both treatment groups, improving by 20 % in the harpagophytum group and by 8 % in the placebo group. Statistical comparison of the treatment groups just missed the designated level of significance ($p<0.05$). A significant difference ($p<0.01$) was found, however, in the number of patients who were free of pain (9 of 54 in the devil's claw group vs. 1 of 54 in the placebo group) (Chrubasik et al., 1996). Another placebo-controlled double-blind study was performed in 100 patients with various signs and symptoms of rheumatic disease (activated osteoarthritis, low back pain, rheumatoid involvement of soft tissues). The daily dose was 2.5 g of extract, equivalent to approximately 5 g/day of the crude drug. After 30 days of treatment, 41 patients in the placebo groups still complained of pain versus 7 patients in the harpagophytum groups (Schmelz et al., 1997).

Another placebo-controlled, double-blind study was performed in 197 patients with chronic low back pain. Daily doses of 600 mg or 1200 mg of a special extract containing 50 mg or 100 mg of harpagoside were compared with placebo over a 4-week period. The main outcome measure was the number of patients who were free of pain without additional analgesic medication. The numbers of pain-free patients at the end of the treatment period were 3 in the placebo group, 6 in the group taking 600 mg/d of the

extract, and 10 in the group taking 1200 mg/d (p < 0.05) (Chrubasik et al., 1999).A further double-blind, placebo controlled study was intended to investigate the effects of
Harpagophytum on sensory, motor and vascular mechanisms of muscle pain. In addition to clinical efficacy and tolerability, possible action mechanisms were analysed by
means of experimental algesimetric methods. The study was performed on patients
with slight to moderate muscular tension or slight muscular pain of the back, shoulder
and neck. The verum group received 2x480 mg/day, of Harpagophytum extract. The
duration of the therapy was 4 weeks. Data recording at 14-day intervals was made using
a visual analogue scale, pressure algometer test, recording of antinociceptive muscular
reflexes, muscle stiffness test, EMG surface activity, muscular ischaemia test, clinical
global score and subjective patient and physician ratings. A total of 31 patients in the
verum group and 32 in the placebo group were treated. After four weeks of treatment
there was found to be a clear clinical efficacy of the verum on the clinical global score
and in the patient and physician ratings. Highly significant effects were found in the
visual analogue scale, the pressure algometer test, the muscle stiffness test and the muscular ischaemia test. No difference from placebo was found in the recording of
antinociceptive muscular reflexes or in the EMG surface activity. Tolerability was good;
no serious adverse effects occurred (Goebel et al., 2001).

The 1998 Commission E monograph states that devil's claw is indicated for anorexia, indigestion (the herb is a bitter!), and for the supportive treatment of degenerative
musculoskeletal disorders (Blumenthal et al., 1998). Gastric and duodenal ulcers are
cited as contraindications. A daily dose of 1.5 g of the crude drug is recommended for
anorexia and 4.5 g for joint ailments. For anorexia, the European Scientific Cooperative
on Phytotherapy (ESCOP) recommends a dose equivalent to 1–3 g of the crude drug 3
times daily; this is approximately twice the dose recommended in the Commission E
monograph (ESCOP, 2003).

8.4.2 Willow Bark, Ash, Aspen

The use of willow bark preparations to treat upper respiratory infections was discussed
critically in Sect. 4.2.1.4. As for their anti-inflammatory use, a notable placebo-controlled, double-blind study was recently performed in 78 patients with activated osteoarthritis of the hip and knee. Following a washout phase, the patients in the test-drug
group took 1400 mg/day of a willow bark extract, equivalent to 240 mg of salicin. They
were told not to use any other analgesics or antirheumatic drugs. The main target criterion was improvement in the WOMAK pain score from the beginning to the end of
the 14-day treatment period. Intention-to-treat analysis of the main criterion showed a
significant (p<0.05) superiority of the willow bark therapy over placebo. A similar
result was found in a number of WOMAK subscores, a pain scale, and a limitation-of-
motion scale. Adverse effects were fewer in the willow bark group than the placebo
group (17 vs. 28). In a concomitant study in 10 healthy subjects, a maximum salicylic
acid serum level of 9.8 μmol/L was measured 4 hours after the ingestion of 1.4 g of willow bark extract. Similar levels would have been expected to occur after a single oral
dose of 40 mg of acetylsalicylic acid. The author concluded that the salicylate in willow

bark extract could not account for the observed effect by itself and that willow bark must therefore contain additional anti-inflammatory and analgesic principles (Schmidt, 1998).

Two additional studies were conducted in patients with nonspecific back pain. An open study was carried out in which two groups of 114 patients each were randomly allocated to receive either a willow bark extract containing 240 mg of salicin or 12.5 mg of a COX-2 inhibitor (rofecoxib) for 4 weeks. Outcomes were measured with the Arhus index. After 4 weeks of treatment, the total index had improved by approximately 20 % and its pain component by approximately 30 %. There were no statistical differences between the treatment groups (Chrubasik et al., 2001). In a double-blind study, 210 patients with low back pain were randomly assigned to receive an oral dose of willow bark extract containing 120 mg or 240 mg of salicin, or a placebo (0 mg). Patients with severe pain were also allowed tramadol as a rescue medication. The main outcome measures were the number of patients who were pain-free after 4 weeks and the frequency of tramadol use. The pain-free patients numbered 4 in the placebo group (6 %), 15 in the group taking 120 mg/d (21 %), and 27 in the group taking 240 mg/d (39 %) (p < 0.001). Significantly more patients in the placebo group required tramadol than in the low-dose and high-dose willow bark groups (Chrubasik et al., 2000).

The leaves and bark of the European aspen (*Populus tremula*), like ash bark (*Fraxinus excelsior*) and willow bark, contain salicylates. Extracts from European aspen leaves and bark, as well as a combined preparation containing extracts from aspen leaves, aspen bark, ash bark, and goldenrod, display analgesic and anti-inflammatory effects in typical animal models. The only published clinical studies deal with a combination product with the brand name Phytodolor®. This product was used in a total of 25 clinical trials, four of which were placebo-controlled studies in patients with rheumatoid and degenerative joint diseases, and most of the studies confirmed efficacy. In the more than 1100 patients participating in the studies, the incidence of adverse effects was three times lower than in parallel groups treated with synthetic antirheumatic drugs (Jorken and Okpanyi, 1996). But due to methodologic deficiencies and uncertainty as to the contributions made by specific active components, Commission E discounted the therapeutic efficacy of European aspen bark in its 1992 monograph. Commission E has not evaluated the combinations product in a separate monograph, and a critical meta-analysis of the therapeutic studies has not been published.

The analgesic use of willow bark in patients with flu-like infections is discussed in Sect. 4.2.2.

8.4.3 Nettle Tops

A 1987 Commission E monograph states that preparations of nettle leaves and tops and nettle root (*Urtica* species) are approved for use in the supportive treatment of rheumatic complaints. The recommended average daily dose is 8–12 g of the crude drug or an equivalent extract dosage (Blumenthal et al., 1998). One nettle-based product is listed among the 100 most commonly prescribed phytomedicines in Germany, and its sales have increased markedly in recent years (see Tables A2 to A4). This nettle leaf extract has been tested in an ex vivo/in vitro study of 20 osteoarthritis patients and 20 healthy volunteers. Cytokine secretion was stimulated in heparinized whole blood from each subject, and then the cytokine concentration was determined in the supernatant. The patients and the healthy subjects took approximately 1.4 g of the nettle leaf extract daily for 21 days. The stimulated cytokine concentrations measured in blood samples from the patients and healthy subjects at 7 and 21 days were significantly reduced compared with baseline levels, which the authors interpreted as an anti-inflammatory effect (Obertreis et al., 1997). The same product was tested in a 3-week observational study in 8955 patients. Only 1.2 % of the patients experienced adverse reactions, consisting of 57 gastrointestinal complaints (0.64 %), 12 allergic reactions (0.13 %), and 6 cases of pruritus (0.07 %) (Ramm and Hansen, 1997). An open pilot study was also done to test the therapeutic efficacy of a nettle leaf powder in acute arthritis. Two groups of 20 patients each took either 200 mg of diclofenac or 50 mg of diclofenac plus 50 g of nettle power daily for 2 weeks. The target parameters were the acute-phase plasma protein level (CRP) and a self-evaluated and physician-evaluated scale for clinical complaints. Measured by these criteria, the outcomes in both treatment groups were nearly identical. The authors concluded that nettle leaf preparations potentiated the effect of nonsteroidal anti-inflammatory drugs (Chrubasik et al., 1997).

8.4.4 Boswellin

An oleo-gum-resin from the Indian frakincense tree (*Boswellia serrata*, family Burserace)is used in the Ayurvedic system of medicine as a folk remedy for osteoarthritis, rheumatism, gout, and psoriasis. The boswellic acids contained in the resin have anti-inflammatory properties, which have been demonstrated in a number of animal models (Ammon, 1996; Singh et al., 1996; Shao et al., 1998; Wildfeuer et al., 1998). A special extract from the oleo-gum-resin of *B. serrata* was tested from 1985 to 1990 in 11 clinical studies in a total of 260 patients with rheumatoid arthritis (survey in Etzel, 1996) and one study was conducted in 50 patients with ulcerative colitis (Gupta et al., 1997). Due to methodologic deficiencies, however, the results of these studies have not been sufficient to prompt approval of a medicinal product based on boswellin in Germany. Qualified clinical studies are still needed to confirm the encouraging results of the preliminary studies. A controlled, double-blind crossover study was recently done in 30 patients with osteoarthritis of the knee who received daily doses of 1000 mg of a *B. serrata* extract or a placebo for 8 weeks. The patients taking the extract showed significant improvements in pain, swelling, and limited range of motion, but there was no improvement in radiographic findings (Kimmatkar et al., 2003).

8.5 Treatment of Pain

The practice of rubbing essential oils and rubefacients into the skin to relieve pain is deeply rooted in folk medicine. Conifer oils, camphor, capsaicin preparations, peppermint oil, wintergreen oil, and rubbing alcohol are commonly used for this purpose. At the time the corresponding Commission E monographs were prepared, no controlled therapeutic studies on these preparations had been published. Available empirical evidence suggested that these remedies had a similar mechanism of action, i.e., soothed pain by the counterirritation of organ-associated skin areas (head zones) via the corresponding spinal neurons. Since 1990, however, a large number of controlled studies have been performed in patients and volunteers, with particular emphasis on peppermint oil and capsaicin preparations. The results of these studies have provided more specific information on mechanism of action and therapeutic efficacy for both of these medicinal herbs.

8.5.1 Peppermint Oil and Tension Headache

In a double-blind crossover study, ethanol solutions containing 10 % peppermint oil or eucalyptus oil were compared with placebo solutions in 38 healthy volunteers. The solution was applied topically to the frontotemporal area, and then the time-course of cold sensation was measured by opposite-side comparison, using thermoelectrodes and a visual analog scale. Only the peppermint oil, not the eucalyptus oil, stimulated the cutaneous cold receptors for longer than 30 minutes. This effect is attributed to an activation of the cold-sensitive A-delta fibers, which can inhibit the deep pain that is mediated by C fibers and may play a key role in the pathogenesis of headache (Bromm et al., 1995; Göbel et al., 1995b).

Based on these neurophysiologic studies, another group of authors performed a placebo-controlled, double-blind study to test the efficacy of the same peppermint oil and eucalyptus oil preparations in experimental ischemic and heat-induced pain. Thirty-two healthy subjects participated in the study, which has a crossover design. The 4 different test preparations were applied to a large skin area on the forehead and temples using a small dose-metering sponge. Peppermint oil in ethanol had a significant effect on experimentally induced pain sensation, whereas eucalyptus oil did not (Göbel et al., 1994, 1995a).

The same group of authors (Göbel et al., 1996) later performed 4 placebo-controlled, double-blind crossover studies to compare the efficacy of peppermint oil with acetaminophen and acetylsalicylic acid. Three of these studies were done in patients with tension headaches (most common form of headache, with a lifetime prevalence of about 30 % of the population), and one was done in patients suffering from migraine headaches. In all studies the headache episodes were treated according to a randomly assigned sequence using a double-blind format. Each attack was treated by giving the patient two capsules of an oral medication (placebo or 1 g acetaminophen or 1 g acetylsalicylic acid) and by the cutaneous application of a 10 % peppermint oil preparation or a placebo solution labeled as peppermint oil. The main study criterion was clinical pain intensity as a function of time after application or ingestion of the test medications. Pain intensity was determined and logged using a self-assessment scale in a headache diary. "Significant clinical improvement" was the main variable for statistical evaluation and was graded on a 0–4 scale according to headache intensity: severe (grade 4), moderate (grade 3), mild (grade 2), very mild (grade 1), or no headache (grade 0). Pain intensity, debilitation due to headache, and the use of substitute medications were evaluated as secondary criteria.

The principal results of the 4 studies are summarized in Table 8.2. In all, 190 protocols could be evaluated from patients with tension headache and 102 protocols from patients with migraine. While most of the patients with tension headache showed statistically significant improvement in response to peppermint oil therapy compared with placebo, or showed no difference compared with acetaminophen or acetylsalicylic acid, the migraine patients showed no significant differences when treated with placebo, peppermint oil, or acetaminophen. These studies indicate that peppermint oil, when applied topically to the forehead and temples in a 10 % ethanol solution, is comparable to acetaminophen and acetylsalicylic acid in reducing the intensity of tension headache pain. Peppermint oil is not effective for migraine headaches, however. Some typical results from the studies of Göbel et al. are shown graphically in Fig. 8.9.

8.5.2 Capsicum (Cayenne Pepper) for Local Pain Relief

Aqueous alcoholic or oily preparations of the fruits of various species of *Capsicum* are traditional topical remedies for arthritis, rheumatic complaints, and various kinds of pain, particularly when used in the form of alcohol extracts. The key active constituents are the capsaicinoids, especially capsaicin, whose content in the various species ranges from 0 to about 1.5 %. When applied topically, capsaicin preparations incite an initial response consisting of erythema, pain, and warmth. This is followed by an extended period of insensitivity marked by a reversible desensitization of afferent nerve fibers. While the erythema, pain, and warmth subside within a few hours, the antinociceptive effects can persist for a period of hours to weeks. With repeated use, the vascular and sensory responses to the agent decline and are eventually extinguished (Hänsel et al., 1992d; Baron, 2000).

Table 8.2.
Studies by Göbel et al. (1996, 1998 a, b) on the efficacy of peppermint oil in the treatment of tension headache and migraine. All the studies were placebo-controlled and had a crossover design.

Number of patients	Indications	Test substances	Key parameters
41	Tension headache	10 % peppermint oil vs 1 g acetaminophen	PI ***, PD *
105	Tension headache	10 % peppermint oil vs 1 g acetaminophen	BKS **, PI **, SCI ***, Sub n.s.
102	Migraine	10 % peppermint oil vs 1 g acetaminophen	SCI n.s., PI n.s., PD n.s., Sub n.s.
44	Tension headache	10 % peppermint oil vs 1 g acetylsalicylic acid	SCI ***, PI ***, PD n.s., Sub n.s.

Abbreviations: PI = pain intensity, **SCI** = significant clinical improvement in pain intensity, **PD** = pain-related debilitation, **Sub** = use of substitute medications. * = p < 0.05, ** = p<0.01, *** = p < 0.001 (comparing peppermint oil against placebo)

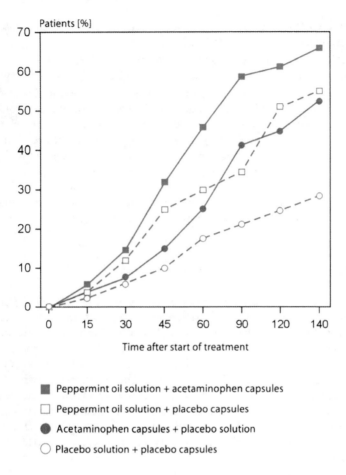

Figure 8.9. ▲ Relative percentage of 105 patients with tension headache who showed significant clinical improvement in headache intensity (= reduction of pain intensity from grade 4, 3, or 2 to grade 1 or 0) at various times after the start of treatment (Göbel et al., 1998 a).

Based on information available at the time, the 1990 Commission E monograph on capsicum (paprika) stated that semisolid preparations (0.02–0.05 % capsaicinoids), liquid preparations (0.005–0.01 % capsaicinoids), and plasters were indicated for "painful muscle spasms involving the shoulder, arm, or spinal region in adolescents and school-age children." The monograph stated that capsicum should not be used on damaged skin or in patients hypersensitive to capsicum preparations. It should not be applied topically for longer than two days due to the risk of sensory nerve damage, and an interval of at least 14 days should be allowed between treatments (Blumenthal et al., 1998). As noted in the following paragraph, these time restrictions are no longer considered valid.

In the years since publication of the 1990 Commission E monograph, a number of controlled clinical studies have been published on the use of topical capsaicin-contain-

Table 8.3.

Placebo-controlled studies with capsaicin cream (0.025 %) [a] or 0.075 % [b] capsaicinoids q.i.d.) in patients with diabetic polyneuropathy, postherpetic neuralgia, or rheumatic disorders.

First author, year (test preparation	Patients (true	Duration	Results
Diabetic polyneuropathy			
Chad, 1990 (b)	24/22	4	PGA n.s., PI n.s., PR *
Scheffler, 1991 (b)	28/26	8	PI *, PR *
Capsaicin study group, 1991 (b)	138/139	8	PGA *, PI *, PR **
Tandan, 1991 (b)	11/11	8	PGA *, PI n.s., PR n.s.
Postherpetic neuralgia			
Bernstein, 1989 (b)	16/16	6	PGA *, PI *, PR **
Drake, 1990 (a)	15/15	4	PR n.s.
Watson, 1993 (b)	75/69	6	PGA *, PI *, PR *
Ellison, 1997 (b)	99/99	8	PGA ***, PR **
Rheumatic disorders			
Deal, 1991 (a)	52/50	4	PGA *, PR *
Schnitzer, 1992 (a)	23/28	9	PI *

Abbreviations: PGA = physician global assessment, **PI** = pain intensity, **PR** = pain relief; **(a)** = cream containing 0.025 % capsaicin, **(b)** = cream containing 0.075 % capsaicin; * = $p < 0.05$, ** = $p < 0.01$, *** = $p < 0.001$, **n.s.** = not significant.

ing preparations for neuralgiform and rheumatic complaints and for pruritus due to various causes. These studies were based on treatment periods ranging from 2 to 8 weeks. The results of 9 placebo-controlled studies are shown in Table 8.3. A 0.075 % capsaicin cream was used in most of the studies. Capsaicin appears to be superior to placebo, especially in patients with diabetic polyneuropathy or postherpetic neuralgia. There were no side effects serious enough to warrant discontinuation of treatment, but there were occasional reports of a burning or pricking sensation or an inflammatory reaction at the application site. These complaints persisted for about 2 weeks and then resolved without sequelae. There was no evidence of neurotoxic injury in any of the studies. It was concluded that these safety aspects Clinical trials on capsicum preparations and pure capsaicin are reviewed in Blumenthal et al. (2003).

8.5.3 Feverfew and Butterbur for Migraine Prevention

Feverfew (*Tanacetum perthenium*) is a plant of the family Asteraceae that grows to a height of 30–80 cm. It is strongly aromatic and has a camhpor-like smell. Probably originating in the eastern Mediterranean region, the plant has been cultivated in Europe for centuries and in North and South America since the 19th century. One of the key constituents of the herb is believed to be parthenolide (minimum content 0.2 %). Dioscorides recommended feverfew as an antipyretic in the first century C.E., and it has been used in England as a remedy for toothache and headache since the 1700's. Interest in its use was revived in the late 1970's when newspaper accounts in the United Kingdom noted that migraine sufferers were chewing small amounts of the leaves to prevent or to moderate the intensity of such attacks. This prompted several initial clinical investigations of the plant, and additional ones are continuing to be conducted.

The identity of the active principle in feverfew is presently controversial. It has long been assumed to be parthenolide, based on the ability of that sesquiterpene lactone to inhibit the release of serotonin from blood platelets. That process is viewed as involving Michael addition to the α, β-unsaturated lactone moiety of parthenolide of systemic nucleophiles such as cysteine, which have been demonstrated in the laboratory to participate in such a reaction. In fact, the government of Canada has established a minimum of 0.2 % parthenolide as a quality criteria for the commercial product. The widespread acceptance of parthenolide as the dominant active principle of feverfew has now been characterized as "a rush to judgment" (Awang, 1998).

Assuming its reproducibility, a study conducted in The Netherlands (De Weerdt et al., 1996) seems to have cast doubt on the parthenolide hypothesis. It involved capsules filled with a dried ethanolic extract of feverfew on microcrystalline cellulose, each containing 0.5 mg of parthenolide. The double-blind cross-over study involved 50 patients to whom the capsules containing the herbal extract or a placebo were administered for 4 months. In the 44 patients who completed the study, there were no differences in number of attacks or lost working days.

The ineffectiveness of the ethanolic extract, in spite of an adequate concentration of parthenolide, would apparently call for a reassessment of the role of that sesquiterpene lactone in migraine prophylaxis. One view holds that other constituents, including volatile oil components such as *trans*-chrysanthenyl acetate might play a role, but this requires verification. In the meantime, it seems prudent to restrict the use of this botanical to preparations of the dried whole leaf of an appropriate variety of the plant. Usual dose ranges from 25–125 mg daily as a migraine prophylactic. Utility of feverfew in the acute phase of the attacks has not been demonstrated.

Efficacy for this indication has been tested in 4 controlled studies. The first such trial (Johnson et al., 1985) was a double-blind, placebo-controlled study of 17 migraine sufferers who had been consuming the herb for at least 3 months. Eight of these continued to take 25 mg of feverfew leaf twice daily, and the 9 others were switched to placebo. In the latter group, there was a significant increase in frequency and severity of the migraine attacks, and nausea and vomiting were more common.

A subsequent double-blind, placebo-controlled cross-over study (Murphy, 1988) involved 72 patients who had not previously taken feverfew. The leaf was administered in the form of 82 mg capsules, each containing 0.54 mg of parthenolide. Cross-over occurred after 4 months, but results were assessed every 2 months. Again, treatment with feverfew was associated with a significant decrease in frequency and severity of the attacks. A third double-blind, placebo-controlled cross-over study (Palevitch et al., 1997) of 4 months duration on 57 patients yielded similar positive results. Another clinical study (Pattrick et al., 1989) designed to investigate the utility of feverfew in treating patients with rheumatoid arthritis did not yield clearly beneficial results.

Two reviews of all the 4 studies concluded that feverfew may be effective in treating migraines, but that more clinical studies are needed to establish its efficacy (Vogler et al., 1998; Pittler et al., 2000). The safety of feverfew, even on long-term consumption, has never been questioned. Continuous ingestion by large numbers of people for periods up to 10 years did not cause any chronic toxicity. Occasional mouth ulcers have been reported, but the only clinical study in which this side effect was analyzed reported a significantly greater frequency in patients consuming the placebo (dried cabbage leaves) than in those using feverfew (Murphy et al., 1988). Persons allergic to other members of the Asteraceae (daisy family) should be cautious in consuming feverfew.

The development of a standardized extract of the rhizome of purple butterbur (*Petasites* hybridus L.) has led to a new clinical approach to the management of migraine headache (Donald and Brown, 2003).

Two randomized, placebo-controlled, double-blind clinical trials tested the efficacy of the standardized butterbur extract (Petadolex®, Weber & Weber International GmbH & Co., Germany) in the treatment of migraines. In the first trial, 60 migraine patients (mean age 28.7 years) were randomized to receive either 50 mg of Petadolex or placebo two times per day for 12 weeks (Grossmann and Schmidrams, 2000). Starting at the fourth week of treatment, the Petadolex group had a significant reduction in the number of migraine attacks compared to the placebo group ($P < 0.05$). Compared to the placebo group, those taking Petadolex had a 60 percent reduction in the number of migraines by week 12. The number of migraine days was also reduced significantly in the Petadolex group (3.4 ± 1.6 at baseline to 1.7 ± 0.9 days after 12 weeks) compared to placebo (3.0 ± 1.3 to 2.6 ± 1.2 days, $P < 0.05$). While the duration and intensity of migraines was significantly reduced at 8 weeks in the Petadolex group ($P < 0.05$), the difference compared to placebo was not significant at week 12. The mean number of accompanying symptoms (e.g., nausea, vomiting) was significantly reduced in the Petadolex group compared to placebo ($P < 0.01$). No adverse events were reported at the end of the 12-week trial.

The second trial randomized 202 migraine patients (ages 19–65 years) to receive either 50 mg of Petadolex, 75 mg of Petadolex, or placebo two times per day for 12 weeks following a four-week baseline run-in period (Lipton et al., 2002). The primary endpoint, frequency of migraine attacks per four weeks, was reduced by 38 percent, 44 percent, 58 percent, and 51 percent in patients treated with 150 mg/day of Petadolex after 1 (baseline), 2, 3, and 4 months respectively. The 100 mg/day group had a reduction of 24 percent, 37 percent, 42 percent, and 40 percent, while the placebo group was 19 percent, 26 percent, 26 percent, and 32 percent, respectively. Treatment differences between those taking 100 mg/day of Petadolex were not significant compared to placebo. However, those taking 150 mg/day had a significant reduction in migraine count over 3 months of treatment compared to placebo ($P < 0.001$). The number of patients who had a 50 percent reduction in mean migraine attack frequency per month relative to baseline were considered therapy responders. The mean percent of responders in the 150 mg/day group (68 percent) was significantly greater than those taking placebo (49 percent) ($P \leq 0.05$). The mean three-month assessment of headache intensity also favored the Petadolex 150 mg/day group compared to placebo ($P = 0.01$). Eighty participants reported 131 adverse events – 23 patients in the placebo group and 29 patients and 28 patients in the 100 mg and 150 mg groups, respectively. The most frequently reported adverse events in patients taking Petadolex were gastrointestinal complaints with burning being the most common complaint (reported by approximately 20 percent of patients taking Petadolex).

Side effects are rare with the use of the PA-free extract and have consisted primarily of mild gastrointestinal complaints (nausea, burping, and stomach pain) with rare reports of vomiting, diarrhea, and skin rash. In a recent safety report on standardized butterbur root extract, documentation of adverse events from 1976 to June 30, 2002 found a total of 75 reports of suspected adverse reactions from Germany and 18 spontaneous reports from other countries received by the manufacturer. Only 19 reports were determined to be possibly causally related to the administration of the medication and 8 reports to be probably causally related to the medication by thorough evaluation by German pharmacovigilance guidelines and standard operating procedures. One case of cholestatic hepatitis was diagnosed as a hypersensitivity reaction with a probable causal reaction to butterbur. Butterbur should not be used during pregnancy or lactation due to lack of safety studies, nor should it be used by those who have suffered from hepatitis or other liver ailments (Danesch and Rittinghausen, 2003).

8.6 Formulations

Recurrent Herpes Simplex

Virtually all agents with a protein-coagulating and astringent action can improve the symptoms of a herpes lesion. Thus, claims such as "eau de cologne works wonders for fever blisters" (Medical Tribune of 24 Jan 1992) are entirely plausible. Eau de cologne consists of 90 % alcohol.

Rx	Eau de cologne	30.0 mL
	Directions: Dab externally onto affected area.	

Alternative:

Rx	Ethanol 90 %	30.0
	Citronella oil	1 drop
	Directions: Dab externally onto affected area.	

Noninfectious Dermatitis

Applied to acutely inflamed areas and small wounds, astringents tighten and dry the superficial cell layers, forming a protective barrier against bacterial invasion and soothing inflammatory symptoms. Herbal astringents contain tannins as their active principle (see Table5-4).

Sample formula for acute eczema:

Rx	Tannic acid	1.0 (to 3.0)
	Purified water to	100.0
	Directions: Use externally; dilute with water and apply as a compress.	

The following formula can be used in sitz baths for hemorrhoidal conditions and for anogenital fissures and erosions:

Rx	Tannic acid	5.0
	Glycerol to	100.0
	Directions: use externally; dilute 1:10 with water.	

Protective and Cooling Ointment

Jojoba wax, a plant product, can be used in place of spermaceti, which is no longer available. The wax is a clear, pale yellow, oily fluid expressed from ripe seeds of the jojoba shrub (*Simmondsia chinensis*). A modified protective and cooling ointment to replace the older soothing ointment described in the *German Pharmacopeia* 10 can be formulated as follows:

Rx	Yellow wax	3.5
	Jojoba wax (liquid)	4.0
	Peanut oil	30.0
	Purified water to	50.0
	Mix and use externally.	

Pain and Spasms

Rubbing alcohol, known in Germany as *Franzbranntwein* (literally, "France burnt wine") was formerly a byproduct of cognac production and is now made by mixing diluted alcohol with essential oils or aromatic tinctures. It has multiple uses in the treatment of muscle pain and spasms. An old pharmaceutical formula is given below:

Rx	Aromatic tincture	0.4
	Ethyl Nitrite Spirit	0.5
	Rhatany tincture	6 drops
	Ethanol (90 vol. %)	100.0
	Distilled water to	200.0

The rhatany (*Krameria triandra* and *K.* spp., Krameriaceae) tincture gives the product a cognac color. Modern products that are marketed (in Germanyu) under the name *Franzbranntwein* may be green or colorless. They usually contain juniper berry oil, spruce needle oil, dwarfpine oil, menthol, camphor, and thymol. Both the essential oils and the alcohol have a rubefacient (hyperemia-inducing) action: alcohol in concentrations higher than 50 % causes mild skin irritation and acts as an antiseptic. Rubbing alcohol is rubbed into the skin to induce local hyperemia for muscle and joint pain, muscle soreness, strains, or bruises; it is also used in sports medicine and for connective-tissue massage. German rubbing alcohol is sold in various strengths (38–45 % v/v) and may be pure or blended with camphor or spruce needle oil. In the United States, rubbing alcohol consists of denatured 70 % ethanol or 70 % isopropanol.

8.7 Drug Products

Herbal remedies used as described in this chapter are subdivided in the 2003 *Rote Liste* into three different categories based on their indications: "Analgesics and Antirheumatics," "Anti-inflammatory Agents," and "Dermatologic Agents." Because the indications overlap, some of the chamomile preparations in the *Rote Liste* are also listed under the heading of "Gastrointestinal Remedies."

 References

Aertgeerts P, Albring M, Klaschka F, Nasemann T, Patzelt-Wnczler R, Rauhut K, Weigel B (1985) Vergleichende Prüfung von Kamillosan Creme gegenüber steroidalen (0,25 % Hydrocortison, 0,75 % Fluocortinbutylester) und nichtsteroidalen (5 % Bufexamac) Externa in der Erhaltungstherapie von Ekzemerkrankungen. Z Hautkr 60: 270–277.

Ammon HPT (1996) Salai Guggal – Boswellia serrata: from a herbal to medicine to a specific inhibitor of leukotriene biosynthesis. Phytomedicine 3: 67–70.

Ammon HPT, Kaul R (1992) Pharmakologie der Kamille und ihrer Inhaltsstoffe. Dtsch Apoth Z 132 (Suppl 27): 3–26.

Awang DVC (1998) Prescribing therapeutic feverfew (Tanacetum parthenium (L.) Schultz Bip., syn. Chrysanthemum parthenium (L.) Bernh.) Int. Med 1: 11–13

Bamford JTM (1985) Atopic eczema unresponsive to evening primrose oil (Linoleic and Gamma-linolenic acids. J Am Acad Dermatol 13: 959–965.

Baron R (2000) Capsaicin and nociception: from basic mechanisms to novel drugs. Lancet 356: 785–6.

Bassett IB, Pannowitz DL, Barnetson RSC (1990) A comparative study of tea-tree oil versus benzoyl peroxide in the treatment of acne. Med J Aust 153: 455–458.

Bernstein JE (1989) Topical capsaicin treatment of chronic postherpetic neuralgia. J Am Acad Dermatol 21: 265–270.

Berth-Jones J, Brown A (1993) Placebo-controlled trial of essential fatty acid supplementation in atopic dermatitis. Lancet 341: 1557–60.

Blumenthal M, Busse WR, Goldberg A, Gruenwald J, Hall T, Riggins CW, Rister RS (eds.). Klein S, Rister RS (trans). (1998) The Complete German Commission E Monographs – Therapeutic Guide to Herbal Medicines. American Botanical Council, Austin, Texas. *www.herbalgram.org*.

Blumenthal M, Hall T, Goldberg A et al. (eds). (2003) The ABC Clinical Guide to Herbs. Austin, TX: American Botanical Council.

Bromm B, Scharein E, Darsow U, Ring J (1995) Effects of menthol and cold on histamine-induced itch and skin reactions in man. Neurosci Lett 187: 157–160.

Buck DS, Nidorf DM, Addino JG (1994) Comparison of two topical preparations for the treatment of onychomycosis: Melaleuca alternifolia (tea tree) oil and chlotrimazole. J Fam Pract 38: 601–605.

Budeiri D, Li Won Po D, Donan JC (1996) Is evening primrose oil of value in the treatment of premenstrual syndrome? Controlled Clin Trials 17: 60–8.

Capsaicin Study Group (1991) Treatment of painful diabetic neuropathy with topical capsaicin. A multicenter, double-blind, vehicle-controlled study. Arch Intern Med 151: 2225–2229.

Carson CF, Riley TV (1995) Antimicrobial activity of the major components of the essential oil of Melaleuca alternifolia. J Appl Bact 78: 264–269.

Chad DA (1990) Does capsaicin relieve the pain of diabetic neuropathy? Pain 42: 387–388.

Chrubasik S, Conradt C, Black A (2003) The quality of clinical trials with Harpagophytum procumbens. Phytomedicine. 10: 613–23

Chrubasik S, Eisenberg E, Balan E et al. (2000) Treatment of low back pain exacerbations with willow bark extract: a randomized double-blind study. Am J Med 109: 9–14.

Chrubasik S, Enderlein W, Bauer R, Grabner W (1997) Evidence for antirheumatic effectiveness of Herba Urticae dioicae in acute arthritis: a pilot study. Phytomedicine 4: 105–108.

Chrubasik S, Junck H, Breitschwerdt H, Conradt CH, Zappe H (1999) Effectiveness of Harpagophytum extract WS 1531 in the treatment of exacerbation of low back pain: a randomized, placebo-controlled, double-blind study. European Journal of Anaesthesiology 16: 118–129.

Chrubasik S, Künzel o, Model A, Conradt C, Black A (2001) Treatment of low back pain with a herbal or synthetic anti-rheumatic: a randomised controlled study. Willow bark extract for low back pain. Rheumatology 40: 1388–93.

Chrubasik S, Wink M (1998) Traditional herbal therapy for the treatment of rheumatic pain: preparations from devil's claw and stinging nettle. Pain Digest 8: 94–101.

Chrubasik S, Wink M (Hrsg) (1997) Rheumatherapie mit Phytopharmaka. Hippokrates Verlag Stuttgart.

Chrubasik S, Zimpfer CH, Schütt U, Ziegler R (1996) Effectiveness of Harpagophytum procumbens in treatment of acute low back pain. Phytomedicine 3: 1–10.

Danesch U, Rittinghausen R. Safety of a patented special butterbur root extract for migraine prevention. Headache 2003; 43: 76–8.

De Weerdt GJ, Bootsman HPR, Hendriks H (1996) Herbal medicines in migraine prevention. Randomized double-blind placebo-controlled cross-over trial for a feverfew preparation. Phytomedicine 3: 225–230.

Deal CL (1991) Treatment of arthritis with topical capsaicin – a double-blind trial. Clinical Therapeutics 13: 383–395.

Del Beccaro MA (1994) Malaleuca oil poisoning. J Toxicol Clin Toxicol 32: 461–4.

Donald J, Brown ND (2003) Standardized Butterbur Extract for Migraine Treatment: A Clinical Overview. HerbalGram 58: 18–19.

Drake HF, Harries AJ, Gamester RE, Justin D (1990) Randomized double-blind study of topical capsaicin for treatment of postherpetic neuralgia. Pain 5 (Suppl.): 58.

Edwards A, Atma-Ram A, Thin RN (1988) Podophyllotoxin 0,5 % VS, podophyllin 20 % to treat penile warts. Genetnourin Med 64: 263–265.

Ellison N, Loprinzi CL, Kugler J, Hatfield AK, Miser A, Sloan JA, Wender DB, Rowland KM, Molina R, Cascino TL, Vukov AM, Dhaliwal HS, Ghosh C (1997) Phase III placebo-controlled trial of capsaicin cream in the management of surgical neurpathic pain in cancer patients. Journal of Clinical Oncology 15: 2974–2980.

Erdös A, Fontaine R, Friehe H, Durand R, Pöppinghaus T (1978) Beitrag zur Pharmakologie und Toxikologie verschiedener Extrakte sowie des Harpagosids aus Harpagophytum procumbens DC. Planta Med 34: 97–108.

Ernst E, Chrubasik S (2000) Phyto-antiinflammatories. A systematic review of randomized, placebo-controlled, double-blind trials. Rheumatic Disease Clinics of North America 1: 13-27.

Ernst E, Huntley A (2000) Tea tree oil: a systematic review of randomised clinical trials. Forsch Komplementärmed 7: 17–20.

ESCOP (2003) Monographs of the medicinal uses of plant drug. Thieme Stuttgart New York, 2003

Etzel R (1996) Special extract of Boswellia serrata (H 15) in the treatment of rheumatoid arthritis. Phytomedicine 3: 91–94.

Fleurentin J, Mortier F (1997) Entzündungshemmende und analgetische Wirkungen von Harpagophytum procumbens und H. zeyheri. In: Chrubasik S, Wink M (eds) Rheumatherapie mit Phytopharmaka, Hippokrates Verlag Stuttgart: 68–76.

Frohne D (1992) Solanum dulcamara L. – Der Bittersüße Nachtschatten. Portrait einer Arzneipflanze. Z Phythother 14: 337–342.

Gehring W, Bopp R, Rippke F, Gloor M (1999) Effect of topically applied evening primrose oil on epidermal barrier function in atopic dermatitis as a function of vehicle. Arzneim-Forsch/Drug Res 49(II): 635–642.

Göbel H, Fresenius J, Heinze A, Dworschak M, Soyka D (1996) Effektivität von Oleum menthae piperitae und von Paracetamol in der Therapie des Kopfschmerzes vom Spannungstyp. Nervenarzt 67: 672–681.

Gobel H, Heinze A, Ingwersen M, Niederberger U, Gerber D (2001) Effects of Harpagophytum procumbens LI 174 (devil's claw) on sensory, motor und vascular muscle reagibility in the treatment of unspecific back pain. Schmerz 15: 10–18.

Göbel H, Schmidt G, Dworschak M, Stolze H, Heuss D (1995a) Essential plant oils and headache mechanisms. Phytomedicine 2: 93–102.

Göbel H, Schmidt G, Soyka D (1994) Effect of peppermint and eucalyptus oil preparations on neurophysiological and experimental algesimetric headache parameters. Cephalalgia 14: 228–234.

Göbel H, Stolze H, Dworschak M, Heinze A (1995b) Oelum menthae piperitae: Wirkmechanismen und klinische Effektivität bei Kopfschmerz vom Spannungstyp. In: Loew D, Rietbrock N (eds) Phytopharmaka in Forschung und klinischer Anwendung. Steinkopff Verlag, Darmstadt: 177–184.

Grossmann M, Schmidrams H (2000) An extract of Petasites hybridus is effective in the prophylaxis of migraine. Int J Clin Pharmacol Ther 38: 430–5.

Gupta I, Parihar A, Malhotra P, Singh GB, Lüdtke R, Safayhi H, Ammon HPT (1997) Effects of Boswellia serrata gum resin in patients with ulcerative colitis. Eur J Med Rs 2: 37–43.

Hänsel R, Keller K, Rimpler H, Schneider G (1992) Hagers Handbuch der pharmazeutischen Praxis. 5th Ed., Vol. 4, Drogen A–D. Springer-Verlag, Berlin Heidelberg New York: 817–831 (a); 342–357 (b); 272–280 (c); 660–680 (d).

Hänsel R, Keller K, Rimpler H, Schneider G (1993) Hagers Handbuch der pharmazeutischen Praxis. 5th Ed., Vol. 5, Drogen E–O. Springer-Verlag, Berlin Heidelberg New York: 367–384 (a); 929–936 (b); 476–479 (c); 747–750 (d).

Hausen HM, Busker E, Carle R (1984) Über das Sensibilisierungsvermögen von Compostitenarten. VII. Experimentelle Untersuchungen mit Auszügen und Inhaltsstoffen von Chamomilla recutita L. Rauschert und Anthemis cotula L., Planta Med 50: 229–234.

Hölzer I (1992) Dulcamara-Extrakt bei Neurodermitis und chronischem Ekzem. Ergebnisse einer klinischen Prüfung. Jatros Dermatologie 6: 32–36.

Hörmann HP, Korting HC (1994) Evidence for the efficacy and safety of topical herbal drugs in dermatology: Part I: Anti-inflammatory agents. Phytomedicine 1: 161–171.

Hörmann HP, Korting HC (1995) Allergic acute contact dermatitis due to Arnica tincture self-medication. Phytomedicine 4: 315–317.

Isaac O (1992) Die Ringelblume. Botanik, Chemie, Pharmakologie, Toxikologie, Pharmazie und therapeutische Verwendung. Wissenschaftliche Verlagsgesellschaft mbH Stuttgart.

Jakovlev V, Isaac O, Flaskamp E (1983) Pharmakologische Untersuchungen von Kamillen-Inhaltsstoffen. VI. Untersuchungen zur antiphlogistischen Wirkung von Chamazulen und Matricin. Planta Med 49: 67–73.

Johnson ES, Kodam NP, Hylands DM, Hylands PJ (1985) Efficacy of feverfew as prophylactic treatment of migraine. Br Med J 291: 569–573.

Jorken S, Okpanyi SN (1996) Pharmakologische Grundlagen pflanzlicher Antirheumatika. In: Loew D, Rietbrock N (eds) Phytopharmaka II, Forschung und klinische Anwendung. Steinkopff, Stuttgart: 115–126.

Kimmatkar N, Thawani V, Hingorani L, Khiyani R (2003) Efficacy and tolerability of Boswellia serrata extract in treatment of osteoarthritis of knee – a randomized double-blind placebo-controlled trial. Phytomedicine 10: 3–7.

Knoch HG (1991) Hämorrhoiden I. Grades: Wirksamkeit einer Salbe auf pflanzlicher Basis. Münch Med Wschr 31/32: 481–484.

König D, Berg A, Keul J, Schäfer W, Zahradnik HP (1999) Prävention und Therapie mit essentiellen Fettsäuren. Bedeutung der Gamma-Linolensäure für die Pathogenese von prämenstruellem Syndrom, Migräne und Präeklampsie. Schweiz Zschr GanzheitsMedizin 11: 130.

Korting HC, Schäder-Korting M, Hart H, Laux P, Schmid M (1993) Anti-inflammatory activity of hamamelis distillate applied topically to the skin. Influence of vehicle and dose. Eur J Clin Pharmacol 44: 315–318.

Korting HC, Schäder-Korting M, Klövekorn W, Klövekorn G, Martin C, Laux P (1995) Comparative efficacy of hamamelis distillate and hydrocortisone cream in atopic exzema. Eur J Clin Pharmacol 48: 461–465.

Lampert ML, Andenmatten C, Schaffner W (1998) Mahonia aquifolium (Pursh) Nutt. Zeitschrift für Phytotherapie 19: 197–128.

Laux P, Oschmann R (1993) Die Zaubernuß – Hamamelis virginiana L. Z Phytother 14: 155–166.

Lecomte A, Costa JP (1992) Harpagophytum dans l'arthrose. Etude en double insu contre placebo. 370 2 Le magazine: 27–30.

Lipton RB, Gobel H, Wilkes K, Mauskop A (2002) Efficacy of Petasites (an extract from Petasites rhizome) 50 and 75 mg for prophylaxis of migraine: Results of a randomized, double-blind, placebo-controlled study. Neurology 58 (Suppl 3): A472

Loew D (1997) Capsaicinhaltige Zubereitungen – Pharmakologie und klinische Anwendung. In: Chrubasik S, Wink M (eds) Rheumatherapie mit Phytopharmaka. Hippokrates Verlag Stuttgart: 149–160.

Loew D (1997) Pharmakologie und klinische Anwendung von capsaicinhaltigen Zubereitungen. Zeitschrift für Phytotherapie 18: 332–340.

Loew D, Möllerfeld J, Schrödter A et al. (2001) Investigations on the pharmacokinetic properties of Harpagophytum extracts and their effect on eicosanoid biosynthesis in vitro ex vivo. Clin Pharmacol Ther 69: 356–364.

Maiche AG, Gröhn P, Mäki-Hokkonen H (1991) Effect of chamomile cream and almond ointment of acute radiation skin reaction. Acta Oncol 30: 395–396.

Manku MS, Horrobin DF, Morse NL et al (1984) Essential fatty acids in the plasma phospholipids of patients with atopic eczema. Br J Dermatol 110: 643–648.

Mennet-von Eiff M, Meier B (1995) Phytotherapie in der Dermatologie. 9. Schweizerische Tagung für Phytotherapie. Z Phytother 17: 201–210.

Michler B, Arnold CG (1996) Pyrrolizidinalkaloide in Beinwellwurzeln. Deutsche Apotheker Zeitung 136: 2447–2452.

Morse PF, Horrobin DF, Manku MS, Stewart JCM, Allen R, Littlewood S, Wright S, Burton J, Gould DJ, Holt PJ, Jansen CT, Mattila L, Meigel W, Dettke TH, Wexler D, Guenther L, Bordoni A, Patrizi A (1989) Meta-analysis of placebo-controlled studies of the efficacy of Epogam in the treatment of atopic eczema. Relationship between plasma essential fatty acid changes and clinical response. Br J Dermatol 121: 75–90.

Murphy JJ, Heptinstall S, Mitchell JRA (1988) Randomized double-blind placebo-controlled trial of feverfew in migraine prevention. Lancet ii: 189–192.

Nissen HP, Blitz H, Kreysel HW (1988) Profilometrie, eine Methode zur Beurteilung der therapeutischen Wirksamkeit von Kamillosan-Salbe. Z Hautkr 63: 184–190.

Obertreis B, Teuscher T, Behnke B, Schmitz H (1997) Pharmakologische Wirkungen des Brennesselblätterextraktes IDS 23. In: Chrubasik S, Wink M (Hrsg) Rheumatherapie mit Phytopharmaka, Hippokrates Verlag Stuttgart: 90–96.

Olson C (1997) Australian Tea Tree Oil Guide. Kali Press, Pagosa Springs, Colorado, p 12.

Palevich D, Earon G, Carasso R (1997) Feverfew (Tanacetum parthenium) as a prophylactic treatment for migraine: a double-blind placebo-controlled study. Phytother Res 11: 508–511.

Patrick KFM, Kumar S. Edwardson PAD, Hutchinson JJ (1996) Induction of vascularisation by an aqueous extract of the flowers of Calendula officinalis L. the European marigold. Phytomedicine 3: 11–18.

Pattrick M, Heptinstall S, Doherty M (1989) Feverfew in rheumatoid arthritis: a double-blind, placebo-controlled study. Ann Rheum Dis 48: 547–549.

Pittler MH, Vogler BK, Ernst E (2000) Efficacy of feverfew for the prevention of migraine (Conchraine Review). In: The Conchrane Library Issue 3, 2000. Oxford: Update Software.

Ramm S, Hansen C (1997) Brennesselblätter-Extrakt: Wirksamkeit und Verträglichkeit bei Arthrose und rheumatischer Arthritis. In: Chrubasik S, Wink M (Hrsg) Rheumatherapie mit Phytopharmaka, Hippokrates Verlag Stuttgart: 97–106.

Rubel DM, Freeman S, Southwell IA (1998) Tea tree oil allergy: What is the offending agent? Report of three cases of tea tree oil allergy and review of the literature. Aust J Dermatol 39: 244–7.

Saho Y, Ho CT, Chin CK, Badmaev V, Ma W, Huang MT (1998) Inhibitory activity of boswellic acids from Boswellia serrata against human leukemia HL-60 cells in culture. Planta Med 64: 328–331.

Saller R, Berger T, ReicWing J, Harkenthal M (1998) Pharmaceutical and medicinal aspects of Australian tea tree oil. Phytomedicine 5: 489–95.

Scheffler NM (1991) Treatment of painful diabetic neuropathy with Capsaicin 0.075 %. J Am Ped Med Ass 81: 288–293.

Schempp CM, Windeck T, Hezel S,. Simon JC (2003) Topical treatment of atopic dermatitis with

St. John's wort cream – a randomized, placebo-controlled, double-blind half-side comparison. Phytomedicine 10 Suppl 4: in press 31–37.

Schempp CM, Winghofer B, Lütke R et al. (2000) Topical application of St. John's Wort (Hypericum perforatum L.) and of its metabolite hyperforin inhibits the allostimulatory capacity of epidermal cells. Br J Dermatol142: 979–84.

Schilcher H (Hrsg) (1987) Die Kamille. Handbuch für Ärzte, Apotheker und andere Naturwissenschaftler. Wissenschaftliche Verlagsgesellschaft mbH Stuttgart.

Schmelz H, Hämmerle HD, Springorum HW (1997) Analgetische Wirkung eines Teufelskrallenwurzel-Extraktes bei verschiedenen chronisch-degenerativen Gelenkerkrankungen. In: Chrubasik S, Wink M (eds) Rheumatherpaie mit Phytopharmaka. Hippokrates Verlag Stuttgart: 86–89.

Schmid BM (1998) Behandlung von Cox- und Gonarthrosen mit einem Trockenextrakt aus Salix purpurea x daphnoides. Placebokontrollierte Doppelblindstudie zur Kinetik, Wirksamkeit und Verträglichkeit von Weidenrinde. Dissertation der Fakultät für Chemie und Pharmazie der Eberhard-Karls-Universität Tübingen.

Schnitzer TH, Morton C, Coker S, Flynn P (1992) Effectiveness of reduced applications of topical capsaicin (0.025 %) in osteoarthritis. Arthritis and Rheumatism 35: 123.

Singh GB, Singh S, Bani S (1996) Anti-inflammatory actions of boswellic acids. Phytomedicine 3: 81–85.

Sorkin B (1980) Hametum-Salbe, eine kortikoidfreie antiinflammatorische Salbe. Phys Med Rehab 21: 53–57.

Steffen C, Menzel J (1983) Enzymabbau von Immunkomplexen. Z Rheumatol 42: 249–255.

Stewart JCM, Morse PF, Moss M, Horrobin DF, Burton JL, Douglas WS, Gould DJ, Grattan CEH, Hindson TC, Anderson J, Jansen CT, Kennedy CTC, Lindskow R, Strong AMM, Wright S (1991) Treatment of severe and moderately severe atopic dermatitis with evening primrose oil (Epogam): a multi-centre study. Journal of Nutritional Medicine 2: 9–15.

Tandan R (1992a) Topical Capsaicin in painful diabetic neuropathy. Diabetes Care 15: 8–18.

VanEimeren W, Biehl G, Tuluweit K (Hrsg) (1994) Therapie traumatisch verursachter Schwellungen. Adjuvante systemische Therapie mit proteolytischen Enzymen. Georg Thieme Verlag Stuttgart New York.

Vogler BK, Ernst E (1999) Aloe vera: a systematic review of its clinical effectiveness. Br J Gen Pract 49: 823–8.

Vogler BK, Pittler MH, Ernst E (1998) Feverfew as a preventive treatment for migraine: a systematic review. Cephalgia 18: 704–8.

Vogt HJ, Tausch I, Wöbling RH, Kaiser PM (1991) Melissenextrakt bei Herpes simplex. Allgemeinarzt 14: 832–841.

Watson CPN, Evans RJ, Watt VR (1988) Postherpetic neuralgia and topical capsaicin. Can J Neurol Sci 15: 197.

Wegener T (1998) Die Teufelskralle (Harpagophytum procumbens DC) in der Therapie rheumatischer Erkrankungen. Zeitschrift für Phytotherapie 19: 284–294.

Wegener T (2000) Devil's Claw: From African Traditional Remedy to Modern Analgesic and Antiinflammatory. HerbalGram 50: 47–54.

Wenzel P, Wegener T (1995) Teufelskralle. Ein pflanzliches Antirheumatikum. Dtsch Apoth Z 135 (13): 1131–1144.

Whitaker DK, Cilliers J, de Beer C (1996) Evening primrose oil (Epogam) in the treatment of chronic hand dermatitis: disappointing therapeutic results. Dermatology 193: 115–20.

Wiesenauer M, Lüdtke R (1996) Mahonia aquifolium in patients with psoriasis vulgaris: an intraindividual study. Phytomedicine 3: 231–235.

Wildfeuer A, Neu IS, Safayhi H, Metzger G, Wehrmann M, Vogel U, Ammon HPT (1998) Effects of boswellic acids extracted from an herbal medicine on the biosynthesis of leukotrienes and the course of experimental autoimmune encephalomyelitis. Arzneimittel-Forschung/Drug Res 48: 668–674.

Willuhn G (1995) Phythopharmaka in der Dermatologie. Z Phytother 16: 325–342.

9 Agents that Increase Resistance to Diseases

Herbal remedies fit very naturally into the natural and holistic system of medicine. As a result, all physicians and laypersons do not appreciate the kind of compartmentalized, organ-based approach to herbal healing that is followed in this book. Indeed, there are two classes of herbal remedies that do not fit into an anatomically oriented scheme: adaptogens and immune stimulants. Adaptogens are agents that are reputed to increase the body's resistance to physical, chemical, and biological stressors. Immune stimulants are agents that activate the body's nonspecific defence mechanisms against infectious organisms, particularly viral and bacterial pathogens.

9.1 Adaptogens

The life of every human being is marked by periods of increased physical and psychological demands. Recurring stresses of this kind generally are not harmful and are even beneficial to health, provided they are within manageable limits. But the degree of tolerance for these stresses varies greatly from one individual to the next. Also, every individual is subject to a life cycle in which overall stress tolerance is maximal from about 20 to 30 years of age. It is estimated that, by age 70, stress tolerance is diminished by approximately one-half (Hofecker, 1987). Critical peak stresses that are handled easily by a healthy young person may become disruptive in one who is debilitated due to age or illness. Irritable stomach, gastric ulcer, and irritable colon are but a few of the secondary disorders that may arise as a result of these critical stresses.

Adaptation syndromes are observed not only in the everyday practice of medicine but also have been investigated in various animal models. Selye (1946) showed in his classic study that previous exposure to a stressor can increase resistance not just to that particular stressor but to other noxious agents as well. In rats, for example, it was found that prior exposure to various stressors such as heat, cold, exertion, or trauma prevented the inflammation of the cecum that was normally induced by the intravenous injection of histamine. Prior exposure to psychological stressors also made rats more resistant to challenges such as papain injection, which normally causes a fatal degree of myocardial necrosis (Bajusz and Selye, 1960).

Hormonal influences are known to play a major role in the pathophysiology of adaptation diseases. For example, rats are normally immune to infection by *Mycobacterium tuberculosis* but become susceptible when treated with immunosuppressive doses of cortisone (20 mg/day). When somatotropic hormone (6 mg/day) was administered concurrently with the cortisone doses, the animals retained their immunity to *M. tuberculosis* infection (Schole et al., 1978). This led the authors to conclude that hormones like cortisone whose secretion is augmented by stressful stimuli can act synergistically with other hormones to maintain homeostasis when the levels of the stress-related hormones bear a specific relation to the concentrations of the other hormones.

A number of substances of microbiologic (Farrow et al., 1978; Kaemmerer and Kietzmann, 1983) or plant origin (Brekhman and Dardymov, 1969; Ciplea and Richter, 1988; Wagner et al., 1994) have shown adaptogenic effects in experimental animals. Most of these effects were measured in live, healthy animals, and the differences relative to controls were significant only in animals that were exposed to various stresses. The antistress effect was nonspecific for the nature of the stress, i.e., the effect did not depend on whether the stress was an infection, a toxin, radiation, trauma, or was physical or psychological in nature. The underlying mechanism of this effect has not been elucidated in animals or in man. Following Selye's line of reasoning, it can be assumed that such substances help the body cope with stressful situations by expanding the adaptation phase while delaying or preventing the exhaustion phase.

9.1.1 Ginseng

Ginseng root and its preparations have had an established place in the traditional healing arts of eastern Asia for more than 2000 years. Furthermore, ginseng has generated what may be the most extensive body of scientific literature ever published on a medicinal herb. Two survey works on ginseng cited and abstracted no fewer than 482 (Ploss, 1988) and 151 (Sonnenborn and Proppert, 1990) books and papers on the use of the herb. A recent book summarizes in extensive detail the growing body of chemical, toxicological, pharmacological and clinical literature on Asian ginseng and ginsenosides (Court, 2000).

9.1.1.1 Plant, Crude Drug, and Constituents

The species *Panax ginseng* is the source of Asian ginseng root (Fig. 9.1). Ginseng is native to Korea and China, growing at altitudes of about 1000 m, but today it is extremely rare in the wild. As demand for the plant increased (by consumers that included the Chinese imperial court), the first ginseng plantations were established some 800 years ago (Hyo-Won et al., 1987). Today the plant is cultivated in Korea, China, and eastern Siberia. *Panax ginseng* is a perennial herb (family Araliaceae) with fleshy, pale yellow, often multibranched roots that have an aromatic odor and a bittersweet taste. The root

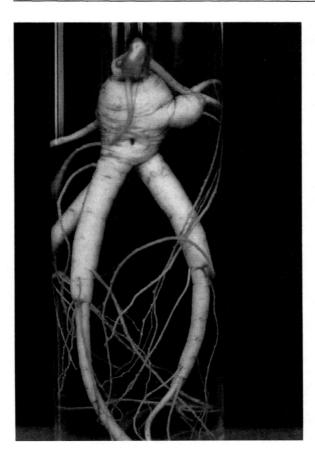

Fig. 9.1. ◄ Ginseng root (from a plant approximately 6 years old).

plant takes about 6 years to mature (although most cultivated ginseng is harvested at 4 years), the stem reaching a height of 60–80 cm. Ginseng powders and extracts are made from the dried roots, which contain 2–3 % glycosidal saponins known as ginsenosides. At least 30 ginsenosides have been chemically identified and given special designations (R followed by a subscript small letter and often a numeral as well, e.g., R_C, Rg_1). American ginseng (*P. quinquefolius*) is native to eastern North America and is cultivated in the United States and Canada. Almost the entire crop is exported to China where it is very popular; it is now extensively cultivated there as well. Roots of the different species are distinguished by their different saponin patterns. Ginseng also contains about 0,05 % volatile substances that are soluble in ether (volatile oil) (Obermeier, 1980; Youn, 1987; Sonnenborn and Proppert, 1990). In the following sections, the discussion is limited to studies of Asian ginseng.

9.1.1.2 Pharmacology and Toxicology

Volumes have been written on the effects of ginseng extracts and ginseng saponins (ginsenosides). Among the effects demonstrated by animal experimentation are the following: CNS-stimulating effects; protective effects against various harmful agents such as ionizing radiation, infections, and toxins (lead salts, alloxan); protection from exhausting physical and psychological stresses; effects on carbohydrate and lipid metabolism and on RNA and protein biosynthesis; and immune-stimulating effects. It is difficult to draw any inferences from these studies regarding the efficacy of ginseng in humans. Neither the mode of administration (usually intraperitoneal) nor the dosage are comparable to ordinary ginseng usage in humans. Ginseng extracts act on the human intestinal flora by promoting the growth of bifid bacteria while selectively inhibiting certain clostridial strains (Ahn et al., 1990). The anabolic (growth-promoting) effects observed in animal tests may also result from indirect effects of ginseng on the intestinal flora.

Acute toxicity studies were performed in mice and rats, and studies on acute to chronic toxicity (20–180 days) were conducted in rats, chickens, and dwarf pigs. Ginseng was tested for teratogenicity in pregnant rats and rabbits and for mutagenicity (carcinogenicity) in the Ames test. None of these studies showed any evidence of an increased toxicological risk (Ploss, 1988).

9.1.1.3 Clinical Studies in Humans

The results of a total of 37 clinical studies were published between 1968 and 1990, 22 during the period 1980–1985. Fifteen of the studies were controlled, and eight were double-blind. The studies covered a total of 2562 cases, including 973 healthy subjects (19 studies), 238 of whom were athletes, 943 geriatric patients (7 studies), 527 patients with various metabolic disorders (5 studies), and a total of 159 postmenopausal women (2 studies). The usual duration of treatment was 60–120 days. Powdered root preparations were administered in doses of 400–1200 mg/day and extract preparations in doses of 200–600 mg/day.

When the results of these studies were evaluated, it was found that subjects in 13 of the studies (1572 cases) showed improvements in mood while on treatment with the ginseng preparation. Seventeen studies (846 cases) also demonstrated improvements in physical performance. Improved intellectual performance was reported in 11 studies, and improvements in various metabolic parameters were noted in another 10 studies. All the studies emphasized the absence or near absence of side effects relating to ginseng therapy. There was only one reported instance of tachycardia. The results were statistically evaluated in only about half the studies. On the whole, it is unlikely that the design and conduct of these studies would conform to current scientific standards (study surveys in Ploss, 1988; Sonnenborn and Proppert, 1990; WHO, 1999; Blumenthal et al., 2003). A systematic review identified only a few high-quality studies showing evidence of increased physical and cognitive performance with ginseng (Vogler und Pittler, 1999). On the opposite side are recent studies in which gains in physical performance could not be demonstrated with ginseng, at least in young, healthy volunteers (Engels et al., 1996; Morris et al., 1996; Allen et al., 1998; Bahrke and Morgan, 2000). A recent article suggests that use of ginseng in traditional Chinese medicine (TCM) and in pharmacological studies in China were dosed significantly higher than the normal doses used in western clinical trials (i.e., about 200 mg per day of the extract standardized to 4 percent ginsenosides), and that therefore some of the western trials that have yielded negative results might produce more positive outcomes at higher doses (Dharmananda, 2002). More clinical trials testing ginseng at various dosage levels appear to be warranted.

9.1.1.4 Indications, Dosages, Risks, and Contraindications

The 1991 Commission E monograph on ginseng root states that the herb is used "As tonic for invigoration and fortification in times of fatigue and debility, for declining capacity for work and concentration", and as an aid to convalescence (Blumenthal et al., 1998). The recommended daily dosage is 1–2 g of the crude drug. A dosage of 200–600 mg/day is recommended for extracts, based on the results of clinical studies. The Commission recommends limiting the duration of treatment to 3 months, as the possibility of hormone-like or hormone-inducing effects cannot be ruled out. Reports of possible addiction problems, blood pressure elevation, nervousness, sleeplessness, and increased libido (Palmer et al., 1978; Siegel, 1979, 1980) have now been thoroughly discredited. For example, the Siegel study (1979) was uncontrolled and the "adverse effects" were found in only 10 percent (14) in a total of 133 subjects. The advers effects reportedly associated with use of the various heterogeneous products that were collectively referred to as "ginseng" were all related to the concomitant consumption of large amounts of caffeine; such adverse effects – e.g., nervousness, irritability, insomnia, elevated blood pressure, morning diarrhea – are all related to the frequent consumption of relatively large amounts of caffeine (Blumenthal, 1991). A recent systematic review and analysis of the published clinical trials and adverse reactions and purported herb-drug interactions – including 82 clinical trials on ginseng as a monopreparation (mostly a standardized extract) and 64 studies on ginseng combination preparations, plus 2 epidemiological studies – concluded that use of Asian ginseng is well-tolerated, with most adverse effects being mild and reversible, though some serious events have been reported (Coon and Ernst, 2002). The authors reported that due to the difficulty of establishing causality, the lack of rigorously collected data on adverse effects, the frequent use of ginseng in combination with other ingredients, and the potential for contamination, adulteration and mislabeling of some commercial ginseng products in the past, the published adverse event information should be interpreted with caution.

Further, it should be noted that all previous reports of adverse effects regarding the use of ginseng (e.g., Siegel, 1979) originated in English-speaking countries where ginseng preparations are sold as food products (i.e., dietary supplements) and were previously not subject to quality or dosage controls compared to the more pharmaceutically-oriented standards for ginseng employed in countries like Germany and Switzerland (Ploss, 1988; Sonnenborn, 1990; WHO, 1999).

9.1.2 Eleutherococcus Root

This herb, often called "Siberian ginseng" but preferably referred to as eleuthero, consists of the dried root of *Eleutherococcus senticosus*, a shrub of the family Araliaceae that grows to 2–3 m; it is native to Siberia and northern China and is botanically related to Asian ginseng (*P. ginseng*). (The term "Siberian ginseng" is no longer legally allowed in the U.S., where the term "eleuthero" must be used on herbal dietary supplements (107th Congress, 2002; Blumenthal, 2002). The slender shrub is distinguished by its very thin, woody spines about 5 mm in length. The dried root of eleutherococcus has a sharp, aromatic, slightly sweet taste. Lignan glycosides of the liriodendrin and coumarin types, including isofraxidin, have been identified as key constituents. Unlike true ginseng, however, eleuthero is not a species of *Panax* and contains only small concentrations of saponins (Bladt et al., 1990).

Eleuthero root was tested and developed in the former Soviet Union during the 1960's as a substitute for ginseng. Pharmacologic studies there demonstrated an effect comparable to or even surpassing that of ginseng root (Brekhman and Dardymov, 1969). As a result, eleuthero root has been listed in the Russian Pharmacopeia as a tonic since the 1960's. It has also found use as an herbal tonic in Western countries since about 1975.

Animal studies on eleuthero extract were comparable in their design and results to the animal tests of ginseng extract. The studies confirmed the protein-anabolic action of both the extract (Kaemmerer and Fink 1980; Zorikow et al., 1974) and of the isolated constituent liriodendrin (Ro et al., 1977). Healthy subjects placed on a 4-week regimen of 10 mL/t.i.d. of an extract with the brand name Eleu-Kokk showed a highly significant increase in immunocompetent cells – principally T-lymphocytes of the helper/inductor type in addition to cytotoxic and natural killer (NK) cells (Bohn et al., 1987). This effect was demonstrated by flow cytometry. The implications of this finding for the clinical use of eleuthero extracts remains unclear (Lovett et al., 1984; Pichler et al., 1985).

In one study, young athletes who took eleuthero extract for 8 days (Asano et al., 1986; n = 6) showed significant gains in physical performance parameters, while another study (Dowling et al., 1996; n = 20) showed no such gains. Two other controlled studies found increases in cognitive performance (Winther et al., 1997) and protective effects against herpes simplex infections (Williams, 1995). But a systematic evaluation of all the controlled studies did not find sufficient data to prove efficacy for any of these indications (Vogler et al., 1999). A review of numerous publications on the pharmacognosy, pharmacology, and clinical use of eleuthero can be found in Betti (2002) and Blumenthal et al. (2003).

The Commission E monograph on *Eleutherococcus senticosus* recommends its use to the same indication as Asian ginseng, i.e., "As tonic for invigoration and fortification in times of fatigue and debility or declining capacity for work and concentration," and as an aid to convalescence (Blumenthal et al., 1998). The recommended daily dose is 2–3 g of the crude drug or an equivalent dose of an extract-based preparation. As with ginseng, the Commission recommends that use be limited to 3 months. Hypertension is noted as a contraindication. There are no known side effects or herb-drug interactions.

9.1.3 Other Adaptogenic Drugs (listed alphabetically)

9.1.3.1 Ashwagandha

Ashwagandha, also known as the winter cherry, is the root of *Withania somnifera*, family Solanaceae. It is probably the most famous of the Ayurvedic botanicals. Sometimes erroneously referred to as "Indian ginseng" because its folkloric use is similar to that of ginseng, Ashwagandha is a small shrub widely distributed throughout the drier regions of India. It is widely used as an adaptogen in the United States, but such employment is supported almost entirely by Indian tradition rather than by science. Several alkaloids, carbohydrates, sterols, and fatty and essential oils have been isolated from the root, but none has been directly linked to the purported use. Ashwagandha has been frequently called "Indian ginseng" – a term denoting its level of respect and multiple tonic-like application in Ayurvedic traditional medicine. However, ashwagandha is NOT related to true ginseng (Panax spp.) as it is in Solanaceae, the nightshade family, while Panax is in the Aralizceae family.

One double-blind clinical trial of Ashwagandha in 141 healthy male volunteers, ages 50–59 years, was conducted over a period of one year (Kuppurajan et al., 1980). At its conclusion, the treated group was found to have statistically significant improvements in hemaglobin, red blood corpuscles, hair melanin, seated stature, and a decrease in serum cholesterol in comparison to the controls. More recently hpoglycemic, diuretic and hypocholesterolemic effects were found in a controlled clinical trials with 12 human subjects (Andallu and Radhika, 2000).

Mishra et al. (2000) reviewed Withania somnifera Dunal (ashwagandha) as a commonly used herb in Ayurvedic medicine. It is an ingredient in many formulations prescribed for a variety of musculoskeletal conditions and as a general tonic to increase energy; improve overall health and longevity; and prevent disease in athletes, the elderly, and during pregnancy. A total of 58 articles were found pertaining to the anti-inflammatory, antitumor, antistress, antioxidant, immunomodulatory, hemopoetic (formation of red blood cells) and rejuvenating properties of ashwagandha. The effectiveness of ashwagandha in a variety of rheumatologic conditions may be due in part to its anti-inflammatory properties, as demonstrated in animal studies. However, only one clinical trial was found that supports the possible use of WS for arthritis. Several animal studies are suggestive of antitumor activity as well as enhancement of the effects of radiation by WS. However, no human studies were included in the review. Several animal studies have found that WS induces a state of nonspecific increased resistance to stress, as measured by an increase in the length of time the animals were able to exercise; reduced stress-induced increases in blood urea nitrogen, blood lactic acid and adrenal hypertrophy. Laboratory studies have found that a root extract of WS stimulates hemolytic antibody responses (creating an immune response in the red blood cells) toward human erythrocytes (red blood cells) indicating immunostimulatory activity. The authors concluded that, while the results from the studies reviewed show promise for the use of ashwagandha as a multi-purpose medicinal agent, the current literature has several limitations. While more clinical trials should be conducted to support its therapeutic use, the lack of systematic toxicity studies is of concern, as is the poor quality of the existing toxicity studies. Nevertheless, insofar as ashwagandha has been one of the most revered and widely used medicinal herbs in the entire system of Ayurveda for several thousand years, its relative long-term safety can be reasonably presumed.

The usual daily dose of the dried powdered root is 3–6 g. The toxicity in therapeutic doses appears minimal. However, high doses of the root in mice (750 mg/kg daily for 15 days) caused serious side effects, including diarrhea, body weight loss, and mortality (Divi et al., 1992). A comprehensive monograph on the chemistry, quality control testing, pharmacology and toxicology and clinical research on ashwagandha has been published recently (Upton and Petrone, 2000).

9.1.3.2 Astragalus

Astragalus, the dried root of *Astragalus membranaceous*, family Fabaceae, is obtained from a perennial plant of medium height native to the drier areas of Northern China and Mongolia. It is now cultivated throughout the world. The drug has a long history of use in China to invigorate vital energy and strengthen bodily resistance. It may therefore be classified as an adaptogen.

Although astragalus has emerged as one of the more important Chinese herbs on the American market, its purported use is based primarily on folklore and in vitro or animal experiments. The few existing clinical studies have involved parenteral administration of the extract (a mode not possible with herbs sold as dietary supplements that are not approved as drugs in the United States) or oral use in combination with other herbs. This renders evaluation difficult.

Whatever activity the plant possesses is thought to derive from a number of contained saponins, complex polysaccharides, and possibly flavonoids. Experiments linking any of these constituents with specific effects of astragalus are lacking. The dose of the drug in traditional Chines medicine is 3–6 g of dried root. Safety of astragalus in normal doses is not associated with any observed adverse effects (McKenna et al., 1998). A thorough review of the quality control parameters and therapeutics of astragalus was recently published (Upton and Petrone, 1999).

9.1.3.3 Cat's Claw

Cat's claw or uña de gato consists of the bark of two species of the genus *Uncaria* (family Rubiaceae). Both *U. tomentosa* and the less common *U. guianensis* are thorny lianas indigenous to tropical South America. The plants are widely collected in Amazonia for shipment to the American and European markets.

Widely used as a folk remedy for a wide variety of conditions by people in South America and by emigrants from those countries, cat's claw is probably best classified at present as an adaptogen. Although there is some in vitro and pharmacologic evidence to support its activity as an immunomodulating, anti-inflammatory, antimutagenic, and antitumor agent, only a few critical clinical trials are available.

Depending on the type of preparation being studied, some of the observed immunologic benefits of cat's claw apparently are produced by the various oxindole alkaloids it contains. Research has now established the existence of two chemotypes of *U. tomentosa*. One contains primarily pentacyclic oxindole alkaloids (POAs, e.g., pteropodine, isopteropodine, isomitraphylline, etc.). These have demonstrated immunostimulant activity. In the other type, tetracyclic oxindole alkaloids (TOAs) rhynchophylline and isorhynchophylline predominate. These have been shown to antagonize the effects of the pentacyclic compounds. Since the two chemotypes are phenotypically identical, most common commercial cat's claw preparations appear to be indiscriminate mixtures which may lack therapeutic utility. The research on the POA-based extract suggests that effective products should contain no more than 0.02 % TOAs (Reinhard, 1997). However, a recent detailed review of the published and some unpublished clinical literature on cat's claw (Blumenthal et al., 2003) determine that up to four different types of preparations are found on the market, and that one of them, a water-based extract of *U. guaianensis* containing no POAs or TOAs, exhibited anti-inflammatory effects in patients with osteoarthritis of the knee [Piscoya et al., 2001] as well as a water based extract *U. tomentosa* (C-Med) showed anti-inflammatory and immunomodulating effects (Lamm et al., 2001; Sheng et al., 2001).

9.1.3.4 Cordyceps

Cordyceps in its wild form is the small blade-shaped fruiting body of a parasitic fungus, *Cordyceps sinensis* (Berk.) Sacc., family Clavicipitaceae, that grows on the larvae of moths, particularly in the mountainous regions of China and Tibet. It has been extensively used in China as a cure-all and tonic for nearly 250 years.

The naturally occurring fruiting bodies are scarce, so a number of hyphal isolates capable of mycelial growth in saprophytic culture have been obtained from them. These have quite different morphological forms and have been given different scientific names by mycologists. The one utilized to produce the commercial cordyceps product sold in the United States is designated *Paecilomyces hepiali* Chen (strain Cs-4). The activity of the fungus apparently resides in the polysaccharide and nucleoside fractions, but definitive conclusions are not yet possible (Zhu et al., 1998).

A number of clinical trials with Cs-4 in various conditions have been conducted in China on a total of more than 2000 patients. The quality of these studies, some of which were blinded, is quite variable. Zhang et al. (1995) carried out a double-blind placebo controlled study of the effects of 3 g of Cs-4 daily on 358 elderly people with various symptoms of senescence. Statistically significant subjective improvements in patients consuming Cs-4 compared to the placebo were found in the alleviation of fatigue, cold intolerance, dizziness, frequent nocturia, tinnitus, hyposexuality, and amnesia.

A study, lasting 26 ± 3 months, examined the effectiveness of Cs-4 as an adjuvant treatment in patients suffering from congestive heart failure (Chen 1995). In 64 patients, the addition of 3–4 g daily of Cs-4 resulted in a significant improvement in the quality of life as measured by standard methods, in comparison to those taking only conventional treatment for the condition. The results of other clinical trials measuring increased efficacy of oxygen utilization and free radical scavenging activity, improved sexual function, and reduction of blood lipids have been summarized by Zhu et al., (1998). It must be noted that all of the clinical trials on cordyceps to date have emanated from China; none has been conducted in Europe or the United States.

Cordyceps is employed as an adaptogen (tonic). The dosage range is 3–9 g daily of either the natural fruiting bodies or the saprophytically cultivated mycelium, or equivalenct doses based on extracts. Occasional side effects include dry mouth, skin rashes, diarrhea, and drowsiness. As is the case with various other herbs, it tends to inhibit blood platelet aggregation.

9.1.3.5 Gotu Kola

Gotu kola (*Centella asiatica*, occasionally still referred to in the literature by its former binomial, *Hydrocotyle asiatica*) of the family Apiaceae consists of the leaves of a slender, creeping plant which grows in swampy tropical areas, particularly in India and Sri Lanka. It has been found to contain several pentacyclic triterpene acids, such as asiatic and madecassic, and their glycosides, asiaticoside and madecassoside. Two factors probably influence the plant's scientifically undocumented reputation as a longevity promoter and a strengthener and revitalizer (adaptogen) of the human body.

In Sri Lanka, the plant is often eaten by elephants which are noted for their longevity among beasts. Further, the kola designation is often confused with the kolanut, the caffeine containing cotyledon of *Cola nitida*, widely used as a stimulant in various beverages. Actually, one study has shown that in small animals, the drug had just the reverse effect, producing calmative effects similar to those of diazepam (Diwan et al., 1991).

A number of pharmacological and clinical studies have shown that gotu kola does exert a beneficial effect on the trophism of connective tissue and favors the cicatrization of wounds. These uses have been summarized (Anon., no date) but are not relative to its use as an adaptogen. The drug is available for this purpose in a number of dosage forms, including tablets and capsules for internal use as well as creams and ointments for topical application.

Forty healthy subjects aged 18-45 years were administered a one-time dose of either 12 g gotu kola powder (Nature's Way, Canada Ltd.) mixed into 300 mL grape juice or 300 mL plain grape juice (matched for color, taste and smell). ASR, heart rate, blood pressure and mood data were recorded at baseline, and at 30, 60, 90 and 120 minutes after ingestion. The startle response was statistically significantly lower 30 and 60 minutes after ingestion of gotu kola compared to placebo, with an effect size of 0.48 and 0.77, respectively indicating some anxiolytic activity. There was no difference between placebo and treatment for later times or at baseline. There was no difference for heart rate or blood pressure, and no difference in mood response except for self-rated energy level. The authors note, however, that anxious, fearful and nervous mood ratings were low in the subjects at baseline. All treatments were well tolerated. This study represents the first double-blind, placebo-controlled experiment with gotu kolu in humans (Bradwein et al., 2000).

The usual dose of gotu kola is 600 mg three times daily. In 1998, Drugs Directorate in Canada banned the sale of the herb, apparently on the basis of an older study that a 0.1 % solution of asiaticoside in benzene applied weekly for 20 months to hairless mice produced one sarcoma in 57 test animals. However, this was not a significant increase in comparison to the controls with benzene which is a known carcinogen (Laerum and Iversen, 1972). McGuffin et al. (1997) have classified gotu kola as an herb that can be safely consumed when used appropriately. The fresh leaves are known to be used as a salad green and there are few reports of toxicity associated with gotu kola.

9.1.3.6 *Rhodiola rosea*

Rhodiola rosea is a perennial plant, native to the northern polar circle and high alpine regions of Europe, Asia and North America, that grows to a height of about 60 cm. Preparations made from the root of *Rhodiola rosea* are used in Siberia and certain regions of Scandinavia to increase resistance to infections. The herb was systematically researched in the former Soviet Union, and more than 180 works on phytochemical, pharmacologic, and clinical studies have been published since 1960. Similar in activity in some ways to *Eleutherococcus*, *Rhodiola rosea* is believed to have stress-reducing and performance-enhancing properties in addition to antioxidant and cardioprotective effects. A survey work was recently published on the results of some 20 recent therapeutic trials in humans (Brown et al., 2003). For example, a randomized double-blind study was done in 20 students who took two daily doses of 550 mg of rhodiola root extract or a placebo during their 3-week examination period. Validated test procedures were run at the start and end of the treatment period to assess psychomotor function, mental work capacity, and self-rated general well-being. All three of these criteria showed significant differences in favor of the group that received rhodiola (Spasov et al., 2000). There are over 17 species in the genus *Rhodiola* but the vast majority of animal research and human clinical trial have been conducted specifically on *R. rosea*. *Rhodiola rosea* is chemically distinct compared to other species in the genus *Rhodiola*, as determined by the presence of three cinnamyl alcohol-vicianosides – rosavin, rosin and rosarin – collectively referred to as "rosavins" (Brown et al., 2003).

Rhodiola rosea has not been evaluated by Commission E, and products based on this herb are not currently marketed in Germany.

9.1.3.7 Botanical Antioxidants (Grape Seed, Green Tea, Pine Bark)

Botanical antioxidants assist the body in resisting various pathologic conditions, especially those associated with aging, and are therefore classified as chemoprotective agents, a type of adaptogen. Polyphenolic oligomers of the flavanoid type were formerly referred to as nonhydrolyzable or condensed tannins. Because most result from a condensation of 2 or more flavan-3-ols, they are also called catechin tannins. However, marketers realized that the tannin designation has little selling power, so they began to refer to these compounds by a bewildering variety of common chemical names, including oligomeric proanthocyanidins (OPC's), procyanidin oligomers (PCO's), proanthocyanidins, procyanidins, leucoanthocyanins, polyphenols, or even "pycnogenols" (an inappropriate name based on the trademark for the leading, patented maritime pine bark extract, i.e., Pycnogenol®).

These compounds occur widely in the plant kingdom. The most prominent commercial sources are: extract of grape seed (*Vitis vinifera*) concentrated 100 fold and standardized to contain 80–85 % procyanidins; green tea leaves (*Camellia sinensis*) which in the unprocessed (i.e., unfermented) form contain up to 30 % procyanidins but which are often concentrated and decaffeinated to yield an extract containing 60–97 % of the compounds; extract of the bark of the maritime pine (*Pinus pinaster*) concentrated to contain about 85 % procyanidins. Certainly these three products differ slightly in identity and quantity of their specific polyphenols, including the degree of oligomerization. However, the products have never been tested one against the other to determine the relative antioxidant activity, so it seems appropriate to assume their physiologic and therapeutic effects are generally similar. Where specific differences occur, these will be noted.

9.1.3.7.1 Pharmacology and Toxicology

A mass of evidence obtained on small animal and in vitro studies supports the effectiveness of procyanidins as potent antioxidants, free-radical scavengers, and inhibitors of lipid peroxidation. Clinical studies of acceptable quality providing evidence of the utility of the compounds in treating specific conditions are, however, relatively few. Procyanidins are also active inhibitors of collagenase, elastase, hyaluronidase, and β-glucuronidase, all of which are involved in the degradation of the main structural components of the extravascular matrix. By this mechanism, procyanidins help maintain normal capillary permeability. Antimutagenic activity in *Saccharomyces cerevisiae* strain S288C has also been demonstrated for these compounds. Procyanidins act synergistically with vitamin C and potentiate the activity of that vitamin in wound healing and in the elimination of excess cholesterol. The polyphenolics of green tea, particularly the relatively potent (–)-epigallocatechin gallate (EGC_g), have been found to possess antitumor properties. These combined activities, all related directly or indirectly to the antioxidative properties of procyanidins, account for much of their therapeutic utility, including protection against pathologies such as cancer and atherosclerosis, normally associated with the aging process.

Tests in experimental animals have shown that procyanidins are well tolerated and devoid of toxic effects. The calculated LD_{50} in rats and mice exceeds 4000 mg/kg. The compounds are also devoid of mutagenic and teratogenic effects.

9.1.3.7.2 Clinical and Epidemiological Studies

Among the few clinical trials with procyanidin-rich grape seed extract for the treatment of specific conditions are two dealing with their effect on the symptoms of chronic venous insufficiency. A double-blind study of 50 patients treated with 150 mg/day of grape seed extract for 1 month found subjective and objective improvements were more rapid and longer lasting than in patients treated with 450 mg/day of the bioflavonoid diosmin. Another double-blind placebo-controlled study of 92 patients with the same symptoms found that 300 mg/day of the GSE administered for 28 days resulted in improvements in 75 % of the patients in comparison to only 41 % for the placebo group. Clinical trials of varying quality on ophthalmologic conditions, including resistance to glare, ocular stress, and retinal functionality, all showed favorable results following treatment with procyanidin-rich grape seed extract (Bombardelli and Morazzoni, 1995).

An epidemiological study of the effect of dietary flavonoids on the risk of lung cancer and other malignant neoplasms was conducted by Knekt et al. (1997). The subjects consisted of 9,959 Finnish men and women aged 15–19 years who were initially cancer free. Food consumption during the past year was estimated by the dietary history method. Dietary patterns continued to be monitored during the 24-year follow-up period. During that time, a total of 1,148 cancer cases was diagnosed among the participants. An inverse association was observed between the intake of dietary flavonoids and the incidence of all types of cancer combined.

A similar study on the risk of pancreatic and colorectal cancers in green tea drinkers was conducted in Shanghai by Ji et al. (1997). A total of 2,266 patients, aged 30–74, with cancers of the colon, rectum, and pancreas were interviewed about their dietary habits (including tea consumption), medical history, and life styles. The results were matched with findings from 1,552 healthy individuals. Among regular tea drinkers (1 or more cups per week for at least 6 months), there was an overall lower risk of rectal and pancreatic cancers in men. But in women regular tea consumption was associated with a reduction in colon cancer as well. Dose responses were observed in both men and women. Additional clinical trials to support these and other observations are urgently required and numerous have been conducted in recent years with similarly promising results. A comprehensive review of green and black tea clinical trials has been published recently (Blumenthal et al., 2003).

9.1.3.7.3 Indications and Dosage

Available clinical evidence tends to support the effectiveness of procyanidins and procyanidin-rich extracts in treating venous insufficiency and conditions associated with alteration of blood rheology and capillary fragility. In addition, epidemiological studies have provided evidence to support the utility of the compounds in cancer prevention. Claims of effectiveness for attention deficit/hyperactivity disorder and arthritis are anecdotal and require scientific verification. The exact degree of utility of procyanidins, and other antioxidants as well, in protecting against stress, cancer, various inflammatory conditions, and cardiovascular disease, remains to be determined. The enormous worldwide consumption (particularly in green tea, considered the world's second most consumed beverage, next to water) and apparent general lack of toxicity lead to the conclusion that these compounds do little harm and may do significant good, particularly as adjuncts to a healthy life style (Mitscher et al., 1997).

Procyanidin-rich preparations are marketed in the form of capsules or tablet containing extracts ranging from 80–97 % polyphenols. Dosage recommendations vary widely from 100–500 mg/day initially to 50–100 mg/day for maintenance purposes. A typical cup of green tea contains between 300–400 mg of polyphenols.

9.2 Immune Stimulants

Immune stimulants are agents that increase the activity of the immune system. Unlike vaccines, however, immune stimulants have no antigenic relationship to specific pathogens. Consequently, their action is nonspecific and is believed to result from the stimulation of cell-mediated immune factors (macrophages, granulocytes, leukocytes) and of mediators that are released by the cellular immune system (Fig. 9.2). When immune stimulants are used, therefore, there is always a risk of physiologic suppression of the immune response, leading to an exacerbation of chronic inflammatory processes. There is a danger that the desired stimulation of host immune defences could activate previously quiescent autoimmune processes (Haustein, 1995).

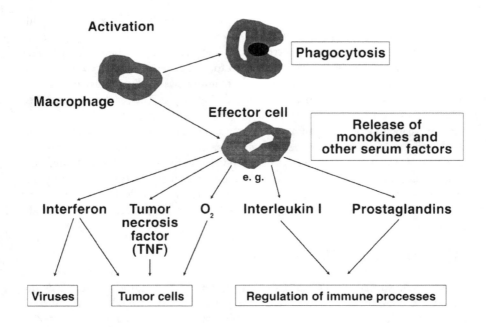

Fig. 9.2. ▲ Nonspecific stimulation of cell-mediated host defenses.

The term immune stimulation is often used in phytotherapy in place of the traditional designation "stimulation and modulation (adaptation) therapy." Nonspecific stimulation therapy consists of inciting a focal or general reaction (inflammation, fever), stimulating the immune system, and/or modulating the autonomic nervous system in order to enhance the performance of natural regulatory processes.

In practice, species of two botanical genera stand out among the immune-stimulant herbs: coneflower (*Echinacea* spp.) and mistletoe (*Viscum album*). Other herbs have assumed a degree of importance – boneset (*Eupatorium perfoliatum*), wild indigo (*Baptisia tinctoria*) and arbor vitae (*Thuja occidentalis*) – but these have been clinically documented as effective only in combination products that also contain echinacea. Preparations made from birthwort (*Aristolochia clematitis*) and Venus flytrap (*Dionaea muscipula*), once used in Germany as immune stimulants, are now banned due to their carcinogenic risks, while all plants in the genus *Aristolochia* have been banned by both herb industry initiatives and government actions due to the presence of the nephrotoxic and carcinogenic aristolochic acid.

9.2.1 Coneflower (Echinacea)

Based on a total of four monographs published by Commission E in 1989 and 1992, two types of coneflower preparation can be recommended and prescribed in Germany today: alcoholic extracts made from the root of the pale purple coneflower (*Echinacea pallida*) and juices expressed from the fresh aerial parts of the purple coneflower (*E. purpurea*). It is noteworthy that until about 1990, the root of *E. pallida* appears to have been regularly confused with that of the species *E. angustifolia* (Bauer and Wagner, 1988). Both species were formerly recognized as sources of the official drug in the United States. Since the last Commission E monograph was published in 1992 there have been additional trials published with positive results conducted with various monopreparations and combination products containing the *root* of *E. purpurea* and/or *E. angustifolia* (Blumenthal et al., 2003)

9.2.1.1 Plant, Crude Drug, and Constituents

The genus *Echinacea* encompasses nine species in several varieties. The first species to be used medicinally was the narrow-leaved purple coneflower (*E. angustifolia*) which may have been confused with the pale purple coneflower (*E. pallida*). These plants are native to eastern North America, where they grow to 40–60 cm and were used by the original inhabitants as a traditional wound-healing remedy and cure-all. European settlers introduced the plant to Europe in the early 1900's. Attempts to cultivate these two species were unsuccessful, so the common purple coneflower (*E. purpurea*) was grown instead and used for pharmaceutical products (Fig. 9.3).

Echinacea pallida root contains characteristic constituents such as echinacein, echinolone, and echinacoside in addition to water-soluble polysaccharides, some of which have exhibited immune-stimulating effects.

The juice of *E. purpurea* is expressed from the fresh flowering plants. Forty parts of juice contain water-soluble extractive from 100 parts of the fresh plant. The chemical composition of the expressed juices is not precisely known; it does contain water-soluble polysaccharides and alkamides but no cichoric acid (Proksch, 1982; Stimpel et al., 1984).

A comprehensive review of the constituents and pharmacology of the echinacea herbs can be found in Bauer and Wagner (1990); two recent critical reviews of clinical trials were conducted by Barrett et al. (1999) and Barrett (2003); a comprehensive clinical monograph of published by Blumenthal et al. (2003), and comprehensive monograph on chemistry, test methods, pharmacology, clinical trials and related data on *E. purpurea* root was recently published by the American Herbal Pharmacopoeia (Upton, 2004).

9.2.1.2 Pharmacology and Toxicology

More than 70 publications have dealt with the pharmacologic effects of echinacea preparations. Most of the studies dealt with the stimulant effects of echinacea on immunocompetent cells in animals and humans. For example, in vitro studies were conducted on the phagocytic activity of human granulocytes incubated with yeast particles, and in vivo studies dealt with the phagocytosis of carbon particles by hepatic and splenic macrophages. Various echinacea preparations, either alone or combined with other herbal extracts (boneset, wild indigo, thuja), were found to stimulate phagocytic activity, as were a number of isolated fractions and pure compounds derived from echinacea

Fig. 9.3. ▶ Common purple cone-flower (*Echinacea purpurea*).

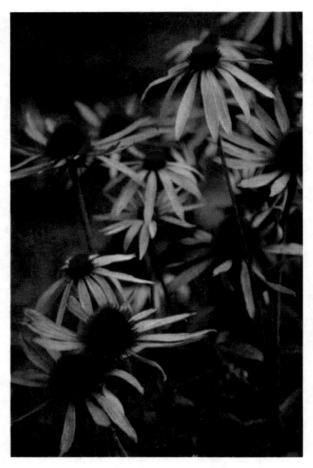

herbs. It was also shown that certain echinacea polysaccharides stimulated the release of interleukin 1, tumor necrosis factor, and interferon (Bauer and Wagner, 1990; Wagner and Jurcic, 1991; Bauer, 1997).

Isolated echinacea polysaccharides had LD_{50} values greater than 2500 mg/kg when administered intraperitoneally in mice, indicating that their toxicity is very low (Bauer and Wagner, 1990). Studies on the genotoxicity of echinacea preparations have been done on two commercial products, one of which is a combination product containing echinacea with other immune-stimulating plant extracts (known commercially as Esberitox®). The results, which have not yet been published, were evaluated in a 1992 summary report for what was formerly known as the German Federal Health Agency (now the Federal Institute for Drugs and Medical Devices). The expert who reviewed the report concluded that adequate mutagenicity tests had been conducted, especially for preparations made of *E. purpurea*, and that no negative results have been found in vitro, indicating a very low probability of tumor-initiating effects. The report also noted that the risk of tumor-promoting effects cannot be assessed at that time due to a lack of in-vivo research on that action (Schulte-Hermann, 1992).

9.2.1.3 Studies on Therapeutic Efficacy

Melchart et al. (1994) published a meta-analysis of 26 controlled clinical trials (18 randomized, 11 double-blind) on the immune-stimulant effects of echinacea. Six of these studies used a total of three single-herb extracts, and 20 used a total of 4 combination products. In all four combination products, echinacea extract (*E. angustifolia* or *E. pallida*) was the main quantitative ingredient and the most likely key active principle. The studies were evaluated by scoring each of 16 criteria and totalling the final scores. Only 8 studies achieved more than 50 % of the maximum possible total score. The best study, which achieved 70 % of the maximum possible score, used a combination product with the brand name Resistan® (Melchart et al., 1994); (this product is no longer available).

Most of the studies dealt with upper respiratory infections, and the best results were obtained for this indication. Six studies, all randomized and placebo-controlled, showed significant improvements in clinical symptoms, and one study indicated a shortened duration of illness. The studies had similar designs and treatment periods, and here we shall summarize the results of the most highly rated study (Dorn, 1989) to serve as an example: In a double-blind protocol, 100 patients with acute flu-like infections took 30 mL of the echinacea preparation or a placebo on the first and second days of treatment; then the dosage was reduced to 15 mL/day on days 3 through 6. The patients were examined on admission (term 1), at 2–4 days into the regimen (term 2), and at 6–8 days (term 3). Seven cold symptoms (lethargy, limb pain, headache, rhinitis, cough, sore throat, and pharyngeal redness) were rated for severity using a semiquantitative scoring system (Fig. 9.4). As one might expect, the scores declined rapidly during the roughly 8-day observation period in both the echinacea- and placebo-treated

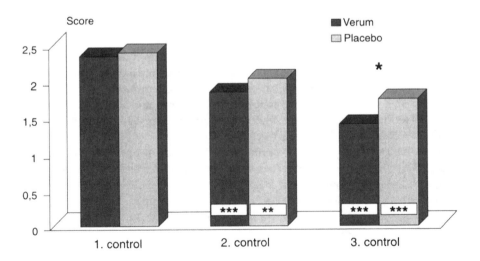

Fig. 9.4. ▲ Change in average severity of a typical flulike infection from admission (1st examination) to days 2-4 of treatment (2nd examination) and days 6-8 of treatment (3rd examination). Dark columns: echinacea preparation; light columns: placebo. Each column represents the mean values for 50 patients in a randomized double-blind study. * = p < 0.05;** = p < 0.001 (Dorn, 1989).

groups. The difference in the scores relative to the third and final examination was statistically significant for all seven symptoms in the echinacea group but for only three of the symptoms in the placebo group (p<0.01–0.001). The results suggest that taking a suitable echinacea preparation when symptoms first appear can, in favorable cases, shorten the duration of a common cold by approximately 1/4 to 1/3 (i.e., from about 10 days to 7 days).

The same combination product used in the Dorn study (1989) (Resistan) was tested for possible prophylactic benefit as an herbal immune stimulant. In a placebo-controlled double-blind study, 646 students at the University of Cologne were placed on a prophylactic course of treatment for at least 8 weeks during the 1989–1990 winter semester to test the possible effect of the product on the frequency of colds. A total of 609 subjects (303 echinacea and 306 placebo) completed the study. A total of 363 of the subjects had had more than three flulike infections during the previous 12-month period and were designated as the "infection-prone" subgroup. Comparison with the placebo indicated 15 % fewer primary infections and 27 % fewer recurrent infections overall in the subjects who took echinacea. The infection-prone subgroup experienced a 20 % reduction in total number of colds relative to the placebo. In contrast to the study population as a whole, the reduction achieved in the infection-prone subjects was statistically significant (p<0.05; Schmidt, 1990).

Since Melchart et al. (1994) published their meta-analysis, another placebo-controlled double-blind study has been published on the effects of a commercial product made from the expressed juice of *Echinacea purpurea* (brand name Echinacin®) in 120 patients with acute upper respiratory infections. The duration of treatment was 10 days. The improvement rates with regard to symptoms and duration of illness were significantly higher in patients taking the echinacea preparation than in placebo-treated controls (Hoheisel et al., 1997). Another study tested the efficacy of three different *E. purpurea* extracts in a total of 59 patients with acute upper respiratory infection. The patients received a daily dose of 40 mg or 280 mg of a whole-plant extract or 180 mg of a root extract for a period of one week. The efficacy of the three preparations was rated on the basis of a total complaint score (12 symptoms) and compared with a placebo. The score decreased by 29 % in the placebo group, by 45 % in the root extract group, and by 63 % and 64 % respectively in the groups that took 40 mg and 280 mg of the whole-plant extract. The results with the whole-plant extract were significantly superior to treatment with a placebo (Brinkeborn et al., 1999).

Meanwhile, two other placebo-controlled studies on the prophylactic use of echinacea did not yield positive results. In one study, 300 subjects received an extract of *E. augustifolia*, an *E. purpurea* extract, or a placebo for 12 weeks. The time to onset of a new upper respiratory infection averaged 66 days, 69 days, and 65 days in the respective groups. Only a subjective rating of treatment response by the test subjects indicated a significant superiority of the echinacea extracts over the placebo (Melchart et al., 1998). Another study tested the prophylactic efficacy of a fluidextract of *E. purpurea* in 109 infection-prone patients (i.e., subjects who had more than three upper respiratory infections in the previous year). The extract was taken for 8 weeks, during which time 65 % of the patients in the echinacea group contracted an acute upper respiratory infection compared with 74 % of the patients who took a placebo (Grimm and Müller, 1999).

As early as the 1950's, studies were done on the effects of echinacea preparations in patients with gynecologic and urologic infections. Although some of these studies had serious methodologic deficiencies in the evaluation of drug efficacy, the relatively large numbers of patients make the studies valuable from the standpoint of evaluating drug safety. One meta-analysis of these studies found that preparations made from the expressed juice of E. purpurea were particularly well tolerated by all age groups when taken orally. In a multicenter study covering a total of 1231 patients, only about 5 % of the participants reported nonspecific and relatively mild side effects such as unpleasant aftertaste or occasional nausea or abdominal pain during a treatment period of 4–6 weeks (Parnham, 1996).

A recent large trial 524 healthy male and female children (2 to 11 years old) an echinacea syrup was tested for its effects in treating symptoms associated with upper respiratory tract infections (URIs) (Taylor et al., 2003). Effects were documented by parents via a daily log of symptoms over a 4-month period. The echinacea preparation (made from the dried fresh-pressed juice of E. purpurea aerial parts) did not produce a reduction in severity or duration of symptoms. However, the researchers reported an unexpected trend of less second and third infections: there was a significantly lower ($P = 0.015$) incidence of URIs in children in the echinacea group (52.3 %) who had at least one URI than in the placebo group (64.4 %). This was termed a "window of protection" – suggesting a possible immune-stimulating effect of echinacea that has been observed in other trials and widespread clinical use.

Two recent reviews of controlled clinical studies confirmed the good tolerance of echinacea but did not find adequate documentation of its efficacy. Giles et al (2000) reviewed 12 studies on the treatment or prevention of upper respiratory infections. The studies prior to 1997 mostly confirmed efficacy, but some of the studies had significant methodologic problems. Three of five studies published since 1997 were confirmatory, but two others, including the largest study (Melchart et al., 1998), were not. The current Cochrane Review of 8 therapeutic trials and 8 prophylactic trials in a total of 3396 patients (Melchart et al., 2001) does not warrant a clear recommendation for the use of echinacea preparations in patients. Barrett (2003) reaches the same conclusion in another review of the pharmacology and clinical aspects of echinacea therapy.

9.2.1.4 Indications, Dosages, and Risks

Commission E revised its monographs on echinacea preparations in 1992, giving a positive rating only to alcoholic root extracts of the pale purple coneflower (E. pallida) and pressed juice from the aerial parts of the common purple coneflower (E. purpurea). Root extracts are indicated "for the supportive treatment of flu-like infections" and echinacea juices for the "supportive therapy for colds and chronic infections of the respiratory tract and lower urinary tract" (Blumenthal et al., 1998). It is recommended that neither preparation be used for more than 8 weeks. This 8-week duration limit has been misunderstood by some as being evidence of the Commission's recognition of potential toxicity of echinacea preparations when used longer than 8 weeks. This is certainly not the case. The Commission decided upon the 8-week duration based on its assessment that if symptoms for the approved indications did not resolve within 8-weeks, then more aggressive therapy was probably needed, requiring intervention by a health professional (Blumenthal et al., 2003)The recommended dose of root extract (1:5 tincture with 50 % ethanol) is equivalent to 900 mg of crude drug daily. A dose of 6–9 mg/day is recommended for echinacea juice. Because echinacea may act at the oropharyngeal level (immune stimulation of tonsillar lymphoid tissues), it is possibly best administered in the form of a liquid preparation or buccal tablet. Due to the potential for stimulating autoimmune process, echinacea is contraindicated by systemic diseases such as tuberculosis, leukoses, multiple sclerosis, collagen disorders, and other autoimmune diseases; however, these contraindications are speculative and theoretical and are not based on any reported case histories.(Blumenthal et al., 2003).

9.2.2 European Mistletoe

Rudolf Steiner introduced the use of mistletoe extracts for the treatment of cancer in 1916. Steiner is best known as the founder of anthroposophy, which is not a science but a philosophy. This historical background would seem to imply that treatment with mistletoe preparations has no place in a rational, scientifically oriented system of phytotherapy. However, efforts have been made to test the effects and efficacy of mistletoe preparations by means of orthodox pharmacologic studies and clinical trials. The following discussions are based purely on evidence furnished by modern testing and evaluation procedures.

9.2.2.1 Plant, Constituents, and Actions

European mistletoe (*Viscum album*, Fig. 9.5) is a semiparasitic evergreen shrub of the family Loranthaceae that extracts water and mineral salts from the host plant but is autotrophic for CO_2. Three subspecies are distinguished by differences in host specificity: broadleaf mistletoe, which grows on all European broadleaf trees except beech, preferring apple trees and poplars; fir mistletoe, which grows on silver fir; and pine mistletoe, which grows on pines, larches, and occasionally on firs.

Immunopharmacologic studies indicate that the lectins in mistletoe are the most important active principles; their effects include the stimulation of T-lymphocytes. The compound designated lectin 1 was found to induce macrophage cytotoxicity in experimental animals. It also stimulated the phagocytosis of various immune cells (Hajto et al., 1989, 1990 a). The lectin content of various mistletoe parts and preparations is highly variable, however, and further progress in this area depends on the manufacture of optimized preparations. A mistletoe extract standardized for mistletoe lectin is now marketed in Germany under the brand name Lektinol. Tests with this product have demonstrated dose-dependent immune-stimulating effects in vitro and in vivo, consisting of immune-cell stimulation, increased cytokin secretion, and cytotoxic effects on various types of tumor cell (Joller, 1996; Beuth et al., 1997; Mengs, 1997; Vehmeyer, 1998; Weber et al., 1998). The lectin-optimized mistletoe extract, which has also shown initial efficacy in the treatment of tumor patients (see 9.2.2.2), is capable of restoring a solid scientific foundation to mistletoe therapy. Besides the lectins, some importance is also ascribed to the acid polysaccharides in mistletoe, which stimulated complement-

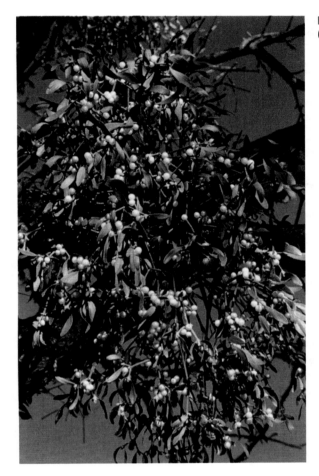

Fig. 9.5. ◄ European mistletoe (*Viscum album*).

system activation and showed other activating effects in vitro (Wagner and Jordan, 1986; Beuth et al., 1992; Gabius et al., 1994).

The mistletoe preparations marketed in Germany are based on the fresh leaves, branches, and berries of European mistletoe. Different products use different processing, methods, and some show a definite anthroposophic influence. Some products (e.g., Plenosol, Helixor) are produced by a relatively simple method that essentially yields an aqueous whole-plant extract. With other products (e.g., Iscador), the anthroposophic origins are unmistakable. One- to two-year-old shoots of the mistletoe shrub, complete with stems, leaves, buds, flowers, and berries, are processed in a fresh condition within 24 h after gathering. First, a kind of juice is prepared by grinding the plant parts, adding distilled water, and crushing the mixture between rollers to produce an aqueous extract in which 1 part extract weight corresponds to 1 part mistletoe weight. This extract is subjected to anaerobic lactic acid fermentation for 4–6 weeks. It is then diluted 1:5, and summer viscum juice is mixed with winter viscum juice to yield a 10 % Iscador stock solution that is further diluted to make injectable solutions of varying strength. The ampoules may be sterilized by heat or by filtration, depending on the legal require-ments in the country of manufacture.

9.2.2.2 Clinical Efficacy Studies

Almost 50 clinical studies have been conducted on mistletoe preparations during the last 30 years. All involved parenteral administration, usually by subcutaneous injection. Given the heterogeneity of the preparation methods, only the results for specific prod-ucts can be meaningfully summarized. Surveys can be found in Keine (1989) and Hau-ser (1993).

Eleven controlled clinical studies on mistletoe preparations were reviewed in a,com-prehensive meta-analysis (Kleijnen and Knipschild, 1994). The authors used a scoring system based on 10 quality criteria to evaluate the study outcomes. The results of this meta-analysis, including types of tumor, products used, and statistical results, are sum-marized in Table 9.1. The authors rated the overall scientific quality of the studies as weak. None of the studies employed a double-blind design. One study was considered to be adequately randomized. The most highly rated study (Dold et al., 1991) was a mul-ticenter study, commissioned by the German Federal Insurance Institute for Employees, in which the effect of Iscador was compared with a multivitamin preparation used as a placebo. The study involved 408 patients with a histologically confirmed diagnosis of advanced, non-small-cell bronchial carcinoma. The patients treated with Iscador had an average survival of 9.1 months, compared with 7.6 months for patients treated with the placebo. At 2 years, 11,5 % of the Iscador patients and 10,1 % of the placebo patients were still alive. The differences in average and 2-year survival were not statistically sig-nificant. The quality of life scores also showed no statistical differences, although the Iscador patients reported an improvement of general well-being significantly more often than the placebo patients. Nevertheless, the authors of this study did not believe

Table 9.1.

Meta-analysis of 11 controlled studies on mistletoe preparations in the treatment of cancer (after Kleijnen and Knipschild, 1994).

First author	Type of cancer	Product name	Statistical result	Total score
Dold, 1991	Bronchial carcinoma	Iscador	0	8,5
Douwes, 1986	Colorectal carcinoma	Helixor	Trend	6,0
Salzer, 1991	Bronchial carcinoma	Iscador	Trend	5,5
Douwes, 1988	Colorectal carcinoma	Helixor	Significant	5,0
Salzer, 1978, 1980	Bronchial carcinoma	Iscador	Significant	5,0
Salzer, 1979, 1983, 1988	Gastric carcinoma	Iscador	Trend	4,5
Fellmer, 1966, 1968	Gastric carcinoma	Iscador	Trend	4,0
Gutsch, 1988	Breast carcinoma	Helixor	Significant	4,0
Heiny, 1991	Breast carcinoma	Eurixor	Significant	3,5
Salzer, 1987a	Breast carcinoma	Iscador	Trend	3,0
Majewski, 1963	Genital carcinoma in women	Iscador	Trend	1,0

that the outcome was sufficient to warrant a general recommendation for this therapy in patients with non-small-cell bronchial carcinoma.

Two studies were performed with an extract standardized to mistletoe lectin 1. In a prospective cohort study in 884 patients with various types of malignant tumors including breast and colon cancers, significant improvements in a validated quality-of-life score were obtained with a dosage of only 2.5 g/kg body weight administered by subcutaneous injection over a trial period of 3 months. With regard to tolerance, 92 % of the patients and 94 % of the physicians rated the tolerance of the test preparation as good to excellent. Adverse side effects consisted of four cases each of erythematous skin rash, itching, or local inflammation at the injection site (Finelli et al., 1998).

In an open study, 477 patients who had undergone head and neck tumor resections were randomly assigned to two groups. One group received a standardized mistletoe preparation in addition to other therapeutic measures for a period of approximately 4 years, and the second group received no adjuvant treatment. The primary outcome measure was survival time. Secondary measures were recurrence rates and quality of life. The study showed no significant intergroup differences in any of the criteria tested (Steuer-Vogt, 2001).

9.2.2.3 Indications, Dosages, and Risks

Commission E published its monograph on European mistletoe in 1984. Although most of the controlled clinical studies (Table 9.1) were completed after that date, they did not yield any fundamental new discoveries. The 1984 monograph states that *Viscum album* is useful "For treating degenerative inflammation of the joints by stimulating cuti-visceral reflexes following local inflammation brought about by intradermal injections. As palliative therapy for malignant tumors through non-specific stimulation" (Blumenthal et al., 1998). These applications are based entirely on the intra- or subcutaneous administration of the drug. The dosages should conform to manufacturer's recommendations. Iscador injectable ampules are supplied in up to 10 different concentrations, which are increased in increments during one treatment cycle, starting with the lowest concentration. They are also recommended for sequential regimens involving treatment with several subspecies (broadleaf, fir, and pine mistletoe); this reflects the anthroposophical origin of this therapy, which is only marginally related to orthodox scientific medicine.

Because the preparation is administered parenterally, it is contraindicated by protein hypersensitivity. Chronic, progressive infections such as tuberculosis also contraindicate the therapy due to the potential for immune effects. The monograph notes several possible side effects: chills, high fever, headache, chest pain, orthostatic hypotension, and allergic reactions.

9.2.3 Medicinal Yeasts

Yeast was used medicinally by the ancient Egyptians and later by the Greeks and Romans. Yeast has always been a popular folk remedy in beer-producing countries, where it has been used as a mild laxative, an antidiarrheal for enteral infections and poisonings, and as a preventive remedy for boils, acne, and eczema.

Dried brewer's yeast (medicinal yeast) is described in the German Pharmacopeia as a bottom-fermented yeast consisting of cells that can no longer replicate but which still retain most of their enzymatic activities. Because they are derived from fungal cultures (*Saccharomyces cerevisae*), brewer's yeast preparations can be classified as phytomedicines. Crude bottom-fermented brewer's yeast has a high content of hop constituents, and the bitter principles must be removed from the yeast before it is processed further for medicinal purposes. By dry weight, brewer's yeast contains 50–60 % nitrogen compounds (proteins, nucleic acids, free amino acids, and biogenic amines), 15–37 % carbohydrates, and 4–7 % fats and lipids, chiefly phospholipids.

The therapeutic use of brewer's yeast is based largely on folk medicine and empirical healing. Several pharmacologic studies showed an increased phagocytic index for peritoneal macrophages in mice (Schmidt, 1977) and a decreased severity of experimental infections in mice and rhesus monkeys (Sinai et al., 1974). Dietary yeast supplementation promoted the more rapid clearing of edema in children with kwashiorkor (severe malnutrition), an effect presumably due to the content of B vitamins in the yeast (Gervais, 1973).

The 1988 Commission E monograph on medicinal yeast states that it is used for "loss of appetite and as a supplement for chronic forms of acne and furunculosis" (Blumenthal et al., 1998). The average recommended dose is 6 g/day. As for side effects, the monograph notes that medicinal yeast can occasionally cause migraine attacks in susceptible patients and that the ingestion of fermentable yeast can cause flatulence.

9.2.4 Goldenseal

One of the most popular herbs in the United States, consistently on the short list of best sellers and accounting for about 4 % of total herbal sales there, is goldenseal, the dried rhizome and roots of *Hydrastis canadensis*. Introduced to early European settlers by the Native Americans, the botanical contains a number of highly colored isoquinoline alkaloids, principally berberine (0.5–6 %) and hydrastine (1.5–4 %) that account for its name.

Long used as a simple bitter and drug of dubious utility, goldenseal was further popularized in the 1980's by members of the counterculture who, based on a misreading of an early work of fiction, erroneously believed that it might mask urine tests for illicit drugs (Foster, 1989). Subsequently, its popularity continued to grow as a purported immune stimulant. It is frequently marketed for this purpose in combination with echinacea. There have never been any clinical studies to support this usage.

Pharmacological studies are also scanty, and most are quite dated. A comprehensive review of goldenseal and its contained alkaloids published 50 years ago (Shideman, 1950) noted that little work had been conducted on this plant in the preceding 40 years; practically nothing of importance has been published since. A recent review by Blumenthal et al. (2003) found no clinical trials conducted on goldenseal available in the modern literature; the review resorted to summaries of clinical studies on berberine to help determine a rational basis for understanding some of the potential clinical pharmacology of ingested goldenseal preparations.

The reputation of goldenseal is based largely upon in vitro studies that have found berberine to act as an antimicrobial. Limited clinical trials also show that the alkaloid may serve as a useful non-systemic antibacterial in the treatment, for example, of diarrhea caused by enterotoxigenic E coli (Rabbani, 1987). However, berberine and related alkaloids are very poorly absorbed from the gastrointestinal tract, so any significant systemic effects such as immune stimulation are precluded (Bergner, 1996–97).

Although the use of goldenseal for any systemic purpose appears to be without scientific merit, the dried rhizome and root are employed in doses of 0.5–1 g three times daily for traveler's diarrhea. Such doses are ordinarily nontoxic, but goldenseal should not be utilized by pregnant women (McGuffin et al., 1997).

The wild plant has been so intensively collected in the United States during recent years that survival of the species is questionable. This has stimulated cultivation efforts which may ultimately result in an adequate supply. However, because any utility goldenseal possesses is almost certainly present in other berberine-containing plants such as barberry (*Berberis vulgaris*) or Oregon grape (*Mahonia aquifolium*), it seems logical to utilize these common plants as sources of that alkaloid instead of the threatened species.

9.3 Therapeutic Significance

Herbal agents that can enhance host defenses nonspecifically fill an important therapeutic niche, especially in outpatient settings where treatment options are extremely limited. This is particularly true of echinacea and mistletoe preparations. With a total of about 1 million prescriptions annually, echinacea preparations are still among the most widely used phytomedicines in Germany. They have been prescribed for patients, including many children, who suffer from frequent recurring infections, particularly of the upper respiratory tract. The goal in such patients is to increase long-term resistance to infection mainly through nonpharmacologic means (e.g., Kneipp applications, exercise, the elimination of harmful agents). Often this approach is unsuccessful. Because there are very few pharmacotherapeutic options for these patients and it appears that echinacea preparations have very little risk potential, a trial with these preparations is justified. Available data, especially from clinical studies, suggest that echinacea products do have some efficacy in stimulating host defenses. Since immune responses are by nature episodic, there seems to be no rationale for the continuous use of these products. That is why the monographs recommend limiting the duration of use to 8 weeks.

Data currently available cannot adequately establish the therapeutic efficacy of traditional mistletoe preparations in a provable, scientific sense. Nevertheless, a large number of positive individual case reports justify the use of mistletoe preparations for the palliative treatment of malignant tumors, inasmuch as orthodox medicine cannot offer suitable therapeutic alternatives. A preparation standardized for mistletoe lectin 1 is currently undergoing clinical trials. This mistletoe preparation appears very promising and offers a means of restoring a sound scientific basis to this practically important therapy.

In contrast to mistletoe preparations for the palliative treatment of malignant tumors, herbal immune stimulants for other indications are no longer covered by health insurance plans in Germany according to the latest drug guidelines (see Table 1.3). The same applies to herbal adaptogens (Asian ginseng and eleuthero). But ginseng preparations still have an important role in physician-assisted self-medication. Eastern empirical medicine, the universal scope of ginseng use, and the relatively comprehensive scientific data base on the actions and efficacy of ginseng all suggest that the temporary use of ginseng products can be beneficial during convalescence and in other states of physical weakness, especially in older patients. The preparation should be taken in a sufficiently high dosage (1–2 g of crude drug or 300–600 mg of extract daily) for a period of no more than several weeks.

In general, despite at least 8 published clinical trials in the areas of immunology and general adaptogenic effects, preparations made from eleuthero have a less traditional and scientific foundation than Asian ginseng. Although this botanical belongs to the same family as ginseng, its constituents are markedly different, indicating the generally low specificity of adaptogenic effects.

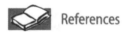 References

107th Congress. Farm Security and Rural Investment Act of 2002. Public Law 107–171 *www.ers.usda.gov/Features/farmbill/.*

Ahn, Y-J, Kim M-I, Yamamoto T, Fujisawa T, Mitsouka T (1990) Selective growth responses of human intestinal bacteria to Araliaceae extracts. Microbial Ecol Health Disease 3: 223–229.

Allen JD, McLung J, Nelson AG, Welsch M (1998) Ginseng supplementation does not enhance healthy young adults' peak aerobic exercise performance. J Am Coll Nutr 17: 462–6.

Andallu B, Radhika B (2000) Hypoglycemic, diuretic and hypocholesterolemic effect of winter cherry (Withania somnifera, Dunal) root. Indian J Exp Biol 38:607–9.

Anon (no date) Centella asiatica. Indena SpA Milan Italy Technical documentation, pp 1–31.

Asano K, Takahashi T, Miyashita M et al. (1986) Effect of Eleutherococcus sentiosus extract on human physical working capacity. Planta Med 3: 175–7.

Bahrke MS, Morgan WP (2000) Evaluation of the ergogenic properties of ginseng. Sports Med 29: 113–33.

Bajusz E, Sellye H (1960) Über die durch Srtreß bedingte Nekroseresistenz des Herzens. Ein Beitrag zum Phänomen der "gekreuzten Resistenz". Naturwissenschaft 47: 520–521.

Barret B, Vohmann V, Calabrese C (1999) Echinacea for upper respiratory tract infection. J Fam Pract 48(8):628–35.

Barrett B (2003) Medicinal properties of Echinacea: a critical review. Phytomedicine 10: 66-86.

Bauer R (1997) Echinacea – Pharmazeutische Qualität und therapeutischer Wert. Zeitschrift für Phytotherapie 18: 207–214.

Bauer R, Wagner H (eds) (1990) Echinacea. Wissenschaftliche Verlagsgesellschaft mbH Stuttgart.

Bergner P (1996-97) Goldenseal and the common cold: the antibiotic myth. Med Herb 8(4): 1, 4–6.

Betti G (2002) Taigawurzel (Eleutherococcus sentiosus) – das pflanzliche Adaptogen zur Steigerung der psychomotorischen, mentalen und physischen Leistungsfähigkeit. J Pharmakol Ther 6: 167–78.

Beuth J, Ko HL, Gabius HJ, Burichter H, Oette K, Pulverer G (1992) Behavior of lymphocyte subsets and expression of activation markers in response to immunotherapy with galactosidespecific lectin from mistletoe in breast cancer. Clin Invest 70: 658–661.

Beuth J, Lenartz D, Uhlenbruck G (1997) Lektinoptimierter Mistelextrakt. Experimentelle Austestung und klinische Anwendung. Zeitschrift für Phytotherapie 18: 85-91

Bladt S, Wagner H, Woo WS (1990) Taiga-Wurzel. Dtsch. Apoth Z 27: 1499-1508.

Blumenthal M (1991) Debunking the "ginseng abuse syndrome." Whole Foods, March:89-91.

Blumenthal M (2002) Farm bill bans use of name "Ginseng" on non-Panax species: "Siberian ginseng" no longer allowed as commercial term. HerbalGram 56:54.

Blumenthal M, Busse WR, Goldberg A, Gruenwald J, Hall T, Riggins CW, Rister RS (eds.). Klein S, Rister RS (trans). (1998) The Complete German Commission E Monographs – Therapeutic Guide to Herbal Medicines. American Botanical Council, Austin, Texas. *www.herbalgram.org*.

Blumenthal M, Hall T, Goldberg A et al. (eds). (2003) The ABC Clinical Guide to Herbs. Austin, TX: American Botanical Council.

Bohn B, Nebe C, Birr C (1987) Flow-cytometric studies with Eleutherococcus senticosus extract as an immunomodulatory agent. Arzneim. Forsch. (Drug Res) 37: 1193-1196.

Bombardelli E. Morazzoni P (1995) Vitis vinifera L. Fitoterapia 66: 291-317.

Bradwein J, Zhou Y, Koszycki D, Shlik J (2000) A Double-Blind, Placebo-Controlled Study of the Effects of Gotu Kola (Centella asiatica) on Acoustic Startle Response in Healthy Subjects. J Clin Psychopharmacol 20:680-684.

Brekhman II, Dardymov IV (1969) New substances of plant origin which increase nonspecific resistance. Ann Rev Pharmacol 9: 419-430.

Brinkeborn RM, Shah DV, Degenring FH (1999) Echinaforce and other echinacea fresh plant preparations in the treatment of the common cold. Phytomedicine 6: 1-5.

Brown RP, Gerbarg PL, Ramazanov Z (2003) Rhodiola rosea – a phytomedicinal overview. HerbalGram 56: 40- 52.

Chen G (1995) Effects of JingShuiBao capsule on quality of life of patients with chronic heart failure. J Adm Trad Chin Med 5: (Suppl.) 40-43.

Coon JT, Ernst E (2002) Panax ginseng: a systematic review of adverse effects and drug interactions. Drug Safety 25(5):323-44.

Court WE (2000) Ginseng: The Genus Panax. Amsterdam: Harwood Scientific Publishers.

Dharmananda S (2002) The Nature of Ginseng: Traditional Use, Modern Research, and the Question of Dosage. HerbalGram 54:34-51.

Divi PU, Sharada AC, Solomon FE, Kamath MS (1992) In vivo growth inhibitory effect of Withania somnifera (ashwagandha) on a transplantable mouse tumor, Sarcoma 180. Ind J Exp Biol 30: 169-172.

Diwan PV, Karwande I, Singh AK (1991) Anti-anxiety profile of manduk parni (Centella asiatica) in animals. Fitoterapia 62: 253-257.

Dold U, Edler L, Mäurer HC, Müller-Wening D, Sakellariou B. Trendelenburg F, et al (1991) Krebszusatztherapie beim fortgeschrittenen nicht-kleinzelligen Bronchialkarzinom. Georg Thieme Verlag, Stuttgart.

Dorn M (1989) Milderung grippaler Effekte durch ein planzliches Immunstimulans. Natur- und Ganzheitsmedizin 2: 314-319.

Dowling EA, Redondo DR, Branch JD et al. (1996) Effect of Eleutherococcus sentiosus on submaximal exercise performance. Med Sci Sports Exerc 28: 482-9.

Engels HJ, Said JM, Wirth JC (1996) Failure of chronic ginseng administration to affect work performance and energy metabolism in healthy adult females. Nutr Res 16: 1295-1305.

Farrow JM, Leslie GB, Schwarzenbach FH (1978) The in vivo protective effect of a complex yeast preparation (Bio-Strath) against bacterial infections in mice. Medita (Solothurn) 8: 37-42.

Finelli A, Limberg R, Scheithe K (1998) Mistel-Lektin bei Patienten mit Tumorerkrankungen. Diagnostik und Therapie im Bild 1998: 2-5.

Foster S (1989) Goldenseal-Masking of Drug Tests From Fiction to Fallacy: an Historical Anomaly. HerbalGram 21:7,35.

Gabius HJ, Gabius S, Joshi SS, Koch B, Schroeder M, Manzke WM, Westerhausen M (1994) From ill-defined extracts to the immunomodulatory lectin: Will there be a reason for oncological application of mistletoe? Planta Med 60: 2-7.

Gervais C (1973) Profitable effect of a lactic yeast in nutrient-deficient Biafran children. Bull Soc Pathol exot 66: 445-447.

Giles JT, Palat CT, Chien SH et al. (2000) Evaluation of echinacea treatment of the common cold. Pharmacotherapy 20: 690–7.

Grimm W, Müller HH (1999) A randomized controlled trial of the effect of fluid extract of Echinacea purpurea on the incidence and severity of colds and respiratory infections. Am J Med 106: 138–143.

Hajto T, Hostanka K, Frei K, Rordorf C, Gabins H-J (1990a) Increased secretion of tumor necrosis factor α, interleukin 1, und interleukin 6 by Heiman mononuclear cells exposed to β-galactoside specific lectin from clinically applied mistletoe extract. Canc Res. 50: 3322.

Hajto T, Hostanka K, Gabius HI (1989) Modulatory potency of the β-galactoside-specific lectin from mistletoe extract (Iscador) and the host defense system in vivo in rabbits and patients. Canc Res 49: 4803.

Hajto T, Hostanka K, Gabius HI (1990b) Zytokine als Lectin-induzierte Mediatoren in der Misteltherapie. Therapeutikon 4: 136–145.

Hauser SP (1993) Mistel – Wunderkraut oder Medikament? Therapiewoche 43(3): 76–81.

Haustein KO (1998) Immuntherapeutika und Zytostatika. In: Schwabe U, Paffrath D (eds) Arznei-verordnungs-Report '98. Springer Verlag, S. 326–331.

Hofecker G (1987) Physiologie und Pathophysiologie des Alterns. Öster Apoth Z 41: 443–450.

Hoheisel O, Sandberg M, Bertram S, Bulitta M, Schäder M (1997) Echinagard treatment shortens the course of the common cold: a double-blind, placebo-controlled clinical trial. European Journal of Clinical Research 9: 261–268.

Hyo-Won B, IL-Heok K, Sa-Sek, H, Byung-Hun H, Mun-Hae H, Ze-Hun K, Nak-Du K (1987) Roter Ginseng. Schriftenreihe des Staatlichen Ginseng-Monopolamtes der Republik Korea.

Ji BT, Chow W-H, Hsing AW, McLaughlin JK, Dai Q, Gao Y-T, Blot WJ (1997) Green tea consumption and the risk of pancreatic and colorectal cancers. Int J Cancer 70: 255–258.

Joller PW, Menrad JM, Schwarz T et al. (1996) Stimulation of cytokine production via a special standardized mistletoe preparation in an vitro human skin bioassay. Arzneimittel-Forschung/Drug Res 46: 649–653.

Kaemmerer K, Fink J (1980) Untersuchungen von Eleutherococcus-Extrakt auf trophanabole Wirkungen bei Ratten. Der praktische Tierarzt 61: 748–753.

Kaemmerer K, Kietzmann M (1983) Untersuchungen über streßabschirmende Wirkungen von oral verabreichtem Zinkbacitracin bei Ratten. Zbl Vet Med A 30: 712–721.

Kiene H (1989) Klinische Studien zur Misteltherapie karzinomatöser Erkrankungen. Eine Übersicht. Therapeutikon 3: 347–353.

Kleijnen J, Knipschild P (1994) Mistletoe treatment for cancer. Review of controlled trials in humans. Phytomedicine 1: 255–260.

Knekt P, Järvinen R, Seppänen R, Heliövaara M, Teppo L, Pukkala E, Aromaa A (1997) Dietary flavonoids and the risk of lung cancer and other malignant neoplasms. Am J Epidemiol 146: 223–230.

Kuppurajan K, Rajagopalan SS, Sitaramen R, Rajagopalan V, Janaki K, Revethi R, Venkataraghavan S (1980) Effect of ashwagandha (Withania somnifera Dunal) on the process of aging in human volunteers. J Res Ayurveda Siddha 1: 247–258.

Laerum OD, Iversen OH (1972) Reticuloses and epidermal tumors in hairless mice after topical skin applications of cantharidin and asiaticoside. Cancer Res 32: 1463–1469.

Lamm S, Shen Y, Pero RW (2001) Persistent response to pneumococcal vaccine in individuals supplemented with a novel water soluble extract of Uncaria tomentosa., C-Med-100®. Phytomedicine 8(4):267–74.

Lovett EJ, Schnitzer B, Keren DF et al (1984) Application of flow cytometry to diagnostic pathology. Lab Invest 50: 115–140.

McGuffin M, Hobbs C, Upton R, Goldberg A (1997). Botanical Safety Handbook. CRC Press, Boca Raton, p. 26.

McKenna DJ (ed) (1998) Natural Supplements. Institute for Natural Products Research, Marine on St. Croix, Minnesota, unpaged.

Melchart D, Linde K, Worku F, bauer R, Wagner H (1994) Immunomodulation with echinacea – a systematic review of controlled clinical trials. Phytomedicine 1: 245–254.

Melchert T Linde K, Fischer P, Kaesmayr J (2001) Echinacea for preventing and treating the common cold (Conchrane Review). In: The Conchrane Library, Issue 1, 2001. Oxford: Update Software.

Mishra LC, Singh BB, Dagenais S (2000) Scientific Basis for the Therapeutic Use of Withania somnifera (Ashwagandha): A Review. Alternative Medicine Review 5:334–346.

Mitscher LA, Jung M, Shankel D, Dou J-H, Steele L, Pillai SP (1997) Chemoprotection: a review of the potential therapeutic antioxidant properties of green tea (Camellia sinensis) and certain of its constituents. Med Res Revs 17: 327–365.

Morris AC, Jacobs I, Kligerman TM (1996) No ergometric effect of ginseng ingestion. Int J Sport Nutr 6: 263–71.

Obermeier A (1980) Zur Analytik der Ginseng- und Eteutherococcusdroge. Dissertation Ludwig-Maximilians-Universität, Munich.

Palmer BV, Montgomery ACV, Monteiro JCMP (1978) Ginseng and mastalgia. Brit Med J 1: 284 (letter).

Pichler WJ, Emmendörfer A, Peter HH et al. (1985) Analyse von T-Zell-Subpopulationen. Pathophysiologisches Konzept und Bedeutung für die Klinik. Schweiz med Wschr 115: 534–55

Piscoya J, Rodriguez Z, Bustamante SA, Okuhama NN, Miller MJS, and Sandoval.(2001) Efficacy and safety of freeze-dried cat's claw in osteoarthritis of the knee: mechanisms of action of the species Uncaria guianensis. Inflammation Research 50:442–448

Ploss E (1988) Panax ginseng C.A. Meyer. Scientific report. Kooperation Phytopharmaka, Cologne.

Proksch A (1982) Über ein immunstimulierendes Wirkprinzip aus Echinacea purpurea. Dissertation, Ludwig-Maximilians-Universität, Munich.

Rabbani GH, Butler T, Knight et al. (1987) Randomized controlled clinical trial for diarrhea due to enterotoxigenic Escherichia coli and Vibrio cholerae. J Infect Dis 155: 979–984

Reinhard K-H (1997) Uncaria tomentosa (Willd.) DC. – cat's claw, un~a de gato oder Katzenkralle. Z Phytother 18: 112–121.

Ro HS, Lee SY, Han BH (1977) Studies on the lignan glycoside of Acanthopanax cortex. J Pharm Korea 21: 81–86.

Schmidt CH (1977) Unspezifische Steigerung der Phagozytoseaktivitäten von Peritoneal-Makrophagen nach oraler Gabe verschiedener Hefepräparationen. Dissertation, Freie Universität Berlin.

Schmidt U, Albrecht M, Schenk N (1990) Pflanzliches Immunstimulans senkt Häufigkeit grippaler Infekte. Plazebo-kontrollierte Doppelblindstudie mit einem kombinierten Echinacea-Präparat mit 646 Studenten der Kölner Universität. Natur- und Ganzheitsmedizin 3: 277–282.

Schole J, Harisch G, Sallmann HP (1978) Belastung, Ernährung und Resistenz. Parey, Hamburg Berlin.

Selye R (1946) The general adaptation syndrome and the disease of adaptation. J Clin Endocrinol 6: 117–130.

Sheng Y, Li L, Pero RW (2001) DNA repair enhancement of aqueous extracts of Uncaria tomentosa in a human volunteer study. Phytomedicine 8:275–282.

Shideman FE (1950) A review of the pharmacology and therapeutics of Hydrastis and its alkaloids, hydrastine, berberine, and canadine. Comm Nat Form Bull 18(102): 3–19.

Siegel RK (1979) Ginseng abuse syndrome: Problems with the panacea. JAMA 341:1614–5.

Siegel RK (1980) Ginseng and high blood pressure. J Am Med Assoc. 243: 32.

Sinai Y, Kaplan A, Hai Y et al. (1974) Enhancement of resistance to infectious disease by oral administration of brewer's yeast. Infection Immunol. 9: 781–787.

Sonnenborn U, Proppert Y (1990) Ginseng (Panax ginseng C.A. Meyer). Z Phythotherapie 11: 35–49.

Spasow AA, Wikman GK, Mandrikow VB, Mirinova IA, Neumoin VV (2000) A double-blind, placebo-controlled pilot study of the stimulating and adaptogenic effect of Rhodiola rosea SHR-5 extract on the fatigue of students caused by stress during an examination period with a repeated low-dose regimen. Phytomed 7: 85–89.

Steuer-Vogt MK, Bonkowsky V, Ambrosch P et al. (2001) The effect of an adjuvant mistletoe treatment programme in resected head and neck cancer patients: a randomized controlled clinical trial. Eur J Cancer 37: 23–31.

Stimpel M, Proksch A, Wagner H et al (1984) Macrophage activation and induction of macrophage cytotoxicity by purified polysaccharide fractions from the plant Echinacea purpurea. Infect Immunity 46: 845–849.

Taylor JA, Weber W, Standish L, et al. (2003) Efficacy and safety of Echinacea in treating upper respiratory tract infections in children. JAMA 290:2824–30.

Upton R, Petrone C (eds) (1999) Astragalus Root: Analytical, quality control, and therapeutic monograph. American Herbal Pharmacopoeia, Santa Cruz, CA.

Upton R, Petrone C (eds) (2000) Ashwagandha Root: Analytical, quality control, and therapeutic monograph. American Herbal Pharmacopoeia, Santa Cruz, CA.

Upton R. (ed.) (2004). Echinacea purpurea Root (Echinacea purpurea (L.) Moench). Analytical, quality control, and therapeutic monograph. American Herbal Pharmacopoeia, Santa Cruz, CA.

Vogler BK, Pittler MH, Ernst E (1999) The efficacy of ginseng. A systematic review of randomised clinical trials. Eur J Clin Pharmacol 55: 567–75.

Wagner H, Jordan E (1986) Structure and properties of polysaccharides from Viscum album (L.) Oncology (Suppl 1): 8–15.

Wagner H, Jurcic K (1991) Immunologische Untersuchungen von planzlichen Kombinations-präparaten. Arzneim.Forsch (Drug Res)41: 1072–1076.

Wagner H, Nörr H, Winterhoff H (1994) Plant adaptogens. Phytomed 1: 63–76.

WHO monographs on selected medicinal plants, Vol.1. World Health Organisation, Geneva 1999, pp 168–82.

Williams M (1995) Immuno-protection against herpes simplex type II infection by eleutherococcus root extract. Int J Altern Compl Med 13: 9–12.

Winther K, Ranlov C, Rein E, Mehlsen J (1997) Russian root (Siberian Ginseng) improves cognitive functions in middle-aged people, whereas Ginkgo biloba seems effective only in the elderly. J Neurol Sciences 150: S90.

Youn YS (1987) Analytisch vergleichende Untersuchungen von Ginsengwurzeln verschiedener Provenienzen. Dissertation, Freie Universität Berlin.

Zhang Z, Huang W, Liao S, Li J, Lui J, Leng F, Gong W, Zhang H, Wan L, Wu R, Li S, Luo H, Zhu F (1995) Clinical and laboratory studies of JingShuiBao in scavenging oxygen free radicals in elderly senescent XuZheng patients. J Adm Chin Med 5 (Suppl.): 14–18.

Zhu J-S, Halpern GM, Jones K (1998) The scientific rediscovery of an ancient Chinese herbal medicine: Cordyceps sinensis part 1. J Alt Comp Med 4: 289–303.

Zorikow PS, Lyapustina TA (1974) Change in a concentration of protein and nitrogen in the reproductive organs of hens under the effect of Eleutherococcus extract. Deposited DOC VINI, 732–774, 58–63, ref Chem Abstracts 86 (1977) 119–732.

Appendix:
The 100 Most Commonly
Prescribed Herbal Medications
in Germany

Figure A1 and Tables A1-A3 review the 100 most frequently prescribed herbal medications in Germany. This information is based on prescription figures for 2002 published in the 2003 *Drug Prescription Report* (Schwabe and Paffrath, 2003). The nomenclature for herbs and herbal products follows the terminology used in the *Rote Liste* 2003. As Table A3 indicates, these 100 herbal products rank among the 2267 most commonly prescribed medications in Germany. Their sales in 2002 totaled 420 million €, compared with total sales of 19,507 billion € for the 2267 most commonly prescribed drugs. Thus, the 100 herbal remedies accounted for 2.15 % of the total drug expenditures that were covered by health insurance programs. Fifty-nine of the 100 most-prescribed phytomedicines are 68 single-herb products (297 million € = 70 % of the herbal drug market), and 32 are combination products (124 million € = 30 %). The latter include 19 two-herb products, 9 three-herb products, 1 four-herb product, 2 five-herb products, and 1 product containing 9 herbs. The leading indications for herbal remedies are listed in order of sales volume in Table A1.

Note that the order of the indications in Table A1 corresponds roughly to the eight chapter headings in this book. Ginkgo preparations are discussed mainly in Chap. 2 (Central Nervous System), and chamomile preparations for external use (pain, rheumatic conditions, bruises) and anti-inflammatory internal use are discussed in Chap. 8 (Skin, Trauma, Rheumatism, and Pain). The 68 most commonly prescribed single-herb products can be reduced to 34 herbs and plant parts, which are listed in order of sales volume in Table A2.

Overall sales figures for the 100 most frequently prescribed phytomedicines declined by 35 % between 1997 and 2002. The percentage decline affected single-herb products, which are desirable in rational phytotherapy, less than combination products. The number of combination products in the top-100 list fell from 41 to 32. In the ranking of indications (Table A1), urologic remedies have advanced by two places since 1997. The products showing the strongest sales increases from 1997 to 2002 (Table A2) are saw palmetto berry extract and pelargonium root extract (first time in the list, ranked 9th),

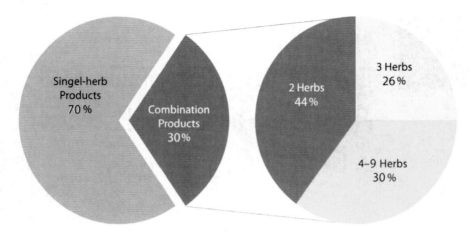

Source: Schwabe and Paffrath, Drug Prescription Report 2003, Springer 2003

Figure A1. ▲ Percentage sales distribution of the 100 most commonly prescribed herbal medications in Germany in 2002, by single-herb and combination products.

while horse chestnut extract and ivy leaf extract (both lacking current research data) have shown the greatest declines.

Table A1.
Distribution of the 100 most commonly prescribed phytomedicines in Germany in 2002, ranked in order of gross pharmacy sales. The numbers in the year columns represent annual sales in millions of euros, N 2002 = number of products available in 2002. Column 1: letter keys for the groups of indications appearing in Tables A2 and A3 below.

	Indications	1994	1997	2000	2002	N 2002
A	Central nervous system disorders	315	236	161	135	25
B	Respiratory disorders	110	76	96	93	25
C	Cardiovascular disorders	116	80	40	31	8
D	Urinary tract disorders	79	76	46	49	11
E	Disorders of the stomach, bowel, liver, or biliary tract	110	57	42	41	11
F	Increasing resistance to diseases	37	37	23	34	4
G	Skin and connective tissue disorders	48	30	20	20	12
H	Gynecologic disorders	10	18	30	17	4
8	All indications	797	645	485	420	100

Table A2.

Seventy of the 100 most commonly prescribed phytomedicines in 2002 were single-herb products. These can be reduced to a total of 34 herbs or active constituents, which are ranked below in order of sales.
Abbreviations: E = extrakt; **P** = powder.

Rank	Herb or active constituent	Products	Indication	Sales in T€
1	Gingko leaves (E)	6	A	73239
2	St. John's wort (E)	10	A	36772
3	Mistletoe (E)	3	F	32729
4	Ivy leaves (E)	4	B	18563
5	Hawthorn leaves and flowers (E)	3	C	15299
6	Saw palmetto berries (E)	3	D	13933
7	Saccharomyces (P)	2	E	13550
8	Nettle root (E)	1	D	10619
9	Pelargonium root (E)	1	B	8715
10	Horse chestnut seed (E)	2	C	8605
11	Thyme (E)	5	B	5795
12	Eucalyptus oil and cineol	2	B	5476
13	Milk thistle fruits (E)	1	E	4535
14	Petasite rhizome (E)	1	A	4108
15	Pumpkin seeds (E)	1	D	4084
16	Chasteberry (E)	2	H	3792
17	Bromelain	1	G	3469
18	Black cohosh rhizome (E)	1	H	3344
19	Chamomile flowers (E)	3	G	3309
20	Valerian root (E)	2	A	2860
21	Colchicum (E)	1	G	2801
22	Grass pollens (E)	1	D	2586
23	Artichoke leaves (E)	1	E	2282
24	Goldenrod (E)	1	D	2072
25	Nettle leaves (E)	1	G	1995
26	Devil's claw (E)	1	G	1956
27	Sage (E)	1	G	1847
28	Comfrey root (E)	1	G	1507
29	Uva ursi leaves (E)	1	D	1246
30	Evening primrose oil	1	G	1241
31	Uzara root (E)	1	E	1103
32	Alexandria senna pods (E)	1	E	1089
33	Witch hazel bark (E)	1	G	890
34	Island moss (E)	1	B	234
	34 herbs or active constituants	**68 single herb products**		**296000**

Table A3.

The 100 most commonly prescribed phytomedicines in Germany in 2002. The numbers in thousands of € per year are based on pharmacy sales prices.

Abbreviations: T = tablet, CT = coated tablet, FT = film tablet, L = liquid, C = capsule, O = ointment or cream, S = suppository, E = extract, P = powder, J = juice, IND = indication code (from Table A1), **A rank** = ranking of phytomedicines by number of prescriptions, **B rank** = ranking of phytomedicines by number of prescriptions among all drug products, **TRx** = thousands of prescriptions, **T€** = thousands of € (gross pharmacy sales)

Brand name (dosage form)	Herbs or active constituents (preparations)	IND	Rank A	Rank B	TRx	T€ per year
Sinupret (CT, FL)	Gentian root (P) Primose flowers (P) Sorrel (P) Elder flowers (P) European Vervain (P)	B	1	18	2769	22660
Gelomyrtol/ -forte (C)	Cineol Limonen α-Pinen	B	2	24	2165	17624
Prospan (T, L)	Ivy leaves (E) (E)	B	3	26	2119	13592
Perenterol (C)	Saccharomyces boulardii (P)	E	4	52	1522	12744
Iberogast (L)	Bitter candytuft (E) Angelica root (E) Chamomile flowers (E) Caraway (E) Milk thistle fruits (E) Lemon balm leaves (E) Peppermint leaves (E) Greater celandine (E) Licorice root (E)	E	5	84	1192	13297
Tebonin (FT, L)	Ginkgo biloba leaves (E)	A	6	178	753	31702
Bronchipret Saft/Tr.	Thyme (E) Ivy leaves (E)	B	7	200	703	3547
Umckaloabo (L)	Pelargonium root (E)	B	8	204	697	8715
Gingium (FT, L)	Ginkgo biloba leaves (E)	A	9	232	655	18595
Soledum Kapseln (C)	Cineol	B	10	249	631	4841
Sinuc (L)	Ivy leaves (E) (E)	B	11	281	572	2797
Remifemin plus (CT)	St. John's wort (E) Black cohosh (E)	H	12	297	550	10082
Crataegutt (C, L)	Hawthorn leaves and flowers (E)	C	13	322	510	12547
Ginkobil Tropf,/ -N Ftbl. (L, FT)	Ginkgo biloba leaves (E)	A	14	474	463	12784
Jarsin (CT)	St. John's wort (E)	A	15	473	378	9643
Korodin Herz-Kreislauf (L)	Hawthorn berries (E) Camphor	C	16	477	376	4334
Sedariston Konzentrat (C)	Valerian root (E) St. John's wort (E)	A	17	522	345	6029
Remifemin (T, L)	Black cohosh (E)	H	18	563	324	3344
Kytta Sedativum F (CT, L)	Valerian root (E) Hop strobiles (E) Passionflower herb (E)	A	19	578	313	4220

Table A3.

(*cont.*)

Brand name (dosage form)	Herbs or active constituents (preparations)	IND	Rank A	Rank B	TRx	T€ per year
Prostagutt forte (C)	Saw palmetto berries (E) Nettle root (E)	D	20	629	289	12752
Hedelix (FL)	Efeublätter (E)	B	21	647	280	1.584
Iscador (L)	European mistletoe (E)	F	22	689	261	14792
Felis (CT)	St. John's wort (E)	A	23	700	257	5660
Neuroplant (C)	St. John's wort (E)	A	24	715	252	6358
Aspecton Saft N (L)	Thyme (E)	B	25	718	250	1777
Tussamag Hustensaft N (L)	Thyme (E)	B	26	761	234	1118
Bronchicum Elixier N (L)	Primrose root (E) Thyme (E)	B	27	782	226	1375
Laif 600 (T)	St. John's wort (E)	A	28	803	221	7281
Rökan (T, L)	Ginkgo biloba leaves (E)	A	29	883	198	8087
Bazoton (FT)	Nettle root (E)	D	30	898	195	10619
Sinufurton Saft (L)	Primrose root (E) Thyme (E)	B	31	929	190	1346
Babix-Inhalat N (L)	Eucalyptus oil Spruce needle oil	B	32	964	181	883
Soledum Hustensaft/ -Tropfen	Thyme (E)	B	33	1002	174	1101
Luvased (CT)	Valerian root (E) Hop strobiles (E)	A	34	1006	173	2043
Sinuforton (C)	Anise oil Primrose root (E) Thyme (E)	B	35	1015	172	1401
Colchicum Dispert (CT)	Colchicum alkaloids (E)	G	36	1023	171	2801
Prostess (C)	Saw palmetto berries (E)	D	37	1038	169	5215
Uzara (L, CT)	Uzara root (E)	E	38	1044	168	1103
Diarrhoesan (L)	Apple pectin Chamomile flowers (E)	E	39	1049	167	1223
Bromelain-POS (T)	Bromelain	G	40	1069	164	3469
Bronchicum Tropfen N (L)	Primrose root (E) Thyme (E)	B	41	905	194	1287
Agnucaston (FT)	Chasteberry (E)	H	42	1116	156	2525
Venostasin retard/ N/S (C, CT, T)	Horse chestnut seed (E)	C	43	1130	154	6082
Kamillosan Lösung (L)	Chamomile flowers (E)	G	44	1164	148	1607
Petadolex (C)	Petasite rhizome (E)	A	45	1170	147	4108
Thymipin N (L)	Thyme (E)	B	46	1178	145	962
Prostagutt mono (C)	Saw palmetto berries (E)	D	47	1185	144	5015
X-Prep (L)	Alexandria senna pods (E)	E	48	1209	140	1089
Kamillenbad Robugen (L)	Chamomile flowers (E, Öl)	G	49	1232	137	1301
Bronchipret TB (T)	Thyme (E) Ivy leaves (E)	B	50	1235	136	1180

Table A3.
(cont.)

Brand name (dosage form)	Herbs or active constituents (preparations)	IND	Rank A	Rank B	TRx	T€ per year
Esberitox N (T, L, Z)	White Cedar Leaf (E) Coneflower root (E) Wild indigo root (E)	F	51	1238	136	1243
Kytta Plasma F/ Salbe F (O)	Comfrey root (E)	G	52	1244	135	1507
Melrosum Husten-sirup N (L)	Thyme (E)	B	53	1249	134	837
Helixor (L)	European mistletoe (E)	F	54	1325	125	7537
Linola Gamma Creme	Evening primrose oil	G	55	1339	124	1241
Bronchoforton N Salbe	Eucalyptus oil Pine needle oil Peppermint oil	B	56	1353	123	1185
Kaveri (FT, L)	Ginkgo biloba leaves (E)	A	57	1364	121	4044
Sedariston Tropfen (L)	Valerian root (E) St. John's wort (E) Lemon balm leaves (E)	A	58	1391	119	1559
Eucabal Balsam S	Eucalyptus oil Pine needle oil	B	59	1394	118	686
Hyperforat (CT)	St. John's wort (E)	A	60	1447	112	1179
Hametum Salbe	Witch hazel (distillate)	G	61	1448	112	890
Euvegal (CT)	Valerian root (E) Lemon balm leaves (E)	A	62	1461	110	2108
Cystinol akut (CT)	Uva ursi (E)	D	63	1469	109	1246
Talso (K)	Saw palmetto berries (E)	D	64	1481	108	3703
Cystinol (L)	Birch leaves (E) Horsetail (E) Goldenrod (E) Uva ursi (E)	D	65	1485	108	908
Prosta Fink forte (C)	Pumpkinseed (E)	D	66	1489	107	4084
Phytodolor/N (L)	Quaking aspen bark and leaves (E) Common ash bark (E) Goldenrod (E)	G	67	1503	106	1502
Sedotussin Efeu	Ivy leaves (E)	B	68	1505	106	590
Transpulmin Balsam E (O)	Cineol Menthol Campher	B	69	1559	102	933
Soledum Balsam Lösung	Cineol	B	70	1566	100	635
Santax S (C)	Saccharomyces boulardii (P)	E	71	1587	99	806
Rheuma-Hek (C)	Nettle leaves (E)	G	72	1616	97	1995
Euvegal Balance (CT)	Valerian root (E)	A	73	1642	95	1379
Teufelskralle ratiopharm (T)	Devil's claw (E)	G	74	1670	93	1956
Sweatosan N (CT)	Sage (E)	G	75	1686	92	1847

Table A3.
(*cont.*)

Brand name (dosage form)	Herbs or active constituents (preparations)	IND	Rank A	Rank B	TRx	T€ per year
Legalon (C)	Milk thistle fruits (E)	E	76	1718	89	4535
Ginkgo Stada (T)	Ginkgo biloba leaves (E)	A	77	1741	87	2071
Carminativum-Hetterich N (L)	Chamomile flowers (E) Peppermint leaves (E) Caraway (E) Fennel (E) Bitter orange peel (E)	E	78	1753	87	572
Texx (T)	St. John's wort (E)	A	79	1775	86	1343
Miroton (CT, L)	False hellabore (CT, L) Lily-of-the-valley (E) Squill (E)	C	80	1793	84	2160
Aescusan 20 (FT)	Horse chestnut seed (E)	C	81	1798	84	2523
Cernilton N (C)	Grass pollen (P)	D	82	1823	82	2586
Orthangin N (C, T, FT)	Hawthorn leaves and flowers (E)	C	83	1827	82	1112
Faros (CT)	Hawthorn leaves and flowers (E)	C	84	1848	80	1640
Lektinol (L)	European mistletoe (E)	F	85	1871	78	10400
Hepar SL (C)	Artichoke leaves (E)	E	86	1919	75	2282
Sedonium (CT)	Valerian root (E)	A	87	1972	72	1481
Hyperesa (C)	Valerian root (E) St. John's wort (E)	A	88	1976	72	1588
Remotiv (FT)	St. John's wort (E)	A	89	1994	70	1601
Esbericum (C)	St. John's wort (E)	A	90	1997	70	1448
Kytta-Cor (T, L)	Hawthorn berries (E) Hawthorn leaves and flowers (E)	C	91	2002	70	1077
Johanniskraut ratiopharm (FT)	St. John's wort (E)	A	92	2042	67	1102
Cystium wern	Fennel oilCamphor	D	93	2093	64	603
Enteroplant (C)	Peppermint oil, Caraway oil	E	94	2112	64	1004
Urol mono (C)	Goldenrod (E)	D	95	2179	61	2072
Helarium (CT)	St. John's wort (E)	A	96	2184	61	1157
Kamillan plus	Chamomile flowers ((E)	F	97	2200	60	401
Agnolyt (C)	Chasteberry (E)	H	98	2206	60	1267
Isla-Moos Pastillen	Island moss (E)	B	99	2208	60	234
Cholagogum F (CT)	Turmeric (E) Greater celandine (E)	E	100	2267	57	1884

Subject Index